HUMAN KINETICS WEB RESOURCE

CW01654599

How to access the supplemental web resource

We are pleased to provide access to a web resource that supplements your *Pilates for Hip and Knee Syndromes and Arthroplasties.* This resource offers guidelines on using Pilates equipment to devise safe programs for clients as well as information on finding qualified Pilates training programs and instructors.

Accessing the web resource is easy! Follow these steps if you purchased a new book:

1. Visit the textbook's Web site at this link: **www.HumanKinetics.com/PilatesForHipAndKneeSyndromesAndArthroplasties.**
2. Click the first edition link next to the book cover.
3. Click the Sign In link on the left or top of the page. If you do not have an account with Human Kinetics, you will be prompted to create one.
4. If the online product you purchased does not appear in the Ancillary Items box on the left of the page, click the Enter Key Code option in that box. Enter the key code that is printed at the right, including all hyphens. Click the Submit button to unlock your online product.
5. After you successfully enter your key code, your online product will appear in the Ancillary Items box. On future visits to the site, all you need to do is sign in to the book's website and follow the link!

➜ Click the Need Help? button on the book's website if you need assistance along the way.

For technical support, send an e-mail to:
support@hkusa.com . . . . U.S. and international customers
info@hkcanada.com . . . . Canadian customers
academic@hkeurope.com . . . . European customers
keycodesupport@hkaustralia.com . . . . . Australian and New Zealand customers

HUMAN KINETICS
The Information Leader in Physical Activity & Health

04-2011

Product: Pilates for Hip and Knee Syn Arthroplasties web resource

Key code: KAPLANEK-YPUAZM-OSG

This unique code allows you access to the web resource.

Access is provided if you have purchased a new book. Once submitted, the code may not be entered for any other user.

Pilates
for Hip and Knee Syndromes and Arthroplasties

Pilates for Hip and Knee Syndromes and Arthroplasties

Beth A. Kaplanek, RN, BSN
Qualified Pilates Instructor ■ Practitioner of Pilates for Rehabilitation

Brett Levine, MD, MS
Orthopaedic Surgeon ■ Rush University Medical Center

William L. Jaffe, MD
Orthopaedic Surgeon ■ New York University Hospital for Joint Disease

Human Kinetics

Library of Congress Cataloging-in-Publication Data

Kaplanek, Beth A., 1952- author.
Pilates for hip and knee syndromes and arthroplasties / Beth A. Kaplanek, Brett Levine, William L. Jaffe.
p. ; cm.
Includes bibliographical references.
ISBN-13: 978-0-7360-9224-1 (soft cover)
ISBN-10: 0-7360-9224-2 (soft cover)
1. Hip joint--Wounds and injuries--Treatment. 2. Knee--Wounds and injuries--Treatment. 3. Pilates method. 4. Arthroplasty. I. Levine, Brett, 1973- author. II. Jaffe, William L., 1938- author. III. Title
[DNLM: 1. Hip Injuries--therapy. 2. Arthroplasty--rehabilitation. 3. Exercise Movement Techniques--methods. 4. Knee Injuries--therapy. 5. Musculoskeletal Diseases--therapy. WE 855]
RD549.K37 2011
617.5'82044--dc22

2010053247

ISBN-10: 0-7360-9224-2 (print)
ISBN-13: 978-0-7360-9224-1 (print)

Copyright © 2011 by Beth A. Kaplanek, Brett Levine, and William L. Jaffe

All rights reserved. Except for use in a review, the reproduction or utilization of this work in any form or by any electronic, mechanical, or other means, now known or hereafter invented, including xerography, photocopying, and recording, and in any information storage and retrieval system, is forbidden without the written permission of the publisher.

Acquisitions Editor: Loarn D. Robertson, PhD; **Developmental Editor:** Amanda S. Ewing; **Assistant Editors:** Antoinette Pomata and Kali Cox; **Copyeditor:** Jocelyn Engman; **Permissions Manager:** Dalene Reeder; **Graphic Designer:** Bob Reuther; **Graphic Artist:** Yvonne Griffith; **Cover Designer:** Keith Blomberg; **Photographer (cover):** Richard LoPinto/© Human Kinetics; **Photographer (interior):** Richard LoPinto/© Human Kinetics; photographs are displaying the Triadball; **Photo Asset Manager:** Laura Fitch; **Visual Production Assistant:** Joyce Brumfield; **Photo Production Manager:** Jason Allen; **Art Manager:** Kelly Hendren; **Associate Art Manager:** Alan L. Wilborn; **Illustrations:** © Human Kinetics; **Printer:** Versa Press

Printed in the United States of America

10 9 8 7 6 5 4 3 2 1

The paper in this book is certified under a sustainable forestry program.

Human Kinetics
Website: www.HumanKinetics.com

United States: Human Kinetics
P.O. Box 5076
Champaign, IL 61825-5076
800-747-4457
e-mail: humank@hkusa.com

Canada: Human Kinetics
475 Devonshire Road Unit 100
Windsor, ON N8Y 2L5
800-465-7301 (in Canada only)
e-mail: info@hkcanada.com

Europe: Human Kinetics
107 Bradford Road
Stanningley
Leeds LS28 6AT, United Kingdom
+44 (0) 113 255 5665
e-mail: hk@hkeurope.com

Australia: Human Kinetics
57A Price Avenue
Lower Mitcham, South Australia 5062
08 8372 0999
e-mail: info@hkaustralia.com

New Zealand: Human Kinetics
P.O. Box 80
Torrens Park, South Australia 5062
0800 222 062
e-mail: info@hknewzealand.com

E5124

Contents

Exercise Finder

Many of the exercises in this book have variations depending on how long postop the exercise is being performed. This exercise finder will let you easily find the exercise you're looking for by time postop. Simply turn to the page listed to find a complete description, with photos, for the exercise in question. The exercise timelines are set in tables to make it easier to create an exercise routine for a syndrome or arthroplasty. The side kick series (SKS) exercises are also broken down by time postop. The second exercise finder is specific for the SKS. Choosing a routine for a hip or knee syndrome from any one of the following categories should be based on the client's core control and available ROM.

PRE-PILATES AND PILATES EXERCISES

Exercise	Pre-Pilates	6 weeks to 3 months	3 to 6 months	6 months and beyond
Abdominal prep	48			
Abduction and adduction	43			
Adductor squeeze	52			
Ankle pump	40			
Breathing	39			
Cancan (modified)			234	234
Corkscrew			182	185
Crisscross		98	174	174
Double-leg kick			198	198
Double-leg stretch		86	163	166
Double straight-leg stretch (lower lift)		94	171	171
Gluteal set	42			
Half roll-down		70	140	140
Half roll-up		75	141	141
Hip circle (modified)			241	241
Hundred		67	135	137
Knee fold	50			
Leg pull (modified)			243	243

(continued)

Exercise Finder *(continued)*

Exercise	Pre-Pilates	6 weeks to 3 months	3 to 6 months	6 months and beyond
Neck pull				207
Neck pull (modified)			204	
Open-leg rocker				179
Pelvic curl	45			
Prone leg lifts	56			
Push-up				260
Push-up (modified)			257	257
Quadriceps set	41			
Rolling like a ball			156	158
Roll-up			143	147
Saw		107	187	187
Serratus push-up				254
Serratus push-up (modified)			251	251
Shoulder bridge			211	211
Shoulder bridge (modified)		117		
Shoulder roll	44			
Side stretch		129	247	247
Single-leg circle		79	150	154
Single-leg kick		113	196	196
Single-leg stretch		83	160	160
Single straight-leg stretch and scissors		88	168	168
Sitting bent-knee lifts	59			
Spine stretch forward		104	177	177
Spine twist			201	201
Supine leg lifts	53			
Swan				193
Swan prep		110	191	
Swimming			238	238
Teaser 1			223	223
Teaser 2			226	226
Teaser 3				231
Teaser prep 1		121	217	217
Teaser prep 2		124	219	219
Toe tap	46			

SIDE KICK SERIES

	LONG LEVER			SHORT LEVER	
Exercise	**6 weeks to 3 months**	**3 to 6 months**	**6 months and beyond**	**6 weeks to 3 months**	**3 to 6 months and beyond**
Body position for long-lever SKS	265	267	267		
Body position for short-lever SKS				303	305
90° bent-knee circle				309	311
90° bent-knee lift and lower				308	310
90° bent-knee rotation					316*
90° bent-knee touch				312	314
90° long-leg circle			297		
90° long-leg lift			296		
Bicycle		287	287		
D-circle		281	281		
Front and back	274	276	276		
Inner-thigh circle	299	302	302		
Inner-thigh lift	298	300	300		
Internal and external rotation	284	285	285		
Lift, lift, lower, lower		293	293		
Little circle	278	279	279		
Parallel leg lift		291	291		
Scissors		289	289		
Up and down	270	272	272		

* 6 months and beyond only for this movement

Preface

In 1997, while hiking down a mountain with my husband, I experienced pain in my right hip that would not go away. Over time, I tried stretching, massage, and over-the-counter medications, but the pain persisted. I decided to get an X ray to see what was wrong. My doctor reviewed my X ray, looked straight into my eyes, and said, "You need a hip replacement." I nearly fell off the table. How could that be? I was too active and too young. I was a fitness instructor and a nurse who enjoyed all kinds of physical activities, including equestrian riding and jumping.

I knew that my life was about to change along with my way of thinking about fitness. I was about to lose a piece of my skeletal system and replace it with a mechanical joint. Did that mean I would have to stop what I loved doing most—exercising and teaching?

In 1999, I was diagnosed with bilateral slipped capital femoral epiphysis, a childhood disorder that can manifest as arthritis in adulthood. Then in August 2001, I had a right hip replacement. My doctor explained that because of my disorder I might eventually need my left hip replaced as well. I realized that finding an exercise regimen to help me maintain my level of fitness without damaging my joints would be an integral part of my continued rehabilitation and future fitness practices.

Exercise is important for many health reasons. For individuals with joint replacements, only low-impact workouts are considered to be safe and to help maintain the integrity of the replacement materials (Klein et al. 2007).

In June 2003, I began studying Pilates, a comprehensive series of exercises and movements with an emphasis on the core musculature. All movements promote strength, stability, and increased range of motion of the joints. Because I enjoyed my Pilates immensely and had such positive results, I decided to seek certification as an instructor. When I visited my surgeon to check on my hips, he asked me what I had been doing. I explained that I had been practicing Pilates and teaching Pilates mat classes. He told me that whatever I was doing, I should keep doing it, since my replacement hip looked great and my left hip had not deteriorated and in fact looked better. He was so impressed with the recuperation and results that he asked if I could put together a Pilates regimen for a journal paper and showcase this form of rehabilitation for people with knee and hip replacements.

In June 2004, I became a certified Pilates instructor and by 2008 I had completed a second program for becoming a practitioner of Pilates for rehabilitation. I've had the opportunity to work with several individuals with joint replacements and syndromes and have witnessed their positive progress. When performed with clear guidelines and principles, Pilates is a very effective form of exercise to increase range of motion and flexibility of the joints, core control, stamina, and stretch. It also provides an overall state of well-being for body and mind. The exercises are easy to modify by making the movements bigger or smaller and changing the flow to meet the individual needs of each client. They do not stress the joints or ligaments but work to strengthen the muscles around them, which is the key to reducing the load on the joint for syndromes or replacements.

To understand further why Pilates is a valuable form of fitness for people with hip and knee syndromes, consider the following background prevalence information. Osteoarthritis of the hip and knee is responsible for almost a million office visits to an orthopaedic surgeon each year and is one of the leading syndromes ultimately leading to joint replacement. Similarly, joint aches (arthralgias) and muscle, tendon, and bursal pains (myalgias, tendinitis, bursitis) frequently require specifically prescribed medical treatment. Often these aches and pains are related to overuse syndromes and can be successfully treated nonoperatively with a short course of oral or topical anti-inflammatory agents and physical therapy. For these patients, it is important to maintain the stretching and strengthening aspects of the physical therapy as a home program after the formal medical treatment terminates. Pilates offers a way to maintain hip and knee function in the form of low-impact strengthening exercises that are readily adaptable to target specific syndromes that may affect the knee or hip and can be incorporated into a home program.

The total number of knee and hip replacements (arthroplasties) being performed in the United States each year is steadily increasing, while the average age of surgical candidates is decreasing (Levine, Jaffe, and Kaplanek 2009). In the United States from 1990 to 2002, the number of primary total hip arthroplasties (THAs) increased 50% per 100,000 persons (193,000 THAs preformed) and the number of total knee arthroplasties (TKAs) tripled (381,000 TKAs performed; Levine et al. 2007; Kurtz et al. 2005; Levine, Jaffe, and Kaplanek 2009). By the year 2030, the number of total hip and total knee replacements is projected to exceed 4 million (Kurtz, Ong, Lau, et al. 2007), and annual hospital costs associated with these procedures are projected to exceed $65 billion by 2015 (Kurtz, Ong, Schmier, et al. 2007).

With the advent of minimally invasive total joint replacement, an interest in rapid rehabilitation protocols and early enrollment in outpatient physical therapy has evolved. A contemporary report has shown early benefits of rapid rehabilitation after minimally invasive total hip arthroplasty (Levine et al. 2007; Berger et al. 2004; Levine, Jaffe, and Kaplanek 2009). In addition, using preoperative and postoperative targeted exercise programs may improve gait adaptations associated with hip and knee osteoarthritis and arthroplasty (Levine, Jaffe, and Kaplanek 2009; Brosseau et al. 2003; Pilot et al. 2006). Joint replacements are on the rise, especially as individuals seek to stay active and maintain good range of motion at their joints without discomfort. Indications for total joint arthroplasty have gradually expanded to encompass younger, more active patients, who in turn are demanding a more rapid and complete return to function as compared with traditional candidates for total joint arthroplasty (Levine et al. 2007; Levine, Jaffe, and Kaplanek 2009). A survey of the members of the Hip Society and the American Association of Hip and Knee Surgeons (AAHKS) showed that Pilates is rated as a sport activity that patients are allowed to participate in after THA (58% allowed without experience and an additional 24% recommended with experience; Klein et al. 2007).

In a preliminary report from the office notes of Dr. William L. Jaffe, an orthopaedic surgeon and adult reconstructive surgeon at New York University Hospital for Joint Disease, 38 patients noted having used Pilates for their rehabilitation after TKA and THA. There were 22 THAs, with an average age of 46.2 years, and 17 TKAs, with an average age of 55.4 years. At 1 year postoperative, a review of patient charts and follow-up calls revealed that 25 patients were extremely satisfied and 13 patients were satisfied with the use and the subsequent outcome of Pilates in their rehabilitation. There were no patients who ranked their experience or outcome as somewhat satisfied or not satisfied (Levine, Jaffe, and Kaplanek 2009).

A postoperative course of physical therapy for knee and hip arthroplasty varies anywhere from 6 to 12 weeks depending on an individual's needs. Pilates is a well-suited form of fitness that can be incorporated into the pre- and postoperative exercise regimen and be continued as a home program. The proposed advantages of utilizing Pilates include improving preoperative function, thereby developing a pathway for return to outpatient exercise and providing a whole-body approach to rehabilitation (Levine, Jaffe, and Kaplanek 2009).

Acknowledgments

To my husband, Chuck Kaplanek, for his ongoing patience, love, and devotion. He is always there for me, supporting my causes and listening to me, as I move forward through my challenges and heal my emotions.

To master instructor, Maggie Amrhein, for her many talents, wonderful personality, and guidance. She has helped me enhance my skills as a Pilates instructor and has continually encouraged me to keep moving forward with my writing on this important project.

To Dina Scafura for her support and help developing the purpose, goals, and objectives of this manual so that all Pilates instructors can learn how to work more safely and efficiently with individuals with knee or hip syndromes.

To my surgeon, Dr. William Jaffe, for inspiring me to continue in the field of Pilates as well as write and complete this manual to benefit the many individuals who are facing or have had a hip or knee replacement.

To Dr. Brett Levine for working with me in the review and writing of this book and for working so hard to get Pilates recognized by the orthopaedic community as a safe and efficacious form of fitness and rehabilitation for patients with hip and knee syndromes or arthroplasty.

To master instructors Michael Fritzke and Ton Voogt for their wonderful Triadball that is used to modify many of the mat and equipment exercises to help individuals with knee and hip syndromes achieve success through movement.

To Power Pilates and Polestar Pilates and their wonderful trainers for helping me to grow, learn, and develop my skills as a qualified Pilates instructor and practitioner of Pilates for rehabilitation.

Also, special thanks to the following people:

Manual Reviewers

Maggie Amrhein, qualified Pilates instructor and professional dancer

Bonnie Heyman, qualified Pilates instructor

Margaret Di Meo, qualified Pilates instructor

Marilyn A. Spoka, paralegal consultant

Dina Scafura, qualified Pilates instructor and personal trainer

Lisa Wark, qualified Pilates instructor

Models

Dina Scafura, qualified Pilates instructor and personal trainer

Maggie Amrhein, qualified Pilates instructor and professional dancer

Beth Kaplanek, registered nurse and qualified Pilates instructor

Richard LoPinto, photographer

Introduction

In preparation for writing *Pilates for Hip and Knee Syndromes and Arthroplasties*, I contemplated the importance of including all the information that would give instructors the theory and reason for applying Pilates exercises as a form of rehabilitation for the client with a hip or knee syndrome or arthroplasty. I began to notice the correlation between the history of Joseph Pilates and his desire to connect with the orthopaedic world and have his teachings recognized by that community as a valuable form of fitness and rehabilitation. In essence, I used Pilates to rebuild my hips, core control, and stability after my hip replacement. Understanding the Pilates principles is essential to applying the method. Otherwise it is just movement without purpose.

The Pilates method is full-body conditioning integrating the body, mind, and spirit as a coordinated whole. It is a unique system of stretching and strengthening exercises developed more than 90 years ago by Joseph Pilates. The exercises strengthen and tone muscles and improve posture, flexibility, range of motion, and balance (Siller 2000). The body and mind work together and gradually integrate the exercise at various levels depending on the individual's needs. Pilates mat work is the backbone of the method. It is a form of fitness that can benefit all people regardless of age or current fitness level. Performing the Pilates exercises consistently and regularly at least 3 times per week, using modifications as needed, is important to experiencing the benefits of the method. *Pilates for Hip and Knee Syndromes and Arthroplasties* bridges the worlds of the physician, physical therapist, and Pilates instructor by laying down the foundation and guidelines for comfortably working with a client with a knee or hip syndrome or joint replacement based on current technology and findings.

This introduction provides a brief history of Joseph Pilates and the Pilates method. It then explains how to use the information provided throughout the rest of the book.

Biographical Sketch of Joseph Pilates

Understanding the history of Joseph Pilates gives credibility to the method and a foundation for the work. You will notice by reading this section that Joseph Pilates was ahead of his time. He wanted his method to be recognized by the medical community as a form of quality of movement for the total body and a restoration of vitality and breath.

Joseph Hubertus Pilates was born in Monchengladbach, Germany, in 1880. However, some records indicate that he was actually born in 1883. Joseph was one of four children. He was a sickly child who had asthma, rickets, and rheumatic fever and was bullied and tormented by his peers. It is possible that this situation caused him to begin his life's work of studying fitness and health to help himself and others.

A family physician gave Joseph an anatomy book, which, according to some people, he devoured. He studied every page, learning about the body and how it moved. He studied nature by hiding in the woods and observing the graceful movements of the animals and the ways they encouraged and nurtured their young. Joseph continued his studies by examining both Eastern and Western forms of fitness, including yoga. By the time he was 14 years old, he had developed his body and was posing for anatomical charts. His rich background of studies, shaped by his experiences, initiated his creation of an innovative system of exercises called *Contrology*, which he continued to develop throughout his lifetime.

In 1912, Joseph left for England to train as a boxer and took employment as a circus performer. In 1914, World War I broke out and Joseph, along with his German nationals, was interned in a camp for enemy aliens. He started in Lancaster, England, where he taught wrestling and self-defense to the detainees. Later, he was moved to the Isle of Man to work with people who were sick and bedridden. This work ultimately led him to hook springs to the bedposts to support the limbs of the people who were bedridden and to utilize this system to move the limbs against the resistance of the springs. He became a type of nurse physiotherapist, developing life-enhancing therapeutic exercises.

World War I ended and Joseph returned to Germany, where he was asked to train the new German military. Disenchanted with the political atmosphere, he decided to leave. Family and friends influenced him to immigrate to the United States. He met his wife, Clara, on his voyage to the United States. Clara played a major role in the development and teaching of the Pilates method. Joseph and Clara opened their first studio in New York City and began attracting a diverse population. The dancing community embraced Contrology, and it soon became the rehabilitation and training for many dancers. Physical therapy as we know it today did not exist back then. If you became injured, you were out of work. For dancers, gymnasts, and athletes, injury could be devastating. Pilates was their connection to physical therapy during these earlier times.

Dr. Henry Jordan, chief of orthopaedics at Lenox Hill Hospital, was a big fan of Joseph's work and referred many of his clients for care. In the 1950s, Joseph worked hard to get the mainstream medical and educational institutions to embrace his work, but unfortunately that did not happen during his lifetime. Joseph knew his work was "50 years ahead of its time" (Pilates Method Alliance 2005, 17).

Many of Joseph's and Clara's students and assistants, now called *first-generation teachers*, carried over the lessons and teachings of Joseph and Clara to others. By 1995, mind–body fitness programs and the medical community were taking notice and pushing the Pilates method forward. In October of 2000, a trademark class-action suit ended, and Pilates became associated with a form of fitness that includes mat and equipment exercises. Today, Pilates is taught in most major countries, and the number of people participating in Pilates increased from 1.7 million in 2000 to 10.5 million in 2004 (Pilates Method Alliance 2005; American Sports Data 2008).

In October of 1967, Joseph Pilates passed away. He would have loved to have seen his teachings and innovations grow in interest daily, not only in the fitness arena but also in the therapeutic community.

Pilates Method and Principles

The Pilates method requires total engagement of the body, mind, and spirit working together in unison. Pilates is a form of fitness that uses the body against resistance, working from head to toe with each flowing movement. The core (powerhouse) is structured around the center of the body and includes the abdominal, gluteal, hip, and low back muscles. Pilates requires strength and control of the core, from which all exercises and movements are initiated and sustained. When Pilates is practiced faithfully 3 or 4 days per week, the body responds with increased awareness, strength, range of motion, joint and spine flexibility, balance, torso stability, and core control.

Pilates is a mind, body, and spirit workout governed by movement principles. It is an exercise system that can be modified to allow anyone from the beginner to the advanced to work effectively. Once you understand the core philosophy of Pilates, you can translate it into any format or fitness routine. Joseph Pilates summed up his exercise regimen precisely: "In 10 workouts you feel different; in 20 you look different; in 30 you will have a whole new body" (Ungaro 2004, 8).

As stated in the 1945 book *Return to Life Through Contrology*, Pilates' philosophy is a vision of health and well-being that gives context to exercise. Pilates' three guiding principles are whole-body health, whole-body commitment, and breath (Pilates Method Alliance 2005; Pilates and Miller 1945).

- **Whole-body health** refers to the development of the body, mind, and spirit in complete coordination with each other. Joseph Pilates wrote that whole-body health could be achieved through exercise; proper diet; good hygiene and sleeping habits; plenty of sunshine and fresh air; and a balance of work, recreation, and relaxation. According to Pilates, "Physical fitness is the first requisite of happiness" (Pilates Method Alliance 2005, 19; Pilates and Miller 1945).
- **Whole-body commitment** pertains to mental and physical discipline, a work ethic, an attitude toward self, and a lifestyle that is necessary to achieve whole-body health. "Faithfully perform your Contrology exercises only four times a week for just three months, you will find your body development approaching the ideal, accompanied by renewed mental vigor and spiritual enhancement" (Pilates Method Alliance 2005, 18; Pilates and Miller 1945).
- **Breath** is an integral part of overall body functioning, increasing volume capacity and oxygenation and leading to other physiological changes. Full and consistent inhalation and exhalation help the circulatory system nourish all the tissues with oxygen-rich blood and carry away impurities and metabolic waste. "Breathing is the first act of life, and the last" (Pilates Method Alliance 2005; Pilates and Miller 1945, 13).

The following additional Pilates principles are used to guide movement:

Concentration is focusing on the exercise while not letting your thoughts wander. It is important to concentrate on the form and to focus on the details and not divert energy into other things.

Centering is the foundation of all the movements. No arm or leg movement should be performed without first stabilizing the core muscles of the body.

Control refers to learning to be in command of movement while initiating it from its correct source and performing it with the correct mindful intent.

Precision is focusing not only on completing an exercise but also on performing it as perfectly as possible.

Breath is correct breathing that affords appropriate oxygenation of the cells while enhancing circulation. Inhalation is used to prepare for the movement, and complete exhalation is used to execute the movement, help activate core support, and intensify the movement.

Flow connects one movement to the next and threads one exercise to the next. Flow develops as you become more familiar with the exercises (Ungaro 2004).

How to Use This Book

Pilates for Hip and Knee Syndromes and Arthroplasties covers the mat work as it relates to the Pilates method. This manual addresses how the mat work can be modified for hip and knee syndromes as well as for pre- and postoperative rehabilitation of clients with hip or knee replacements, formally known as *arthroplasties*. It is the intent of this book to show the adaptability of the method as a key form of fitness and rehabilitation for these populations, especially during the first postoperative year.

The goals of this book are to (1) further introduce Pilates to the orthopaedic community as a safe and efficacious form of fitness and rehabilitation to restore function, strength, and balance to the motivated client with a knee or hip syndrome or arthroplasty and (2) help qualified Pilates instructors feel comfortable working with a client with a knee or hip syndrome or arthroplasty by setting up protocols with specific modifications for these populations. Most instructors have no idea what modifications or guidelines to follow when working with a client who has undergone a joint replacement. Basic modifications are taught during the training program; however, not enough information is covered in most programs to help the instructor feel comfortable working with a client with a joint syndrome or replacement. The information and the setup of the exercises in *Pilates for Hip and Knee Syndromes and Arthroplasties* create a foundation to work from in order to select an effective exercise formula for clients with hip or knee syndromes or replacements. During the first postoperative year, the foundation is set for the future, allowing the muscles and ligaments time to heal and strengthen.

When working with a client with a syndrome, it is important to select a program that allows the individual to work successfully within a range of motion without pain. When working with a client with a recent joint replacement, it becomes extremely important to build a foundation upon which the client can over time return to a safe range of motion with full function. Working effectively, building core strength, and staying within safe parameters allow for a gradual return to normal life activities and sports.

Pilates for Hip and Knee Syndromes and Arthroplasties begins by reviewing the anatomy of the hip and knee and the surgical and nonsurgical procedures and guidelines for range of motion pre- and postoperative. Chapters 1 and 2 cover this information. Reviewing the anatomy of the hip and knee, the related syndromes, and the surgical and nonsurgical treatments imparts a better sense as to why certain exercises are applied at various timelines and based on individual needs and available range of motion without pain. The guidelines for range of motion in patients with syndromes or arthroplasty are applied to a series of pre-Pilates movements and Pilates mat exercises, which are covered in chapter 3. A special feature of this book is the way in which the exercises are laid out on postoperative timelines. Chapter 4 covers Pilates exercises that are appropriate for 6 weeks to 3 months postoperative. Chapter 5 covers Pilates exercises that are appropriate for 3 to 6 months and 6 months and beyond postoperative. Chapter 6 presents a comprehensive section on the side kick series in all of the postoperative timelines. Chapter 7 provides sample Pilates mat program sequences for syndromes and pre- and postoperative hip and knee arthroplasty. Exercises from all the postoperative categories can be chosen for a client with a syndrome depending on the available range of motion. Included at the beginning of this book is an exercise finder that takes you directly to each exercise at each postoperation timeline; this makes it easier for you to find and create an exercise program. You do not have to read every chapter of this book in order to utilize the exercise formulas and guidelines for range of motion, although doing so is recommended.

All exercises should be performed under the guidance of a qualified Pilates instructor and with permission from the treating physician. The individual needs, restrictions, and recommendations for range of motion should be specified by the treating physician and followed accordingly. Reading *Pilates for Hip and Knee Syndromes and Arthroplasties* does not qualify an individual to be proficient in rehabilitation and Pilates. You should always stay within the scope of your qualifications based on your degree or certification.

Every exercise in this book is photographed at each postoperative milestone. Every exercise is also described in detail, making it easy for you to select an exercise and walk your client through the completion of that exercise. Here is what you'll find:

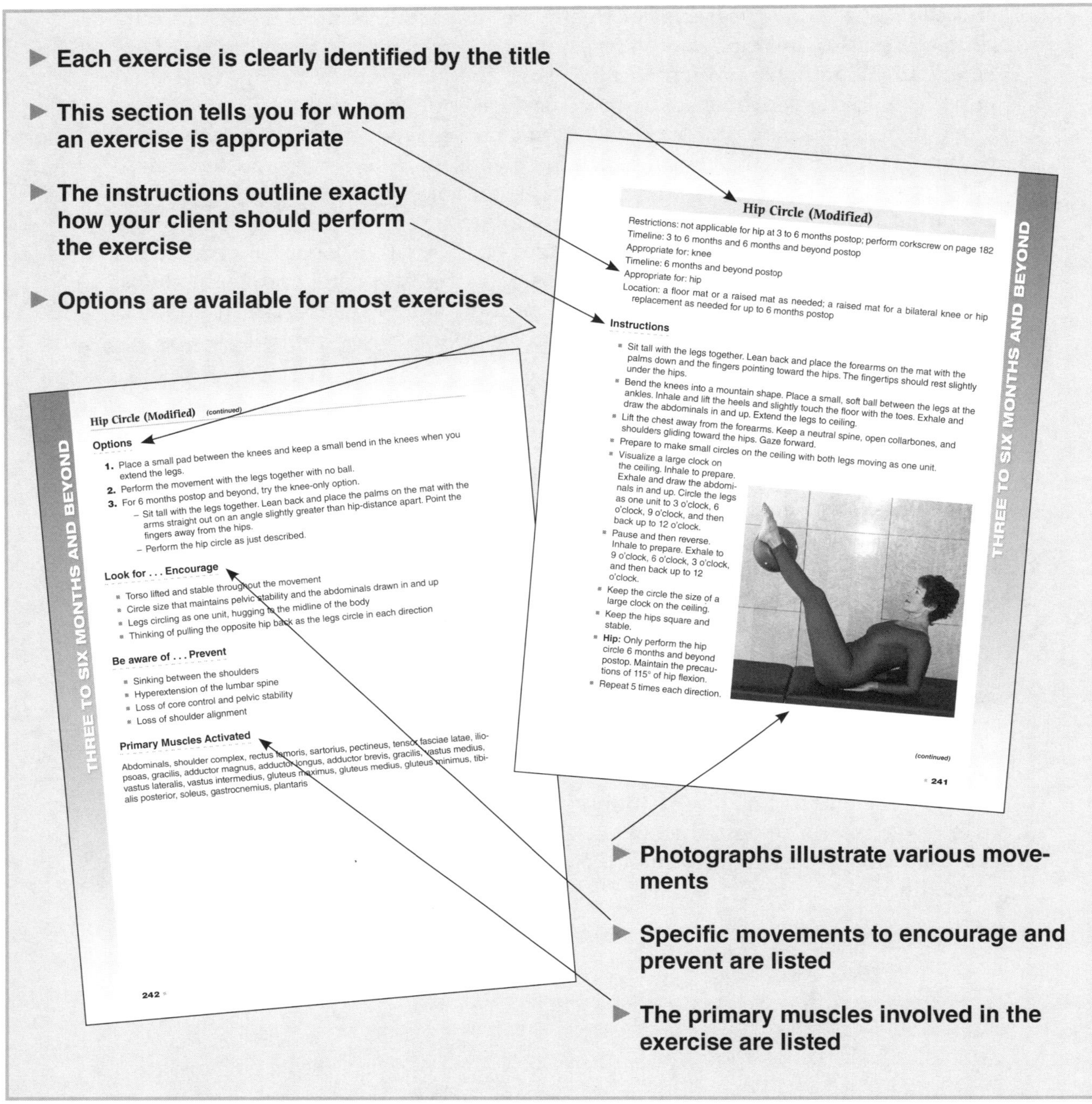
Each exercise is clearly identified by the title
This section tells you for whom an exercise is appropriate
The instructions outline exactly how your client should perform the exercise
Options are available for most exercises
Photographs illustrate various movements
Specific movements to encourage and prevent are listed
The primary muscles involved in the exercise are listed
Hip Circle (Modified)
THREE TO SIX MONTHS AND BEYOND

PART I

Hip and Knee Anatomy, Syndromes, and Treatments

Each year hip and knee disorders are responsible for thousands of visits to orthopaedic doctors, primary care physicians, and emergency rooms. Chapters 1 and 2 review the anatomy of the hip and knee, discuss the most common hip and knee syndromes, and briefly describe some of the general nonoperative and operative treatments.

> ⚠ All exercises should be performed under the guidance of a qualified Pilates instructor and with referral from the operative physician. The client's needs, restrictions, and ROM recommendations should be specified by the physician and followed accordingly. These guidelines may vary from the protocols that follow, and the protocols should be modified based on the individual's needs and the surgeon's preferences.

This manual also includes specific Pilates mat exercises to address several of the syndromes reviewed in these early chapters. These exercises can be implemented in a regular fitness or rehabilitation program to increase core strength and stability, range of motion, and flexibility. In addition, for several of the syndromes reviewed in this part of the book, chapter 7 lists sample Pilates mat program sequences.

chapter 1

The Hip

A comprehensive knowledge of the anatomy of the hip is crucial to understanding and indentifying normal and pathological states of the hip joint, muscles, tendons, and ligaments. This chapter gives a detailed review of this basic anatomy of the hip and the actions of its controlling muscles. Having this information in hand will help you comprehend and relate to the discussion on hip syndromes and the review of nonsurgical and surgical interventions addressed in later chapters. Combining the relevant anatomy and physiology of the hip joint affords a better understanding as to why certain exercises are suggested within various timelines to treat hip syndromes. Stretching and strengthening the appropriate muscle groups are the crux of treating soft tissue injuries and pathology of the hip. A well-designed treatment program should maximize these modalities within specified confines so as to avoid exacerbating the condition being treated while providing a reproducible and sustainable regimen for clients.

Hip Anatomy

The hip joint is a synovial joint formed by the articulation of the spherical femoral head and the cuplike acetabulum, which together make up a functional ball-and-socket joint. The acetabulum develops during childhood and early adolescence and involves the union of three bones: the ilium, ischium, and pubis. The conglomerate of this bony structure is referred to as the *innominate bone* or *pelvis*. The pelvis is responsible for supporting the majority of the body weight and forms a complex articulation with the spine at the sacroiliac joint (Wunderbaldinger et al. 2002; Magee 2008).

The hip joint maintains excellent inherent stability due to the bony anatomy and the relative depth of penetration of the femoral head into the acetabulum. The

See the insert at the back of the book for illustrations of hip anatomy.

ball and socket are covered by a white glistening material called *articular cartilage* that allows the joint surfaces to smoothly and painlessly glide over each other during normal activities. The labrum is a cartilaginous ring attached to the outer rim of the acetabulum. This structure provides additional depth to the acetabulum and is of paramount importance to the stability of the hip joint. Labral tears are often seen in athletes, dancers, and people with hip dysplasia. Femoral acetabular impingement (FAI) syndrome may also be associated with acetabular labral tears and hip pain, clicking, and feelings of instability.

The bony anatomy of the hip is reinforced by several strong ligaments, a fibrous capsule, and the surrounding musculotendinous units. The relevant bony structures, muscles, and tendons work in concert to provide the seamless functionality essential for standing, walking, and running. These activities all require a functional range of motion (ROM) and adequate strength of the adjacent muscles. Physical restrictions and pathological contractures of the hip can limit these movements and in turn place abnormal stresses on the surrounding structures such as the lumbar spine, contralateral hip, and knees.

The fibrous joint capsule attaches circumferentially around the rim of the acetabulum and at the base of the femoral neck, near the intertrochanteric line anteriorly and at the level of the midfemoral neck posteriorly. Synovial fluid is produced by the specialized cells that line the inside of the hip joint. This layer is typically quite thin, but pathological inflammation may lead to an overproduction of joint fluid and a hypertrophic synovitis. The capsule serves to confine this fluid within the joint, and the fluid allows the articular surfaces to be lubricated and nourished appropriately. Osteoarthritis, which is degeneration of the articular cartilage, essentially irritates the joint and leads to an overproduction of inflammatory cells and fluid that causes swelling and pain within the joint.

Three strong extracapsular ligaments surround the joint capsule and serve to prevent hip dislocation and support normal joint function: (1) the iliofemoral ligament, (2) the ischiofemoral ligament, and (3) the pubofemoral ligament. The iliofemoral ligament is considered to be the strongest and acts as a checkrein to prevent excessive hip extension. This ligament also plays a role in the upright posture of the hip. The ischiofemoral ligament is the weakest and winds tightly on extension, helping to stabilize the hip in extension. The pubofemoral ligament protects against excessive abduction of the femur and also limits extension. All three ligaments limit medial (internal) rotation of the femur (Magee 2008). The ligamentum teres is an intracapsular ligament that attaches to the acetabular notch and to a depression, or fovea, on the superomedial aspect of the femoral head. It is stretched with hip dislocation or subluxation and early in life is crucial to the blood supply to the femoral head (Calais-Germain 2007).

There are multiple muscles involved in the stability and function of the hip joint. The following lists group these muscles according to their actions (Magee 2008, 672):

Flexion

- Psoas
- Iliacus
- Rectus femoris
- Sartorius
- Pectineus
- Adductor longus
- Adductor brevis
- Gracilis

Extension

- Biceps femoris
- Semimembranosus
- Semitendinosus
- Gluteus maximus

Gluteus medius (posterior portion)
Adductor magnus (ischiocondylar part)

Abduction

Tensor fasciae latae
Gluteus minimus
Gluteus medius
Gluteus maximus
Sartorius

Adduction

Adductor magnus
Adductor longus
Adductor brevis
Gracilis
Pectineus

Lateral Rotation

Gluteus maximus
Obturator internus
Obturator externus
Quadratus femoris
Piriformis
Gemellus superior
Gemellus inferior
Sartorius
Gluteus medius (posterior portion)

Medial Rotation

Adductor longus
Adductor brevis
Adductor magnus
Gluteus medius (anterior portion)
Gluteus minimus (anterior portion)
Tensor fasciae latae
Pectineus
Gracilis

Hip Syndromes and Nonoperative Treatments

The most common hip syndromes and ailments include trochanteric bursitis; iliopsoas disorders; hip osteoarthritis; ligament tears; snapping hip syndrome; fractures of the femoral neck, intertrochanteric area, and subtrochanteric area; osteonecrosis (avascular necrosis) of the femoral head; congenital hip dysplasia; slipped capital femoral epiphysis; labral tears; and FAI. Many of these conditions can be treated nonoperatively, and not all of these disorders ultimately require total hip arthroplasty (THA). When nonoperative treatment no longer provides adequate relief of symptoms related to intra-articular pathology for performing activities of daily living, only then does THA become a viable option.

Conservative (nonoperative) treatments for the hip include rest, hot and cold therapy, topical agents, analgesics, nonsteroidal anti-inflammatory agents (NSAIDs), intra-articular corticosteroid injections, acupuncture, nutritional supplements (glucosamine and chondroitin combinations), physical therapy, and exercise. These treatments should be maximized before considering surgical intervention. In many degenerative disease processes, such as osteoarthritis and inflammatory arthropathies, the conservative approach is used in order to buy time before surgical intervention becomes necessary. Hip injections are generally a combination of a local anesthetic agent (lidocaine or Marcaine) and a corticosteroid. These injections are administered under fluoroscopic guidance and are limited to 3 or 4 per year. Too many injections may cause weakness of the connective tissues surrounding the joint as well as deterioration of the articular cartilage, making the treatment less effective over time. If more than four injections are needed annually, then alternative treatments need to be explored.

The most common hip syndromes, such as trochanteric bursitis, iliopsoas tendinitis, and snapping hip syndrome, can be treated without surgery. These syndromes are often associated with subtle injuries or overuse. Many times the onset of pain and disability correlates with a change in workout or job activities or with the start of new hobbies or activities. Each year, these treatable conditions are responsible for several hundred thousand office visits to an orthopaedist. For the purposes of this book, this chapter focuses on the following common hip syndromes: trochanteric bursitis, iliopsoas disorders, and osteoarthritis.

Trochanteric Bursitis

There are many bursae adjacent to the hip joint; there is some debate as to the exact number and locations of these bursae. The trochanteric bursa is a common source of pain, and this pain is often referred to as *greater trochanteric pain syndrome* (*GTPS*; Shbeeb and Matteson 1996). GTPS is often described as lateral hip pain and commonly affects middle-aged and elderly patients, with a female predominance (Bird et al. 2001). The onset of the syndrome may correlate with a traumatic incident but is often insidious. Lateral hip pain may radiate down to the outside of the knee (Shbeeb and Matteson 1996). Patients report pain associated with sleeping on the affected side as well as with activity and prolonged sitting. Physical examination findings typically include antalgic gait, pain on palpation over the greater trochanter, crepitation or snapping with ambulation, normal hip ROM, and pain with resisted abduction or with passive extension and adduction (iliotibial band tightening).

The location of the greater trochanteric bursa tends to overlap GTPS with other musculoskeletal disorders such as gluteus medius or minimus tears and tendinitis, lumbar spine disease, intra-articular hip disease and disorders, rheumatoid arthritis, postsurgical inflammation secondary to hardware, and other local bursal syndromes, either iliopsoas or ischial (Archibeck 2007). The trochanteric bursa lies deep to the fascia lata on the side of the hip, overlying a portion of the gluteus medius, greater trochanter, and vastus lateralis complex (Archibeck 2007). In one report more than 63% of patients with clinically presumed trochanteric bursitis were found to have concomitant injury to the gluteus medius tendon on magnetic resonance imaging (MRI; Bird et al. 2001). Typically, the diagnosis is made based on the clinical examination and history; however, plain radiographs, MRI, computed tomography (CT), bone scan, and sonography may be used in the diagnosis of refractory or ambiguous cases.

The most common treatment modality for trochanteric bursitis is nonoperative and includes oral or topical anti-inflammatory agents, traditional physical therapy focusing on iliotibial (IT) band stretching and abductor strengthening, ultrasound, and massage. In refractory cases a localized injection consisting of a local anesthetic and corticosteroid may be given directly to the GTPS source. Injections may be administered every 3 to 4 months and serve as a diagnostic and therapeutic modality. Typically, 60% to 70% of patients experience significant relief of their symptoms with an appropriately placed corticosteroid injection (Ege Rasmussen and Fano 1985; Shbeeb and Matteson 1996). On the rare occasion surgical excision of the bursa, removal of the trochanteric prominence, or a release or lengthening of the IT band may be needed; however, permanent pain relief is unpredictable. Before surgical intervention, the diagnosis of trochanteric bursitis should be verified to prevent operative treatment of an incorrect diagnosis.

At this time, use of the Pilates method has not been documented for the treatment of trochanteric bursitis. A sample of a recommended Pilates program sequence for GTPS is listed in chapter 7 on page 336. A warm-up consisting of breathing, pelvic curl, knee fold, adductor squeeze, and abdominal prep helps to prepare the patient for the more strenuous regimen that follows. The first series of Pilates exercises focuses on core strengthening and consists of the hundred, half roll-up, and full roll-up. As trochanteric bursitis is often part of a larger pain syndrome, the following exercises are recommended to help with general hip and low back strengthening and stretching: single-leg circle, rolling like a ball, single-leg stretch, double-leg stretch, scissors, lower lift, spine stretch forward, corkscrew, saw, swan, single-leg kick, teaser prep 1, swimming, and bridging. In treating trochanteric bursitis it is recommended to focus on hip abductor strengthening and IT band stretching and to include several movements from the side kick series (SKS)—such as little circle, internal and external rotation, 90° bent-knee lift, 90° bent-knee circle, and inner-thigh lift—with appropriate padding under the hip. This series is akin to formal physical therapy stretching and strengthening exercises. Topical or oral anti-inflammatory agents and local massage may still be recommended to aid in the resolution of GTPS.

Typically, GTPS responds to 4 to 6 weeks of targeted therapy. When pain persists longer than this time interval, the client should seek further treatment with a physician. This treatment may include an injection or formal physical therapy. People prone to recurrent GTPS should incorporate this Pilates series into their weekly workout regimen as a preventative measure.

Iliopsoas Disorders

Inflammation of the iliopsoas bursa or tendon is not an uncommon cause of anterior hip (groin) pain and snapping (Johnston et al. 1998). This pain syndrome is often related to osteoarthritis or rheumatoid arthritis of the hip, local hip synovitis, or tendon irritation over the anterior ridge of a prominent or retroverted metallic cup following THA (Grindulis 1986; Toohey et al. 1990). Diagnosis of iliopsoas pathology is based on the history, which often includes groin pain or snapping. Physical examination often demonstrates pain with resisted hip flexion or snapping with extension and hip rotation. A mass in the groin can occasionally be palpated, as can an internal snapping with hip extension and inward rotation from a flexed, adducted, and externally rotated position (Archibeck 2007).

Further evaluations to confirm the diagnosis include ultrasound, MRI, CT, or bursography; plain radiographs typically are negative. One report documented ultrasound as the most cost-effective diagnostic test and MRI as the most accurate (Archibeck 2007; Wunderbaldinger et al. 2002). Nonoperative management of iliopsoas syndrome is the treatment of choice and consists of rest, oral and topical anti-inflammatory agents, stretching, and strengthening. As in GTPS, corticosteroid injections are helpful in cases refractory to more conservative measures. An exercise regimen of hip rotation exercises and stretching has been reported to be successful in treating iliopsoas syndrome (Johnston, Lindsay, and Wiley 1999).

In cases developing after THA, anterior iliopsoas impingement and tendinitis may be the source of pain in up to 4.3% of patients. Postsurgically this pain is often associated with a prominent or malpositioned acetabular component, with retained cement, with excessively long screws, or with an overhanging femoral collar (Heaton and Dorr 2002; Lachiewicz and Kauk 2009). The diagnosis is based on clinical and radiographic evaluation of the postoperative patient. Local injection of the iliopsoas tendon or bursa can be used to confirm the diagnosis. Treatment involves nonoperative management as described, surgical release of the tendon, or revision hip surgery as deemed necessary (Heaton and Dorr 2002).

Use of the Pilates method in treating iliopsoas syndrome has not been documented at this time. This manual lists a series of exercises that can be used to strengthen the core and stretch the anterior structures of the hip and in effect treat iliopsoas syndrome. The exercises discussed are similar to those initiated in a formal physical therapy regimen and serve as an alternative to attending prescribed therapy sessions. The protocol is similar to that for trochanteric bursitis and focuses on core strengthening and hip flexor strengthening and stretching. Therefore, after the warm-up, an emphasis should be placed on the hundred, half roll-down, single-leg circle, rolling like a ball, single-leg stretch, double-leg stretch, scissors, lower lift, corkscrew, saw, swimming, and bridging. Using topical or oral anti-inflammatory agents and local massage to aid in the resolution of iliopsoas syndrome is also recommended. Typically, iliopsoas syndrome responds to 4 to 6 weeks of targeted therapy. When pain persists longer than this time interval, the client should seek further treatment with a physician. This treatment may include injection or formal physical therapy. People prone to iliopsoas tendinitis or bursitis should incorporate this Pilates series into their weekly workout regimen prophylactically.

Hip Osteoarthritis

Osteoarthritis of the hip is a very common disorder. It is estimated that 185,000 THAs were performed in 2002 for degenerative hip conditions (Kurtz et al. 2005). It is also estimated that 43 million Americans have osteoarthritis. There is a linear association with advancing age. Diagnosis is made on a clinical history of groin pain, difficulty with rotational activities of the hip (such as putting on socks and shoes and getting in and out of a car), and pain related to activity. Physical examination often demonstrates groin pain with attempted hip rotation as well as significantly restricted rotational motion of the hip; limited internal rotation and an external rotation contracture are most common. A flexion contracture of the hip is not uncommon and is associated with contracted anterior hip structures, including the hip capsule and hip flexors. Excessive hip contracture can lead to increased stress on the lumbar spine that is often compensated by an exaggerated lumbar lordosis.

Often, plain radiographs are all that are necessary to diagnosis hip osteoarthritis, as joint space narrowing, osteophyte formation, subchondral sclerosis, and cyst formation can be readily seen on plain X rays. More advanced imaging studies typically are not necessary to establish the correct diagnosis. Nonoperative treatment modalities include oral or topical anti-inflammatory agents, weight loss, use of assistive devices, and low-impact stretching and strengthening exercises. A more rigorous exercise program usually is not well tolerated in patients with osteoarthritis. The sample Pilates sequence in chapter 7 (see p. 339) involves a series of low-impact stretching exercises that may be helpful in maintaining well-being and fitness as well as ROM at the hip joint. As the pain progresses and the ROM decreases with advancing osteoarthritis, the Pilates exercises should be modified to accommodate these limitations while still maintaining a healthy lifestyle. When the pain interferes with activities of daily living, disrupts sleep patterns, or becomes incapacitating, the patient should seek physician care.

Operative Treatments

Surgical interventions for hip pathology and syndromes may include arthroscopy, THA, and hip resurfacing. Each intervention is described briefly so as to provide a general understanding of the depth and invasiveness of each procedure and the limitations and restrictions that may be required during the recovery from surgery.

Hip Arthroscopy

Hip arthroscopy involves making small surgical incisions, or portals, that afford access to the hip joint. A pencil-size arthroscope is then advanced into the hip joint to survey the damage and intra-articular pathology. The arthroscope is essentially a video camera that transmits the image of the hip to a television monitor and allows the surgeon to examine the inside of the hip. Hip arthroscopy is used for young, active adults with a history of hip pain and a diagnosis amenable to treatment via this method. The most common treatments with hip arthroscopy are removal of loose bodies, removal or repair of torn portions of the labrum, debridement of bony areas associated with FAI, and treatment of articular cartilage tears. This procedure is technically difficult to perform and should be done by a trained sport or hip specialist. The postoperative recovery time is less than that of open procedures, but restrictions may apply based on the injury or pathology being treated.

Total Hip Arthroplasty

Hip replacement surgery is reserved for patients with end-stage degenerative joint disease that may be related to a variety of conditions such as osteoarthritis, rheumatoid arthritis, avascular necrosis, posttraumatic arthritis, and so on that lead to pain refractory to conservative measures. Figure 1.1 illustrates the hip before and after THA. Hip replacement surgery is an elective procedure and should be performed only if all other forms of treatment have failed and the patient can no longer function at an acceptable level. As an elective procedure, THA should be performed when the person is clinically, radiographically, and mentally prepared for surgery.

Modern technology has advanced in the field of hip replacements, and current implants last longer and perform better than their predecessors did. A person's age, level of fitness, and health determine the type of replacement and the technique used during the surgery. Fixation of THA implants to the bone has changed greatly in the past decade. A move toward cementless fixation has occurred, as it is believed that cementless fixation maximizes component longevity and prevents future loosening. In general, younger patients and patients with good bone quality receive a hip that is biologically fixed (press-fit technique), while a cemented hip is reserved for the elderly or for patients with osteoporosis. The press-fit technique is based on the premise that the implant will be slightly larger than the prepared bone and will be impacted into place. The surface of the implant has small pores or ridges into which bone will grow. Some implants are coated with a bioactive material such as hydroxyapatite that hastens fixation of the implant to the adjacent bone.

When cemented implants are used, bone cement (polymethylmethacrylate) is mixed and pressurized into the canal of the femur. The implant is then placed into the cement mantle. In a matter of minutes the cement sets up and hardens, producing an implant that is securely fixed to the bone. The cement acts as a grout, filling

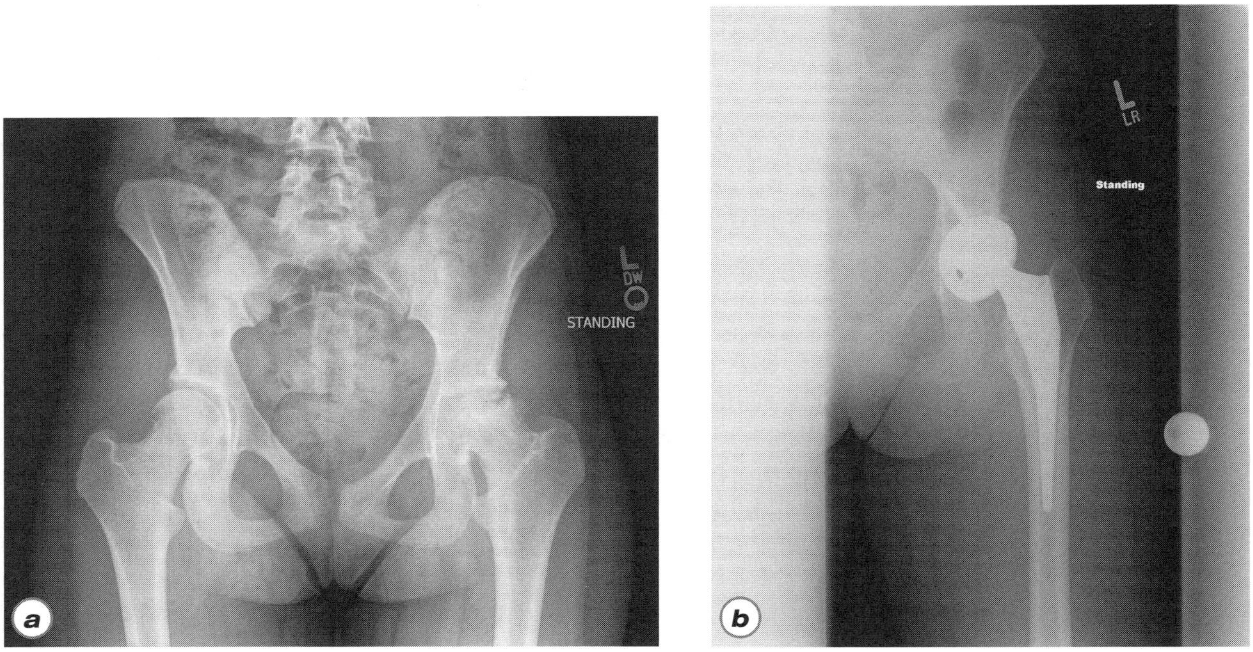

FIGURE 1.1 X ray showing *(a)* a normal right hip and a severely degenerative left hip secondary to osteonecrosis of the femoral head and *(b)* the left hip following THA.
Courtesy of Brett Levine

in spaces, and does not have adhesive properties. It tends to lose fixation over time; as patients age the femoral canal expands away from the formally well-fixed cement mantle. A secondary concern with cement fixation is a relative hypotension generated by pressurizing the cement into the canal during component implantation. However, despite these concerns there are many reports of successful cemented implants at intermediate and long-term follow-up.

The purpose of hip replacement surgery is to remove the damaged and worn parts of the native hip joint—the hip socket, acetabulum, and femoral head—and replace them with smooth, artificial implants. The replaced joint restores the patient's ability to ambulate and maintain flexibility without pain. The hip implant comprises four parts that work together to restore the original function of the ball-and-socket joint:

1. A metal hip stem, typically made of a titanium or cobalt-chrome alloy, that is inserted into the top of the femoral canal
2. A metal cup, typically made of titanium, tantalum, or cobalt-chrome alloy, that holds the articular liner
3. A cup liner, typically made of polyethylene, ceramic materials, or a cobalt-chrome alloy, that articulates with the femoral head
4. The femoral head or ball, typically made of cobalt-chrome alloys or ceramic materials, that is attached to the hip stem and inserted into the liner to form the ball-and-socket joint

Notice that there are several types of materials that can be used in a replacement. The surgeon chooses the materials based on the individual's needs and preferences. The materials and surgical techniques being used today have increased the potential life span of a replacement to up to 30 years (Mullins et al. 2007; Wroblewski, Fleming, and Siney 1999).

There are several surgical approaches that can be utilized during THA. Think of them as a variety of doors that can be opened to get to the site of the hip joint and expose the area for a successful replacement. The approaches are called the *anterior, anterolateral, posterior, transtrochanteric,* and *direct lateral approaches* and are named according to the direction and muscular intervals of the surgical dissection. Surgeons utilize the approach they are most comfortable performing as well as base the incision length and invasiveness of the technique on the patient's body mass index (body habitus). Regardless of the selected incision size, approach, or implant materials, a well-done THA with appropriate implant position is what truly makes a difference for the patient. Less-invasive approaches and aggressive early rehabilitation typically benefit patients for the first 6 to 12 weeks; thereafter, the approach or level of invasiveness does not matter, as most patients will be performing at the level of their age- and activity-matched peers.

In the transtrochanteric approach the greater trochanter and its attached muscles are sectioned to expose the hip joint. The view of the hip is best with this approach; however, the greater trochanter has to be reattached at the end of the operation. Fixation and healing of this bony fragment can be difficult depending on the bone quality and the strength of the abductor muscles that insert on the greater trochanter. Postoperative precautions involve restricted abduction and possibly limited weight bearing for the first 6 weeks after surgery. While not frequently used on routine primary THA in the United States, this approach still remains an option for complex and revision surgeries.

In the posterior approach, muscular insertions into the posterior greater trochanter are elevated from the bone for exposure of the hip joint. These muscles are reattached at the end of the procedure and require 6 to 12 weeks to heal after surgery. During this time it is important for the patient to follow the directed hip precautions to prevent instability or dislocation. This approach significantly improves the dislocation rate if a meticulous repair of the posterior capsule and short external rotator muscles is performed.

The other approaches take varying routes through and between the muscles to reach the hip capsule. For the direct lateral approach, a portion of the gluteus medius is divided to access the hip joint and then is repaired at the end of the procedure. With this approach it is advisable to limit resisted hip abduction to allow the repair to heal and to prevent future difficulties with a Trendelenburg gait. Delicate handling of the abductor muscles is necessary to minimize damage and postoperative heterotopic ossification in this powerful muscle mass. The anterolateral and direct anterior approaches avoid direct muscle sectioning and require varying levels of postoperative activity restrictions, ranging from restrictions similar to those for the posterior approach to no limitations at all. While hip stability is inherently higher in these approaches, they are more technically difficult to perform, require more surgical assistants, and, when compared in prospective, randomized trials, may not be more clinically efficacious than the more traditional approaches are.

Once adequate exposure of the hip joint is obtained, the remainder of the surgery follows the same basic steps regardless of the surgical approach. First the joint capsule is incised along with the supporting ligaments to clear the area and expose the femoral head and acetabulum. The hip is dislocated and the femoral head is removed with a saw. Usually the acetabulum is prepared first and reamers are used to remove the remaining cartilage. A healthy bed of bleeding cancellous bone is created and a press-fit or cemented cup is inserted. The femoral canal is prepared with a series of broaches or reamers used to create a uniform space in which to insert a cemented or cementless component.

There are many sizes of acetabular and femoral components so as to maximize the stability and ROM of the joint while maintaining appropriate leg length. Leg length is an important measurement, as care is taken to keep the legs as close to the same length as possible. However, there are times when it is necessary to make the operative leg slightly longer than the contralateral limb to assure appropriate muscle tension and enhance the overall stability of the hip replacement. The muscles may be thought of as springs, and the more tension placed on the muscle, the tauter it will be. Increasing the neck length or offset of the implant applies more tension on these muscles and increases their effectiveness to keep the hip from dislocating. In theory, severe muscle weakness could be a contraindication for a standard THA and may necessitate the need for a more constrained device.

The technique used to close the wound depends on the surgical approach and surgeon preference. In general, many tissues around the hip joint are elevated from the bone and must be repaired adequately. The supporting ligaments are reinserted once the replacement is in place, and then the surgical site is closed. Sutures or staples may be used to close the wound depending on the surgeon's or patient's preferences. It takes 6 to 12 weeks for the joint capsule and adjacent muscle insertions to heal.

Hip Resurfacing

Hip resurfacing is a relatively new procedure in the United States, but it has been used in Europe and worldwide for decades. A few implant devices have Food and Drug Administration (FDA) approval for implantation in the United States at this time. Despite an early enthusiasm for this procedure, recently there has been a trend toward more limited indications. The ideal patient for a resurfacing is a high-demand individual (someone who runs, jumps, and engages in other high-impact activities on a regular basis) who is less than 60 years of age, has osteoarthritis or inflammatory arthritis, and has a desire to return to high-impact activities. While hip dysplasia and osteonecrosis of the femoral head are not contraindications for this procedure, they must be carefully assessed by the operating surgeon in order for the resurfacing to have a successful outcome. Hip resurfacings are most commonly performed in males, as issues with the smaller components implanted in females have arisen over the past 4 to 5 years. A second concern for female patients is their relatively high risk for future osteoporosis and hip fracture. Hip fractures occur in up to one-third of women greater than 65 years old, and since resurfacing preserves the femoral neck, women with hip resurfacing are still at risk for this fragility fracture. On the other hand, for young, physically active patients, hip resurfacing is regarded as a bone-conserving alternative to THA.

The surgical procedure for hip resurfacing is much more intrusive than that of primary THA. Larger incisions are necessary to implant the components, as resurfacing leaves the femoral head intact, unlike in THA, for which the femoral head is removed early in the procedure. In order to safely implant the cup, the femoral head must be moved either in front or in back of the cup depending on the surgeon's approach to the hip. Once the acetabulum is prepared as it is for THA, a single-piece cup is implanted into the cavity. A metal cap is then cemented onto the head of the femur after it is appropriately shaped. The only available articulation for hip resurfacing is metal on metal. Once both components are in place, the closure is similar to that used with THA. The same surgical approaches and restrictions that apply for THA hold for hip resurfacing as well.

There are several advantages and disadvantages to this operation. The main disadvantage is the lack of long-term published data for resurfacing—only 7 to 8 years of follow-up versus up to 30 years for THA. The implants are offered only as a metal-on-metal articulation, which is prohibited in women of childbearing age and relatively contraindicated for patients with renal disease. Metal ion hypersensitivity reactions, although quite rare, have been reported with these cobalt-chrome articulations. On the advantages side are an improved ROM and a lower risk for dislocation with the large femoral head sizes that are used with hip resurfacings. Femoral neck strength improves with time and patients are allowed to run and perform high-impact activities at 1 year following the surgery. Additional advantages to hip resurfacing include preservation of the femoral neck for future surgeries, low wear rates of the metal-on-metal articulations, and successful early results reported with modern implants.

Conclusion

Healthy hips create a good foundation for the core muscles and affect a person's ability to perform activities of daily living and remain active. The importance of muscle strengthening preoperatively cannot be understated, as such exercise improves muscle memory for postoperative recovery, helps maintain a reasonable ROM, and serves a protective role in future injuries. Most important, a well-designed preoperative exercise regimen gives clients a sense of well-being and improves their postrehabilitation time frame. Regardless of the surgical procedure being performed, the overall goal is to maintain muscle strength and motion so that the body is better equipped to handle the daily impact imparted on the hip joints. The Pilates method is a perfect form of fitness to meet these goals and to provide a low-impact exercise regimen that is enjoyable, strengthens the core, and improves and maintains the ROM of the affected and adjacent joints.

chapter 2

The Knee

This chapter reviews the basic anatomy and syndromes of the knee. A fundamental knowledge of knee anatomy is important in understanding the knee pathologies treated on a regular basis. Surgical and nonsurgical interventions pertaining to common syndromes and injuries about the knee are reviewed as well.

As we delve deeper into the actions, origins, and insertions of the muscles, ligaments, and tendons, it becomes more apparent how injuries and overuse syndromes affect the physiological function of the knee joint. It is this knowledge that helps us devise appropriate treatment plans and workout regimens to alleviate and prevent the pain associated with these conditions. The goal of this chapter is to impart this basic information so that the plans for care are clear and concise and yet open for interpretation by those with an intimate knowledge of the anatomy and physiology of the human knee joint. The people caring for these syndromes should be able to see the utility of the Pilates method as it relates to the anatomy of the knee and how this method compares with traditional means of treatment.

Knee Anatomy

The knee is a hinge joint capable of flexion and extension with limited rotational capacity. The complex and controlled rollback of the tibiofemoral articulation allows for a tremendous range of flexion in the normal knee. The knee endures considerable stress from weight bearing, gravity, and the impact of walking, running, and dancing. Sport injuries commonly affect the knee, leading to acute and chronic pain and disability. The knee joint depends more on the adjacent ligaments, tendons, and muscles and less on the configuration and constraints of the bony anatomy for its strength and stability (Magee 2008).

There are four bones that make up the knee complex: (1) the distal end of the thigh, called the *femur*; (2) the proximal end (plateau) of the tibia; (3) the kneecap (patella);

See the insert at the back of the book for illustrations of knee anatomy.

and (4) the fibula, which is a thinner bone that accompanies the tibia down the lateral side of the lower leg. The fibula does not articulate with the knee joint and is not typically involved in common knee syndromes or in replacement surgery. Thus it is not included in the remainder of the discussion.

The three bones that form the knee joint are the distal femur, the proximal tibia, and the patella. The femoral trochlea groove articulates with the patella and the distal femur articulates with the tibia in both flexion and extension. The patella is lax and mobile in full extension and engages the trochlea groove as the knee moves into flexion. There is a spectrum of conditions in which the patella does not articulate correctly in the trochlea groove; these conditions are often associated with hypoplasia or a malformed trochlea groove or an imbalance of the quadriceps muscles that allows the patella to tilt laterally. The distal femur and proximal tibia articulate with the knee extended (creating the extension gap), and the posterior condyles of the distal femur articulate with the tibia during knee flexion (creating the flexion gap). These two gaps are independent of one another and yet need to be balanced and stabilized by the adjacent structures of the knee to assure proper function of the joint. The knee capsule is a fibrous sac that encloses the entire joint cavity. It attaches just above the supracondylar region of the femur and includes the patella and the proximal aspect of the tibia. The joint capsule has a tough fibrous outer membrane and an inner synovial membrane that produces synovial fluid. This viscous liquid lubricates the joint and nourishes the articular cartilage that coats the surfaces of the bones in the joint. Synovial fluid production is often accelerated in pathological conditions associated with inflammation and hypertrophy of the synovium.

The distal end of the femur has two rounded articular surfaces called the *medial* and *lateral condyles* and has a shape resembling that of a rocker. The medial and lateral condyles have a dual radii of curvature configuration that when coupled with the ligamentous restraints of the knee results in the screw-home mechanism (which can be seen as the knee moves from flexion to extension) and the posterior rollback of the femur on the tibia. The proximal aspect of the tibia is divided into two surfaces on either side of the tibial spines (small elevated region in the middle of the tibial plateau). The medial condyle of the tibia is concave and the lateral condyle of the tibia is convex. Both are protected by cartilage and articulate with the posterior aspect of the femoral condyles in flexion and the distal femur in extension. The joint space between the tibia and the femur contains two intra-articular cartilaginous discs called the *menisci* that are affixed to the tibial plateau via the coronary ligaments. The medial meniscus is a C-shaped piece of cartilage that is thicker posteriorly than it is anteriorly. The lateral meniscus has a similar yet more circular shape and is generally of equal thickness throughout. Together the menisci cushion the joint by distributing downward forces outward and away from their points of anchor and thus serve as a means to better distribute the contact forces of the femur on the tibia. The menisci are slightly mobile, the lateral more so than the medial. They aid in lubrication and nutrition of the joint and act as shock absorbers, spreading the stress over the articular cartilage and decreasing cartilage wear. The menisci reduce friction with movement and aid the ligaments and capsule in preventing hyperextension (Magee 2008; Calais-Germain 2007).

The knee joint depends on the intra-articular and adjacent ligaments and muscles to maintain the stability and direct the motion of the knee. The ligaments act as primary stabilizers and guide the movement of the bones in relation to one another. The following are four predominant ligamentous stabilizers of the knee:

1. Medial collateral ligament (MCL)—The MCL is responsible for varus and valgus (side-to-side) stability of the knee. It runs medially distal to the adductor tubercle and extends to the medial surface of the tibia
2. Lateral collateral ligament (LCL)—The LCL is responsible for varus and valgus (side-to-side) stability of the knee. It runs laterally from the lateral epicondyle of the femur to the fibular head.
3. Anterior cruciate ligament (ACL)—The ACL is responsible for the anterior and posterior (front-to-back) stability of the knee. It extends superiorly, posteriorly, and laterally, twisting on itself as it extends from the tibia to the femur.
4. Posterior cruciate ligament (PCL)—The PCL is responsible for the anterior and posterior (front-to-back) stability of the knee. It extends superiorly, anteriorly, and medially from the tibia to the femur.

The cruciate ligaments cross each other and are primary anteroposterior and rotational stabilizers of the knee (Magee 2008; Calais-Germain 2007). The patella attaches to the quadriceps muscles via the quadriceps femoris tendon and is directly attached to the tibial tubercle by the patellar tendon. On the undersurface of the kneecap lies a thick layer of articular cartilage measuring up to 7 millimeters, the thickest area of cartilage in the human skeleton. During flexion and extension different parts of the patella articulate with the femoral trochlea groove. The patella improves the efficiency of extension for the last 30°, with the straight leg being 0°. It functions as a guide for the quadriceps and as a means to potentiate the forces produced by the muscles by creating an ideal lever arm. The patella has a secondary role in protecting the femoral condyles and in serving as a bony shield for the cartilaginous surface (Magee 2008).

There are several bursae located adjacent to the tendons and ligaments surrounding the knee joint. A bursa is a fluid-filled sac that functions as a gliding surface to reduce friction between moving tissues of the body. The four main bursae of the knee are the (1) suprapatellar bursa, (2) subcutaneous prepatellar bursa, (3) infrapatellar bursa, and (4) pes anserine bursa. Typically these bursae are very thin cell layers and serve as a potential space; however, in certain disease states the bursae can become quite thick and hypertrophic and can generate a tremendous amount of fluid in a bursal sac.

The quadriceps and hamstrings are the two major muscle groups aiding in extension and flexion of the knee. The following lists group the movements of the knee with the muscles that direct those motions (Magee 2008, 749):

Flexion

- Biceps femoris
- Semimembranosus
- Semitendinosus
- Gracilis
- Sartorius
- Popliteus
- Gastrocnemius
- Tensor fasciae latae (in 45°-145° of flexion)
- Plantaris

Extension

- Rectus femoris
- Vastus medialis
- Vastus intermedius
- Vastus lateralis
- Tensor fasciae latae (in up to 30° of flexion)

Medial Rotation of Flexed Leg (Non-Weight-Bearing Leg)

- Semimembranosus
- Semitendinosus
- Sartorius
- Gracilis
- Popliteus

Lateral Rotation of Flexed Leg (Non-Weight-Bearing Leg)

- Biceps femoris

Knee Syndromes and Nonoperative Treatments

There are many different syndromes and injuries that can occur at the knee. The knee is vulnerable to injury especially during sport activities. Overuse disorders are common and result in various forms of tendinitis or bursitis. Osteoarthritis, gout, and inflammatory arthritides may lead to advanced destruction of the cartilaginous surfaces of the knee joint. The subcutaneous nature of the knee affords the possibility of significant damage in the setting of a traumatic injury.

Syndromes and injuries associated with the knee include bursitis, gout, tendinitis, osteoarthritis, rheumatoid arthritis, and avascular necrosis as well as sport-related ligament tears, bone avulsion, ligament sprain, patellar dislocation, meniscal tears, ruptured tendons, fractures, IT band syndrome, and patellofemoral syndrome. Many of these injuries and syndromes are amenable to nonoperative management and are treated with short courses of monitored physical therapy. Knee replacement should be considered only when the knee condition is significantly advanced or severely painful such that no other form of treatment provides relief and the degree of impairment affects quality of life.

Conservative (nonoperative) treatments for the knee include rest, hot and cold therapy, topical agents, analgesics, NSAIDs, intra-articular injections (corticosteroids or viscosupplementation), acupuncture, nutritional supplements (glucosamine and chondroitin combinations), physical therapy, and exercise. Knee injections generally are a combination of a numbing agent (local anesthetic) and a corticosteroid and may be administered every 4 months for up to a total of 4 injections per year. Injections can be administered locally to sites of irritation, including bursae and tendon sheaths, or within the knee joint (intra-articular injections). An excessive number of closely spaced injections can destroy the connective tissues surrounding the joint, as well as the articular cartilage, making further use of this treatment counterproductive. If more than 4 injections are needed in a year, then alternative treatments need to be explored.

Another type of injection used to treat knee pain and early osteoarthritis is viscosupplementation. This is an injection of various formularies of hyaluronic acid, a fluid that provides lubrication, shock absorption, and subtle anti-inflammatory benefits. Viscosupplementation is approved by the U.S. FDA for treatment of the early stages of knee osteoarthritis. The series of injections may involve 1 to 7 doses spaced 1 week apart. Most commonly, 3 to 5 injections are required. Recently, a single-injection formulary was introduced into the market to improve the timing and administration of viscosupplementation. The procedure may be repeated over the course of a year as needed. Symptomatic relief of osteoarthritis pain is the goal. This treatment does not cure the disorder, but it can buy time before joint replacement or a more aggressive treatment option becomes necessary.

For the purposes of this book, this chapter focuses on the following knee syndromes: patellofemoral syndrome and chondromalacia of the patella, pes anserinus bursitis, IT band syndrome, suprapatellar tendopathy (tendinitis), infrapatellar tendopathy (jumper's knee), and osteoarthritis of the knee. These syndromes are among the most common cases causing patients to seek the guidance of a physician for injury or pain localized to the knee. The information in the following sections was compiled by literature reviews of Brugioni and Falkel (2004) and Calais-Germain (2007).

Patellofemoral Syndrome and Chondromalacia of the Patella

Patellofemoral pain syndrome encompasses a broad class of syndromes that are characterized by significant and diffuse anterior knee pain (surrounding the patella) and that are exacerbated by activities placing undue stress on the anterior compartment of the knee (such as running, navigating stairs, kneeling, squatting, and rising from a seated position). During these high-stress activities, the forces across the patella can range from 3 to 8 times a person's body weight. While patellofemoral syndrome encompasses the entire constellation of syndromes associated with the anterior compartment of the knee, chondromalacia of the patella describes the softened surface of the articular cartilage of the patella and is a pathological change to the cartilage rather than a condition. Specific numbers are difficult to establish; however, patellofemoral knee pain is responsible for a significant percentage of office visits each year to orthopaedists and general practitioners.

Clinical symptoms include pain around the kneecap that worsens with rising from a seated position, climbing stairs, running, and jumping. There may be a history of patellar dislocation, feelings of knee instability, or a sensation of internal catching. Typically, a specific traumatic event is not identified, but on occasion a direct blow to the patella can be the initiating source of pain. On physical examination, patients often have a genu valgum (knock-knee) deformity, walk with the patellas pointing toward one another (increased femoral anteversion or pigeon-toe gait), and demonstrate crepitation as they flex and extend the knee. The Q angle is formed by the intersection of a line drawn from the anterior superior iliac spine (ASIS) through the middle of the patella with a second line drawn from the tibial tubercle to the middle of the patella. Often this angle is increased in patients with patellofemoral pain and can be associated with patellar instability, chondromalacia of the patella, and patellofemoral arthrosis. When the knee is in extension, the Q angle should be less than 18° and 22° for men and women, respectively.

Conservative management of patellofemoral pain is the treatment of choice and is based on the underlying etiology of the syndrome. The goal is to develop a program to strengthen the quadriceps, particularly the vastus medialis muscle, to assist in proper tracking of the patella. Patella taping and patella sleeve braces may also offer pain relief and comfort. Use of the Pilates method in treating patellofemoral pain has not been documented at this time.

Listed in this manual is a series of exercises that can be used to strengthen and stretch the anterior structures of the knee and possibly treat patellofemoral syndrome. The exercises discussed are similar to those initiated in a formal physical therapy regimen and serve as an alternative option to attending traditional therapy. The sample Pilates program sequence outlined for pes anserinus bursitis can be followed and adapted to treat anterior knee pain. The goal is to start with a pre-Pilates program to work on strengthening the core and establish an appropriate warm-up regimen to include stretching and breathing. Once the core-stabilizing exercises have been completed, the regimen can be modified to focus on stretching the hamstrings and quadriceps using the prone leg lift, single-leg circle, half roll-down into full roll-up, modified shoulder bridge, spine stretch forward, and saw. Quadriceps strengthening can be achieved with the sitting bent-knee lift, quadriceps set, modified leg pull-up, modified hip circle, and a side kick series (SKS) consisting of up and down, front and back, small circles, D-circles, and bicycle. It is recommended to use topical or oral anti-inflammatory agents and local massage to aid in the resolution of patellofemoral pain. Typically, anterior knee pain responds to 4 to 6 weeks of targeted therapy. When the pain persists beyond this time interval, the patient should seek further treatment with a physician. People prone to patellofemoral pain should incorporate this Pilates series into their weekly workout regimen.

Pes Anserinus Bursitis

The pes anserinus bursa lies under the medial hamstring muscles on the medial flare of the tibia just distal to the joint surface. The overlying muscles include the sartorius, gracilis, and semitendinosus—for help remembering the insertion order, use the mnemonic *say grace before tea*. This form of bursitis may stem from an overuse syndrome, particularly in swimmers and long-distance runners who have recently taken up these respective sports. This syndrome can also be associated with medial compartment osteoarthritis and can occur after total knee arthroplasty (TKA), particularly with irritation over the medial edge of an overhanging tibial tray. Typically the pain is present on palpation and can be confused with medial meniscal pathology. There can be swelling, erythema, and calor. Radiographs and MRIs may be obtained to rule out other sources of pain, as often the diagnosis is difficult to pinpoint.

Treatment typically involves conservative measures, including NSAIDs (oral or topical), ice, and activity modification. Often tightness of the knee muscles can be identified and patients can benefit from a generalized knee stretching program. The sample Pilates program sequence described in chapter 7 (see p. 320) is offered as an alternative way to stretch the muscles of the knee and aid in the resolution of pes anserinus bursitis. The following exercises can be quite helpful when incorporated into an exercise routine for pes anserinus bursitis: sitting bent-knee lift, half roll-down, single-leg circle, double-leg stretch, modified shoulder bridge, and an SKS consisting of up and down, inner-thigh lifts, inner-thigh circles, internal and external rotation, 90° bent-knee lower and lift, and 90° bent-knee touch. If the pain generated from the medial side of the knee does not improve over 4 to 6 weeks of gentle stretching with the Pilates method, the patient should seek further treatment or diagnostic imaging by a physician.

Iliotibial Band Syndrome

The IT band is a musculotendinous unit that extends from the side of the hip to the lateral aspect of the knee, inserting on Gerdy's tubercle. This band of tissue may be associated with a tendinitis syndrome or bursitis in long-distance runners and bicycle racers. The irritation typically occurs over the prominence of the lateral femoral epicondyle and is exacerbated by training over mountainous or hilly terrain. Downhill running leads to increased contact of the IT band and the femoral condyle as the knee flexes. In cyclists, this syndrome is associated with pedal devices that lock the foot to the bike, preventing normal rotation of the knee during the cycling motion.

Patients present with lateral knee pain during the aforementioned activities. On examination, the lateral knee pain can be localized to an area over the lateral epicondyle and Gerdy's tubercle with extension of the knee. The pain often occurs as the knee extends from 90° to 30° or 40° before reaching full extension. Treatment consists of rest, ice, compression, and NSAIDs followed by gentle stretching of the knee. While the Pilates method has not been documented as a treatment option for IT band syndrome, a program that stretches the knee while minimizing impact and exacerbating activities is helpful and therapeutic for this syndrome. Use of a Pilates program should initiate after a short (5-7 day) rest, begin slowly, and progress as comfort level progresses. If symptoms do not improve over 4 to 6 weeks, follow-up with a physician for further evaluation is recommended.

The following exercises can be quite helpful when incorporated into a regular Pilates regimen for IT band syndrome: pre-Pilates pelvic curl, knee folds, abduction and adduction, adductor squeeze. Follow these exercises with Pilates movements of hundred, half roll-up, full roll-up, single-leg circle, spine stretch forward, saw, corkscrew, modified hip circle, and a side kick series (SKS) of up and down, front and back, little circle, D-circle, internal and external rotation, and inner-thigh lift and circle.

Suprapatellar and Infrapatellar (Jumper's Knee) Tendopathy

Suprapatellar tendinitis causes pain at the proximal pole of the patella at the insertion of the quadriceps tendon. This pain typically occurs in adult athletes over the age of 40 as part of an overuse syndrome. Pain is associated with resisted extension and passive flexion of the knee. Infrapatellar tendopathy is an overuse syndrome of the younger athlete (18-25 years old). There may be a palpable nodule at the inferior pole of the patella where the pain is generated. Pain is exacerbated by resisted extension and passive flexion of the knee.

Treatment for both syndromes centers around rest, ice, compression, and NSAIDs, followed by a course of graduated stretching exercises. The Pilates mat exercises are readily adaptable to stretching and strengthening the quadriceps and hamstrings. Focusing on the following pre-Pilates and Pilates exercises aids in treating the tendopathy adjacent to the patella: quadriceps set, pelvic curl into shoulder bridge, adductor squeeze, single-leg circle, corkscrew, roll-up, swimming, and an SKS consisting of front and back, little circles, and D-circles. If the peripatellar knee pain does not improve over 4 to 6 weeks of gentle stretching using the Pilates method, then the patient should seek further treatment or diagnostic imaging by a physician. Patients prone to developing infrapatellar or suprapatellar tendopathy should incorporate these exercises into their weekly regimen to prevent recurrence of these syndromes.

Osteoarthritis of the Knee

Knee pain secondary to osteoarthritis is common among adults worldwide. Presently, more than 40 million Americans have osteoarthritis, and this number is anticipated to rise to 60 million over the next decade. *Osteoarthritis* is a generic term that describes multiple etiologies with the common end result of cartilage destruction in a synovial joint. The knee is the most commonly affected peripheral joint, and the prevalence of knee osteoarthritis increases with age. Risk factors for osteoarthritis of the knee can be divided into systemic and local. Systemic risk factors include age, gender, race or ethnicity, dietary factors, smoking, and estrogen deficiency. Local risk factors include obesity, joint mechanics (limb alignment, sensation, and joint laxity), muscle (quadriceps) weakness, occupational stress, physical activity, and injuries. Patients experience pain that may be localized or diffuse throughout the entire knee joint. The pain is typically a dull and intermittent ache that is related to activity and gradually progresses to sharp and more constant pain. Knee stiffness with prolonged sitting or first thing in the morning is common; the stiffness tends to improve as the joint becomes more active during the day. Feelings of instability may result from degeneration and fragmentation of the articular cartilage and menisci. Recurrent swelling, increased deformity (bowing at the knees), and a generalized increase in the size of the knee are often seen as the osteoarthritis progresses. Patients may experience a decrease in ROM and possibly develop a flexion contracture of the knee that manifests as an inability to actively straighten the knee to full extension. As the disease progresses, the ability to walk normally (without assistive devices) and navigate stairs becomes compromised. Consultation with a physician typically takes place when the osteoarthritis or knee pain begins to interfere with activities of daily living or interrupt sleeping habits.

Plain radiographs are typically all that is necessary to diagnose knee osteoarthritis. Joint space narrowing, osteophyte formation, subchondral sclerosis, and cyst formation are readily seen on X ray. More advanced imaging studies are usually not necessary to establish the diagnosis. Nonoperative treatment modalities include oral or topical anti-inflammatory agents, weight loss, use of assistive devices, and low-impact stretching and strengthening exercises. A more rigorous exercise program is usually not well tolerated in patients with osteoarthritis. The sample Pilates sequence in chapter 7 (see p. 323) provides a series of low-impact stretching exercises that may be helpful in maintaining well-being and fitness as well as ROM at the knee. As the osteoarthritis advances, the pain progresses, and the ROM decreases, it is appropriate to modify the Pilates exercises to accommodate these limitations while still helping the patient to maintain a healthy lifestyle. When the pain interferes with activities of daily living, disrupts sleep patterns, or becomes incapacitating, the patient should seek physician care.

Operative Treatments

Surgical interventions for knee issues and syndromes may include arthroscopy or TKA. Following are brief descriptions of each intervention.

Knee Arthroscopy

Knee arthroscopy is a same-day surgical procedure—surgery in the morning and home in the evening—that requires anesthesia and allows the surgeon to debride the damaged areas of the knee. The arthroscopic procedure consists of 2 to 3 slit-like (0.25 inch, or 0.64 centimeter) incisions on the front of the knee that allow the surgeon to insert the instruments, which are approximately the diameter of a pencil. A camera is used to explore the joint and survey the damage to the articular cartilage, menisci, and ligaments. Decisions are then made to debride, shave, trim, and clean the damaged portions of the joint. Basically, the joint surfaces are smoothed over and the soft tissue tears and fibrillation are removed. Areas of cartilage loss can be treated by a microfracture technique in which a picklike instrument is used to create small holes in the uncovered bone. The goal is for these areas to fill in with fibrocartilage and provide some relief from the articulation of bone against bone. After arthroscopic guided microfracture, the postoperative course often includes an extended time of non-weight-bearing activity depending on the surgeon's beliefs. Recently, newer techniques for cartilage and meniscal transplantation are offered to younger patients with relatively small cartilaginous defects. Formal physical therapy is not always recommended postoperatively, but rehabilitative exercises are often helpful in accelerating the recovery process.

Knee Arthroplasty

Knee replacement surgery has been conducted for more than 30 years. Considerable advances in technology, surgical techniques, and perioperative care have taken place over the past decade, making knee replacement surgery more reproducible and reducing the associated morbidity. Expedited therapy protocols and less-invasive surgery have made the early postoperative recovery a little easier and faster. The average age of an individual undergoing a knee replacement is decreasing and is now in the early 60s. Since today's Americans are living longer, the demand for TKA has tripled from 129,000 in 1990 to 381,000 in 2002 (Kurtz et al. 2005). Figure 2.1 shows a normal knee and a knee following TKA.

In general, the incision for a knee replacement is made down the midline of the knee, and the goal is to avoid ending the incision directly over the tibial tubercle. The surgeon must visualize the three bones being operated on: the distal end of the femur, the proximal tibia, and the patella. The soft tissue at the upper end of the tibia is elevated to release soft tissue contractures as needed, and the kneecap is pulled to the side to expose the tibial plateau and femoral condyles. The ligaments of the knee play a paramount role in stabilizing the joint. Care is taken to preserve and keep intact the surrounding ligaments, tendons, and muscles, as they are critical elements for the biomechanics and stability of the knee. Depending on the type of replacement, the PCL is retained or sacrificed, and, in modern-day implants, the ACL is released in all cases.

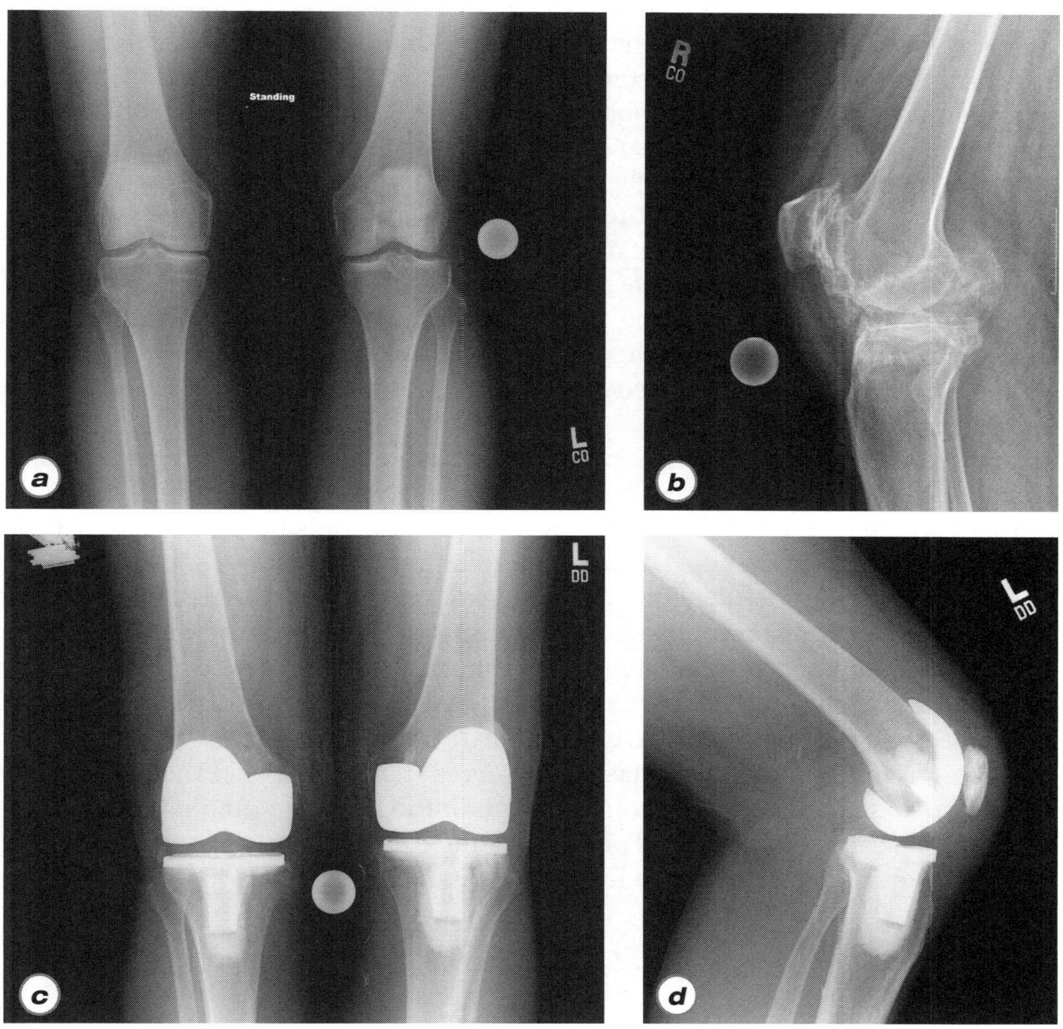

FIGURE 2.1 X ray of *(a)* a normal knee, *(b)* a knee with severe arthritis, *(c)* a total knee replacement, and *(d)* the lateral view of a knee replacement with the knee in flexion.

Courtesy of Brett Levine

Flat surfaces are created (bad bone and cartilage remnants are removed) by sawing off the tibial plateau and the femoral condyles in order to prepare them for acceptance of the replacement materials. Appropriate jigs are utilized to make these cuts to assure that the correct amount of bone is resected for the brand and model of knee replacement being used. In addition, the undersurface of the kneecap (patella), which slides over the surface of the femur, may be resurfaced with a round plastic button. TKA is not exactly an accurate description of the replacement. In reality, the joint is resurfaced and the cartilage surfaces are removed and replaced with metal and plastic components.

The surgical approaches to the knee are the medial and lateral parapatellar, midvastus, subvastus, and quadriceps sparing. Sectioning less muscle and tendon during surgery leads to early ability to perform a straight-leg raise and lowers the risks of lateral releases. However, specific precautions or changes in postoperative rehabilitation do not usually vary with the surgical approach to the knee in primary TKA. Regardless of the approach, the most important aspects are implanting the components in appropriate alignment and providing good ligamentous balancing to assure long-term success.

The implant is either fixed with the press-fit technique or cemented with bone cement that resembles grout. The decision to use the press-fit technique versus cement depends on the age of the patient, the condition of the bones, the surrounding tissues of the joint, and the surgeon preference. Most surgeons cement TKAs; only a minority use all press-fit components at this time. The cementless implants are more expensive than the cemented implants are, but they may offer improved long-term success if the bone adequately grows into the implants. Cementless techniques consist of metal implants with porous surfaces that allow bone to integrate within the prosthesis. Due to the advent of metallic foams with enhanced bone ingrowth characteristics, there has been a recent resurgence in this technology. The cemented procedure allows the client to be weight bearing as tolerated immediately after surgery. In the press-fit (cementless) technique, weight bearing may be restricted for the first 6 weeks, allowing bone to grow into the prosthesis, depending on the implant and surgeon preference.

During the procedure, the surgeon adjusts and assures proper tracking of the kneecap (patella), which is often a preoperative source of pain. A challenge for the surgeon is balancing the tension of the ligaments, as the knee joint is inherently an unstable joint. Without the ligaments, the bones are rolling or sliding on a flat surface with muscles holding the knee together. Therefore, the ligaments that are left intact during knee replacement must be of the proper tension and balance for optimal function.

There are many types of prostheses that the surgeon can use. The choice is made based on the client needs and conditions. The following are several currently available prostheses: mobile bearing knee arthroplasty, posterior stabilized TKA, cruciate-retaining knee arthroplasty (preserves the PCL function), unicompartmental knee replacement (one compartment of the knee is replaced), bicompartmental replacement (medial and patellofemoral compartments are replaced), and patellofemoral replacement (the kneecap is replaced).

Conclusion

The stability of the knee is not due to its bony structure but to the arrangement of the adjacent ligaments and muscles. Reviewing the pertinent anatomy should clarify why specific Pilates exercises are chosen to treat the various knee syndromes.

The knee encounters considerable stress from bearing the weight of the body and performing the activities of daily living as well as undergoes the wear and tear of recreational activities such as walking, running, and sports. A well-designed program to strengthen the muscles around the joint is imperative for improving the longevity of the native structures.

In the setting of a knee syndrome or following surgical intervention it becomes even more important to strengthen the muscles surrounding the knee in order to take unnecessary loads off the joint. A preoperative exercise routine builds the muscle memory that will help improve the postoperative rehabilitation and provides a sense of well-being for the client. Pilates is an ideal form of fitness in this setting, as it is low impact, strengthens the core of the body, and incorporates ROM exercises that assist in strengthening the joint and increasing flexibility.

PART II

Pilates Mat Exercises

Whether you are a qualified Pilates mat instructor, physical therapist, or physician, part II of this book provides the foundation and recommendations for Pilates techniques for hip and knee syndromes and arthroplasties. The quality of the program an individual follows the first year postoperatively for a joint replacement or recovery from a syndrome is the key to a successful return to functional movement.

Chapters 3 through 7 help the instructor with a Pilates mat certification work with a client with a hip or knee syndrome or replacement. (The accompanying web resource gives further information for a Pilates instructor who is fully qualified in using the equipment when working with a client with a hip or knee syndrome or joint replacement.) Chapter 3 begins with a table that lists the classical Pilates movements in the beginning, intermediate, and advanced series. The classical mat work is the base for selecting Pilates movements for the pre- and postoperative rehabilitation of the hip or knee. The classical mat exercises are modified based on the recommended range of motion for hip and knee arthroplasties and syndromes. Chapter 3 also includes the pre-Pilates exercises.

Chapters 4 and 5 break down the mat work into postoperative timelines of 6 weeks to 3 months, 3 to 6 months, and 6 months and beyond. A comprehensive set of the side kick series with variations for each postoperative timeline is displayed in chapter 6. Chapter 7 provides case scenarios and sample Pilates mat program sequences for several knee and hip syndromes. It also provides two complete sample Pilates mat program sequences for clients with TKA and THA at each pre- and postoperative timeline.

! All exercises should be performed under the guidance of a qualified Pilates instructor and with referral from the operative physician. The client's needs, restrictions, and ROM recommendations should be specified by the physician and followed accordingly. These guidelines may vary from the protocols that follow, and the protocols should be modified based on the individual's needs and the surgeon's preferences.

chapter 3

Setting the Foundation

Before you can create a Pilates program for your client, it is important that you know the range of motion (ROM) guidelines and special notes that are applied to the exercises for both the hip and knee, whether it is a syndrome or a joint replacement. All of the exercises in this manual come from Joseph Pilates' original work, combining the method with the specified ROM guidelines for an individual with a hip or knee condition.

This chapter begins with three tables. The first table (table 3.1) displays the classical series of Pilates exercises broken into the beginner, intermediate, and advanced series to show how Joseph Pilates laid out the original formulas of his exercises. The classical formulas make up the base for the next two tables. Table 3.2 addresses the hip and table 3.3 addresses the knee. The exercises are organized into sections based on postoperative timelines of 6 weeks to 3 months, 3 to 6 months, and 6 months and beyond. Note that some of the beginner exercises may not be applicable until 6 months and beyond postoperatively based on surgical restrictions and ROM guidelines.

Following the tables are the baseline recommendations for ROM and pre- and postoperative modifications for the hip and knee. They should be applied to every pre-Pilates and Pilates exercise for individuals with a hip or knee syndrome or replacement, depending on the postoperative timeline and ROM restrictions. In order to show how to get started with the exercises for a client with a hip or knee syndrome or arthroplasty, several case scenarios are included to give guidelines on the application of the exercises. Next are suggested pre-Pilates exercises that prepare the core muscles and ROM and strengthen the body. These exercises prepare the client for the beginner series of Pilates exercises. The pre-Pilates exercises are especially important for the client who has never performed Pilates exercises or is in the very early postoperative stage.

Pilates Mat Tables

Table 3.1 shows the original classical mat exercises performed in the beginner, intermediate, and advanced levels designed by Joseph Pilates (Pilates Method Alliance 2005). This table is presented here because the classical mat work forms the basis for selecting Pilates exercises for the pre- and postoperative rehabilitation of the hip and knee, which are shown in tables 3.2 and 3.3. Today, many of the advanced exercises in the original classical order have been modified for the beginner and intermediate levels and variations have been added to the classical mat programs.

Table 3.2 shows the classical mat order for the postoperative Pilates regimen for THA clients. Rather than organizing the exercises according to the beginner, intermediate, and advanced levels, table 3.2 organizes the exercises according to the postoperative timeline: 6 weeks to 3 months, 3 to 6 months, and 6 months and beyond. The client starts the mat series with a pre-Pilates warm-up, staying within the guidelines for postoperative ROM or specific syndrome precautions. All of these exercises (or modifications) are performed under the guidelines of the hip precautions recommended by the surgeon and dictated by the type of surgery. The exercises in table 3.2 are implemented based on the client's uniqueness, capabilities, surgery type, and tolerances. The individual performing these exercises should advance to the next level only after demonstrating a strong sense of core stability, strength, and flexibility as tolerated.

Table 3.3 shows the classical mat order for the postoperative Pilates regimen for TKA clients. Rather than organizing the exercises according to the beginner, intermediate, and advanced levels, table 3.3 organizes the exercises according

TABLE 3.1 Original Classical Pilates Mat Series

Beginner	Intermediate	Advanced
Hundred	All previous exercises	All previous exercises
Full roll-up	Single straight-leg stretch	Rollover
Single-leg circle	Double straight-leg stretch	Corkscrew
Rolling like a ball	Crisscross	Double-leg kick
Single-leg stretch	Open-leg rocker	Swan dive
Double-leg stretch	Saw	Scissors
Spine stretch forward	Single-leg kick	Bicycle
Side kick	Neck pull	Shoulder bridge
Seal	Spine twist	Jackknife
	Teaser	Hip circle
	Swimming	Leg pull front
		Leg pull
		Kneeling side kick
		Side bend
		Boomerang
		Crab
		Rocking on the stomach
		Control balance
		Push-up

Reprinted, by permission, from Pilates Method Alliance, Inc.®, *The PMA® Pilates Certification Exam: Study Guide* (Miami, FL: Pilates Method Alliance, 2007), 63-71.

TABLE 3.2 Classical Pilates Mat Series for THA Clients

6 weeks to 3 months	3 to 6 months	6 months and beyond
Hundred	All previous exercises	All previous exercises
Half roll-down and half roll-up	Full roll-up	Rolling like a ball
Single-leg circle	Double-leg kick	Open-leg rocker
Single-leg stretch	Corkscrew	Swan
Double-leg stretch	Neck pull (modified)	Neck pull
Single straight-leg stretch	Spine twist	Side kick (variations)
Double straight-leg stretch	Shoulder bridge	Teaser 2 and 3
Crisscross	Side kick (variations)	Cancan (modified)
Spine stretch forward	Teaser 1 and 2	Hip circle (modified)
Saw	Swimming	Leg pull (modified)
Swan prep	Serratus push-up (modified)	Serratus push-up
Single-leg kick	Push-up (modified)	Push-up
Shoulder bridge (modified)		
Side kick (variations)		
Teaser prep 1 and 2		
Side stretch		

The exercises listed for 6 weeks to 3 months are described and photographed in chapter 4, while the exercises listed for 3 to 6 months and 6 months and beyond are described and photographed in chapter 5. All the side kick series exercises are described and photographed in chapter 6.

TABLE 3.3 Classical Pilates Mat Series for TKA Clients

6 weeks to 3 months	3 to 6 months	6 months and beyond
Hundred	All previous exercises	All previous exercises
Half roll-down and half roll-up	Full roll-up	Open-leg rocker
Single-leg circle	Rolling like a ball	Swan
Single-leg stretch	Corkscrew	Neck pull
Double-leg stretch	Double-leg kick	Side kick (variations)
Single straight-leg stretch	Neck pull (modified)	Teaser 2 and 3
Double straight-leg stretch	Shoulder bridge	Cancan (modified or full)
Crisscross	Spine twist	Hip circle (modified or full)
Spine stretch forward	Side kick (variations)	Leg pull (modified)
Saw	Teaser 1 and 2	Serratus push-up
Swan prep	Swimming	Push-up
Single-leg kick	Cancan (modified)	
Shoulder bridge (modified)	Hip circle (modified)	
Side kick (variations)		
Teaser prep 1 and 2		
Side stretch		

The exercises listed for 6 weeks to 3 months are described and photographed in chapter 4, while the exercises listed for 3 to 6 months and 6 months and beyond are described and photographed in chapter 5. All the side kick series exercises are described and photographed in chapter 6.

to the postoperative timeline: 6 weeks to 3 months, 3 to 6 months, and 6 months and beyond. The client starts the mat series with a pre-Pilates warm-up, staying within the guidelines for postoperative ROM and specific syndrome precautions. All of these exercises (or modifications) are performed under the guidelines of the knee precautions recommended by the surgeon. The exercises in table 3.3 are implemented based on the client's uniqueness, capabilities, surgery type, and tolerances. The individual performing these exercises should advance to the next level only after demonstrating a strong sense of core stability, strength, and flexibility as tolerated.

Range of Motion Guidelines for Arthroplasty and Syndromes

This section outlines the ROM guidelines for clients who have undergone primary knee or hip surgery or have developed knee or hip syndromes. These recommendations are to be applied to every pre-Pilates and Pilates exercise for the hip and knee described in this book. The information in this section is based on standard surgical approaches for hip and knee replacement. There are several approaches a surgeon may take. In addition, hip and knee precautions may vary depending upon the type of surgery and surgeon preference; therefore, a client must follow the guidelines and precautions prescribed by the physician, which may vary from those described in this section.

A special note of caution: Any individual with a hip or knee replacement may gradually return to sport activities as directed by the surgeon. Typically, high-impact activities such as singles tennis, running, jumping, high-impact aerobics, and so on should be avoided to prolong the life span of the joint replacement. In general, high-risk sport activities should be reserved for patients with previous experience performing this activity. It is not advisable to initiate the learning curve involved with these activities after joint replacement. For example, a person who played tennis before a joint replacement may want to consider playing doubles versus singles tennis, while a person who never played tennis before the joint replacement may not be advised to start tennis. Similarly, downhill skiing involves significant skill and should be resumed at a lower level of difficulty only by clients with previous experience. High-impact activities and sports that require significant torsional motion need to be restricted or avoided, especially in active people who are looking to resume a high level of competition. Dislocation, fracture, or injury to a replaced joint may lead to subsequent revision surgery and may prolong recovery. It is better to resume a more recreational lifestyle and err on the side of caution when considering a return to sport and high-demand activities.

TOTAL HIP ARTHROPLASTY

Timeline

- 0 to 6 weeks postop
- Based on postoperative precautions for posterior, direct lateral, anterolateral, and anterior surgical approaches

Recommendations

Crossing the midline	No*
Internally rotating the leg	No*
Externally rotating the leg	No*
Crossing the knees while sitting	No*
Flexing the hip (degree of flexion from the chest)	Maximum of 90°*

*May be allowed for the anterior and anterolateral approaches based on surgeon preference. It takes a minimum of 6 weeks for the initial healing of the joint capsule and periarticular muscles.

TOTAL HIP ARTHROPLASTY

Timeline

- 6 weeks to 3 months, 3 to 6 months, and 6 months and beyond postop
- Based on postoperative precautions for posterior, direct lateral, anterolateral, and anterior surgical approaches

Recommendations

Crossing the midline	No greater than 20° for up to 6 months, then as tolerated
Internally rotating the leg	No greater than 20° with knee flexed for up to 6 months, then 30° for 6 months and beyond
Externally rotating the leg	Up to 30° when combined with hip flexion; avoid external rotation and extension of the hip
Crossing the knees while sitting	At 6 weeks, may work on crossing knees while sitting as tolerated
Flexing the hip (degree of flexion from the chest with the client in supine position with the legs in tabletop position—see figure 3.1) ***Note:*** Most individuals with moderate to severe osteoarthritis continue to have limited ROM and work as tolerated but not to exceed prescribed precautions	**1.** 90° to 100° of flexion up to 3 months postop **2.** Work up to 110° of flexion by 6 months postop **3.** Work toward 115° of flexion at 6 months and beyond postop as tolerated
Lifting more than 50 pounds (23 kilograms)	Heavy lifting with a THA is not recommended; specific weight restrictions can be modified based on patient experience and in accordance with previously listed precautions

Note that these precautions are set for a timeline up to one year post joint replacement. Variations in ROM for the first year may occur based on surgeon preferences and surgical approach along with the individual's motivation, size, and fitness level.

It takes up to 3 months for the joint capsule to heal completely after THA. Functional rotation of the hip should be limited to the provided guidelines, as it is important not to pivot into extremes of internal or external rotation when the operative foot is planted firmly on the ground. For instance, clients who have a right hip replacement and want to turn to the right should not step onto the right foot with the body weight to turn right. Instead, they should take care to pick up the right foot and then turn right (i.e., avoid weight-bearing internal rotation of the operative lower extremity).

There are several surgical approaches that surgeons may use. Clients must always follow the precautions prescribed by their surgeon, and these restrictions may vary from the ones provided here. In addition, surgical approaches and bearing surfaces have evolved significantly in recent years. Hip replacement precautions may vary depending on the bearing surface (e.g., metal-metal), surgical approach, and surgeon preference. It is important to discuss these short-term and potentially long-term restrictions with the surgeon.

Figure 3.1 correlates with the ROM recommendations for the postoperative hip. It represents the degrees of hip flexion with the body in supine position. The head is 180° and the feet extended on the mat are 0°. The legs extended to the ceiling are represented by the 90° mark; 90° can also represent the legs in tabletop position with the knees pointing to the ceiling. Flexion greater than 90° represents the legs in tabletop position coming in toward the chest, and flexion of 90° and less represents the legs extended up to the ceiling and out on a diagonal.

- 45° = legs extended out on a diagonal
- 90° = legs extended to ceiling
- 90° = legs in tabletop position with the knees pointing to the ceiling
- 110° = legs in tabletop position with the knees bent and coming in toward the chest, neutral spine
- 115° = the end range of legs in tabletop position with the knees bent and coming in toward the chest, neutral spine for hip arthroplasty at 6 months and beyond
- 125° = legs in tabletop position with the knees bent and coming in toward the chest, neutral spine

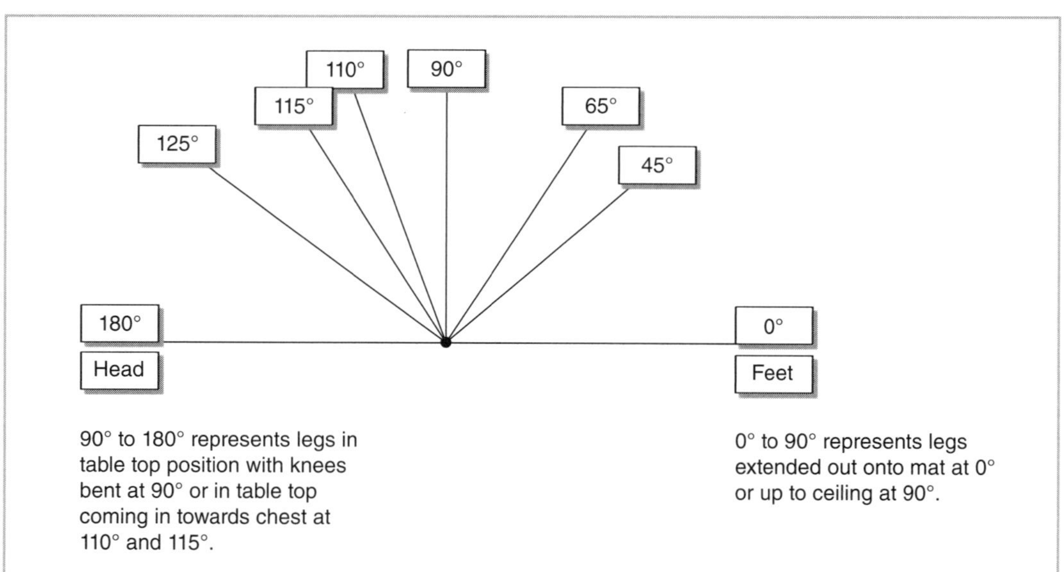

FIGURE 3.1 Degrees of hip flexion with the body in supine position.

TOTAL KNEE ARTHROPLASTY

Timeline

6 weeks to 3 months, 3 to 6 months, and 6 months and beyond postop

Recommendations

Crossing the midline of the body	OK as tolerated
Internally rotating the legs	OK as tolerated
Externally rotating the legs	OK as tolerated
Crossing the knees while sitting	OK
Flexing the knee	OK as tolerated
Heavy lifting	Heavy lifting with a TKA is not advised; specific weight restrictions can vary based on patient experience

The degree of ROM a person has before surgery is an important factor in determining the amount of ROM that the person can regain after surgery (±10°). It takes 6 weeks for the initial healing of the joint capsule to occur, and the healing process continues for up to 3 months. The patient should not pivot into extremes of internal or external rotation when the operative foot is firmly planted on the ground. The patient should not place all of the body weight on the foot of the operative leg to turn toward that direction. For instance, clients who have a right knee replacement and want to turn to the right should not step onto the right foot with the body weight to turn right. Instead, they should take care to pick up the right foot and then turn right (i.e., to avoid extreme pivoting and twisting of the affected extremity).

HIP SYNDROMES

Timeline

The following guidelines apply for the acute stage through rehabilitation.

Recommendations

Crossing the midline	OK as tolerated
Internally rotating the leg	OK as tolerated
Crossing the knees while sitting	OK as tolerated
Degree of range from chest	Based on individual needs
Heavy lifting	During the acute healing phase, heavy lifting is to be avoided; normal weightlifting activities may be resumed as syndrome resolves
In general	Keep legs parallel and hip-distance apart with neutral pelvis

KNEE SYNDROMES

Timeline

The following guidelines apply for the acute stage through rehabilitation.

Recommendations

Crossing the midline of the body	OK as tolerated
Internally rotating the legs	OK as tolerated
Externally rotating the legs	OK as tolerated
Crossing the knees while sitting	OK as tolerated
Heavy lifting	During the acute healing phase, heavy lifting is to be avoided; normal weightlifting activities may be resumed as syndrome resolves
In general	Keep legs parallel with soft knees and hip-distance apart with neutral pelvis

Getting Started With the Pilates Exercises

No two clients begin at the same level pre- or postoperatively when starting a Pilates routine. Each client has a varying ability to concentrate, visualize, feel the movement working from the correct source, and engage the core. Some clients may stay in the pre-Pilates stage for several weeks before being introduced to the beginner Pilates exercises with modifications for their postoperative rehabilitation. Clients with a knee or hip syndrome for which surgery is not performed also vary in ROM and flexibility without pain. Movement without pain is the key to building confidence and the desire to continue to exercise. Start slowly and build the foundation for movement and core development.

In order to give a better understanding of how to begin a Pilates routine, this section presents several examples of client profiles and suggested regimens. This information should help you to see how to begin an exercise regimen for a client with a history of a hip or knee condition. The examples presented here are merely a few of the many profiles that can be encountered. It is always advisable to take a good medical and surgical history from the client and know the client's exercise history, potential, and goals. When choosing an exercise routine for a client with a syndrome, select exercises that are modified to match the client's ability to move without pain and stay within the prescribed precautions noted earlier in this chapter and dictated by the physician's preference for the client. Here are the scenarios:

1. A client comes in to learn Pilates, has no previous Pilates exercise experience, and is 6 weeks postoperative from an arthroplasty.
   - Begin with a selection of pre-Pilates exercises and stay with this system until the client demonstrates the ability to work from the correct source and engage the core.
   - Start the mat exercises for 6 weeks to 3 months after surgery, progressing along an appropriate and well-tolerated time frame.
   - Limit ROM based on the client's ability to engage the core musculature and protect the back.

2. A client comes in to learn Pilates, has a preoperative history of regular Pilates exercise, and is 6 weeks postoperative from an arthroplasty.
   - Warm up from a selection of the pre-Pilates exercises.
   - Start the mat exercises for 6 weeks to 3 months after surgery, progressing along an appropriate and well-tolerated time frame.
   - Apply baseline recommendations for ROM and modifications for 6 weeks postoperative.
3. A client comes in to learn Pilates at 3 to 6 months postoperative from an arthroplasty and has no previous Pilates exercise history.
   - Begin with a selection of pre-Pilates exercises and stay with this system until the client demonstrates the ability to work from the correct source and engage the core.
   - Start the mat exercises for 6 weeks to 3 months postoperative.
   - Limit ROM based on the client's ability to engage the core musculature and protect the back.
   - Advance to the next level (3-6 months postoperative) only when the client can demonstrate correct form and core stability.
4. A client comes in to learn Pilates, has no previous Pilates exercise history, and has a hip or knee syndrome.
   - Begin with a selection of pre-Pilates exercises and stay with this system until the client demonstrates the ability to work from the correct source and engage the core and move without pain.
   - Start exercises in the 6 weeks to 3 months postoperative section. Use yoga blocks, pads, pillows, or towels to support the adjacent joints and help the client to move comfortably without pain.

These four clients provide only a small glimpse of the many case scenarios that you will encounter as a Pilates instructor. Initially, start with the basics and keep the routines simple. Limit the number of repetitions and work within a comfortable level at which the client can experience success with the exercises. Chapter 7 includes several case scenarios with exercise program sequences for knee and hip syndromes as well as knee and hip arthroplasty that can be used as sample programs.

Pre-Pilates Exercises

Pre-Pilates exercises are performed in the early stages of learning Pilates and as a warm-up to a Pilates exercise routine. These are exercises that initiate movement, function, and strength. Many of the exercises resemble those a physical therapist instructs a client to do in the perioperative timeframe. The difficulty of the exercises will vary. In addition, some of the exercises may pertain more to the knee or more to a hip; however, almost all of the pre-Pilates exercises can be performed by clients with knee or hip syndromes or replacements. The pre-Pilates exercises suggested within this section serve to

- warm up the body to prepare it for the Pilates exercise routine,
- begin ROM for a client with no Pilates experience and a knee or hip syndrome, and
- begin ROM for a client with no Pilates experience and a knee or hip arthroplasty.

All of the exercises must be performed using the baseline guidelines for ROM and the modifications for knee and hip syndromes or arthroplasty presented earlier in this chapter (pp. 32-36). In addition, it is important to think about where the exercises should be preformed, especially during the early postoperative days or for clients with a syndrome that limits ROM.

- For a unilateral hip or knee arthroplasty, exercises should be performed on a table or raised mat so that when the client sits down, the hip is slightly higher than the knee *for the first 3 months postoperatively*. For the client with a unilateral knee replacement, the hip and knee can be on the same level. After 3 months, the exercises can be performed on the floor using proper body mechanics for lowering to the mat.
- For the bilateral hip or knee arthroplasty, exercises may have to be performed on a table or raised mat for comfort and ease. After approximately 6 months or less, the client should be able to perform the exercises on the floor using proper body mechanics for lowering to the mat.

Breathing

- Lie supine on the mat with a pillow under the knees and the arms long by the sides of the body (or you can place your hands on each side of the rib cage, as shown here).
- Inhale through the nose and exhale through the mouth as if you were blowing out of a straw. Feel the abdominals flowing in and up, with each exhale melting the navel toward the spine.
- Inhale and expand the lungs, opening the rib cage side to side and through the back *(a)*. Exhale and feel the sides of the rib cage soften and flow in toward the pelvis *(b)*. As you inhale, the rib cage expands. As you exhale, melt the navel toward the spine, drawing the abdominals in and up and softening the ribs.
- While breathing, think of lengthening the body from the top of the head to the base of the spine. Feel and visualize one long line.
- Feel the shoulders gliding away from the ears and toward the hips.
- Open the collarbones as if taffy were strung across the chest.
- Use the breathing to relax the body and center the mind in preparation for the Pilates routine.

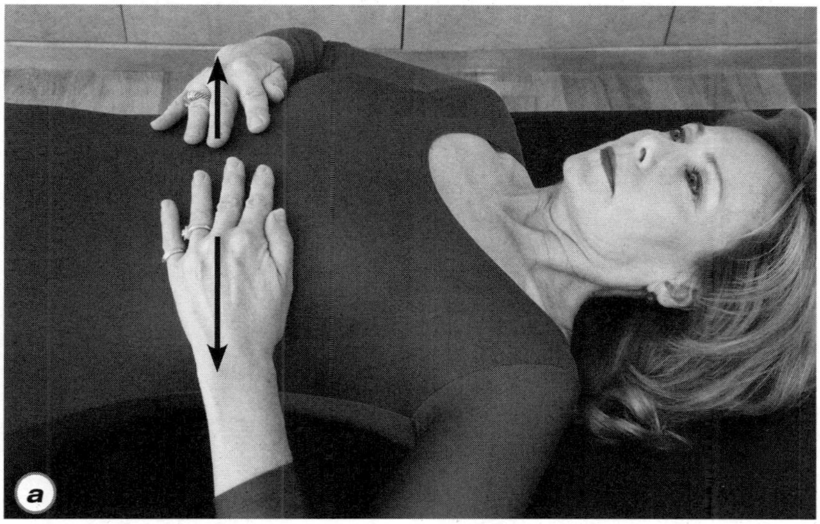

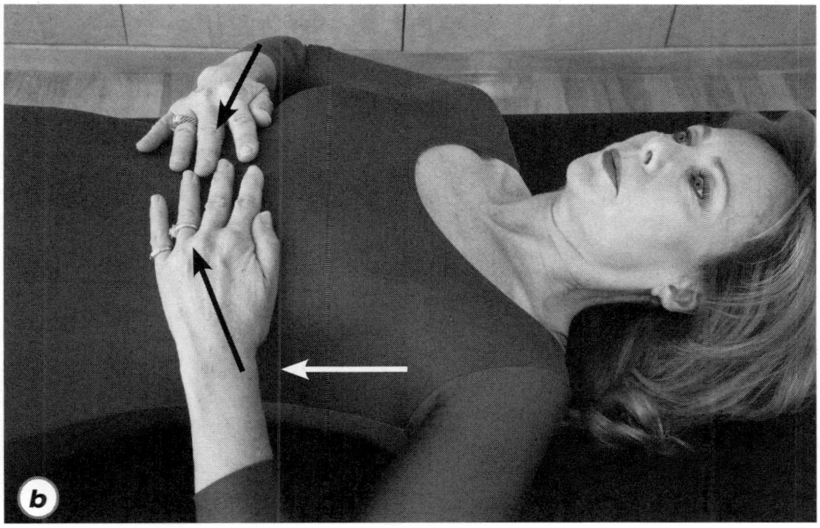

Ankle Pump

- Lie supine on the mat and place a rolled-up towel or mat under the knees. Flex *(a)* and point *(b)* both feet slowly together or one at a time *(c)*.
- Repeat each foot 10 to 20 times or both feet together 10 to 20 times.
- Inhale and exhale in a flowing fashion. Draw the abdominals in to stabilize the core.
- Point the toes and lengthen; flex and bring the toes toward the chest and lengthen the heels to the wall.

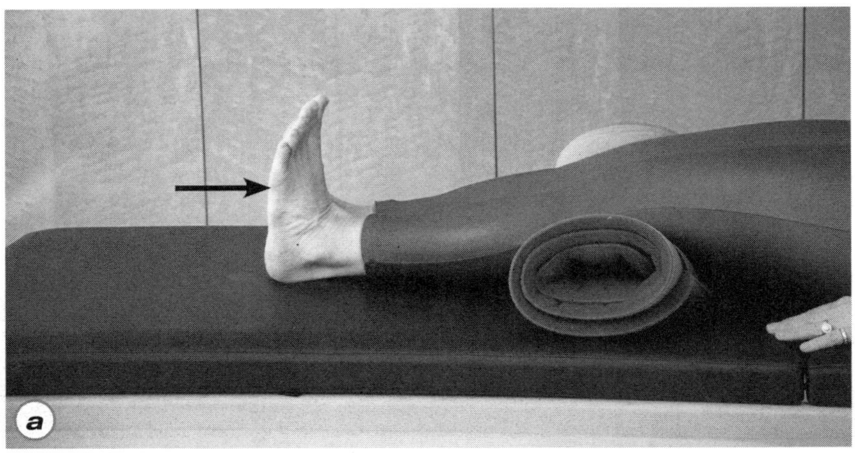

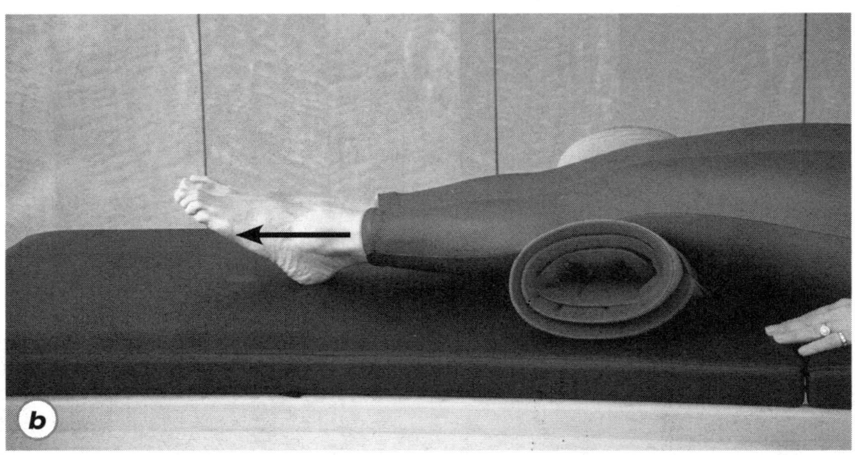

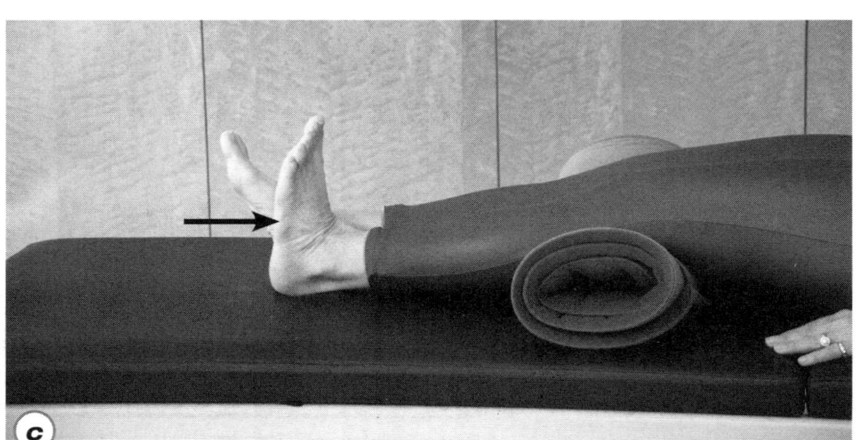

Quadriceps Set

- Lie supine on the mat with a rolled-up towel, mat, or pillow under the knees. Press the backs of the knees against the rolled-up towel or mat and hold for 5 seconds and then release.
- Repeat 10 times per leg.
- Inhale and exhale in a flowing fashion. Draw the abdominals in to stabilize the core.

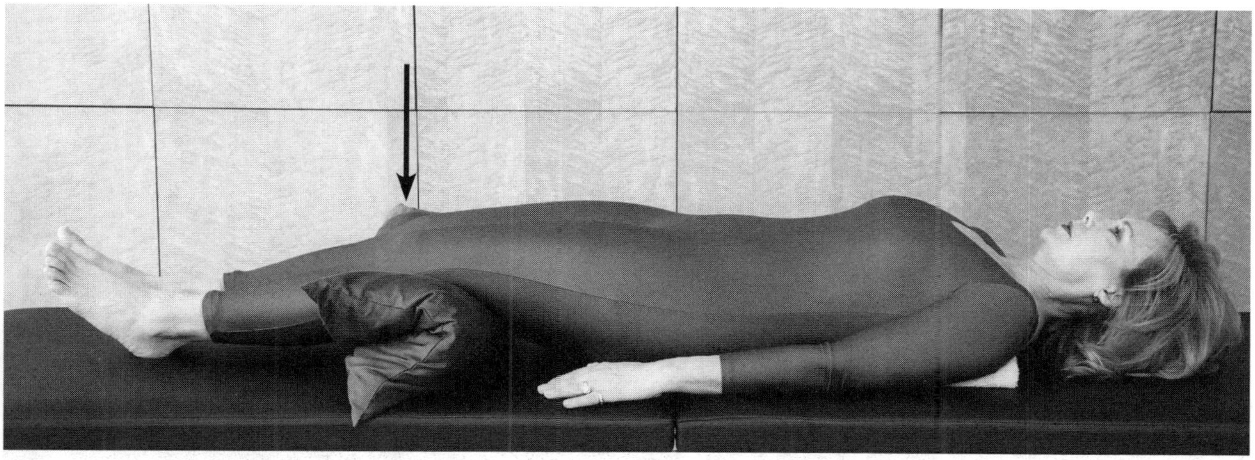

Gluteal Set

- Lie supine on the mat with a rolled-up towel, mat, or pillow under the knees.
- Inhale to prepare; exhale and draw the abdominals in and up and engage the buttocks (gluteus muscles), squeezing them together. The hips will lift a little. Hold for 5 seconds and then release.
- Repeat 5 to 10 times.

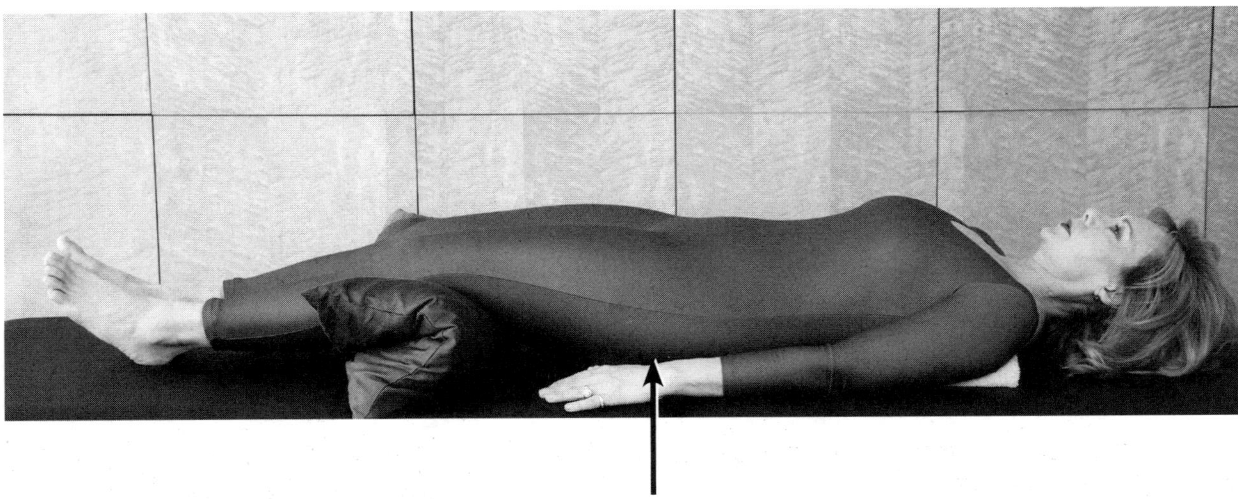

Abduction and Adduction

- Lie supine on the mat with the legs parallel and hip-distance apart. Lengthen out on the mat *(a)*.
- Starting with the left leg (keeping the second toe, ankle, knee, and hip in alignment), exhale and draw the abdominals in and up. Lightly slide the leg out to the left *(b)*. Hold for a count of 3, and then inhale and slide the leg back along the mat toward the right leg as if a magnet were drawing the legs together *(c)*. Try to keep the toe and heel on the same plane. A soft surface will be needed in order to let the heel glide out to the side and back to the start.
- Repeat 5 times and then switch to the right leg and repeat 5 times.

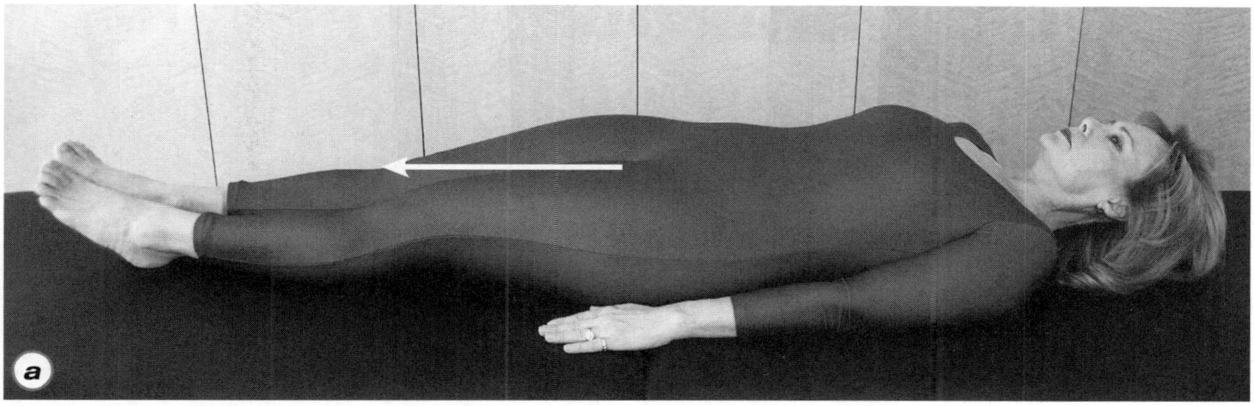
a

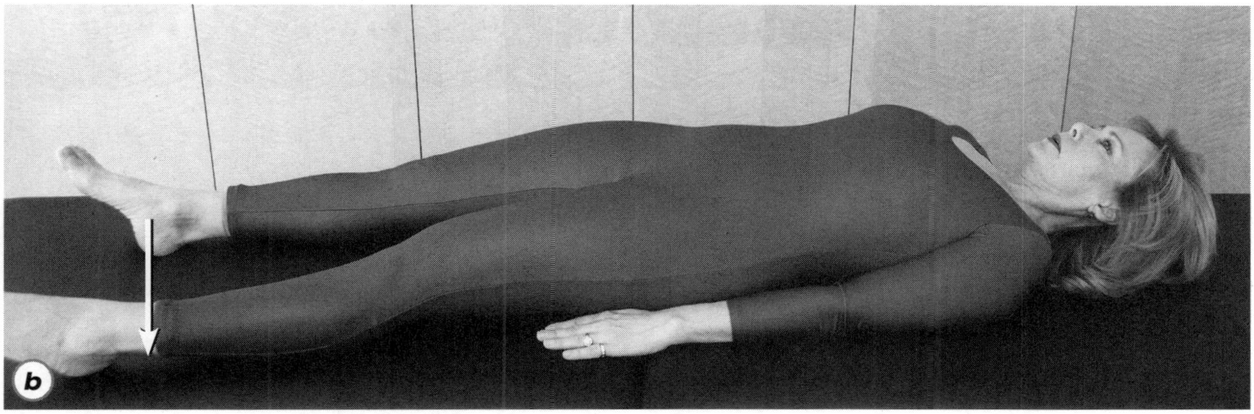
b

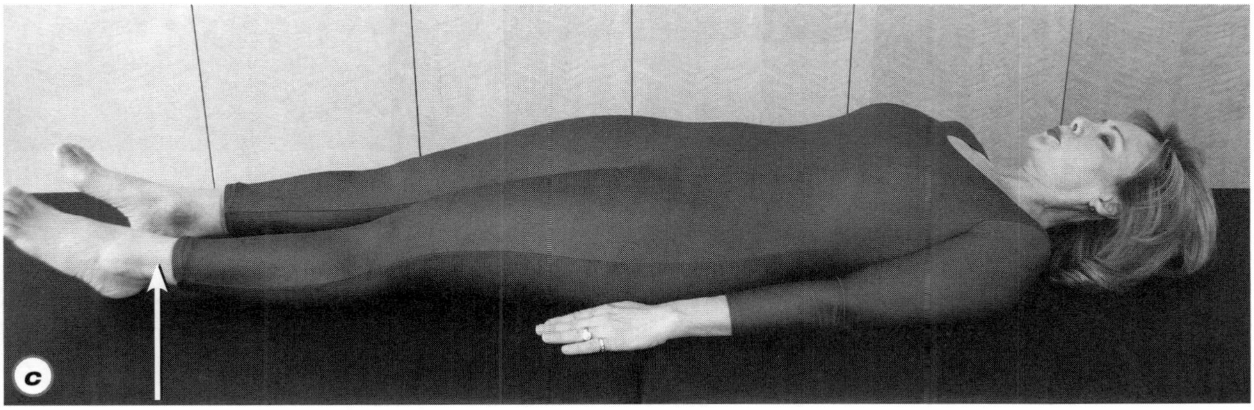
c

Shoulder Roll

- Lie supine on the mat with a pillow or rolled-up towel under the knees. The arms should be long along the sides of the body and the shoulders should be in a neutral position *(a)*.
- Inhale and slide the shoulders up toward the ears *(b)*. Exhale, drawing the abdominals in and up, and press the shoulder blades down toward the mat *(c)* and lengthen toward the hips *(d)* as if suspenders were hooked to the bottoms of the shoulder blades and attached to the hips.
- Stabilize the core by drawing the abdominals in and up, keeping the tailbone long on the mat.
- Repeat 5 times.

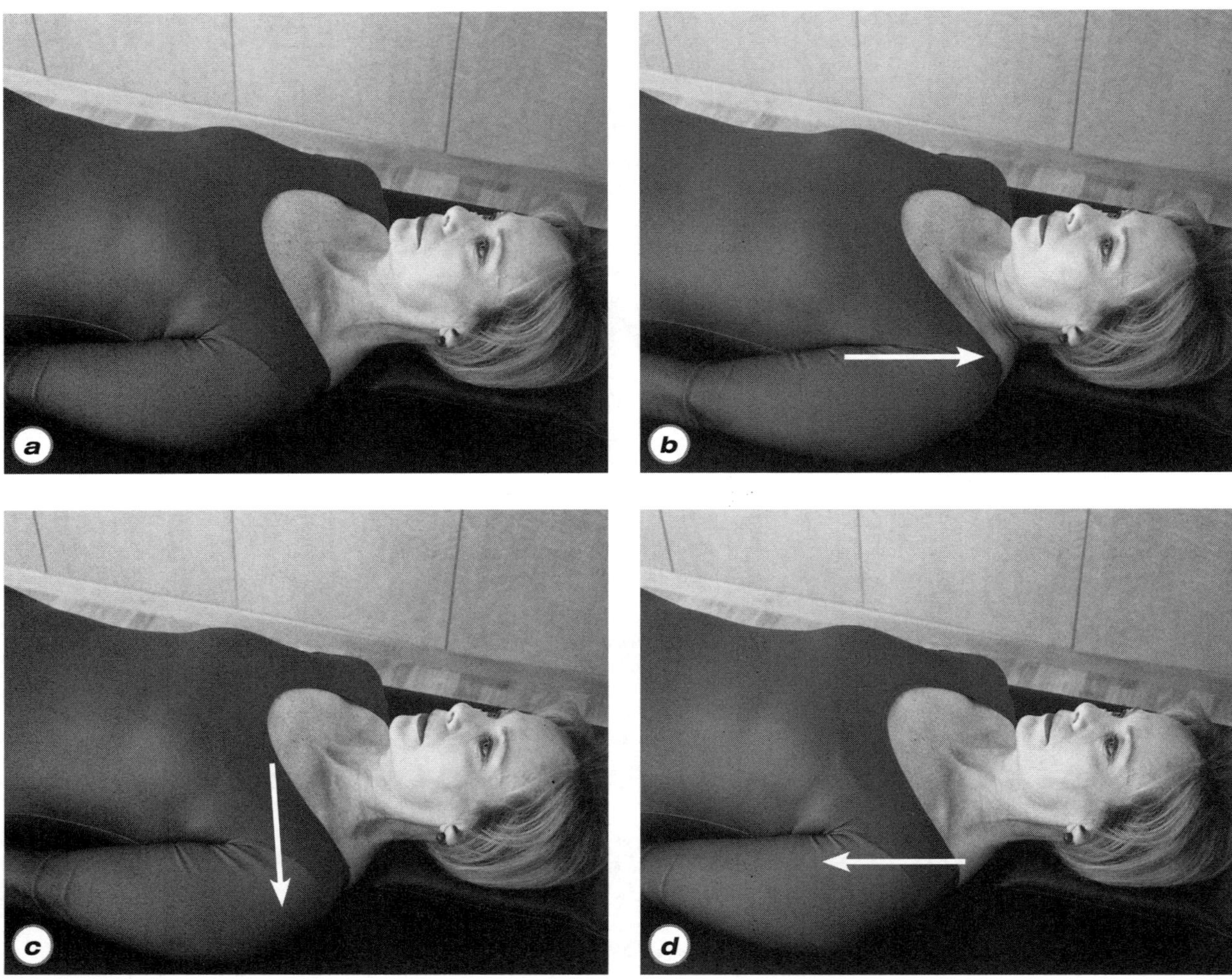

Pelvic Curl

- Lie supine on the mat with the knees bent to create a mountain shape; the legs hip-distance apart; and the second toe, ankle, knee, and hip all lined up *(a)*. Option: Place a small, soft ball between the knees and hug it lightly toward the midline of the body. Lengthen the arms on the mat along each side of the body. (In the photos, the arms are across the chest so that you can see the pelvic curl movement.)
- Place an imaginary marble in the belly button.
- Inhale to prepare, exhale, and curl the tailbone up toward the nose, imprinting the waist into the mat and drawing the abdominals in and up *(b)*. Imagine the marble rolling to the nose.
- Inhale and roll the tailbone back to neutral *(c)*, with the imaginary marble rolling back to the belly button. Exhale and press the tailbone into the mat and tilt the belly button toward the feet, creating a slight arch in the lower back *(d)*. Imagine the marble rolling toward the feet. Inhale, exhale, and curl the tailbone toward the nose, and so on.
- Repeat steps *a* through *d*, massaging the spine in each direction, 5 times.
- Start making the pelvic curl smaller and smaller until you feel the imaginary marble floating around in the belly button, as if it were floating in a pool of water, so that the belly button and pubic bone are on the same plane and creating a neutral spine.

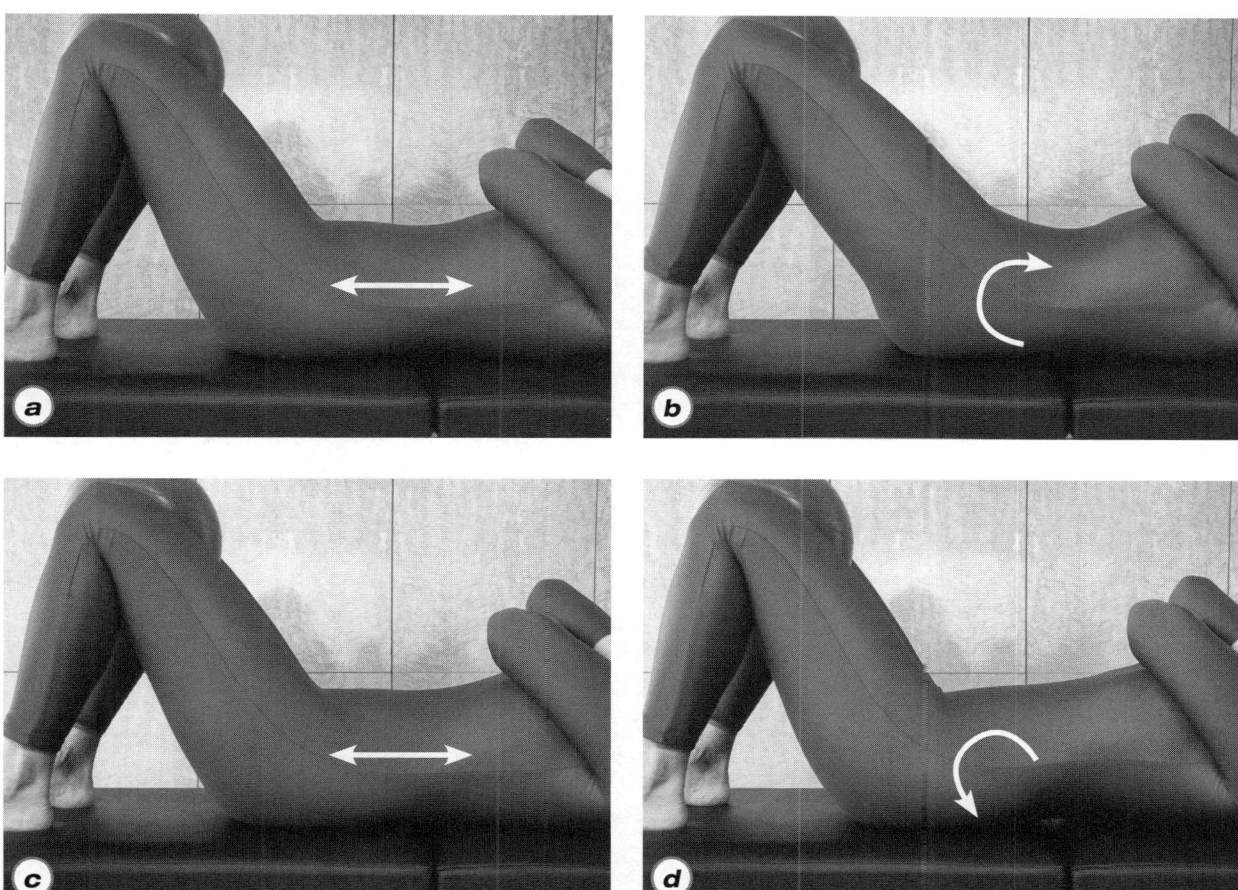

Toe Tap

- Lie supine on the mat, with the knees bent into a mountain shape, the legs hip-distance apart, and the head and shoulders lying flat on the mat or on a soft pad under the head.
- Draw the abdominals in and up, keeping an imaginary marble in the belly button.
- Inhale to prepare, exhale, and bring the left leg into tabletop position *(a)*. The hip should be in line with the knee and the knee should be in line with the ankle.
- Keeping the tabletop position of the leg (don't let the shin lift and lower), exhale and lower the left leg toward the mat—release from the hip with the toe leading. Keep the abdominals engaged at all times and maintain a neutral spine *(b)*. Keep the right leg bent and stable with the movement.
- Lift and lower the left leg 5 times.
- Switch legs and repeat with the right leg, keeping the left leg steady on the mat. Inhale to lift, exhale to lower the leg, and maintain a neutral spine.

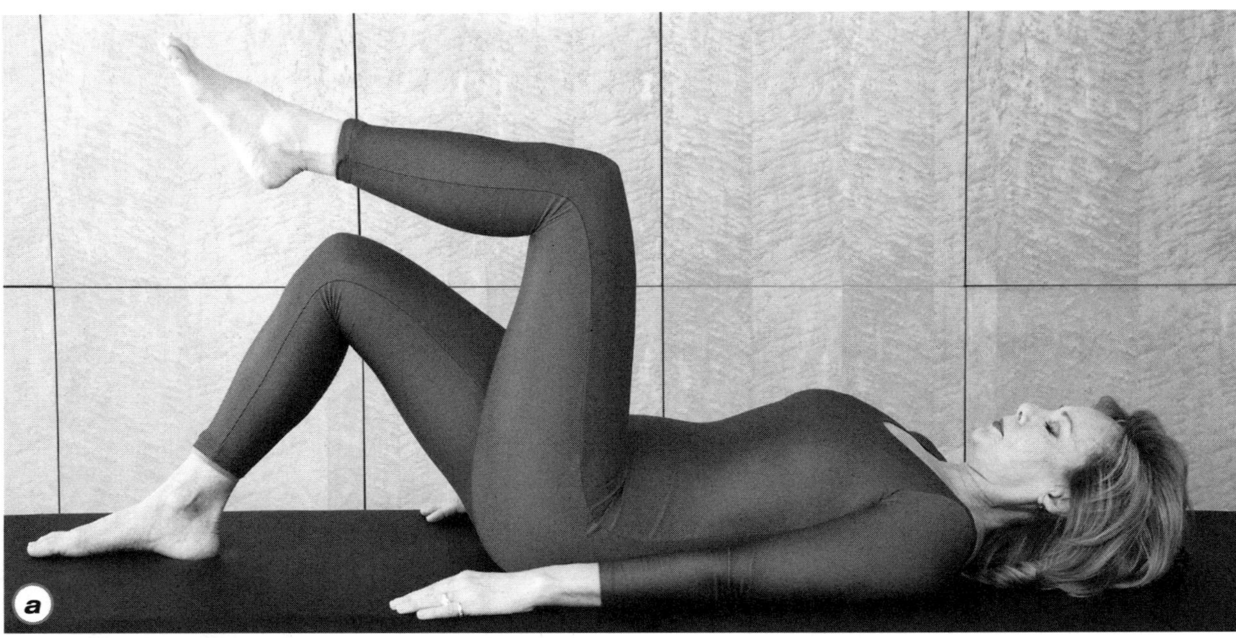

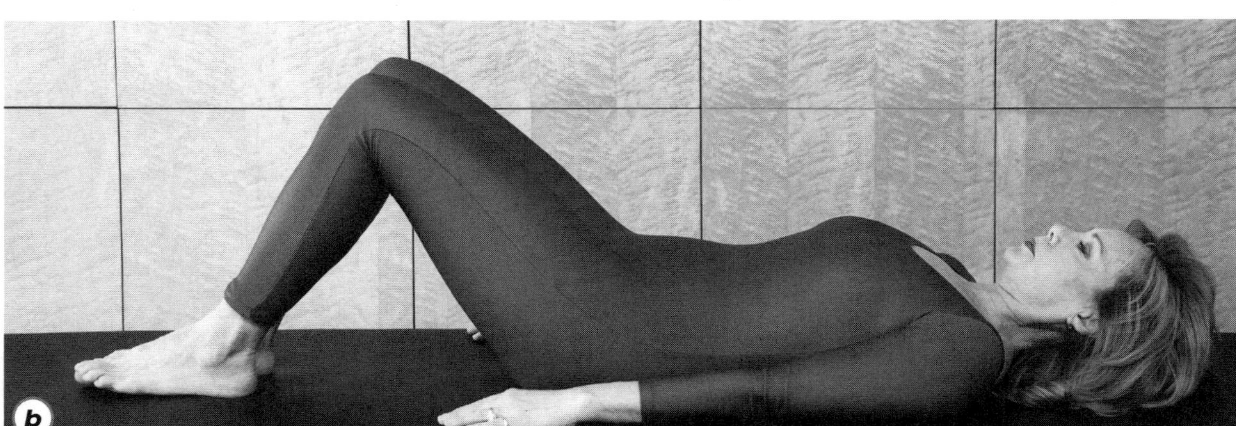

Option

- Bring both legs into tabletop position. The hands should be in a flat diamond shape under the tailbone to protect the lower back *(a)*.
- Lift and lower each leg, switching between right and left each time *(b)*.
- Exhale each time you lower the leg.
  - Keep open collarbones with the shoulders gliding toward the hips and away from the ears. Think of taffy stretched across the collarbones to keep the chest open and suspenders on the bottoms of the shoulder blades to help the shoulders glide to the hips.
  - Focus on keeping the core engaged. It is not important how far you reach the toe to the mat. It is important not to let the lower back lift as the leg lowers and to maintain a neutral spine.
  - As the core strengthens, lengthen both arms along the sides of the body instead of placing the hands in a diamond pattern under the tailbone.

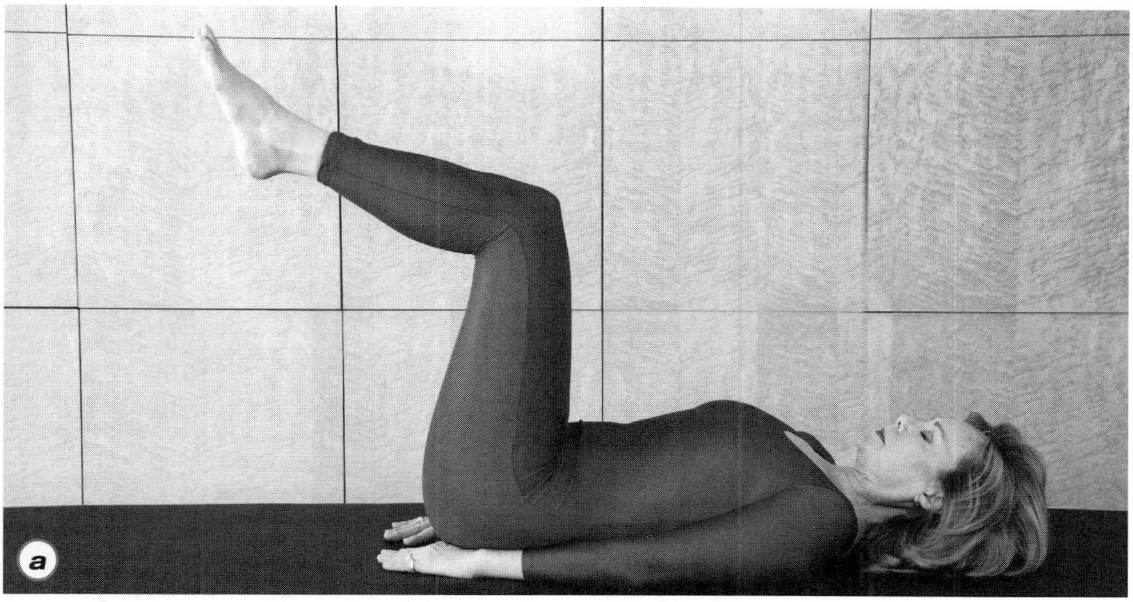

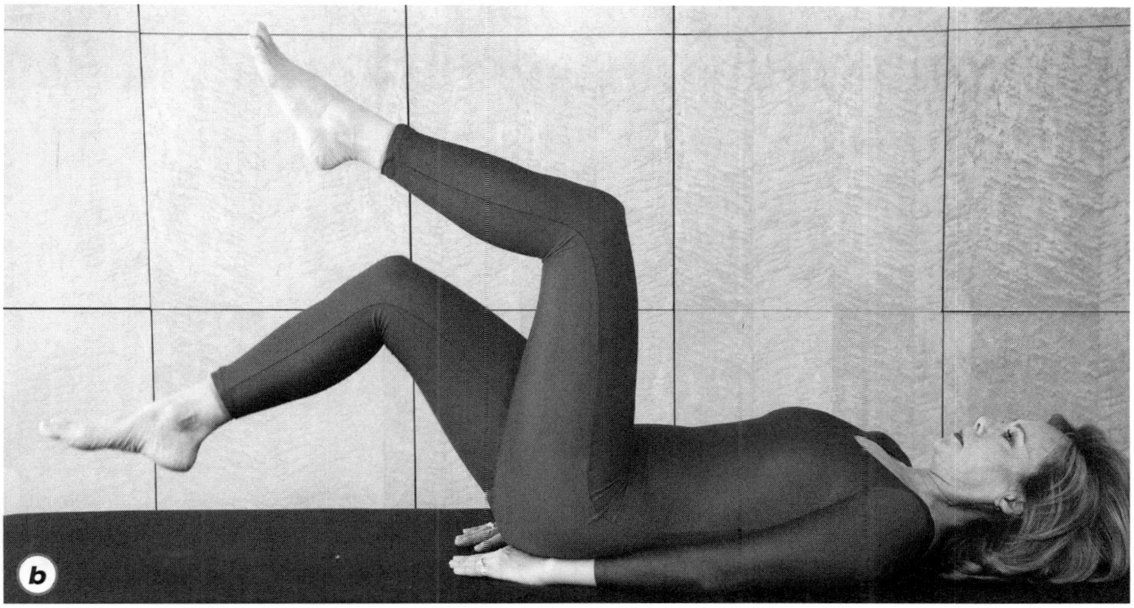

Abdominal Prep

- Lie supine on the mat with the knees bent into a mountain shape, the feet flat on the mat, and the legs parallel and hip-distance apart. Option: Place a small, soft ball between the knees and hug it lightly toward the midline of the body.
- Float both arms toward the ceiling with the palms facing away from the face. The arms are shoulder-width apart *(a)*.
- Inhale to prepare, exhale, and begin to float the arms toward the abdominals, curling the head and shoulders up off the mat to the bottom tips of the shoulder blades. Gaze toward the thighs *(b)*. Hover the arms off the mat in line with the body above the abdominal wall. Keep the tailbone long on the mat.
- Hold for 5 counts, inhale, and slowly lower the head and shoulders down to the mat while floating the arms back to the starting position.
- Repeat 5 times.
- Keep an imaginary tangerine under the chin as the head and shoulders curl up off the mat.

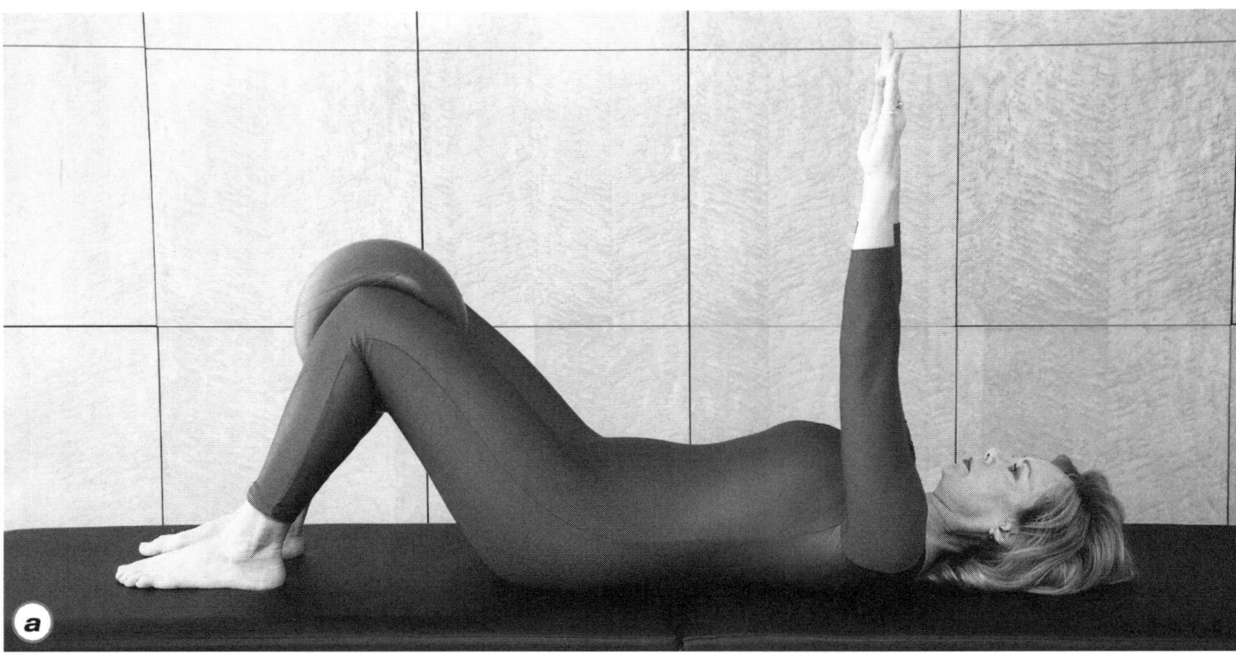

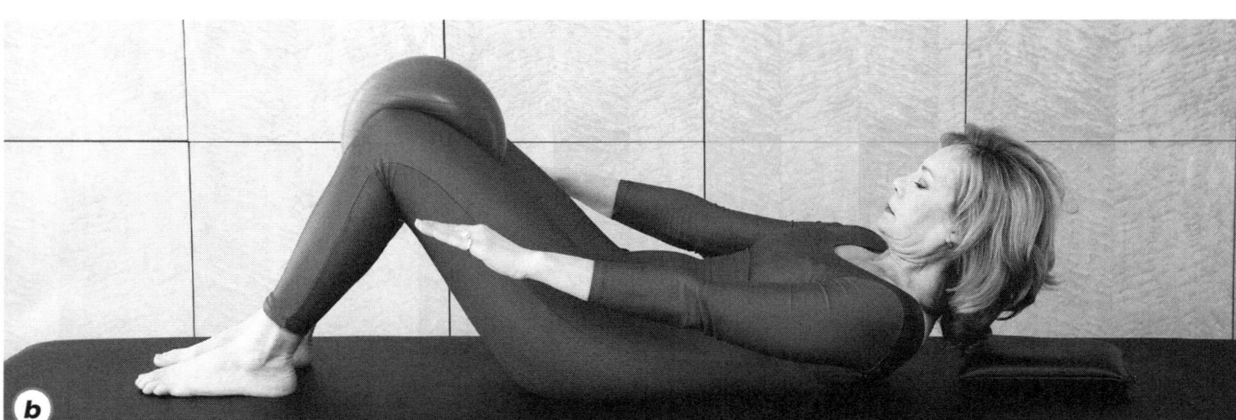

Option

Interlace the fingers of both hands and place the hands behind the head at the base of the skull. Run the thumbs down the sides of the neck to help support the head and neck during the abdominal prep. Try to keep the tailbone long and on the mat while keeping the head and shoulders rounded up off the mat. Maintain a neutral spine.

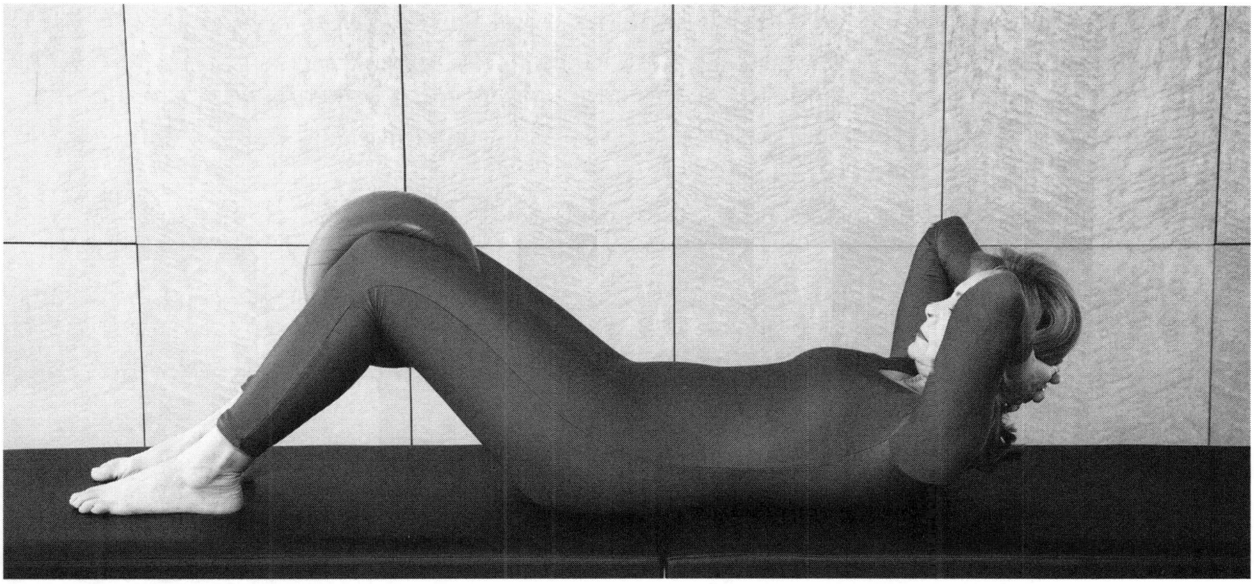

Knee Fold

- Lie supine on the mat with the knees bent into a mountain shape, the feet flat on the mat, the legs slightly apart by a distance about the size of a fist, and the head and shoulders long on the mat *(a)*.
- Starting with the left leg, inhale to prepare, exhale, and let the knee open out to the left side, so that it is externally rotated out to open the hip. The foot will be rotating to the outside lateral edge *(b)*. For the hip, rotate the knee externally to a maximum of 30°.
- Inhale and slide the leg out toward the end of the mat *(c)*, rotate the leg back to a parallel position with the knee and toe on the same line, and then exhale and slide the foot (heel) along the mat back up toward the core by bending the knee back into the start position *(d)*.
- Draw the abdominals in deeply as you return the leg back to the starting position. Keep the core and pelvis stable throughout the entire move. Stabilize the opposite leg with the movement.
- Repeat 5 times and then switch legs.

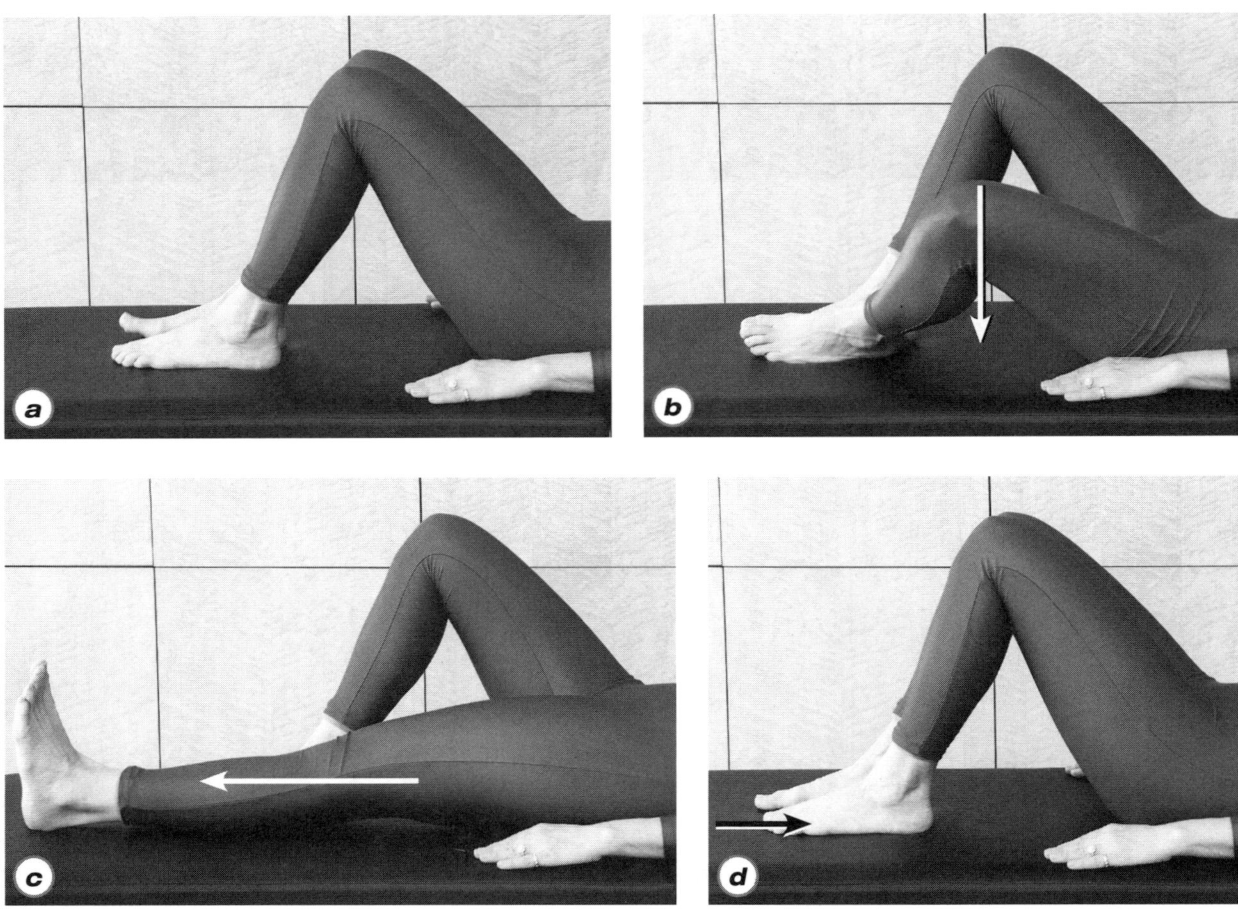

Option

- Let both legs rotate out (external rotation, with the soles of the feet coming together) and slide them out toward the end of the mat. Rotate the legs back to parallel and then slide both legs together to the bent-knee position *(a-e)*.
- For the hip, only rotate the knees externally to a maximum of 30°.
- Use a stable core as the knees ease out to the sides with control.

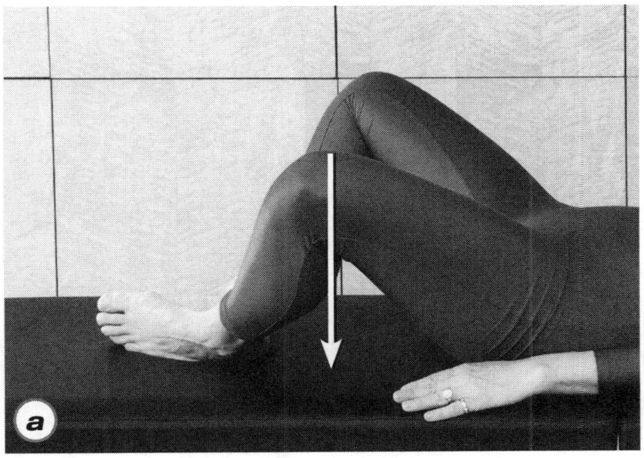
a

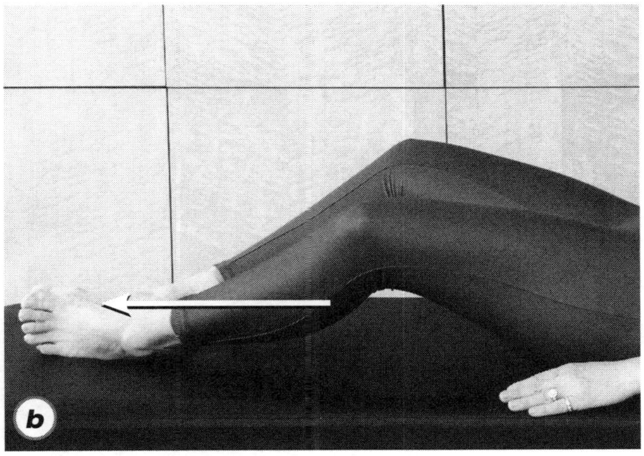
b

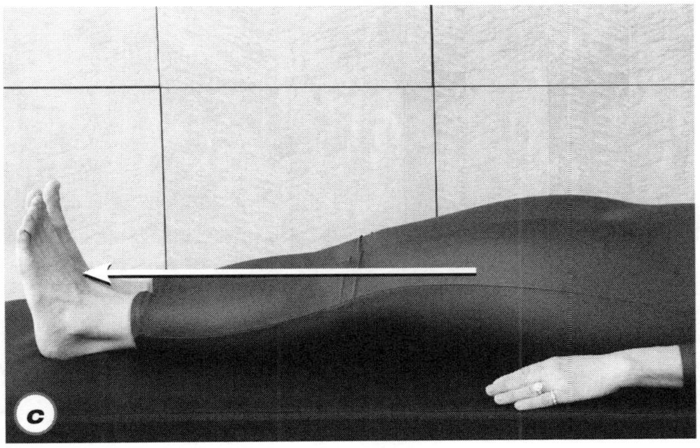
c

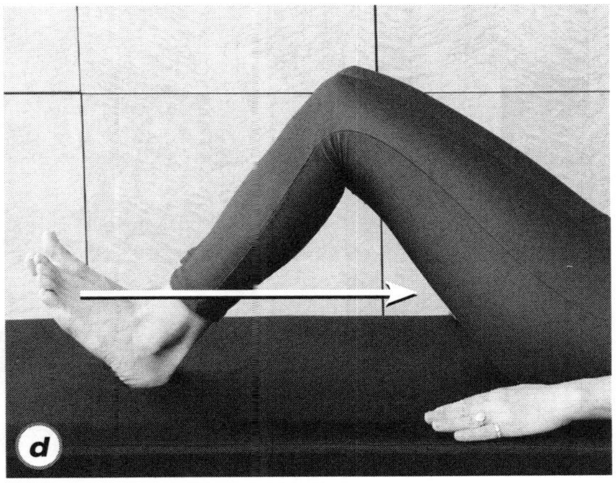
d

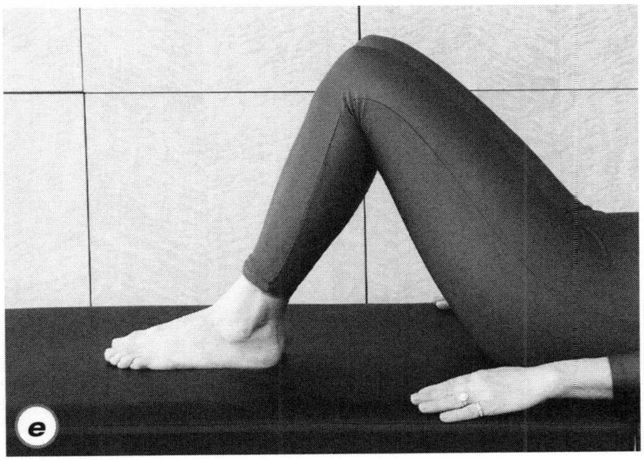
e

Adductor Squeeze

- Lie supine on the mat with the knees bent and the feet flat on the mat. The legs are hip-distance apart.
- Place a small, soft ball between the inner thighs.
- Inhale to prepare, exhale while drawing the abdominals in and up, and squeeze the ball without lifting or curling up the tailbone. Think of engaging only the inner-thigh muscles.
- Hold for a count of 5 and then release without losing the ball.
- Repeat 5 to 8 times.
- Keep the tailbone long on the mat, lengthen the shoulder blades toward the hip points.

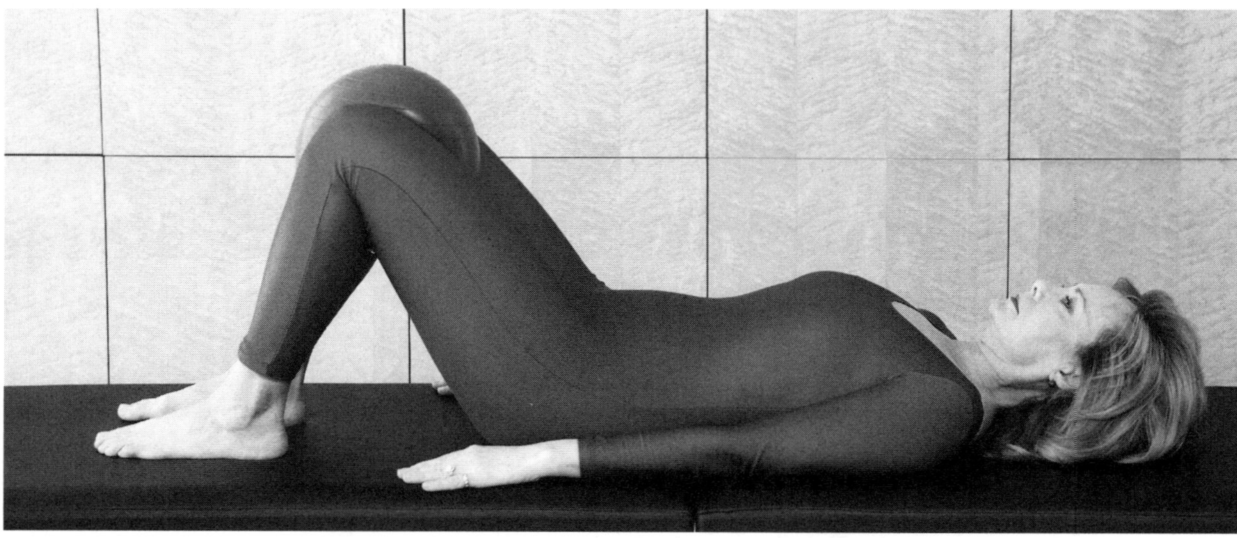

Supine Leg Lifts

- Lie flat on the mat with the legs extended onto the mat with a rolled-up towel, blanket, or pillow under the knees. The arms are long by the sides of the body. Place a pad under the head as needed.
- With the knees slightly flexed, draw the abdominals in and up and keep the torso steady throughout the movement.

Version One: Straight Leg

- Inhale and lift the working leg up to about 45° with a slightly flexed knee *(a)*.
- Exhale and slowly lower the leg back to the mat *(b)*. Keep the second toe, ankle, knee, and hip in alignment.
- Keep a rolled-up towel or mat under the knees.
- Keep the knees slightly flexed or bent into a mountain shape as needed to perform the movement.
- Repeat 6 times on each leg, and work up to 10 repeats.

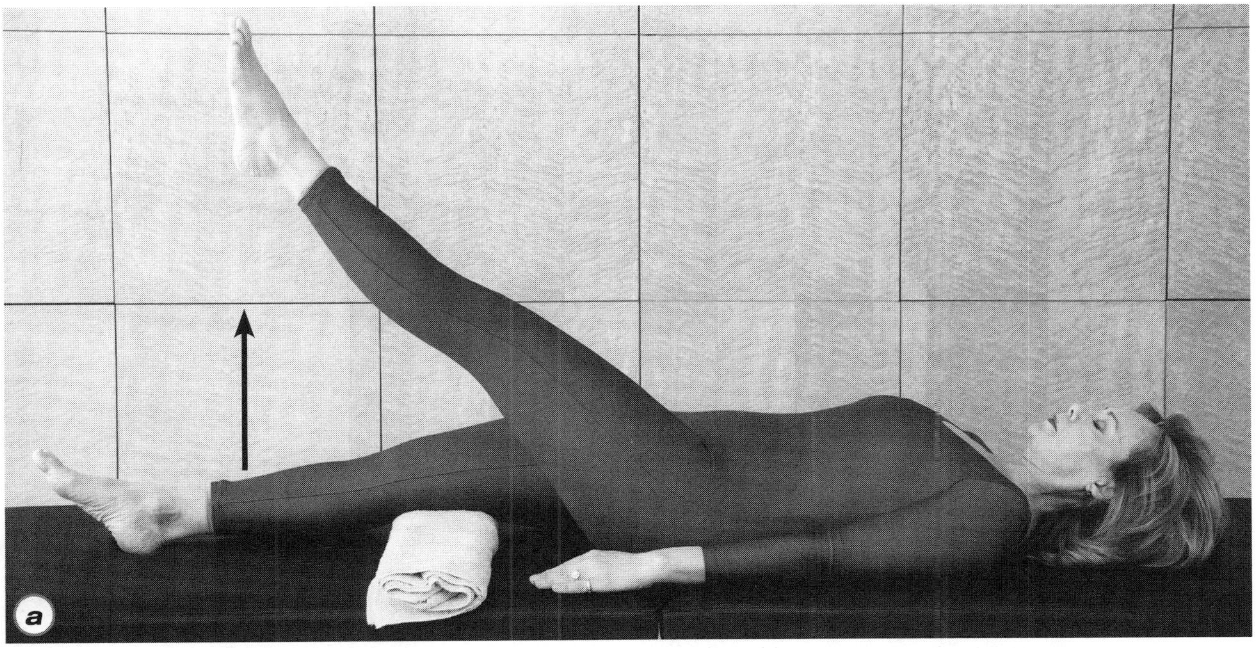

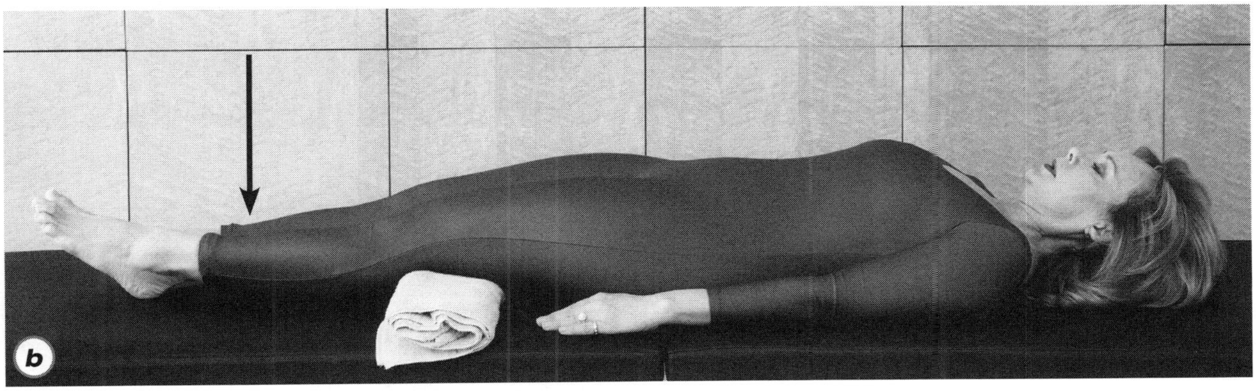

(continued)

Supine Leg Lifts *(continued)*

Version Two: Straight Leg Up, Down, Out, In

- Inhale to prepare, exhale, and lift the working leg *(a)*, lower the leg *(b)*, press the leg out to the side *(c)*, and press the leg in *(d)*. The flow is up, down, out, and in. Keep the leg parallel with no turn out and a slightly flexed knee.
- Keep a rolled-up towel or mat under the knees.
- Keep the knees slightly flexed or bent into a mountain shape as needed to perform the movement.
- Repeat 6 times per leg and work up to 10 repeats.

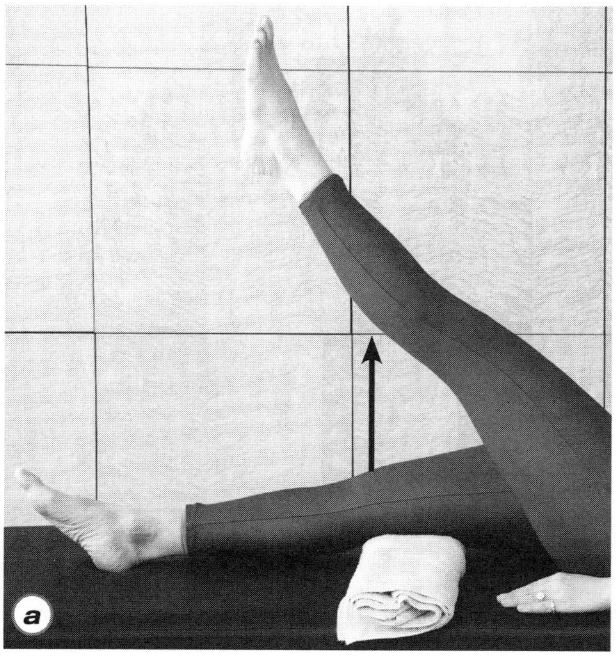

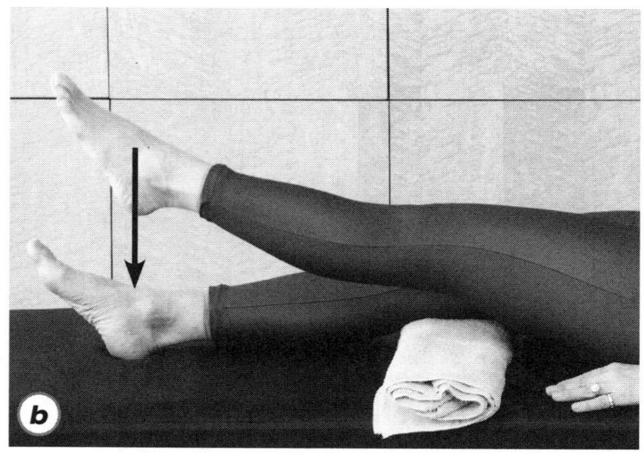

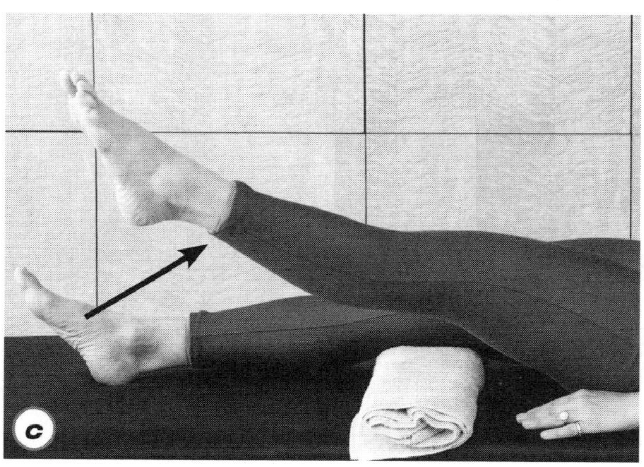

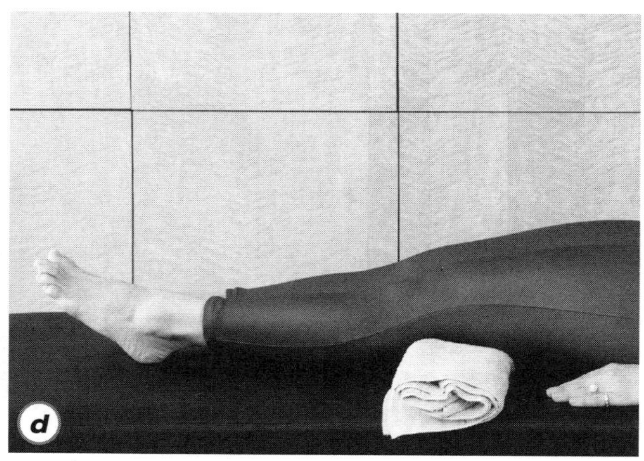

Version Three: Bend In, Lengthen Out

- Lift the working leg *(a)*, bring it into tabletop position and bend the knee in toward the chest *(b)*, extend the leg straight out toward the opposite wall *(c)* Keep the leg up off the mat when you extend the leg out.
- Keep a rolled-up towel or mat under the opposite knee.
- Keep the opposite knee slightly flexed or bent into a mountain shape as needed.
- Bend the knee in toward chest, keeping the tailbone long on the mat.
- For the hip, maintain 90° of hip flexion.
- Repeat 6 times per leg and work up to 10 repeats.

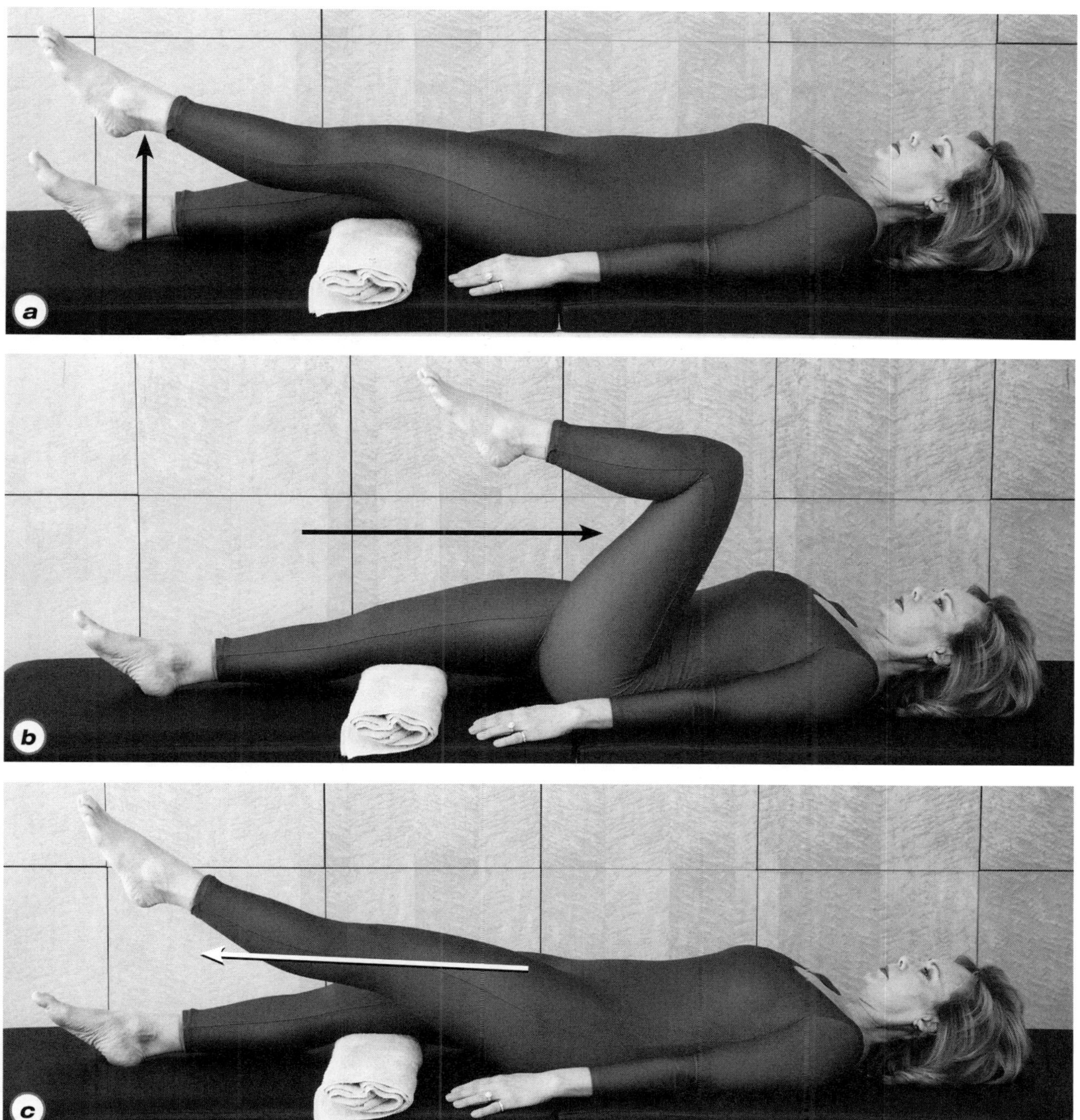

Prone Leg Lifts

- Lie prone on the mat with the legs extended and hip-distance apart. Place a folded towel under the torso and hips.
- Make a pillow with the hands and place the forehead on the pillow. Draw the navel to the spine, keeping the hip points on the mat with the movement.

Version One: Single-Leg Lift

- Inhale, drawing the abdominals in and up, and lift the right leg as high as you can. Engage the gluteus muscles and hamstrings.
- Exhale and slowly lower the leg to the start position.
- Repeat 6 to 8 times.
- Switch and lift the left leg.

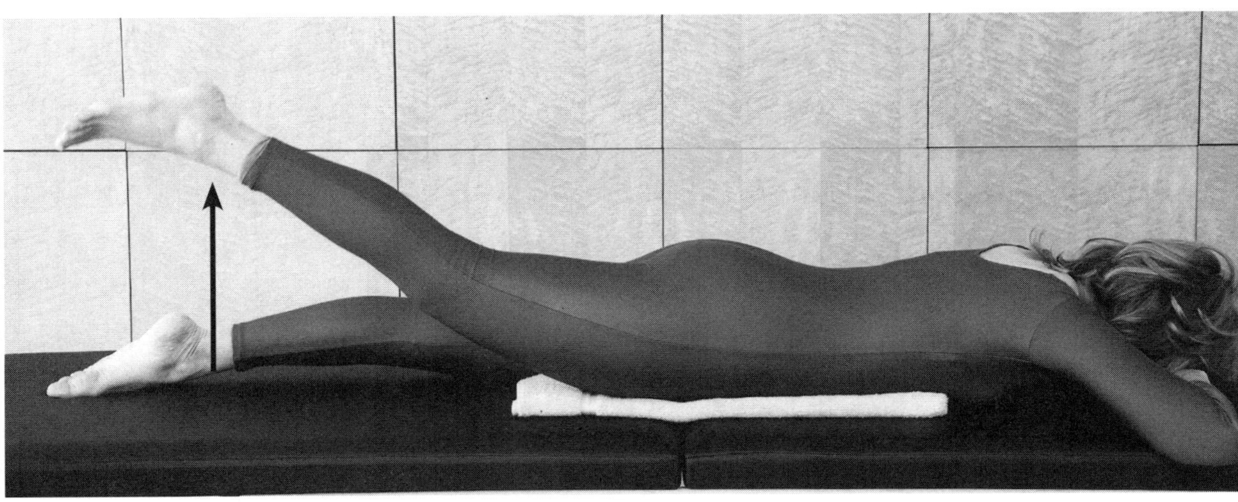

Version Two: Single-Leg Bent-Knee Lift

- Bend the right knee comfortably.
- Lift and lower each leg 6 times.
- Keep the hip points on the mat and the abdominals engaged with the movement.

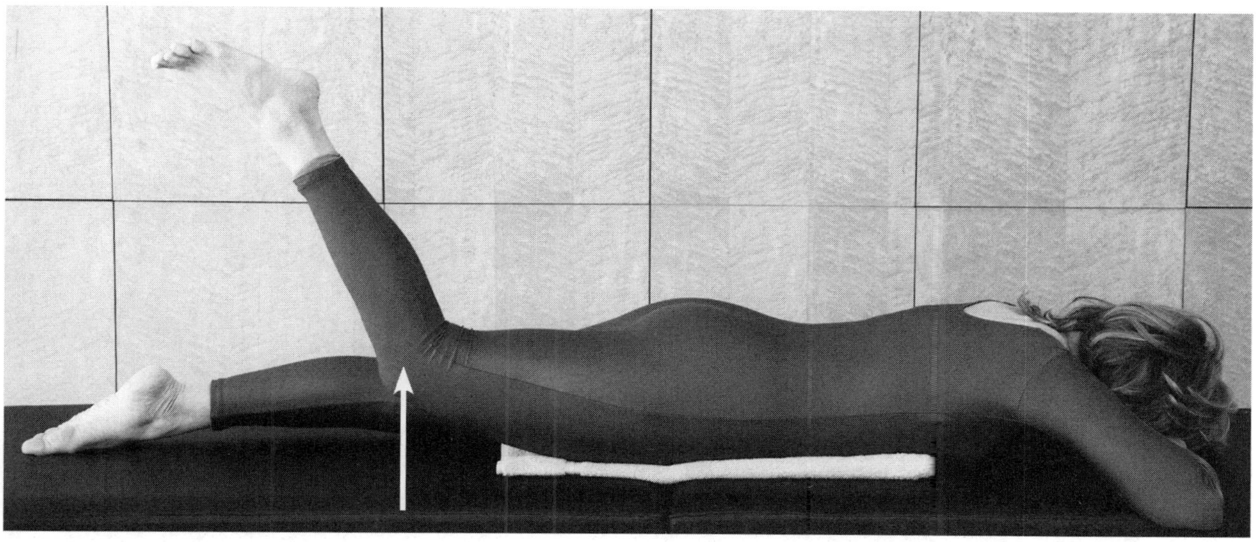

(continued)

Prone Leg Lifts *(continued)*

Version Three: Double-Leg Lift

- Keep the legs straight with slightly flexed knees.
- Lift both legs together and then slowly lower them to the starting position.
- Repeat 6 times.
- Keep the hip points on the mat with the abdominals drawn in and up with the movement.
- Use slow and controlled movement. Inhale to lift, exhale to lower.

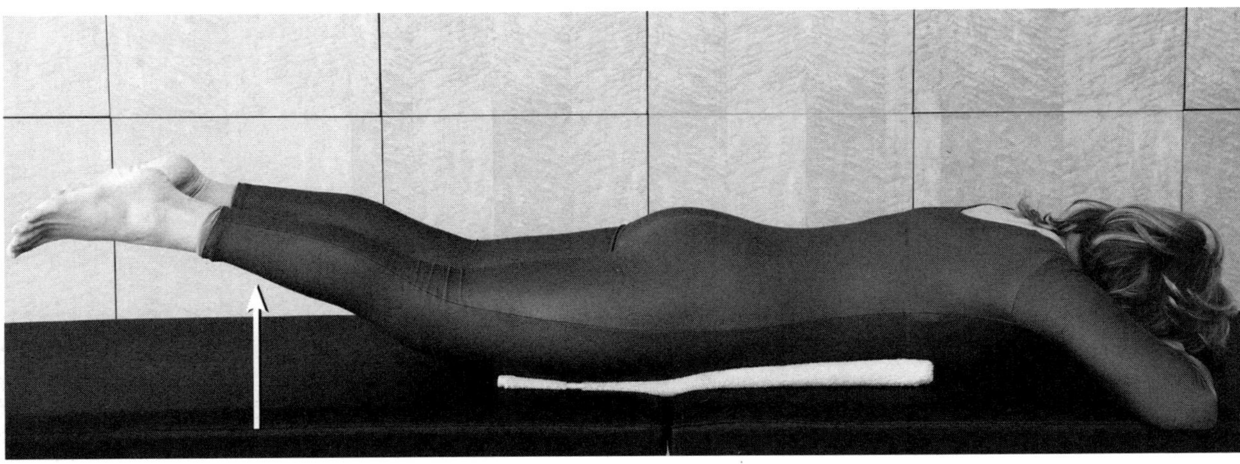

Sitting Bent-Knee Lifts With or Without Resistance

- Sit toward the edge of a chair or raised surface that keeps the hips slightly higher than the knees. (The sit bones should be 3 to 4 inches from the front edge of the chair.) Place the feet on the floor. Use a sturdy pillow or towels to create this position.
- Sit tall with the shoulders back and down and the abdominals drawn in and up.

Version One: Single-Leg Bent-Knee Lift

- Lift the heel of the working leg, engage the abdominals *(a)*, and lift the leg 5 to 6 inches (13-15 centimeters) off the ground *(b)*. Lower back to start, barely touching the toe to the floor during the repeats.
- Inhale to lift and exhale to lower.
- Repeat 8 to 10 times per leg.
- Note: If you feel this exercise more in the hip flexors than in the quadriceps, lean back, place the hands behind the body to support the torso, and then perform the movement. Maintain a neutral spine.

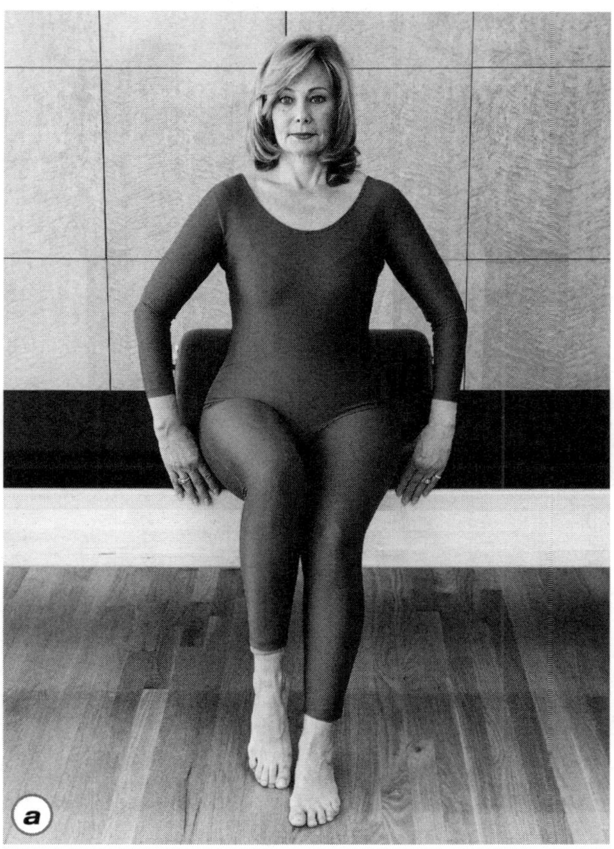
a

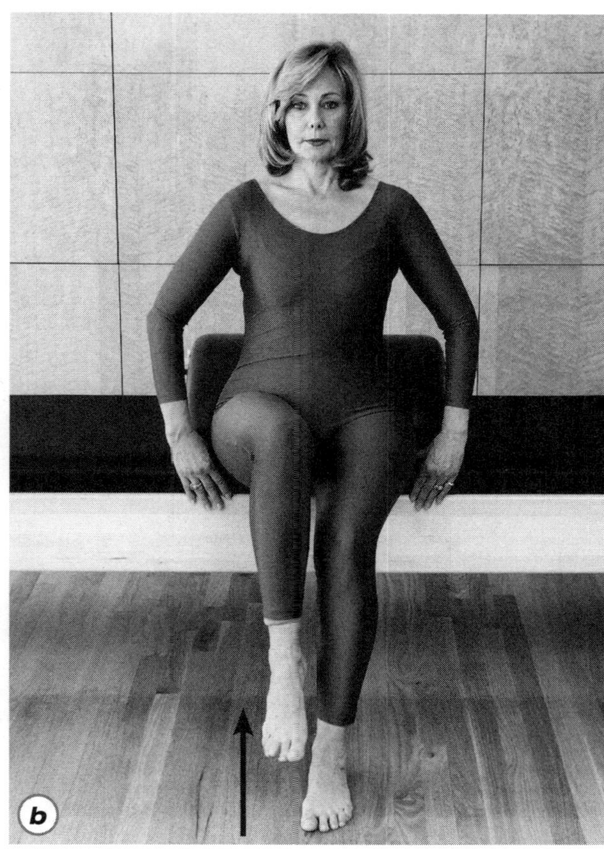
b

Version Two: Single-Leg Bent-Knee Lift: Up, Out, In, Down

- Lift the leg *(a)*, press the leg out to the side *(b)*, return the leg to center *(c)*, and lower the leg *(d)*. The flow is up, out, in, and down.
- Repeat 5 to 8 times per leg.

(continued)

Sitting Bent-Knee Lifts With or Without Resistance *(continued)*

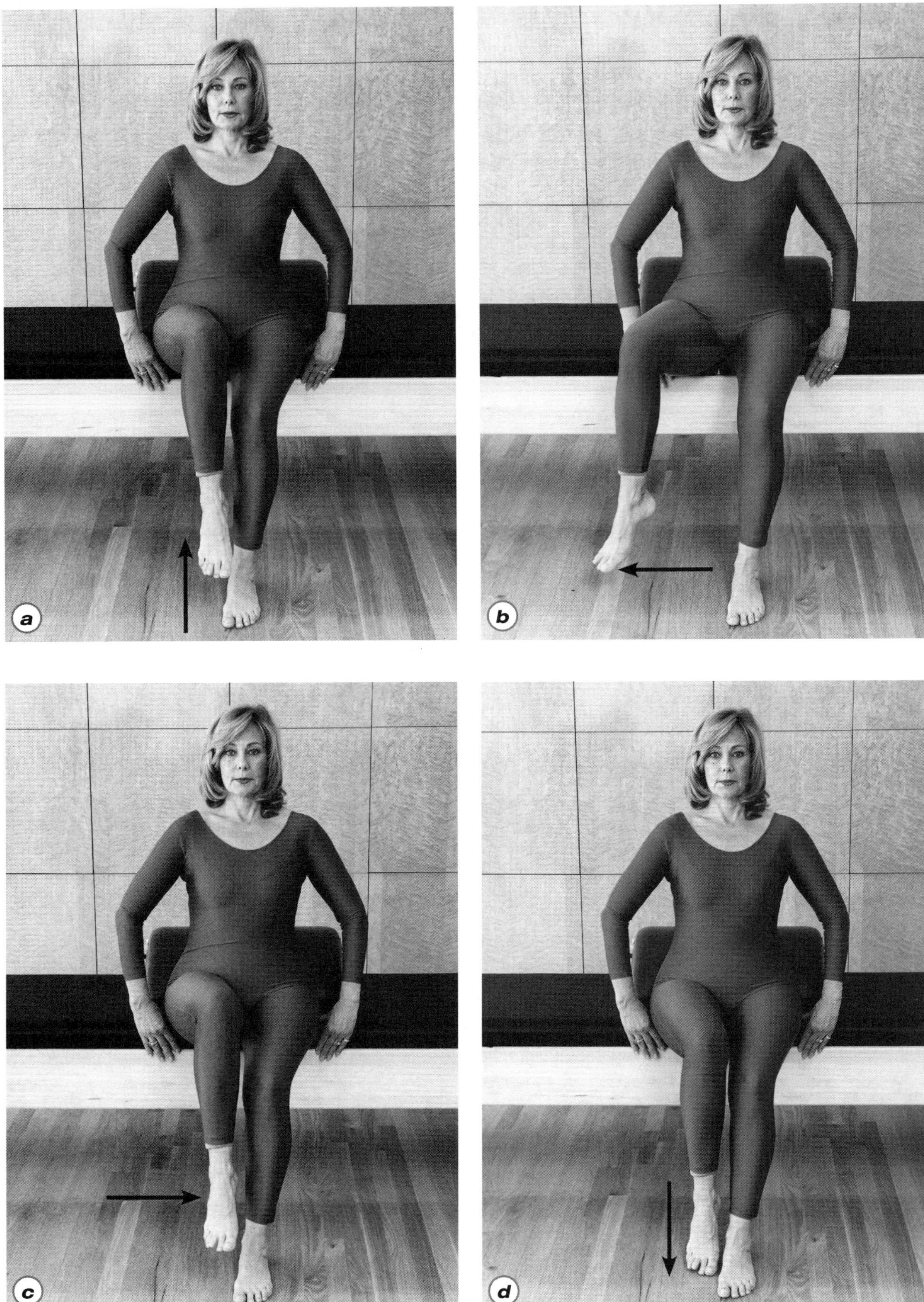

Version Three: Single-Leg Extension

- Lift the leg *(a)* and extend the leg straight out and in *(b)*.
- Repeat the extension up to 8 times.
- Release and lower the leg to the starting position.

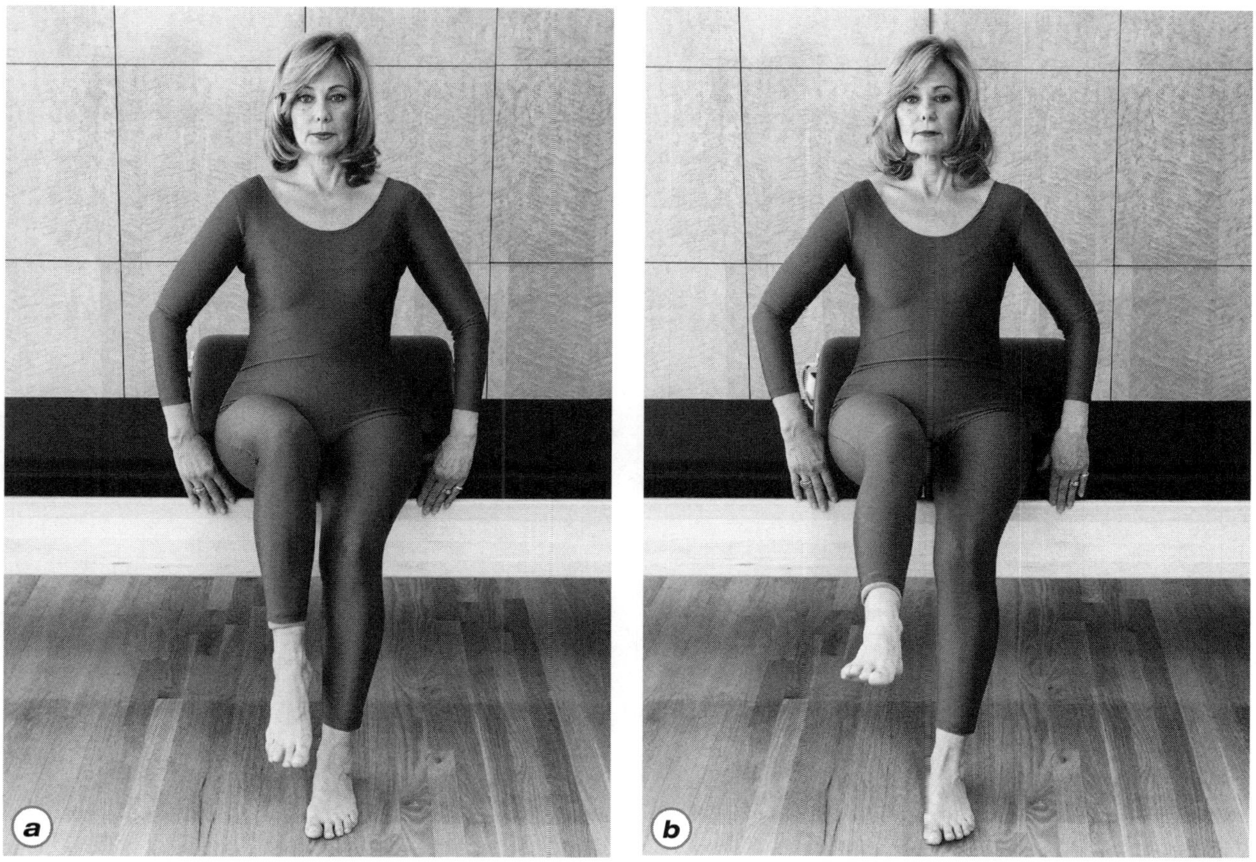

(continued)

Sitting Bent-Knee Lifts With or Without Resistance *(continued)*

Version Four: Sitting Tall Adductor Squeeze

- Sit forward toward the edge of a chair. Place a small, soft ball or Pilates ring between the inner thighs halfway between the groin and the knee. Keep the elbows wide and barely touching the table or chair.
- Sit tall, draw the abdominals in and up, and squeeze the small ball or ring. Hold for 5 counts and then release, holding the ball or ring in place.
- Repeat 5 times.

The following are two options for the sitting tall adductor squeeze:

- Squeeze the ball or ring and then squeeze deeper and pulse for a count of 8; repeat 5 times.
- Hug the ball or ring to the midline, pulse the right leg in toward the ball for 8 counts while holding the left leg steady, and then switch legs.

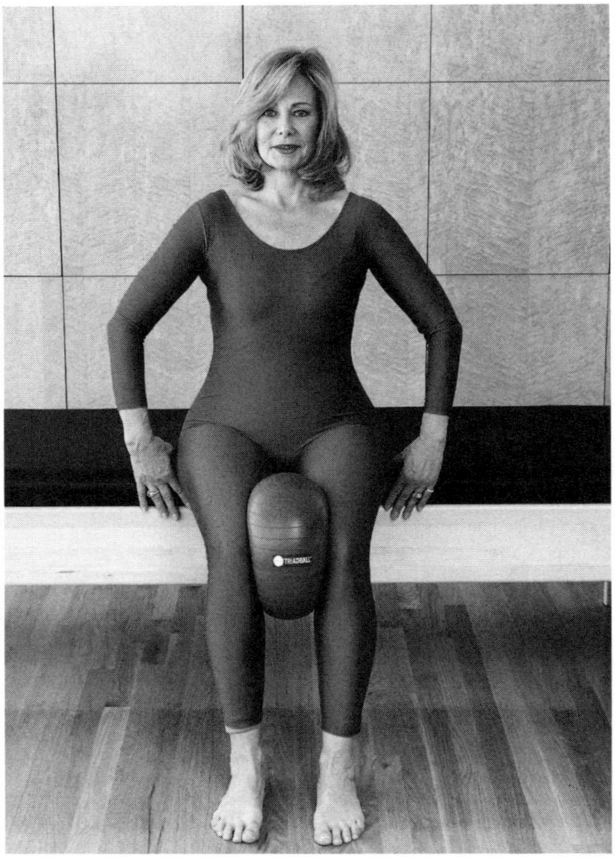

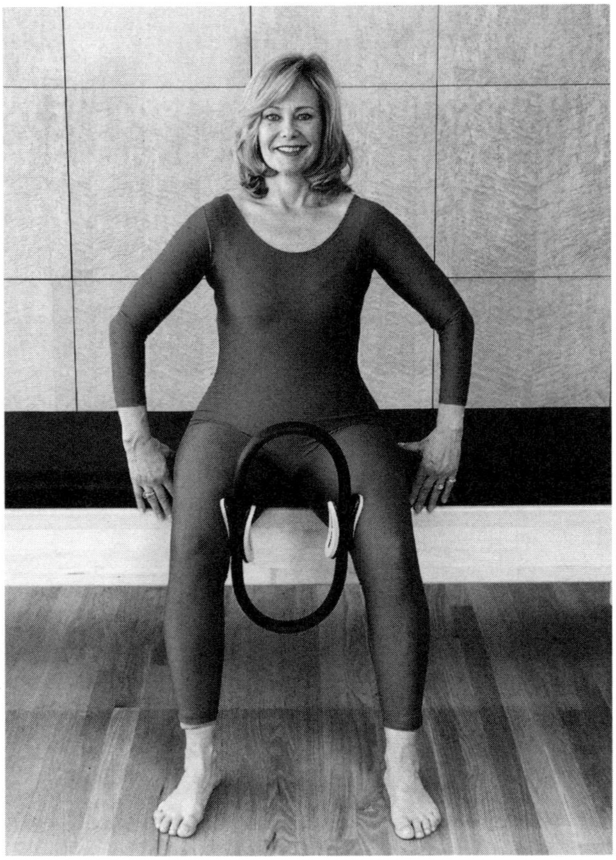

Version Five: Single-Leg Band Lifts

- Place a long exercise band tied into a large loop around the top of the bent knee of the active leg and under the foot of the stabilizing leg.
- Lift the working leg, hold for 3 counts, and then lower slowly. Repeat 7 times per leg.

chapter 4

Pilates Mat Exercises for Six Weeks to Three Months Postoperative

This chapter discusses and illustrates the classical Pilates mat exercises, including modifications and several options, all in keeping with the specified ROM guidelines for clients with hip or knee arthroplasty. Please refer to the ROM guidelines in chapter 3 (pp. 32-36) before starting a mat program. The exercises in this chapter match the first columns in tables 3.2 and 3.3 (p. 31).

Props such as soft balls, towels, pads, and exercise bands are very important tools to assist with the movements. For the arthroplasty client, and sometimes for a client with a syndrome, it is important to perform the movements on a raised mat that is at least hip height. See page 38 in chapter 3 for further guidelines on this.

When working with a client with a syndrome, it is important to select movement modifications that allow the client to move without pain, build core strength and stability, strengthen the muscles surrounding the joints, and improve ROM. Start slowly and reduce the modifications as the client builds core strength and stability.

In many of the exercises, you will see the use of a small, soft ball 8 to 10 inches (20-25 centimeters) in diameter. For the purposes of this book, the Triadball was used in the various exercises and options. The ball should not be fully inflated. It should be firm enough to support the body yet pliable enough to hold and squeeze. When used under the head and neck, the shoulders will be slightly off the mat and the eye line will be at a 45° angle. Make sure the weight of the head is resting on the ball. There should be no tension in the neck (Fritzke and Voogt 2009, 1).

Each exercise presented in this chapter shows the setup and action of the movement with several options. The instructions also include what to look for and encourage and what to be aware of and prevent. The primary muscles of the movement are listed, with emphasis on the muscles that are activated or stabilized from the pelvis, hip, and knee.

All exercises should be performed under the guidance of a qualified Pilates instructor and with referral from the operative physician. The client's needs, restrictions, and ROM recommendations should be specified by the physician and followed accordingly. These guidelines may vary from the protocols that follow, and the protocols should be modified based on the individual's needs and the surgeon's preferences.

Hundred

Timeline: 6 weeks to 3 months postop
Appropriate for: knee and hip
Location: a raised mat, hip height

Instructions

- Lie supine on the mat with the knees bent, the feet flat on the mat, and the arms long by the sides of the body. Place a small, soft ball between the knees. Lightly hug the ball to the midline of the body. Support the head on a small pillow.
- Draw the abdominals in and up (feel the waistband flowing in toward the spine).
- Lift the arms straight up in line with the abdominals.
- Inhale and pump the arms for 5 counts then exhale and pump the arms for 5 counts. With the exhale, scoop deeper into the abdominals.
- Repeat for 5 to 10 breaths.

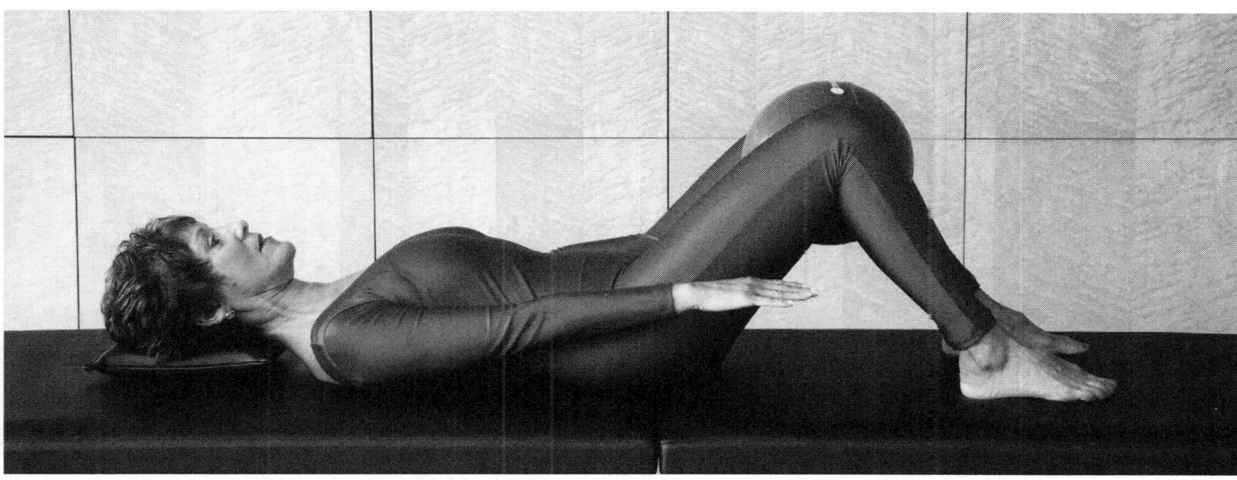

(continued)

Option: Supporting Feet

Place the feet with bent knees on a small barrel, a box, or two study pillows. Keep the legs parallel and hip-distance apart with or without a small, soft ball.

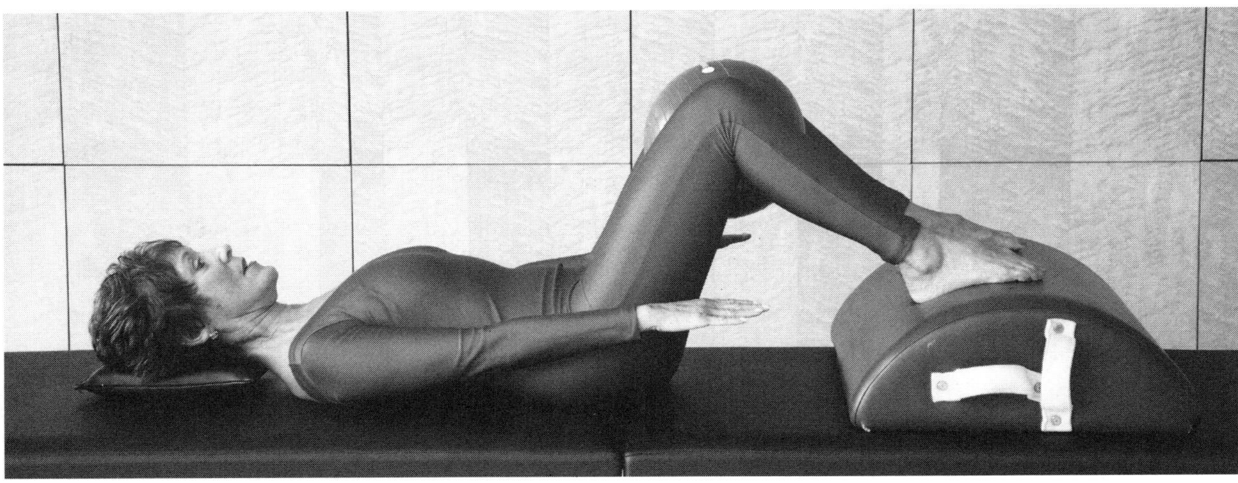

Option: Supporting the Head, Neck, and Shoulders

1. Place a ball 8 to 10 inches (20-25 centimeters) in diameter under the head and neck; see pages 65-66 for instructions for placement.

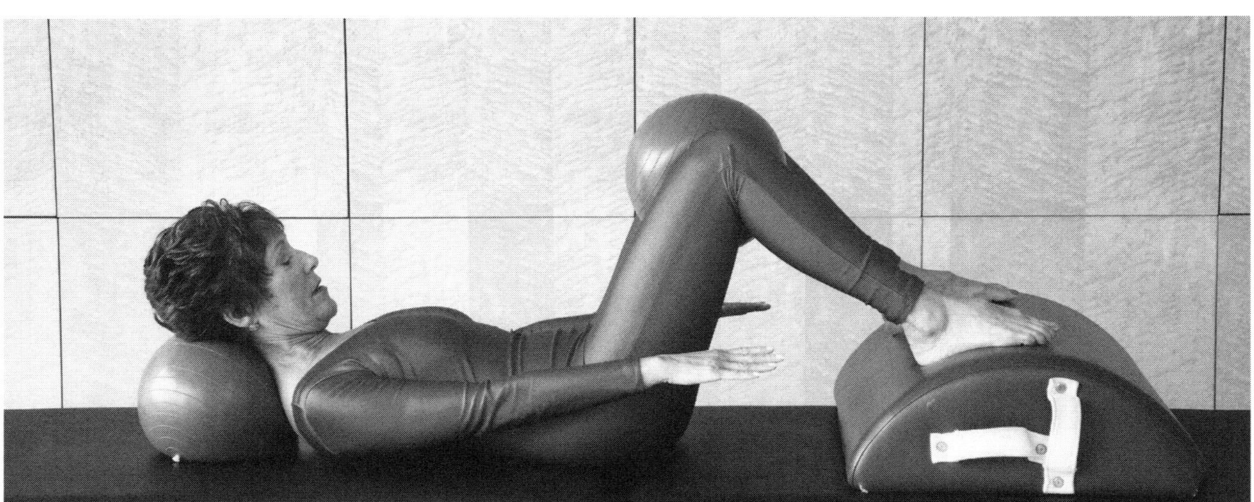

2. Curl the head, neck, and shoulders off the mat. The chin is toward the chest, shoulders rounded up to the bottom tips of the shoulder blades, with an imaginary tangerine between the chin and the chest. Gaze at the thighs.

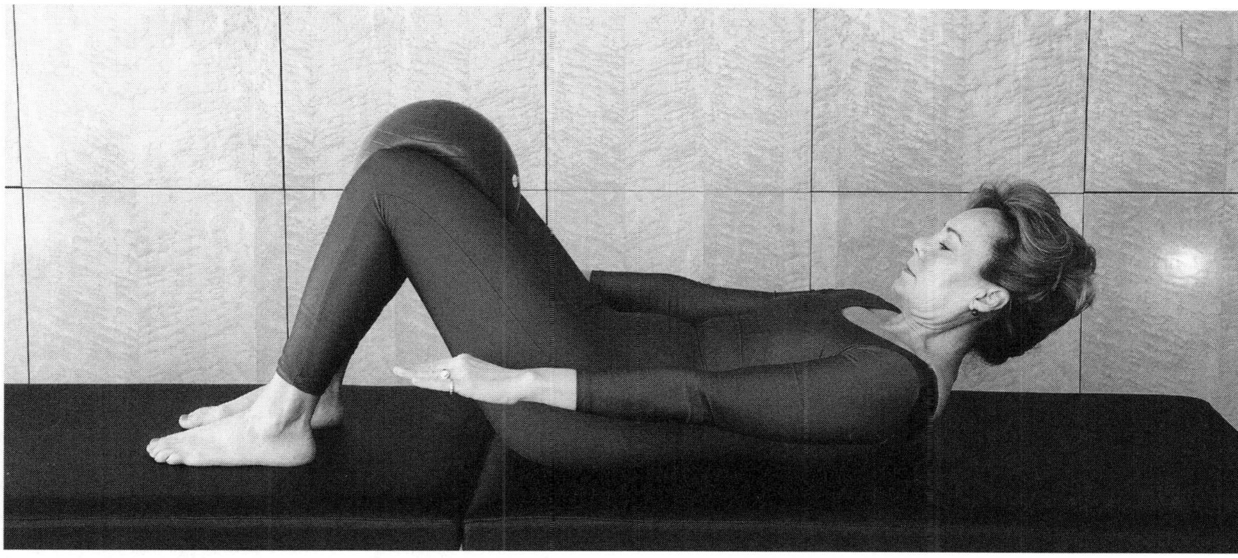

3. Toward the second to third month postop, you may advance, as tolerated, by placing the legs in a tabletop position.

Look for . . . Encourage

- Shoulders gliding toward the hips as if suspenders were hooked to the bottom tips of the shoulder blades and attached to the hips
- Abdominals drawn in and up
- Tailbone long on the mat, maintaining neutral spine
- Straight arms pumping in line with hands as if splashing into water against resistance
- Open collarbones, as if taffy were stretched across the shoulders

Be aware of . . . Prevent

- Pumping the hands up and down
- Arching the lower back (lumbar spine) and losing a neutral spine
- Bulging abdominals

Primary Muscles Activated

Abdominals, anterior scalene, sternocleidomastoid, biceps, triceps, shoulder complex, iliopsoas, rectus femoris, sartorius, pectineus, adductor magnus, adductor longus, adductor brevis, gracilis, biceps femoris, semimembranosus, semitendinosus, popliteus, gastrocnemius, tensor fasciae latae, plantaris

Half Roll-Down

Timeline: 6 weeks to 3 months postop
Appropriate for: knee and hip
Location: a raised mat, hip height

Instructions for Knee

- Sit up on the mat with the knees bent into a mountain shape with a small, soft ball placed between the knees and the hands under the thighs holding with a light touch *(a)*.

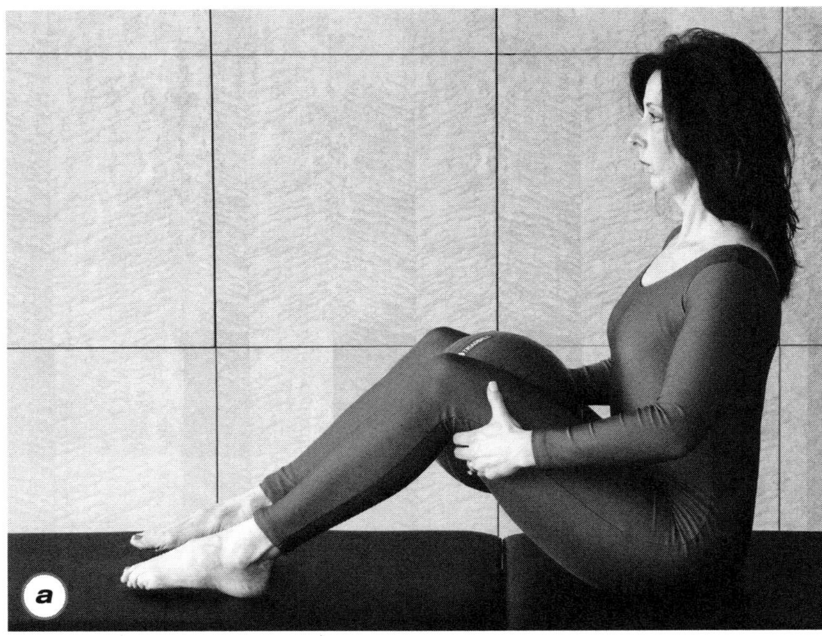

- Bring the chin toward the chest, look toward the thighs, and inhale to prepare. Exhale and roll off the sit bones, drawing the abdominals in deeply and forming a C-curve in the lower spine.

- Continue to exhale and roll down to the length of the arms, hugging the ball between the knees *(b)*.
- Inhale to prepare, exhale, and roll back up. Maintain the flexion in the spine as you round back up to the start *(c)*.
- Repeat 5 to 10 times. Keep the rhythm slow and controlled.
- Note: As you roll toward the mat and back up it may be necessary to tuck the feet under a support strap to provide stability in order to perform the move correctly.

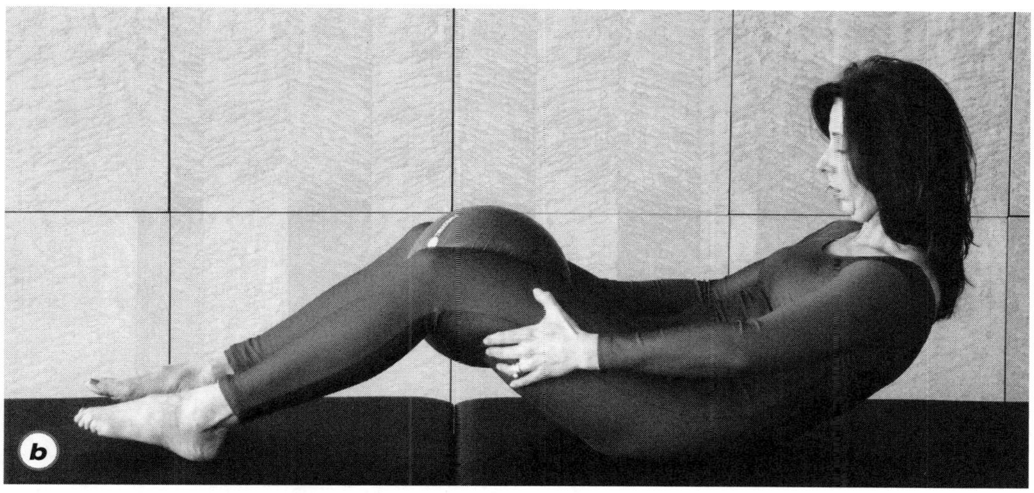
b

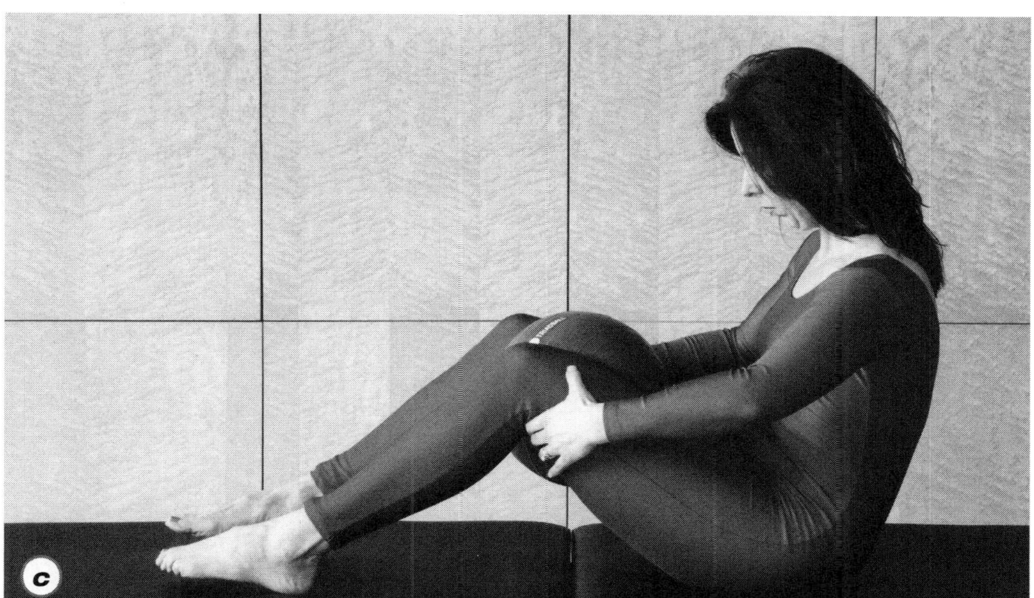
c

(continued)

Instructions for Hip

- Sit up on the mat with a slight bend in the knees (keeping 90°-100° of hip flexion) with a small, soft ball placed between the knees and the hands under the thighs holding with a light touch *(a)*.
- Bring the chin toward the chest, look toward the thighs, and inhale to prepare. Exhale and roll off the sit bones, drawing the abdominals in deeply and forming a C-curve in the lower spine.
- Continue to exhale and roll down to the length of the arms, hugging the ball between the knees *(b)*.

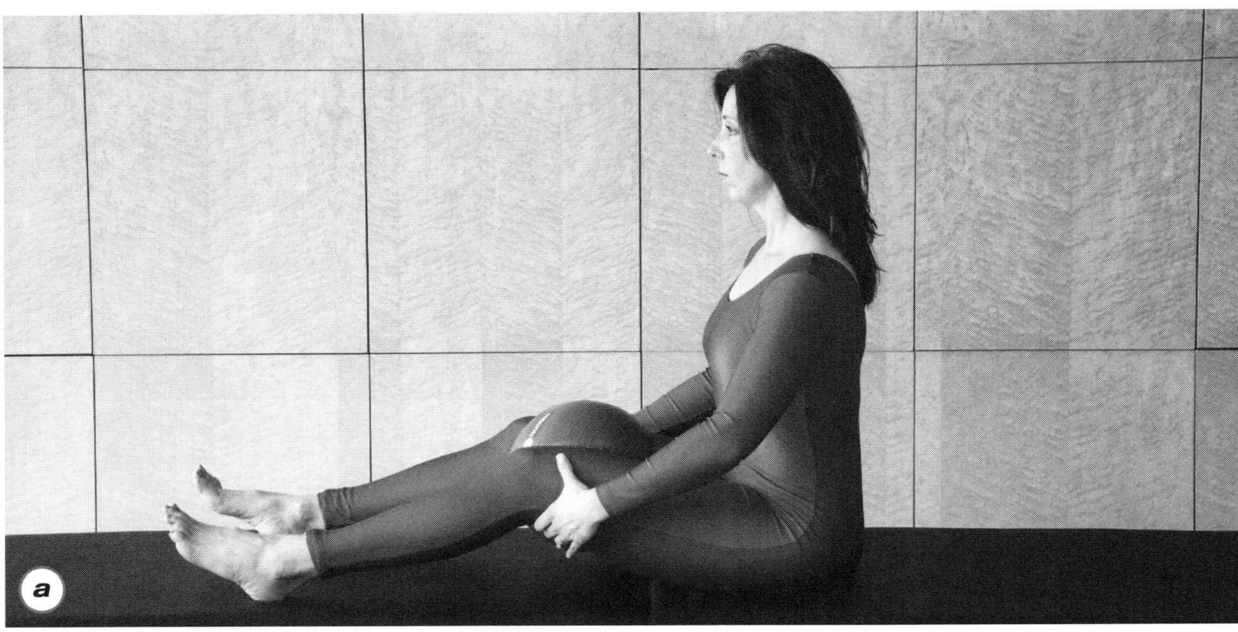

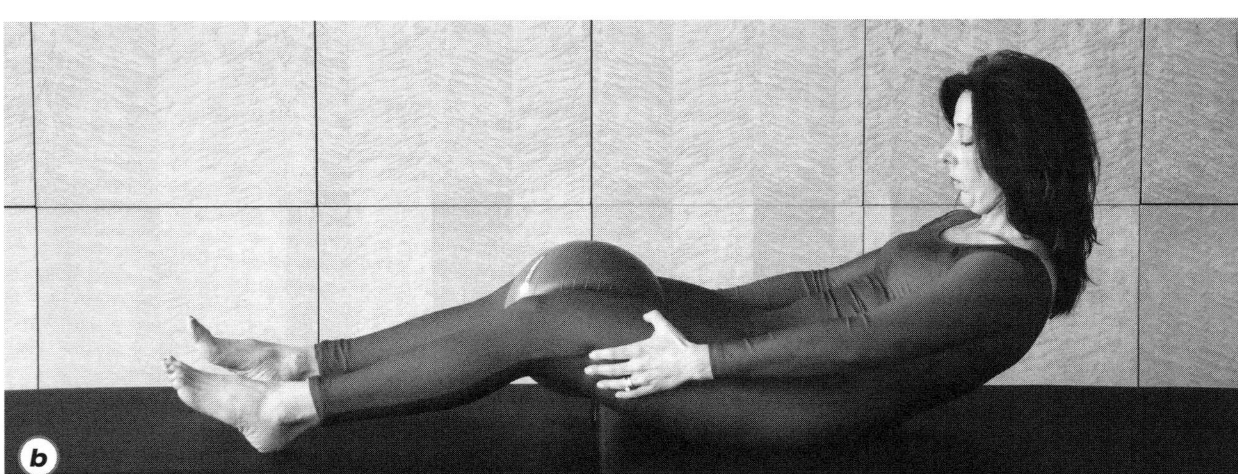

- Inhale to prepare. While exhaling, bring the chin toward the chest and roll back up, keeping the flexion of the spine as you round back up to the start. Maintain 90° to 100° of hip flexion *(c)*.

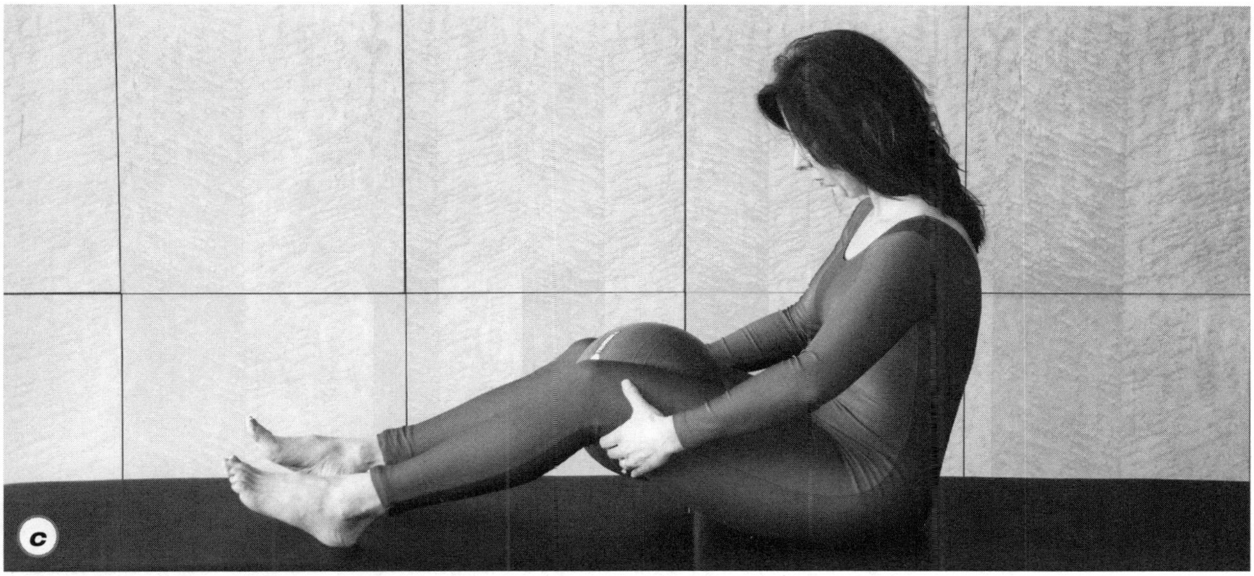

- Repeat 5 to 10 times. Keep the rhythm slow and controlled.
- Note: As you roll toward the mat and back up, it may be necessary to tuck the feet under a support strap to provide stability in order to perform the move correctly.

Instructions for Knee and Hip Together

- Roll down to the length of the arms only if you can maintain control of the movement by not lifting the legs or losing the articulation of the spine.
- Reduce ROM as needed.

(continued)

Option

Place a second ball under the lower back and imprint the lower spine into the ball (roll down only enough to imprint the vertebrae and then roll back up). This option applies to either hip or knee clients.

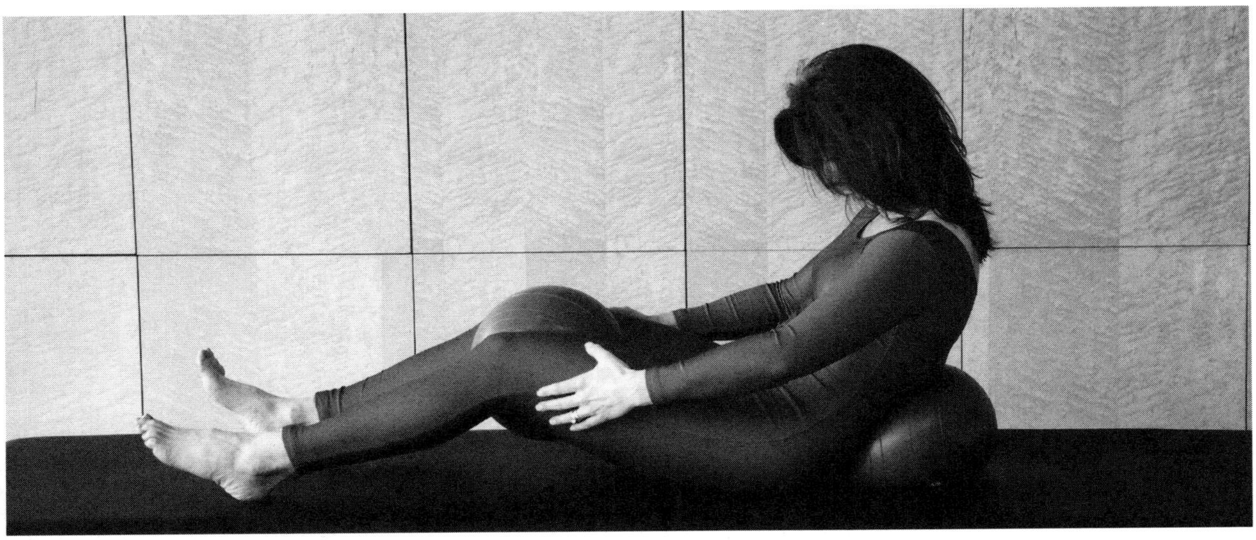

Look for . . . Encourage

- Articulation of each vertebra down to the mat as if each piece of the spine were being imprinted into a bed of wet sand
- A deep scoop in the abdominals
- Shoulders gliding toward the hips as if suspenders were hooked to the bottom tips of the shoulder blades and attached to the hips
- Legs hugged toward the midline of the body

Be aware of . . . Prevent

- Gripping in the hip flexors
- Rolling down or up in segments of the spine

Primary Muscles Activated

Abdominals, iliopsoas, rectus femoris, sartorius, pectineus, gracilis, adductor magnus, adductor longus, adductor brevis, biceps femoris, semitendinosus, semimembranosus, tensor fasciae latae, gastrocnemius, popliteus, plantaris

Half Roll-Up

Timeline: 6 weeks to 3 months postop
Appropriate for: knee and hip
Location: a raised mat, hip height

Instructions for Knee

- Sit up on the mat and bend the knees to a mountain shape. Place a small, soft ball between the knees and place the hands under the thighs, holding with a light touch *(a)*.
- Bring the chin toward the chest, look down into the abdominals, and inhale to prepare. Exhale and roll off the sit bones, scooping the navel to the spine, drawing the abdominals in deeply, and forming a C-curve in the lower spine *(b)*.

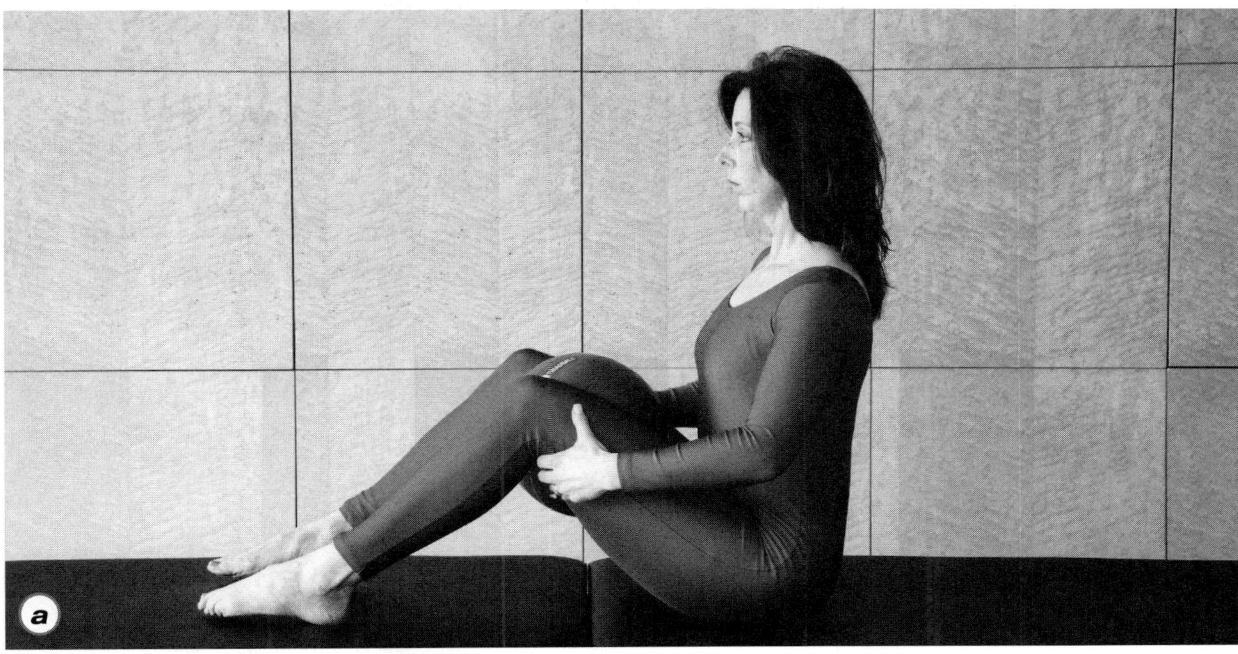
a

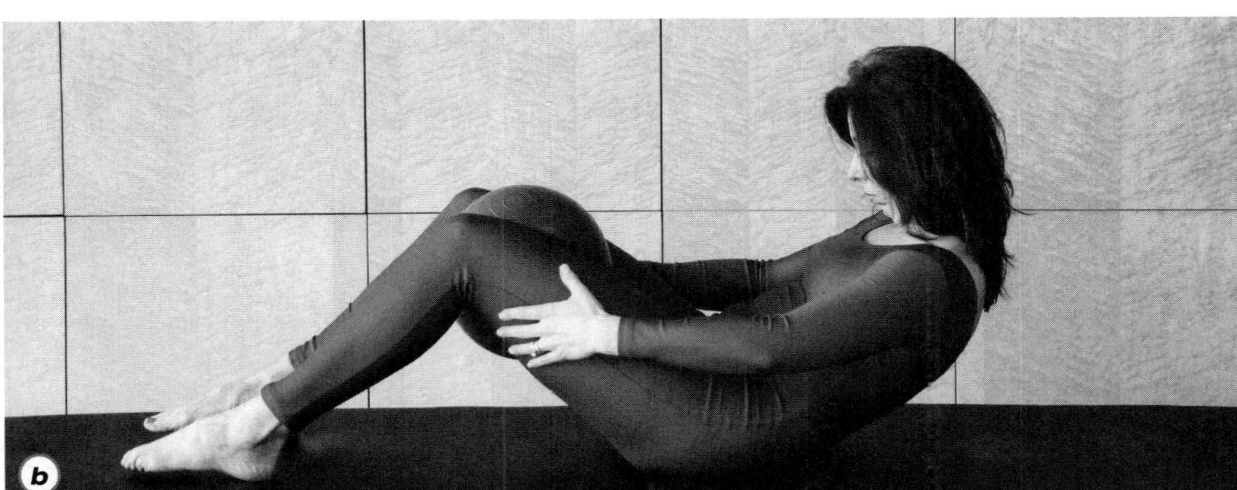
b

(continued)

Half Roll-Up *(continued)*

- While continuing to exhale, roll all the way down to the mat, pressing each vertebra into the mat as if you were imprinting into a bed of wet sand *(c)*.

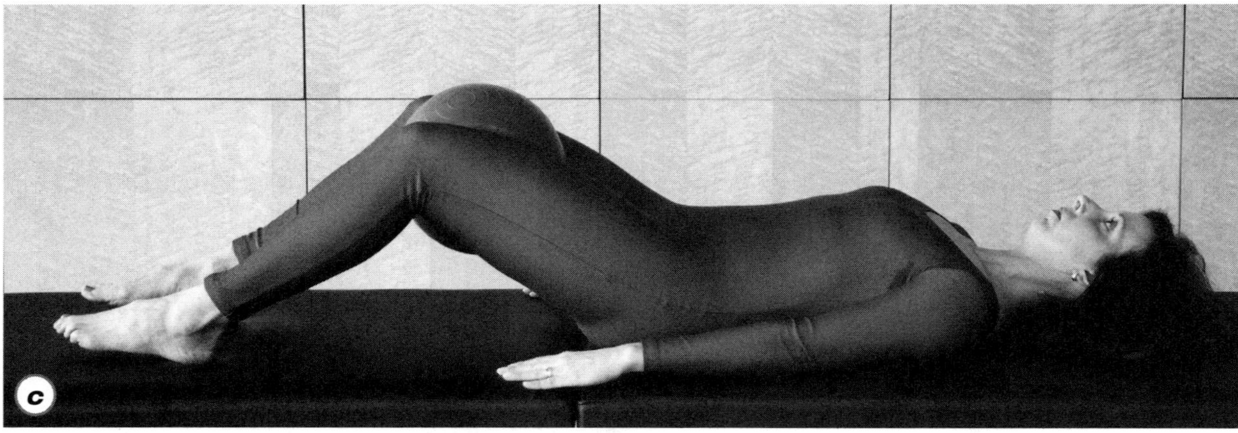

- Inhale to prepare. Exhale, bring the chin toward the chest, place the hands back under the thighs, and use the hands as needed to roll up one vertebra at a time. Maintain flexion of the spine as you round back up to the start.
- Keep a deep scoop in the abdominals.
- Keep the knees in a flexed position as tolerated, hugging the ball to the midline of the body.
- Repeat 5 to 10 times. Keep the rhythm slow and controlled.
- Note: As you roll down and back up, it may be necessary to have the feet under a strap to provide stability in order to perform the move.

Instructions for Hip

- Sit up on the mat with a slight bend in the knees (keeping 90°-100° of hip flexion) and with a small, soft ball placed between the knees and the hands under the thighs holding with a light touch *(a)*.
- Bring the chin toward the chest, look toward the thighs, and inhale to prepare. Exhale and roll off the sit bones, drawing the abdominals in deeply, and forming a C-curve in the lower spine *(b)*.

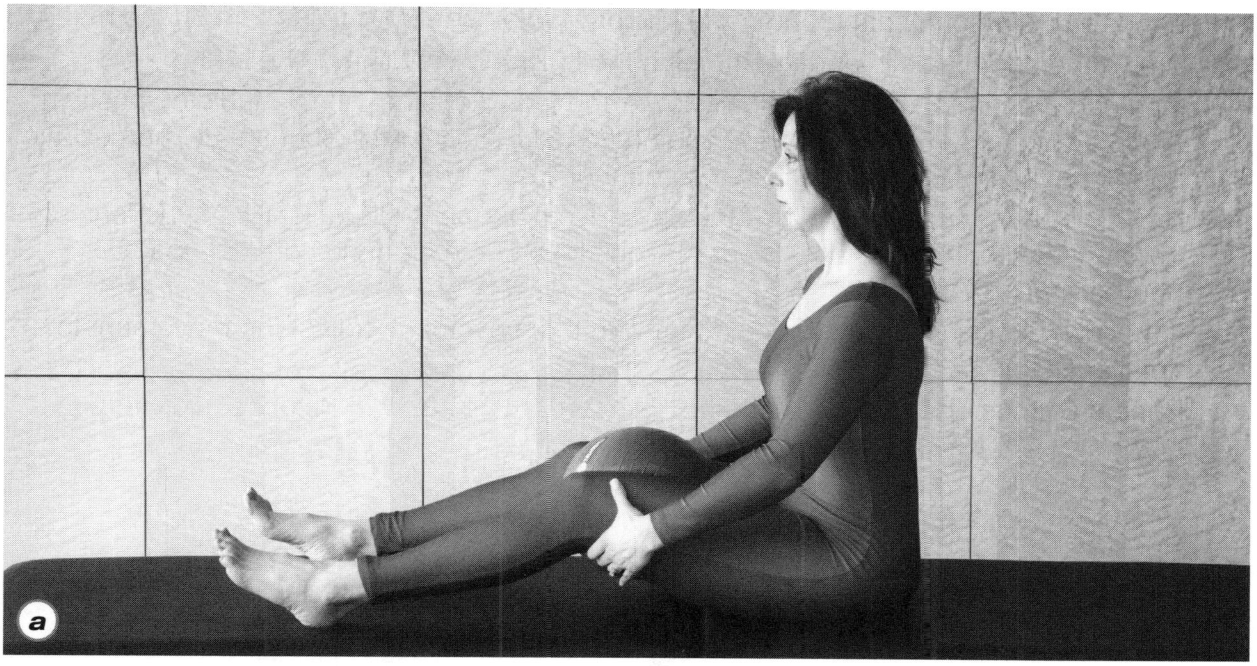

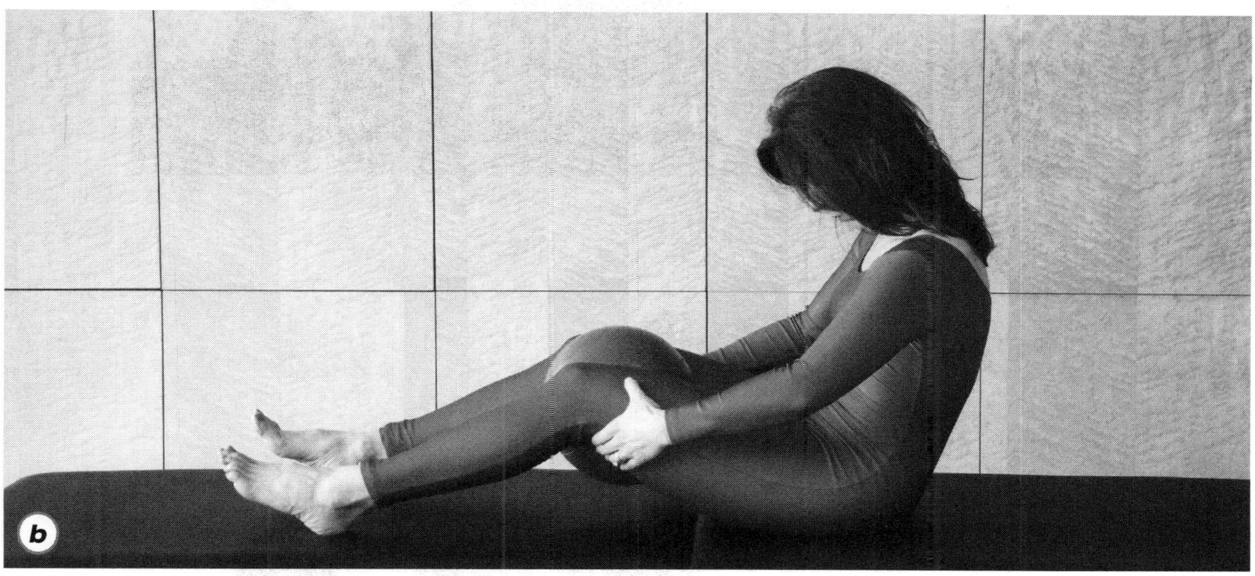

(continued)

- While continuing to exhale, roll down all the way to the mat, pressing each vertebra into the mat as if you were imprinting into a bed of wet sand *(c)*.

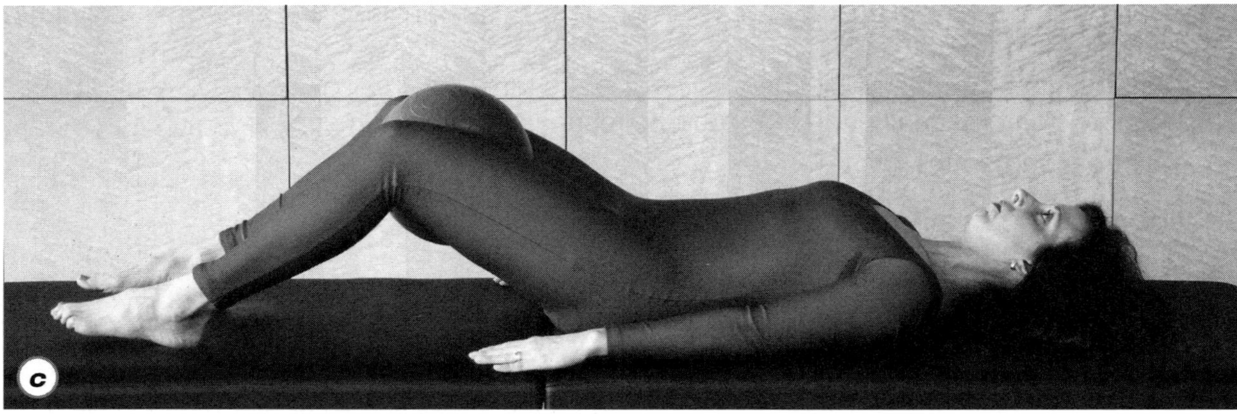
c

- Inhale to prepare. Exhale and bring the chin toward the chest. Place the hands back under the thighs and use them as needed to roll up one vertebra at a time. Maintain the flexion of the spine as you round back up to the start; keep 90° to 100° of hip flexion.
- Keep a deep scoop in the abdominals.
- Keep the knees in a flexed position as tolerated, hugging the ball to the midline of the body.
- Repeat 5 to 10 times. Keep the rhythm slow and controlled.
- Note: As you roll down and back up, it may be necessary to have the feet under a strap to provide stability in order to perform the move.

Look for . . . Encourage

- Articulation of each vertebra down to the mat as if each piece of the spine were being imprinted into a bed of wet sand
- A deep scoop in the abdominals
- Shoulders gliding toward the hips as if suspenders were hooked to the bottom tips of the shoulder blades and attached to the hips
- Legs hugged toward the midline of the body

Be aware of . . . Prevent

- Gripping in the hip flexors
- Rolling down or up in segments of the spine

Primary Muscles Activated

Abdominals, iliopsoas, rectus femoris, sartorius, pectineus, gracilis, adductor magnus, adductor longus, adductor brevis, biceps femoris, semitendinosus, semimembranosus, tensor fasciae latae, gastrocnemius, popliteus, plantaris

Single-Leg Circle

Timeline: 6 weeks to 3 months postop

Appropriate for: knee and hip

Location: a raised mat, hip height

Instructions

- Lie supine on the mat with a pad under the head as needed with a small barrel, pillows, rolled-up towels, or mats under the knees to create a bent-knee position.
- Place an exercise band around the bottom pad of the right foot. Make sure the exercise band is open and flat against the foot.
- Extend the right leg to the ceiling to a maximum of 90° of flexion with *(a)* or without *(b)* a bend in the knee. Keep a light but secure grasp on the exercise band. Hold the band together with both hands, with elbows on the mat and hands held stable on the core.
- Draw the abdominals in and up.
- **Knee:** Inhale to prepare. Exhale and circle the right leg across the midline toward the left hip and down and around to the width of the right shoulder and back to the starting position. Stop at the top. Make small circles that are the size of a basketball.
- **Hip:** Inhale to prepare. Exhale and circle the right leg to the *midline only* and down and around to the width of the right shoulder and stop at the top. Make small circles that are the size of a basketball.
- Circle 3 to 5 times and then reverse direction and circle 3 to 5 times. Change legs and repeat.
- Keep the hips planted on the mat with minimal movement. The goal is to maintain a stable torso throughout the movement.

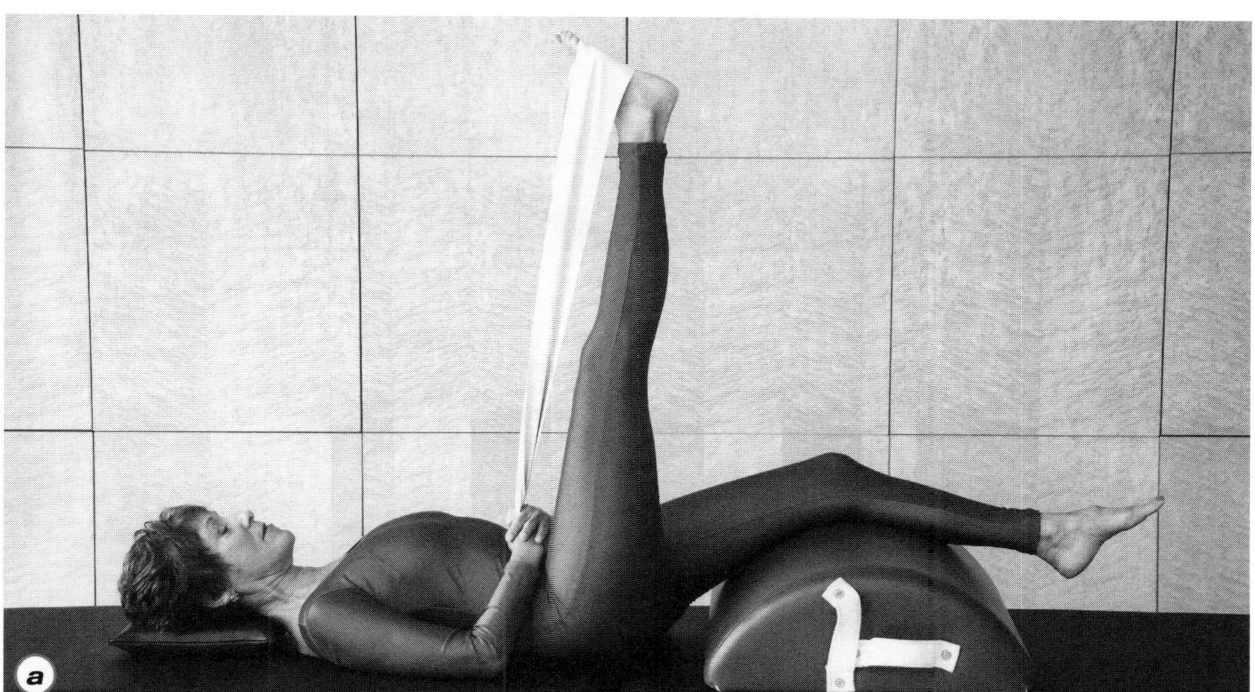

(continued)

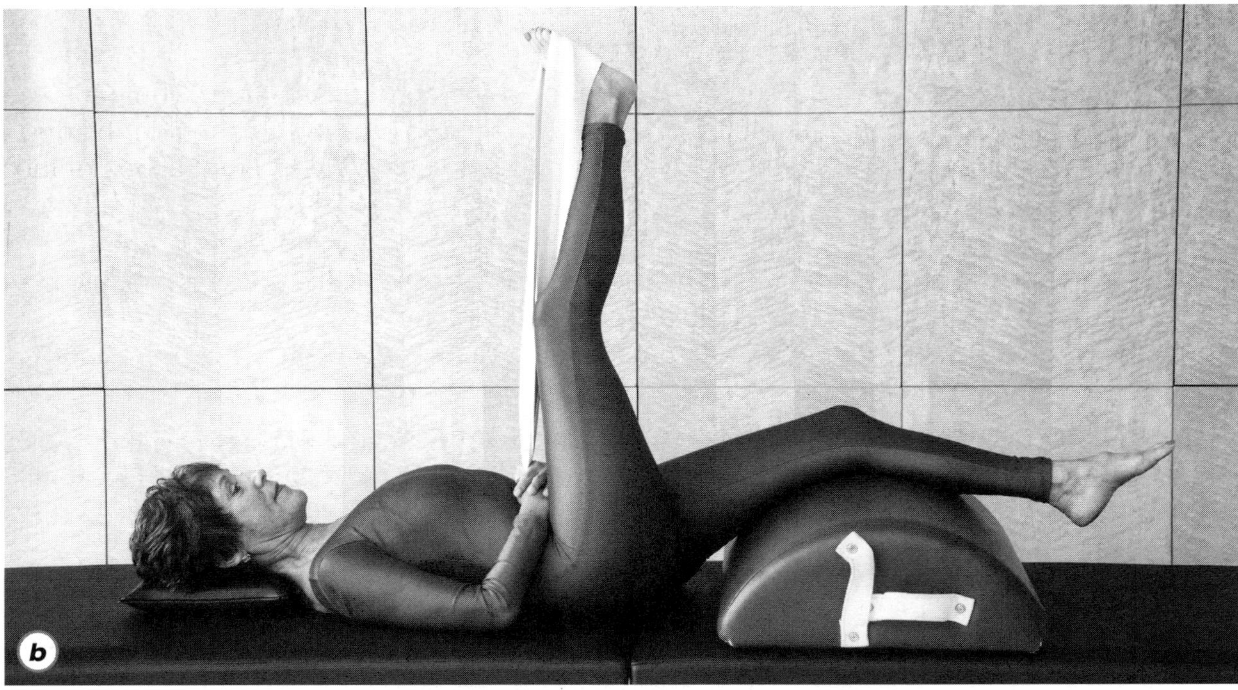

Options

1. Place the working leg into a tabletop position with the exercise band around the pad of the foot and the arms bent with the elbows on the mat holding the exercise band securely in place. Extend the opposite leg over the barrel, pillows, or rolled-up towels.

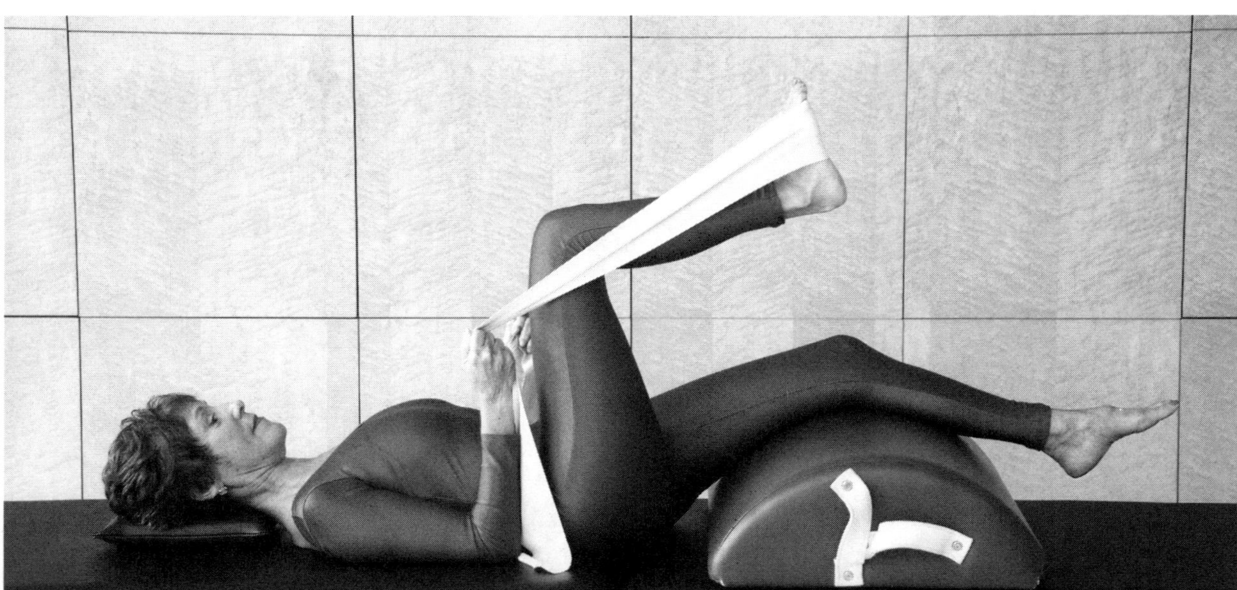

2. Place a small, soft ball under the knee of the working leg, keep a tabletop position, and perform the leg circles. Place a rolled-up towel under the extended leg as needed.

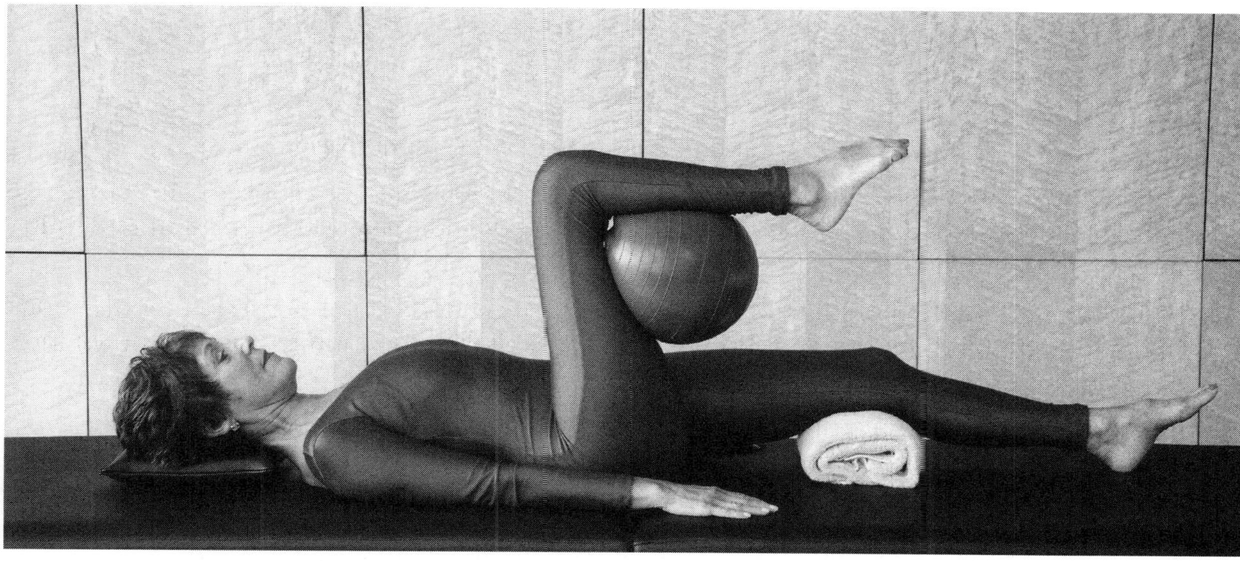

3. Use two soft balls, one behind the knee of the working leg and one under the thigh of the extended leg. Rest the foot of the extended leg lightly on the mat.

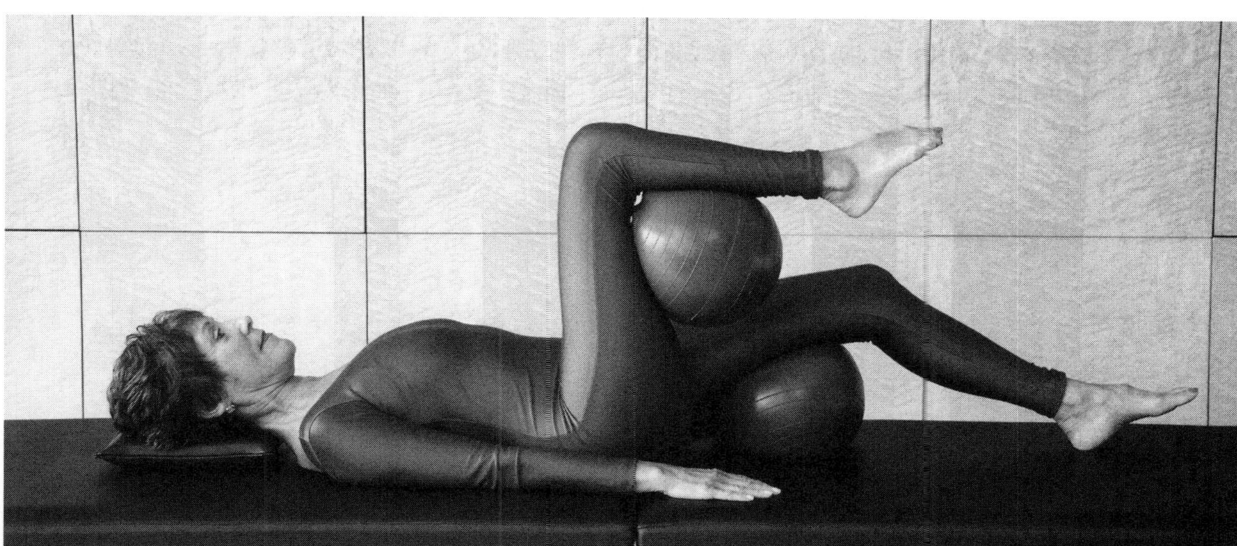

(continued)

Look for . . . Encourage

- Working leg engaged hip to toe
- Shoulders gliding toward the hips as if suspenders were hooked to the bottom tips of the shoulder blades and attached to the hips
- A secure hold maintained on the exercise band
- Stable core and torso and leg working with precision and control
- Open collarbones as if taffy were strung across the shoulders
- Elbows lengthening on the mat toward the feet when using the exercise band
- Arms long by the sides of the body when not using the exercise band
- Disassociation of the head of the femur from the acetabulum (stable pelvis with a flowing movement of the working leg)

Be aware of . . . Prevent

- Lower lumbar spine arching away from the mat and loss of the neutral spine
- Movement of the pelvis and lack of disassociation of the hip from the pelvis

Primary Muscles Activated

The primary muscles activated depend on the chosen option. Abdominals, rectus femoris, vastus medialis, vastus intermedius, vastus lateralis, sartorius, pectineus, iliopsoas, gluteus maximus, gluteus medius, gluteus minimus, biceps femoris, semitendinosus, semimembranosus, tensor fasciae latae, adductor magnus, adductor longus, adductor brevis, gracilis, sartorius, popliteus, gastrocnemius, plantaris

Single-Leg Stretch

Timeline: 6 weeks to 3 months postop
Appropriate for: knee and hip
Location: a raised mat, hip height

Instructions

- Lie supine on the mat with a pad under the head and the legs in tabletop position. Place both hands on each side of the right thigh before the knee.
- **Knee *(a)*:** Lengthen the left leg toward the ceiling and bring the right knee in toward chest as tolerated, keeping the tailbone long on the mat. Scoop the navel to the spine, drawing the abdominals in and up, and switch. Bend the left knee and lengthen the right leg to the ceiling.

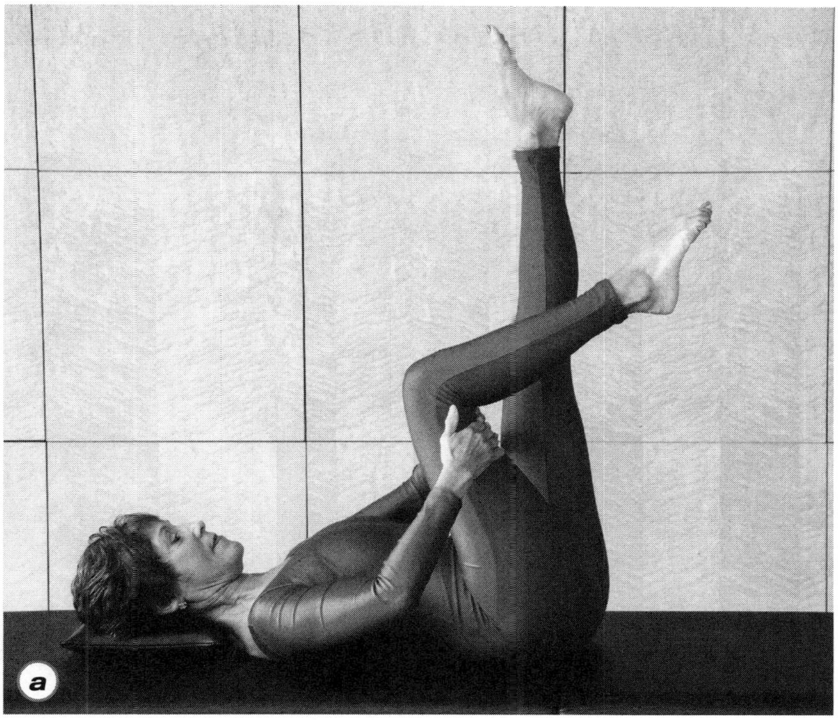
a

- **Hip *(b)*:** Lengthen the left leg toward the ceiling and keep the right knee at 90° to 100° of hip flexion, keeping the tailbone long on the mat. Scoop the navel to the spine, drawing the abdominals in and up, and switch. Bend the left knee and lengthen the right leg to the ceiling.
- Inhale for two leg movements and exhale for two leg movements.
- Repeat 6 times per leg.

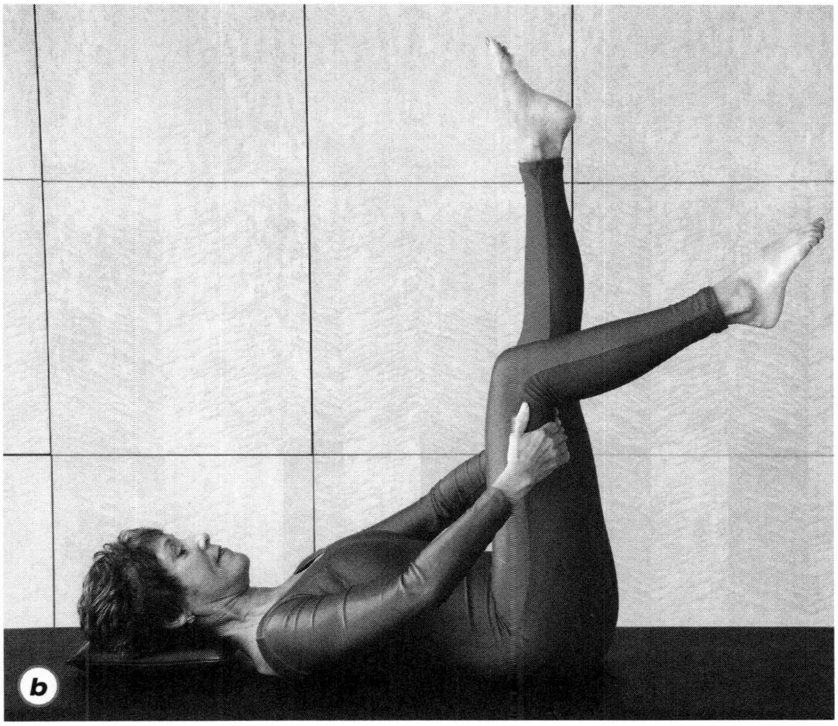
b

(continued)

Options

1. Place a small, soft ball behind the head, neck, and tops of the shoulders. This is appropriate for either the knee *(a)* or the hip *(b)*.

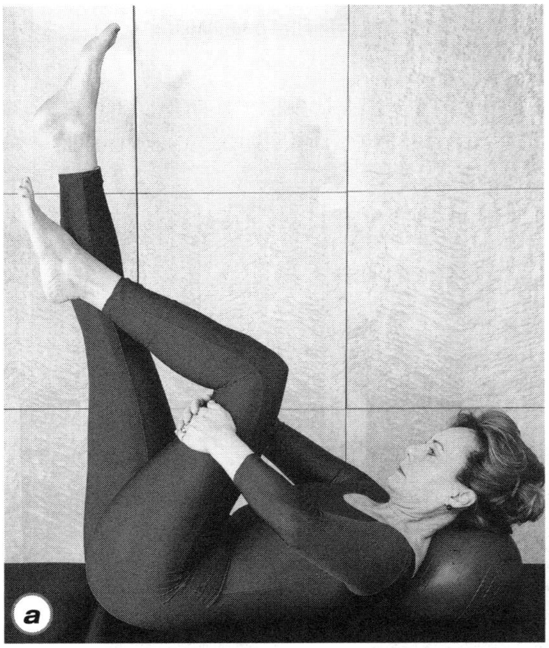
a

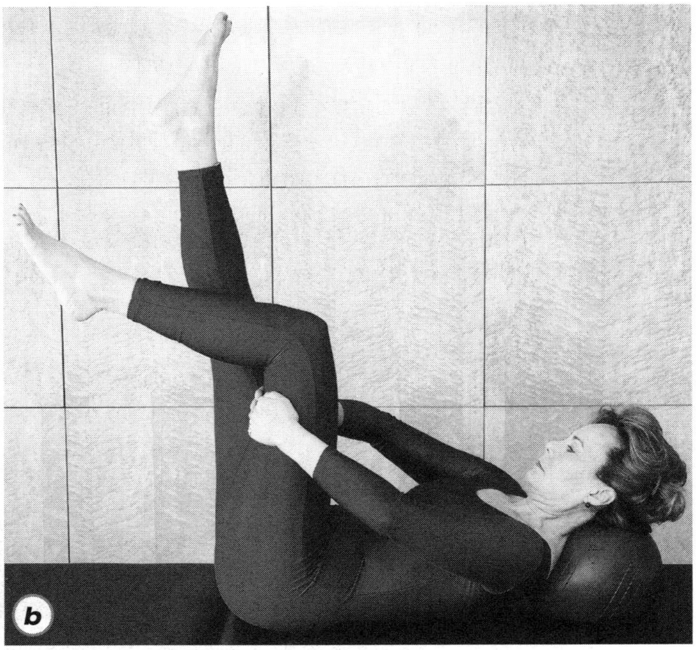
b

2. Curl the head, neck, and shoulders off the mat, looking toward the thighs to perform the movement. Extend the left leg out to 65° as tolerated.

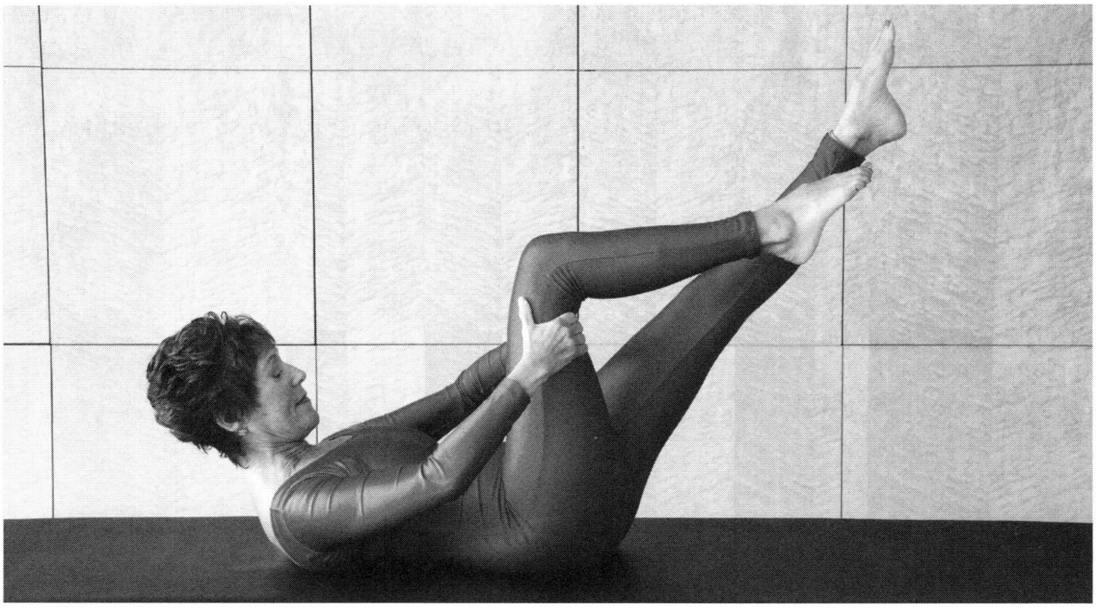

Look for . . . Encourage

- Precision and control as the legs are alternated
- Tailbone long on the mat
- Shoulder blades gliding toward the hips as if suspenders were hooked to the bottom tips of the shoulder blades and attached to the hips
- Abdominals drawn in and up

Be aware of . . . Prevent

- Tension in the head, neck, and shoulders
- Arching (hyperextension) of the lumbar spine away from the mat

Primary Muscles Activated

Abdominals, biceps, triceps, deltoids, anterior scalene, sternocleidomastoid, rectus femoris, vastus medialis, vastus intermedius, vastus lateralis, sartorius, pectineus, iliopsoas, biceps femoris, semitendinosus, semimembranosus, tensor fasciae latae, adductor longus, adductor brevis, gracilis, popliteus, gastrocnemius, plantaris

Double-Leg Stretch

Timeline: 6 weeks to 3 months postop
Appropriate for: knee and hip
Location: a raised mat, hip height

Instructions

- Lie supine on the mat with a pad under the head, the knees bent, and the feet placed on a small barrel or two sturdy pillows. Place a small ball between the knees, hug the legs to the midline of the body, and extend the arms on a diagonal toward the tops of the thighs *(a)*.
- Draw the abdominals in and up.
- Inhale and lengthen both arms back in line with the ears *(b)*.
- Exhale and circle the arms out and around. Lengthen back over the thighs while drawing the abdominals in and up.
- Keep the back ribs on the mat and the abdominals in and up as you extend the arms back.
- Simultaneously squeeze the ball to the midline as the arms circle around to the thighs.
- Keep the tailbone long on the mat.
- Repeat 6 times.

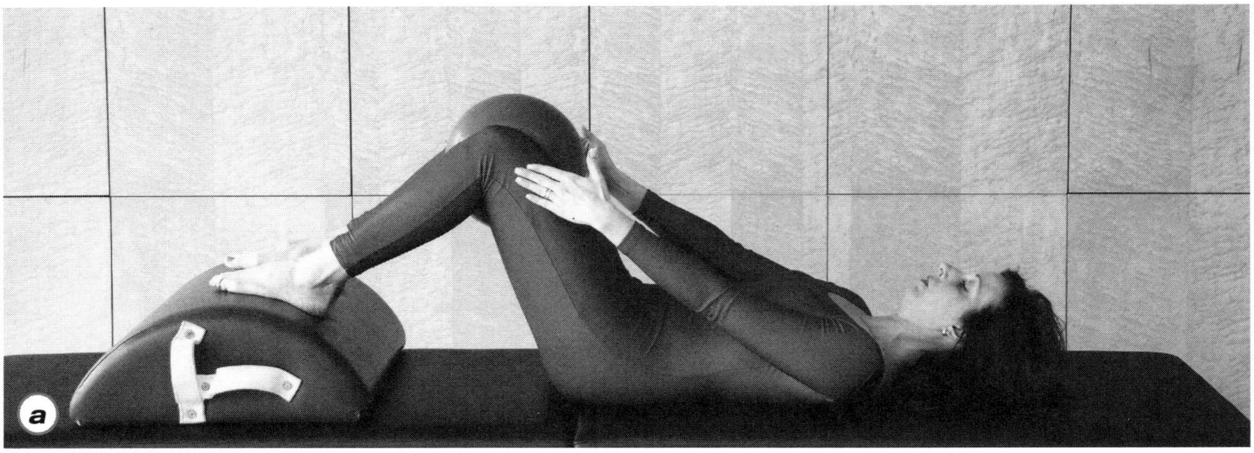
a

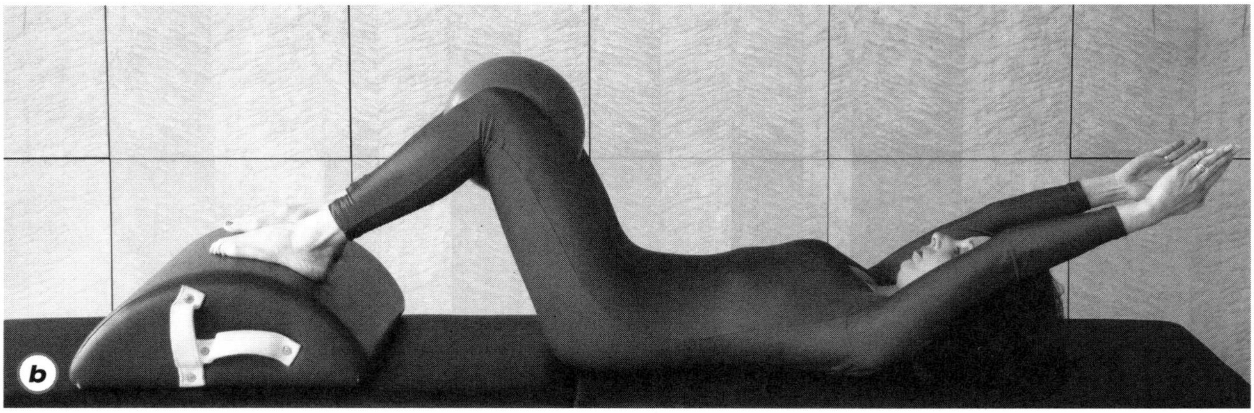
b

Options

1. Place a small, soft ball under the head, neck, and shoulders and perform the movement. See pages 65-66 for instructions of placement of the bal .

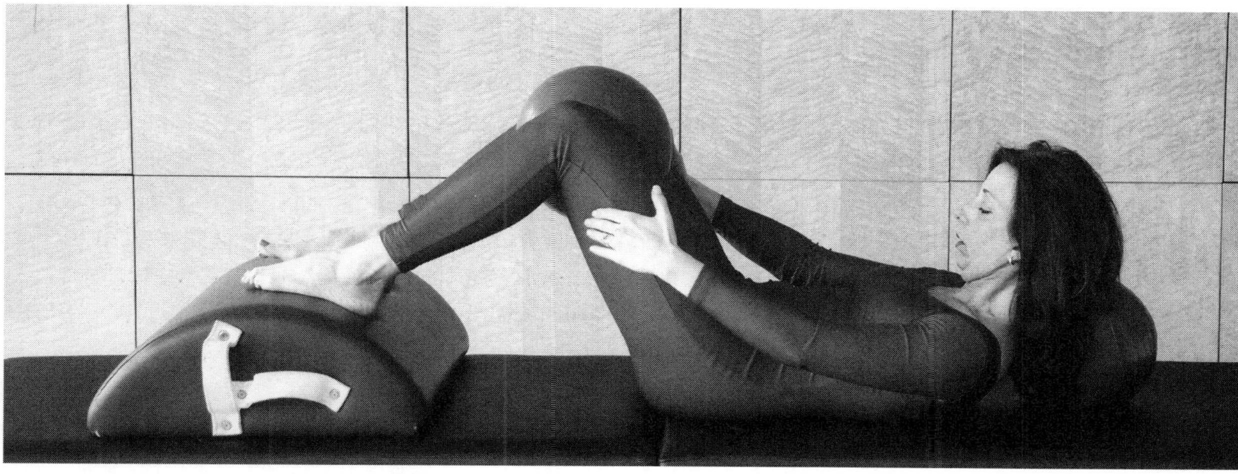

2. Provided that you have awareness and control of the core musculature, curl the head and shoulders up off the mat up to the bottom tips of the shoulder blades. Look toward the thighs and keep a deep scoop to complete the repetitions of the exercise.

Look for . . . Encourage

- Precision of movement
- Shoulders gliding toward the hips as if suspenders were hooked to the bottom tips of the shoulder blades and attached to the hips
- Tailbone long on the mat
- Abdominals drawn in and up

Be aware of . . . Prevent

- Tension in the head, neck, and shoulders
- Shoulders elevated toward the ears

Primary Muscles Activated

Abdominals, biceps, deltoids, anterior scalene, sternocleidomastoid, rectus femoris, sartorius, adductor magnus, adductor longus, adductor brevis, pectineus, gracilis, iliopsoas, biceps femoris, semitendinosus, semimembranosus, gastrocnemius, popliteus, tensor fasciae latae, plantaris

Single Straight-Leg Stretch and Scissors

Timeline: 6 weeks to 3 months postop
Appropriate for: knee and hip
Location: a raised mat, hip height

Instructions

- Lie supine on the mat and place the legs into a tabletop position with a small pad under the head as needed. Place both hands beneath the right thigh before the knee joint.
- **Knee *(a)*:** Extend both legs to the ceiling, keeping the knees slightly bent. Scissor the left leg to 45° with a relaxed foot, drawing the abdominals in and up. Pull the right leg in toward the chest with a gentle double pulse and then switch legs. Perform a double pulse with the left leg while the right leg simultaneously reaches out to 45°. Scoop deep into the abdominals with each action of the leg.

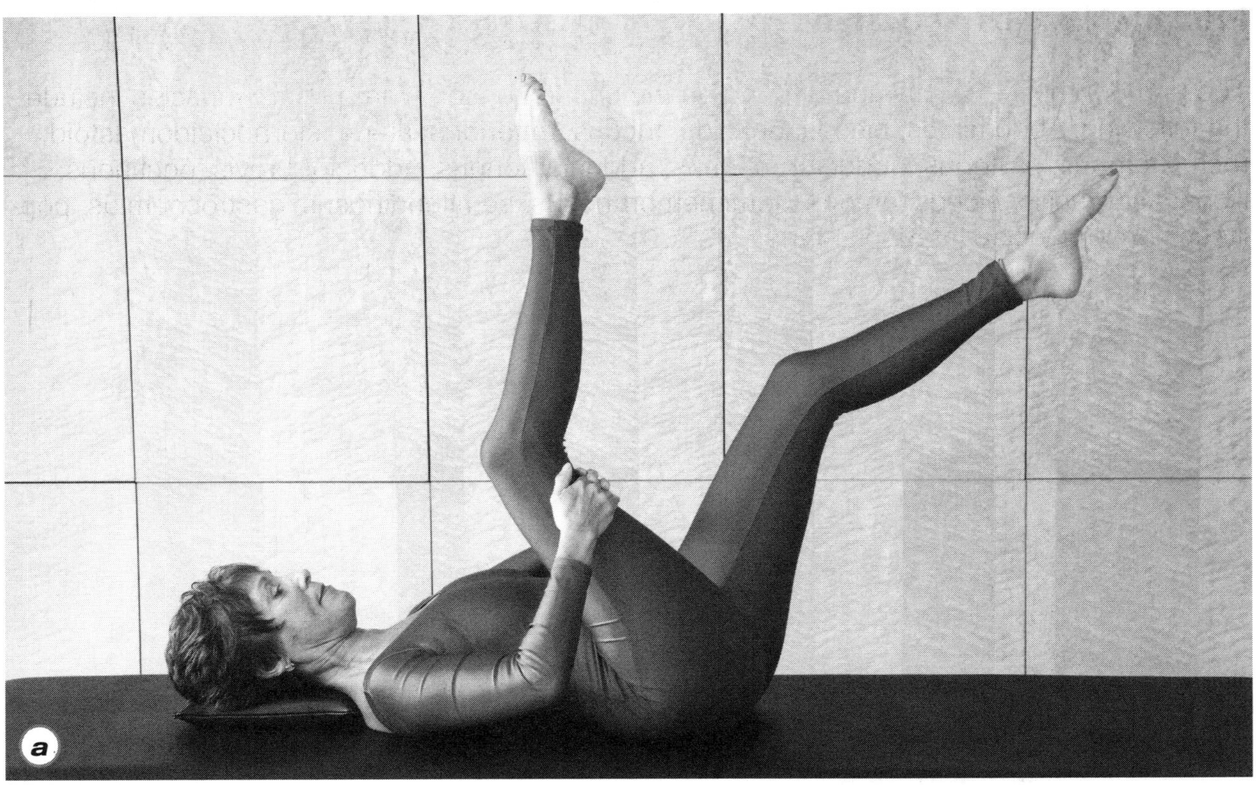

- **Hip *(b)*:** Extend both legs to the ceiling, keeping the knees slightly bent. Scissor the left leg to 45° with a relaxed foot, drawing the abdominals in and up. Pull the right leg in toward the chest with a gentle double pulse, keeping 90° to 100° of hip flexion while the other leg simultaneously reaches out to 45°. Switch legs and perform a double pulse with the left leg while the right leg reaches out to 45°. Scoop deep into the abdominals with each action of the leg.
- Inhale for two leg movements and exhale for two leg movements.
- Repeat 6 times per leg.

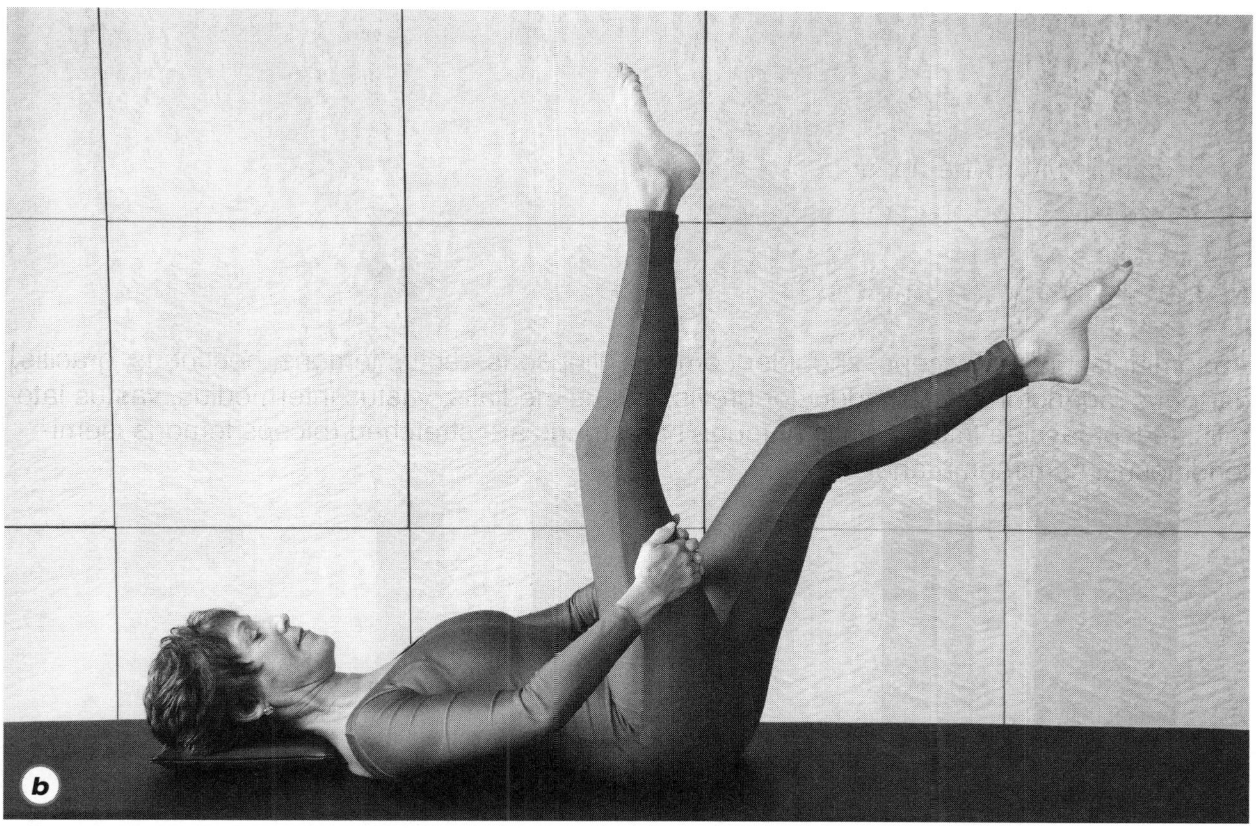

(continued)

Options

1. Provided that you have awareness and control of the core musculature, you can curl the head, neck, and shoulders off the mat up to the bottom tips of the shoulder blades. Look toward the thighs and stay in a deep scoop to complete the repetitions of the exercise. Keep the knees slightly flexed. This is appropriate for either the knees *(a)* or the hips *(b)*.

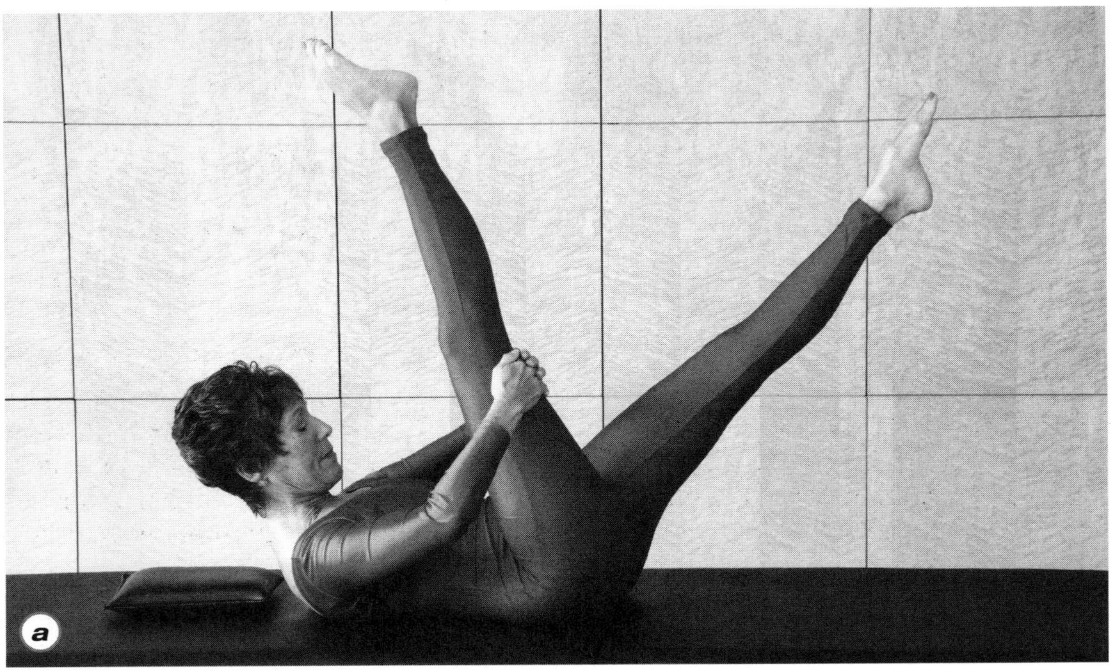

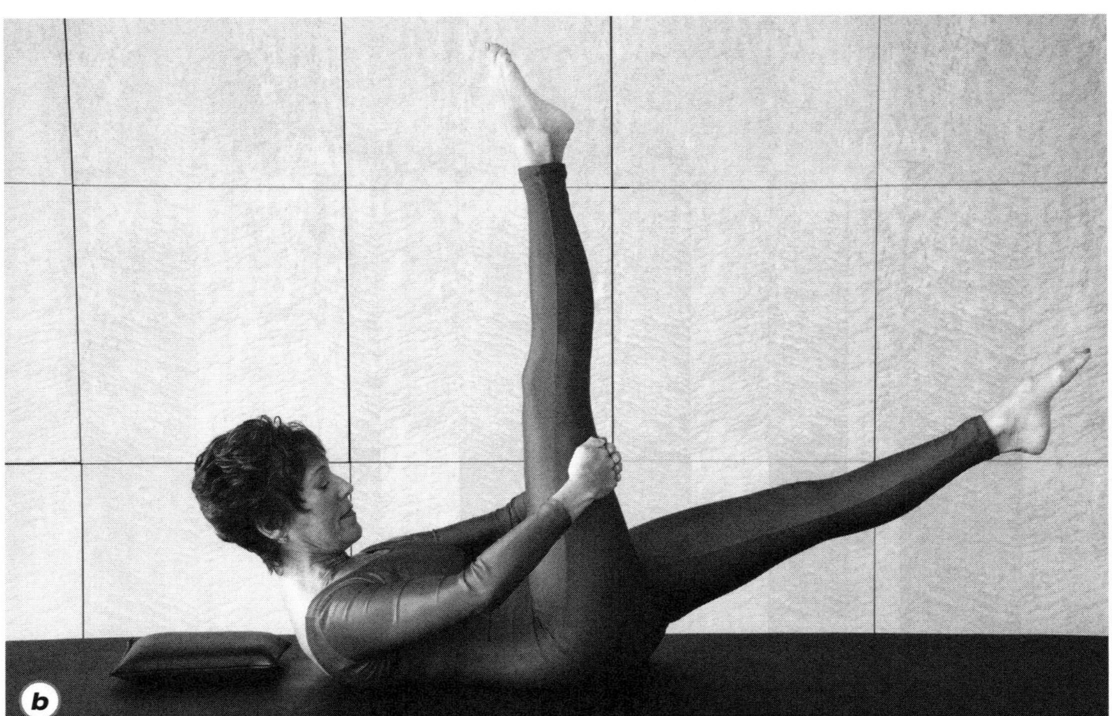

2. Place the hands in a diamond shape under the tailbone. Keep the elbows wide and on the mat and perform the leg portion of the exercise.

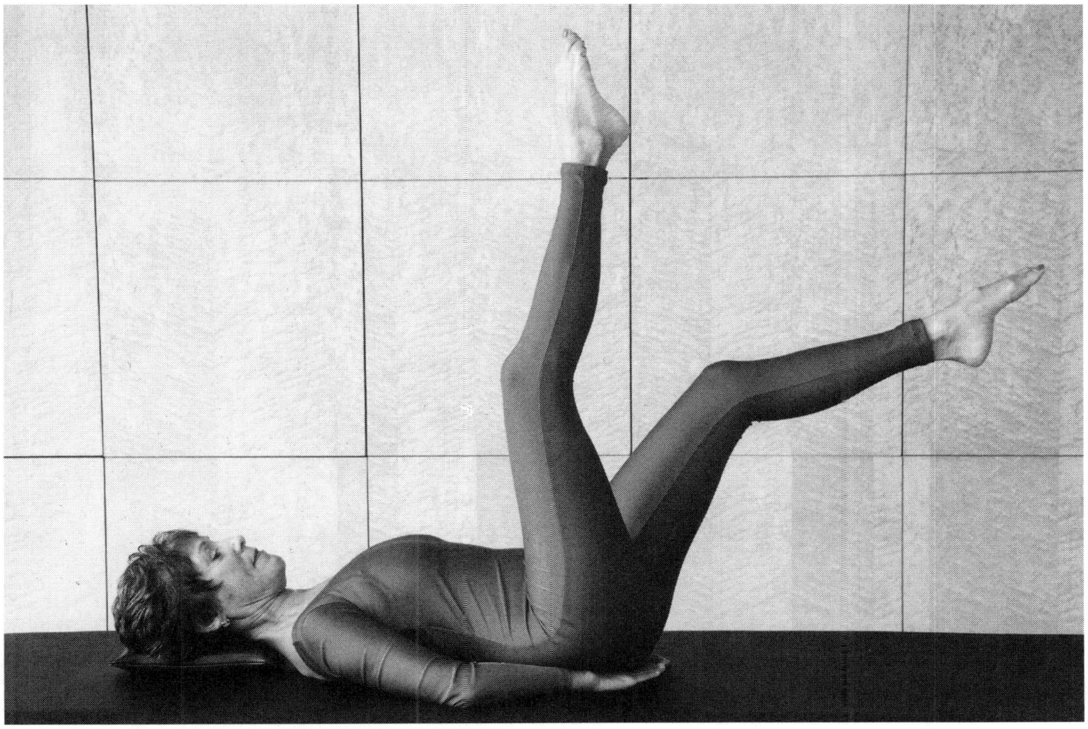

(continued)

Single Straight-Leg Stretch and Scissors *(continued)*

3. Place a small, soft ball under the head, neck, and shoulders. Place the hands in a diamond shape under the tailbone or place them behind the thighs. This modification is appropriate for either the knee *(a)* or the hip *(b)*.

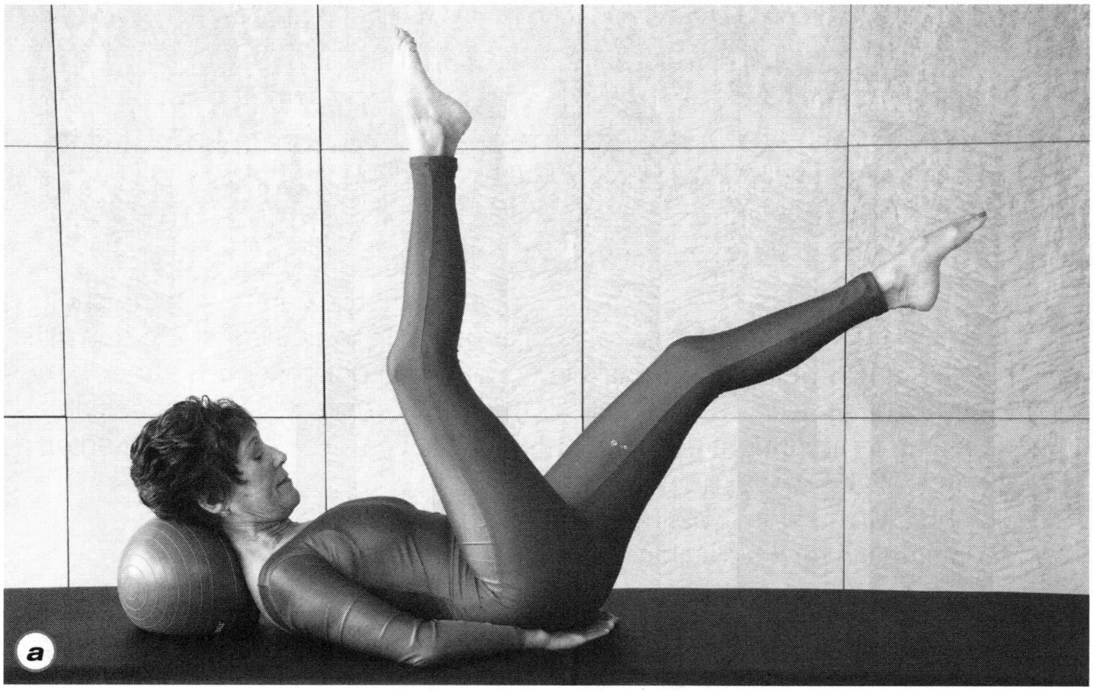

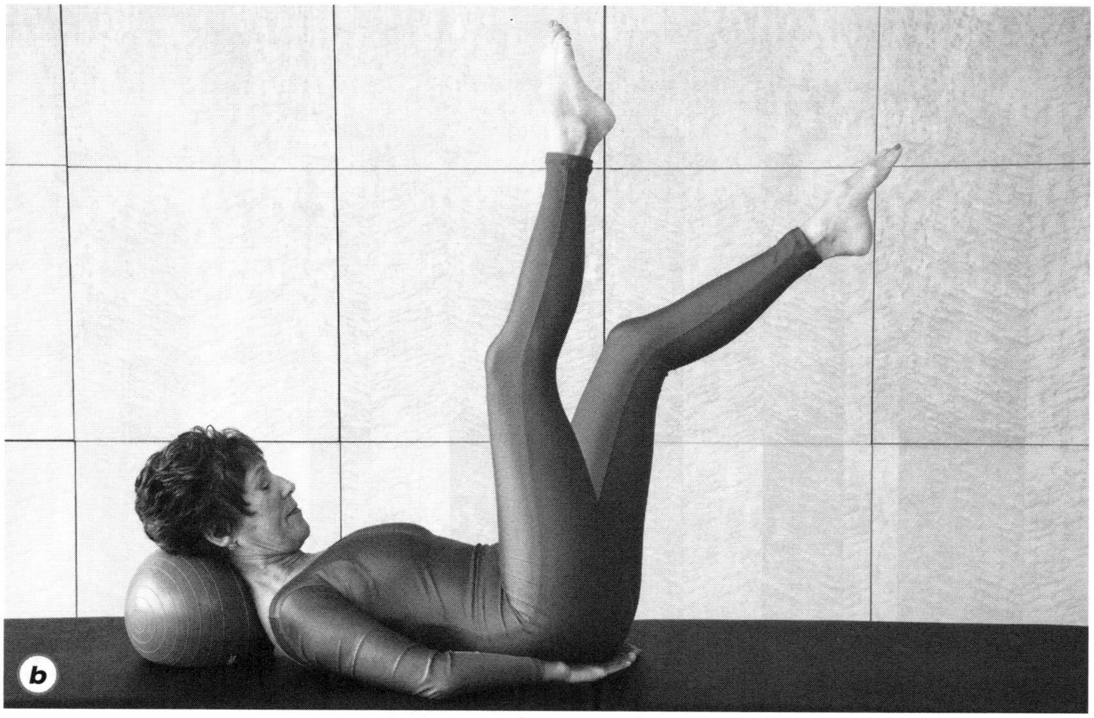

Look for . . . Encourage

- Shoulders gliding toward the tailbone as if suspenders were hooked to the bottom tips of the shoulder blades and attached to the hips
- Open collarbones
- Abdominals drawing in and up
- Legs long with a small bend in the knees, especially if the hamstrings are tight
- Tailbone long on the mat

Be aware of . . . Prevent

- Tension in the head, neck, and shoulders
- Arching (hyperextension) of the lumbar spine

Primary Muscles Activated

Abdominals, biceps, deltoids, anterior scalene, sternocleidomastoid, iliopsoas, rectus femoris, sartorius, adductor longus, adductor brevis, pectineus, gracilis, vastus medialis, vastus lateralis, vastus intermedius, tensor fasciae latae, hamstrings are stretched (semimembranosus, semitendinosus, biceps femoris)

Double Straight-Leg Stretch (Lower Lift)

Timeline: 6 weeks to 3 months postop

Appropriate for: knee and hip

Location: a raised mat, hip height

Instructions

- Lie supine on the mat with the head on a pad as needed and the legs bent into tabletop position. Place a small, soft ball between the knees. Lengthen the arms down by the sides of the body, pressing the arms and hands into the mat *(a)*. As an option, place the hands in a diamond shape under the tailbone, with the elbows wide and on the mat *(b)*.
- Draw the abdominals in and up, hugging the ball to the midline of the body.
- Inhale to prepare. Exhale and slowly lower the legs, keeping them in tabletop position, 5 to 6 inches (13-15 centimeters), hinging from the hips for the count of 3. Then exhale and bring the legs back to 90° on the count of 1.
- Draw the abdominals deeply into the spine. Do not arch the lower back as the legs are lowered toward the mat. Only lower the legs to the point that the core can maintain a neutral spine on the mat.
- If the lower back lifts away from the mat with the movement, adjust the movement to a smaller ROM.
- Repeat 6 times.

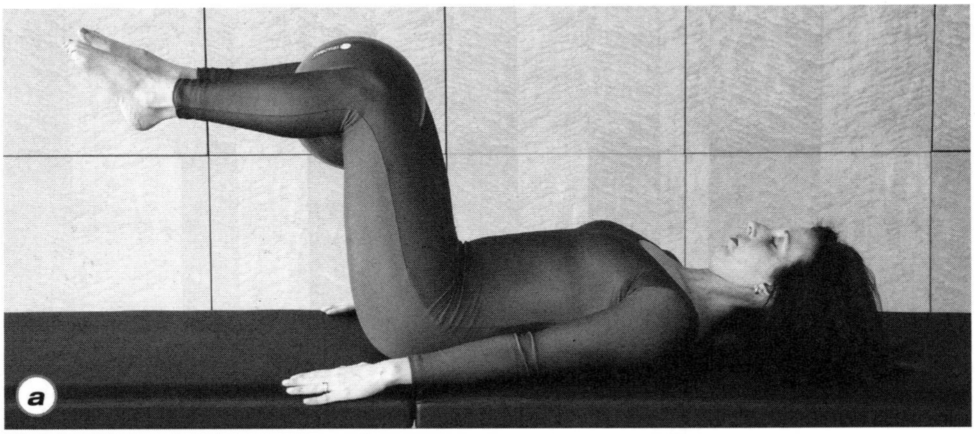

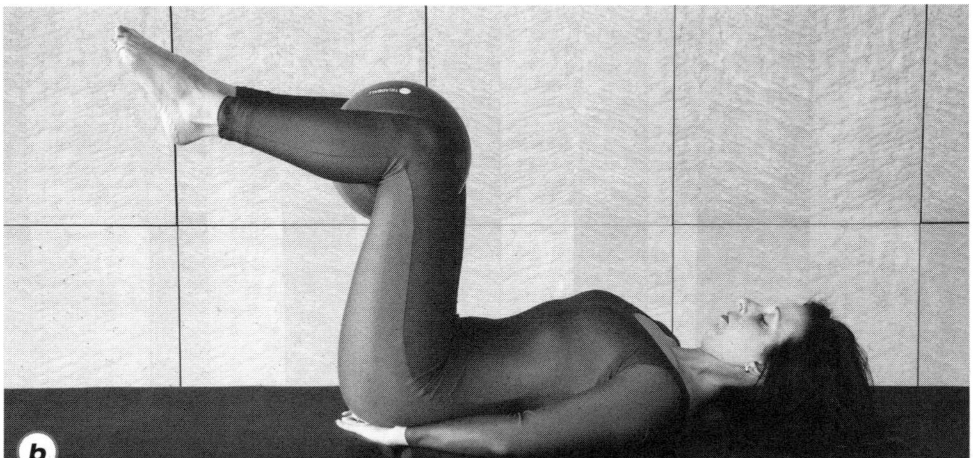

Options

1. Provided that you have awareness and control of the core musculature, you can curl the head and shoulders off the mat up to the bottom tips of the shoulder blades. Look toward the thighs and stay in the deep scoop to complete the repetitions of the exercise.

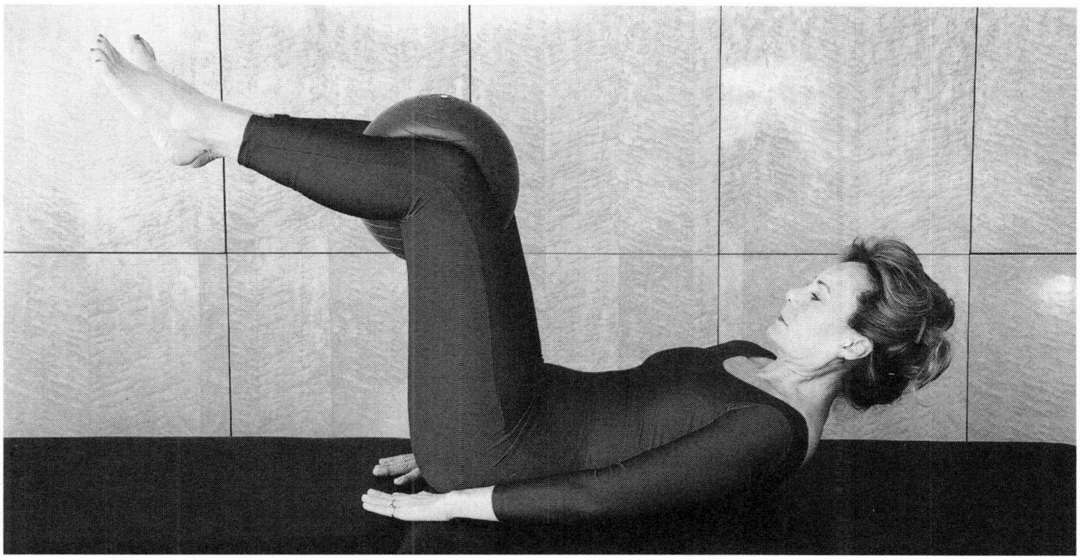

2. Place a small, soft ball under the head, neck, and shoulders to perform the movement. See pages 65-66 for the placement of the ball. Keep legs hip-distance apart or place a second ball between the knees if needed.

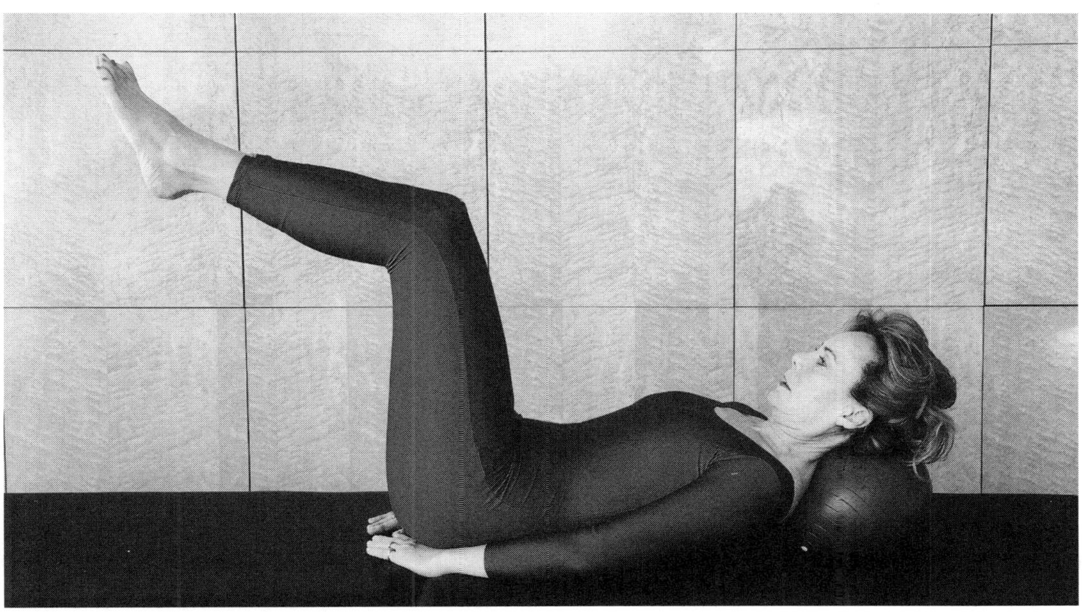

(continued)

Double Straight-Leg Stretch (Lower Lift) *(continued)*

3. Place the legs on a box, a small barrel, or several sturdy pillows and hold a small, soft ball between the legs. Place one hand over the other and place the hands behind the head at the base of the skull with the thumbs running down the sides of the neck *(a)*. Scoop deeply into the abdominals and inhale to prepare. Exhale and curl the head and shoulders off the mat *(b)*. Hold the position for the count of 3, inhale, and lower on a count of 1. Repeat 6 to 8 times.

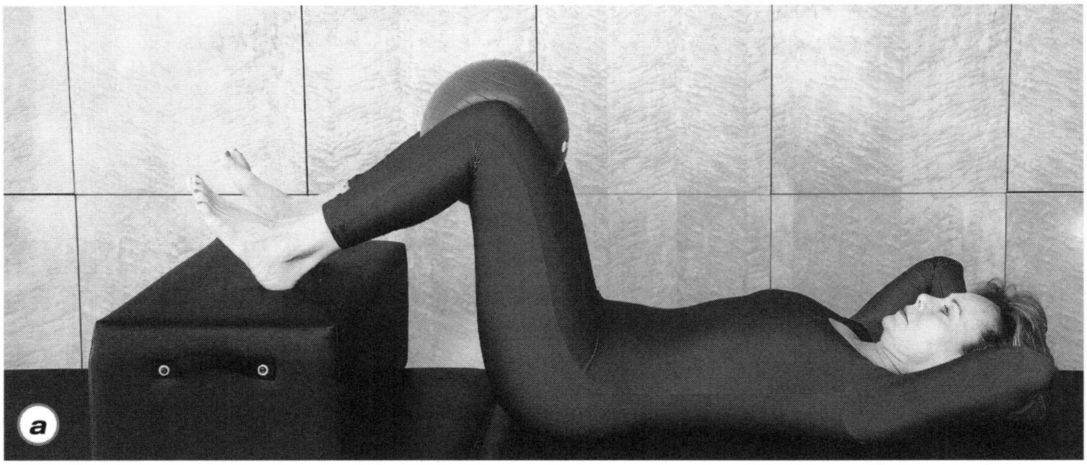

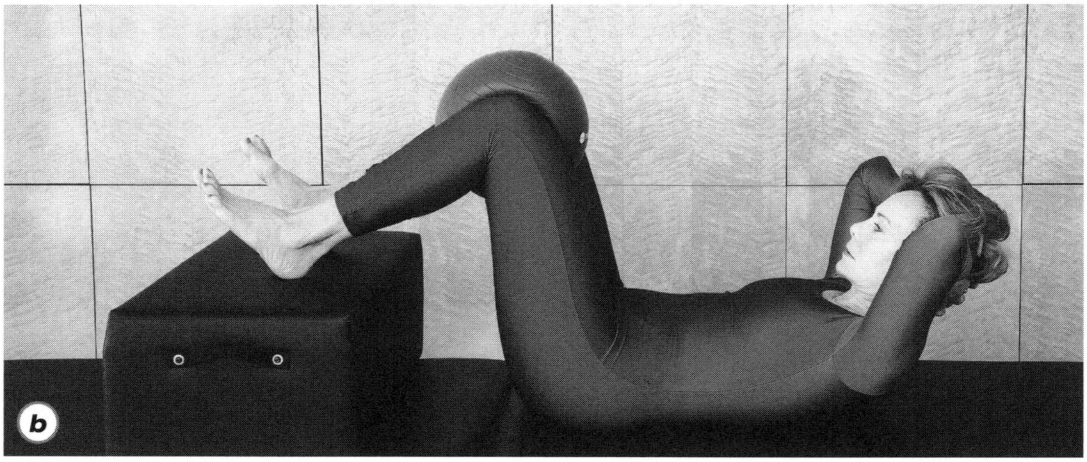

Look for . . . Encourage

- Tailbone long on the mat
- Shoulders gliding toward the hips as if suspenders were hooked to the bottom tips of the shoulder blades and attached to the hips
- Abdominals drawn in and up
- Open collarbones
- Hinging from the hips as the legs lower

Be aware of . . . Prevent

- Tension in the head, neck, and shoulders
- Arching (hyperextension) of the lumbar spine when the legs lower
- Lowering the heels to the floor versus hinging from the hip

Primary Muscles Activated

The primary muscles activated depend on the chosen option. The primary muscles include the following: Abdominals, anterior scalene, sternocleidomastoid, iliopsoas, rectus femoris, sartorius, adductor magnus, adductor longus, adductor brevis, pectineus, gracilis, biceps femoris, semimembranosus, semitendinosus, gastrocnemius, popliteus, tensor fasciae latae, plantaris

Crisscross

Timeline: 6 weeks to 3 months postop
Appropriate for: knee and hip
Location: a raised mat, hip height

Instructions

- Lie supine on the mat with the knees bent, the feet placed on the floor, a barrel or sturdy pillows placed under the knees. Place a small, soft ball between the knees; hug the ball to the midline.
- Place the head and shoulders on the mat. Layer the hands one on top of the other and place them behind the head at the base of the skull with the thumbs running down the sides of the neck. Keep the elbows wide and slightly off the mat.
- Inhale to prepare. Exhale and curl up off the mat to the bottom tips of the shoulder blades, drawing the abdominals in and up. Twist from the waist and bring the left shoulder toward the right hip while extending the left arm to the outside of the right thigh. Press the hand against the thigh and reach. Gaze diagonally forward. Hold for 3 counts.
- Inhale, center the body, and place the left hand back behind the head. Exhale and twist toward the left, extend the right arm to the outside of the left thigh, and hold for 3 counts.
- Repeat 6 sets.
- Lower to start position after each set as needed.
- Work toward staying rounded up for all 6 sets.
- Do not let the tailbone curl up, losing neutral spine, when performing the movement.

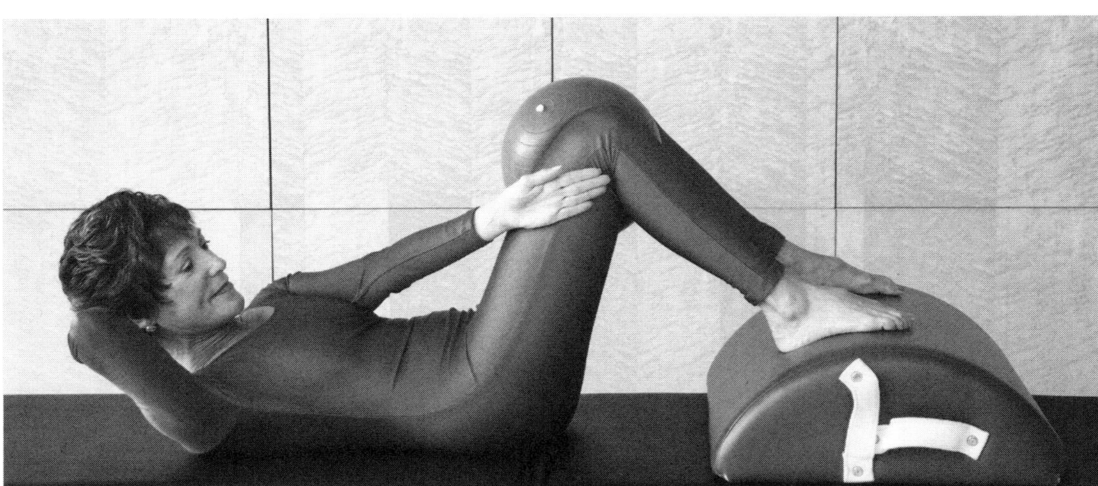

Options

1. Use a ball.
   - Place the feet on the mat and place a small, soft ball between the knees.
   - Place the head and shoulders on the mat. Layer the hands one on top of the other and place them behind the head with the thumbs running down the sides of the neck. Keep the elbows wide and slightly off the mat.
   - Inhale to prepare. Exhale and roll up to the bottom tips of the shoulder blades. Twist from the waist, bringing the left shoulder toward the right hip. Gaze diagonally forward and hold for 3 counts.

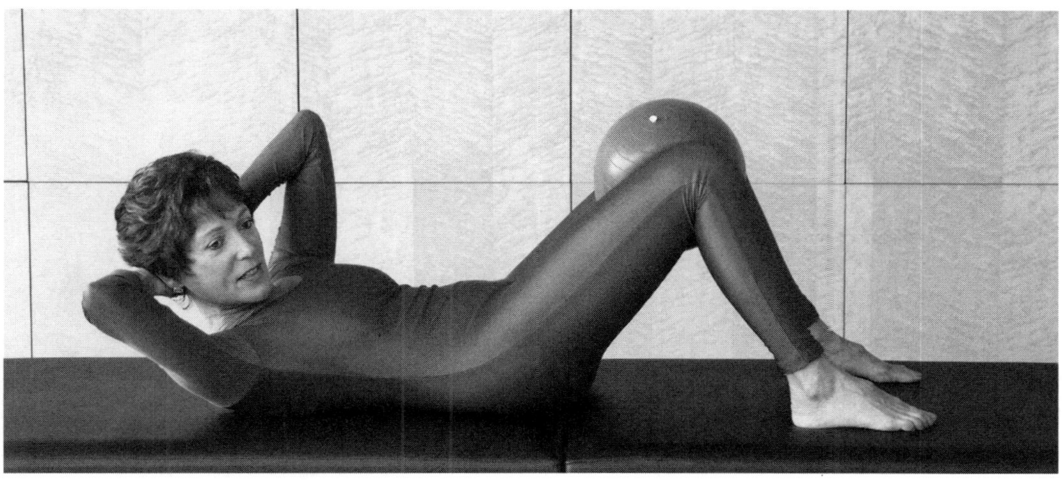

   - Twist to center and roll back down to the mat. Inhale to prepare. Exhale and roll up to the bottom tips of the shoulder blades. Twist from the waist, bringing the right shoulder toward the left hip, and hold for 3 counts. Twist to center and then roll back down to the mat.
   - Hug the ball to the midline of the body during the movement. Repeat for 5 sets.

(continued)

Crisscross *(continued)*

2. Use an exercise band.
   - Fold an exercise band in half and place it behind the head. Leave 3 to 4 inches (8-10 centimeters) of space for the hands to hold the band snugly to perform the movement.
   - Curl up to the bottom tips of the shoulder blades and twist from the waist toward the right hip; gaze diagonally forward. Hold for 3 counts and then switch sides. Repeat for 5 sets.
   - Work at getting the shoulders up off the mat and twisting from the waist.

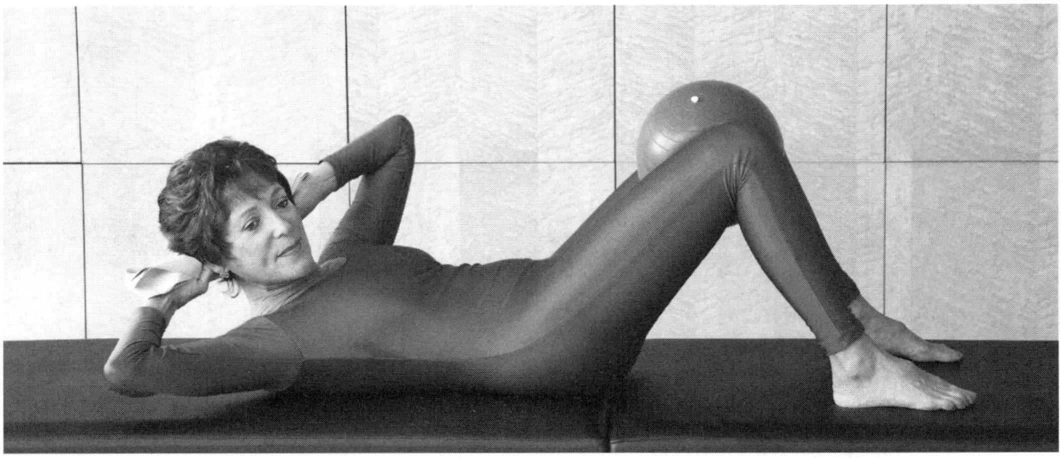

3. Over the course of a month, work toward bringing the legs up to a tabletop position to perform the movement. This option can be done with an exercise band and pad between the knees *(a)* or with an exercise band and ball *(b)*.

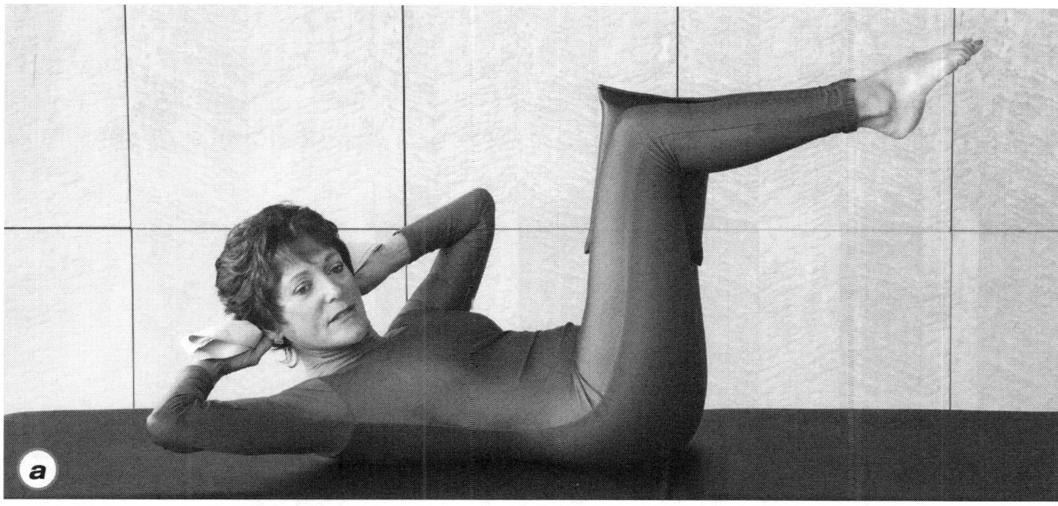

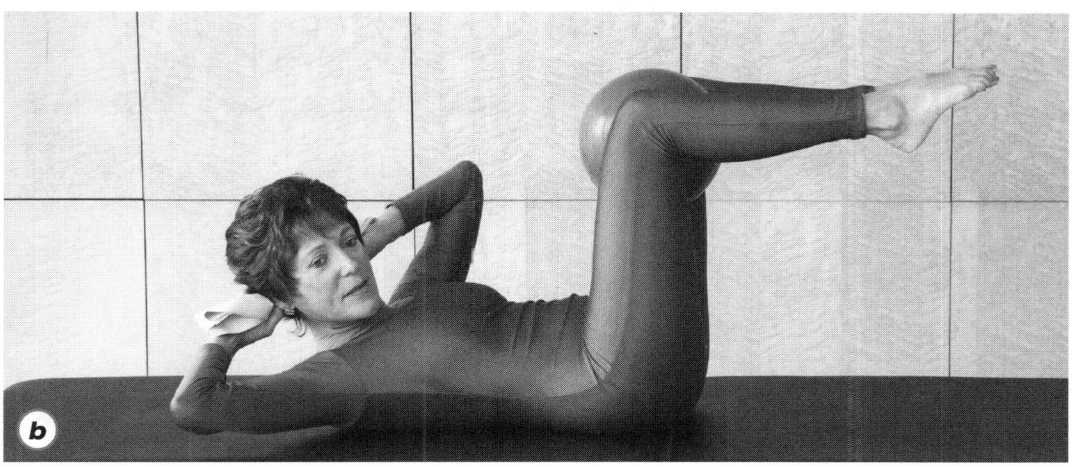

(continued)

4. Use a knee lift.
   - Lie supine on the mat with the knees bent and the feet on the mat.
   - Place the head and shoulders on the mat. Layer the hands one on top of the other and place them behind the head with the thumbs running down the sides of the neck. Keep the elbows wide and slightly off the mat.
   - Inhale to prepare. Exhale and curl the head, neck, and shoulders up off the mat. Simultaneously twist from the waist, bringing the left shoulder toward the right knee as you bring the leg in toward the chest. Gaze diagonally forward. Hold for 3 counts.

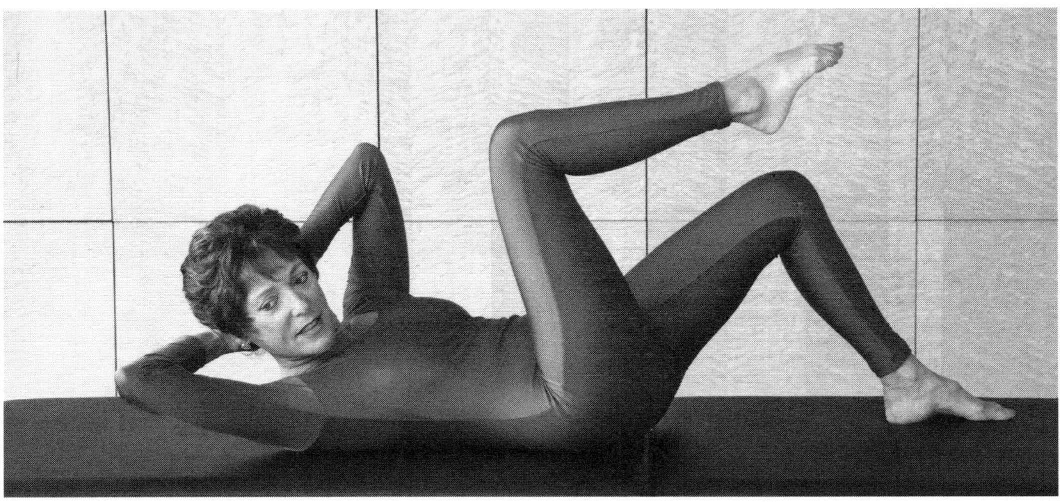

   - Twist to center, roll back down to the mat, and lower the leg.
   - Inhale to prepare. Exhale and roll back up, bringing the right shoulder toward the left knee. Hold for 3 counts. Twist to center and roll back down on the mat and lower the leg.
   - Repeat 5 sets.
   - **Hip:** Keep 90° to 100° of flexion for the first 3 months postop.

Look for . . . Encourage

- The pelvis stable on the mat during the twist
- Twisting from the waist, bringing the obliques toward the opposite hip
- Elbows wide and stable with the twist
- Lifting off the mat up to the bottom tips of the shoulder blades to perform the movement
- Keeping neutral spine with the movement

Be aware of . . . Prevent

- Tension in the head, neck, and shoulders
- Folding the elbow in toward the opposite hip
- Tailbone curling up when the upper body rounds up to the bottom tips of the shoulder blades, losing neutral spine

Primary Muscles Activated

The primary muscles activated depend on the chosen option. The primary muscles include the following: Abdominals, biceps, deltoids, triceps, anterior scalene, sternocleidomastoid, rectus femoris, sartorius, adductor magnus, adductor longus, adductor brevis, pectineus, iliopsoas, gracilis, biceps femoris, semimembranosus, semitendinosus, gastrocnemius, popliteus, tensor fasciae latae, plantaris

Spine Stretch Forward

Timeline: 6 weeks to 3 months postop
Appropriate for: knee and hip
Location: a raised mat, hip height

Instructions

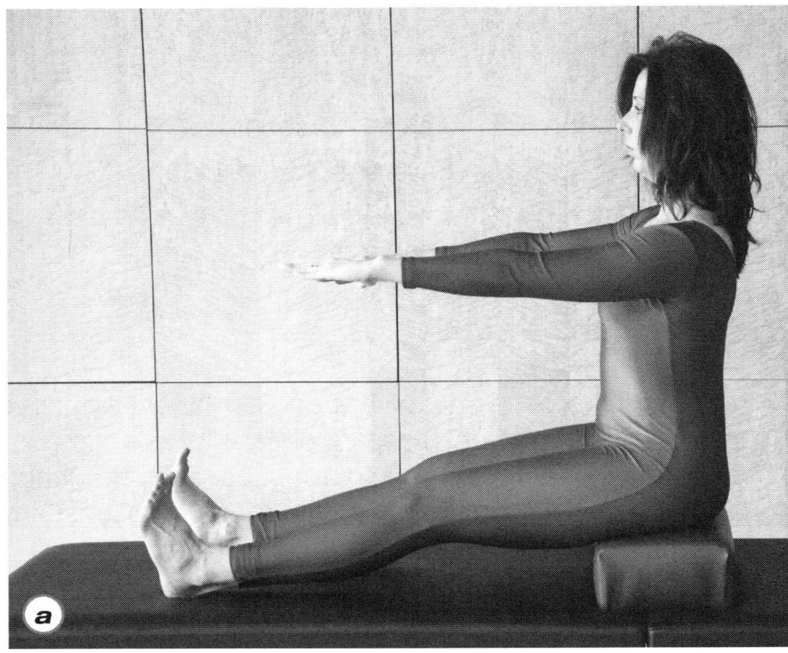

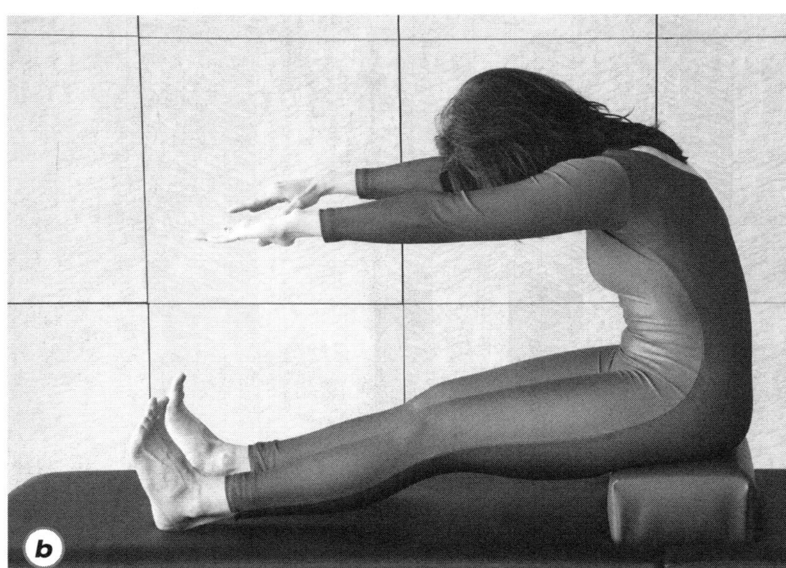

- Sit tall on a moon box or long box to elevate the pelvis above the feet. Extend the legs, keeping them hip-distance apart, with the knees slightly bent and the feet flexed. Lift the arms to shoulder height, keeping them shoulder-width apart and long and parallel to the legs *(a)*.
- Sit tall as if you were sitting up against a wall. Inhale and lift the abdominals in and up. Exhale, bring the chin toward the chest, and round up and over an imaginary large beach ball, creating a large C-curve in the middle of the spine. Keep the shoulder blades gliding toward the hip points and imagine the belly button flowing back toward the spine in opposition to the hands as they reach for the opposite wall *(b)*.
- Inhale and begin to roll back up. Extend the spine and sit tall with the arms long and parallel to legs.
- **Knee:** Keep the knees slightly bent and soft.
- **Hip:** Maintain 90° of hip flexion.
- Repeat 3 to 5 times.

Options

1. Place a small, soft ball under the knees as needed.

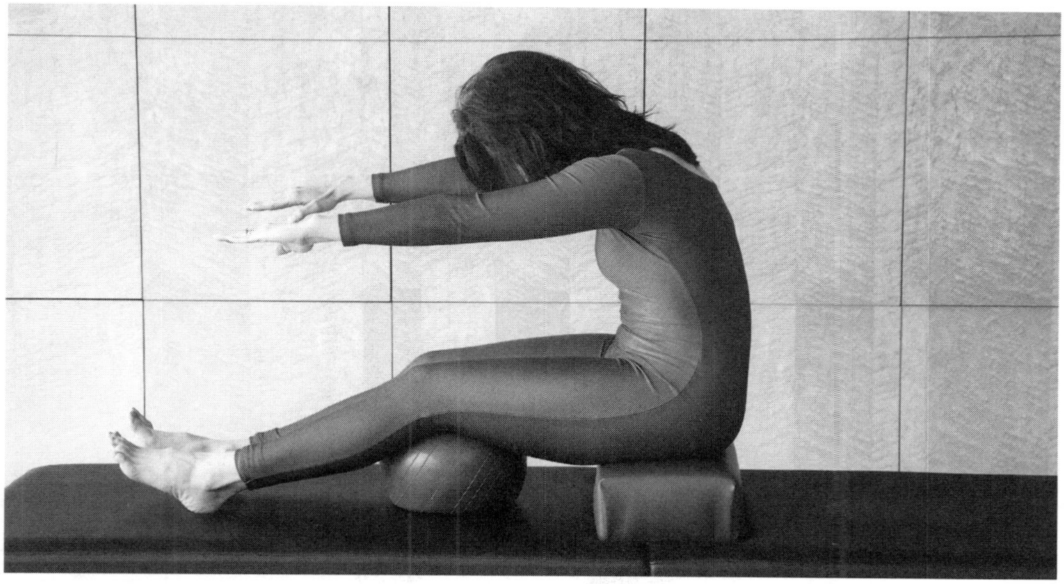

2. Place the hands on the thighs instead of holding them parallel to the floor.
3. Hold a wooden stick to keep the shoulders at shoulder height and shoulder width; press out on the sides of the stick as if you were opening an expandable tension curtain rod.
4. Roll up a mat and use it to sit on instead of using a box to elevate the pelvis.

(continued)

Look for . . . Encourage

- Shoulders gliding toward the hips as if suspenders were hooked to the bottom tips of the shoulder blades and attached to the hips
- Sitting tall as if a string were attached to the crown of the head and extended to the ceiling
- Thinking of lifting up and over a large beach ball
- Waistband flowing in toward the spine
- A feeling of drawing the ribs to the hips when lifting up and over to create a C-curve in the middle of the spine

Be aware of . . . Prevent

- Rounding from the upper back
- Excessive gripping in the hip flexors

Primary Muscles Activated

Abdominals, biceps, triceps, shoulder complex, iliopsoas, rectus femoris, pectineus, gracilis, sartorius, adductor longus, adductor brevis, vastus medialis, vastus intermedius, vastus lateralis, tensor fasciae latae, tibialis anterior, hamstrings are stretched (biceps femoris, semitendinosus, semimembranosus)

Saw

Timeline: 6 weeks to 3 months postop

Appropriate for: knee and hip

Location: a raised mat, hip height

Instructions

- Sit tall on a pad, moon box, or long box to elevate the pelvis above the feet. Extend the legs and open them wider than hip-distance apart. Flex the feet. Stretch out the arms to each side, reaching toward the walls. Lift the arms to slightly below shoulder height and keep them parallel to the floor.
- **Knee:** Keep the knees slightly bent and soft *(a)*.
  - Inhale to prepare. Exhale and twist to the right from the waist. Bring the chin to the chest and reach the left hand, palm facing down, to the outside of the right little toe. Meanwhile, reach the right arm back in opposition. Look toward the back hand *(b)*.
  - Draw the abdominals in and up while drawing the left hip back in opposition.
  - Inhale, roll up to an upright position, and then rotate the spine back to center. The shoulders are above the pelvis.
  - Exhale and switch sides, twisting to the left.
  - Repeat 5 times in each direction.

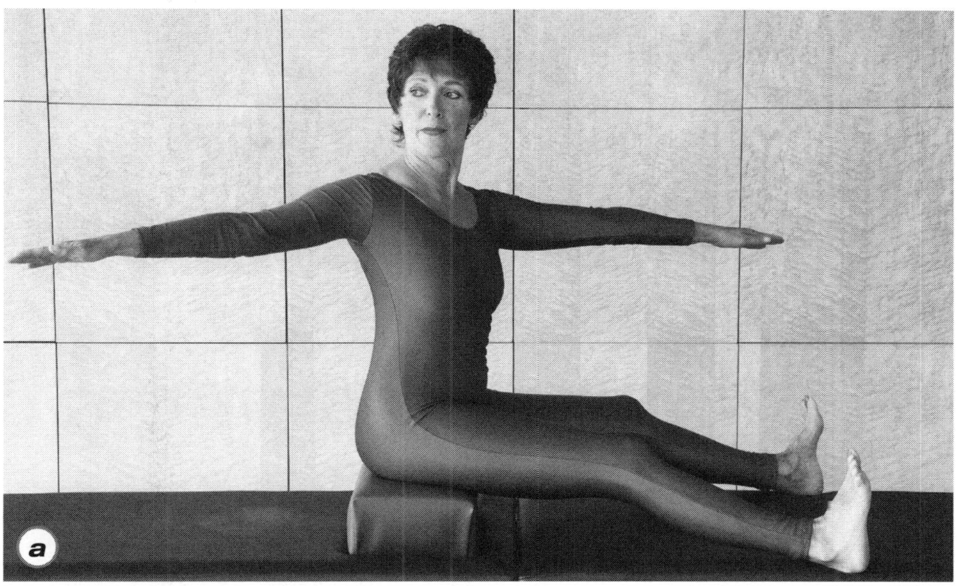

a

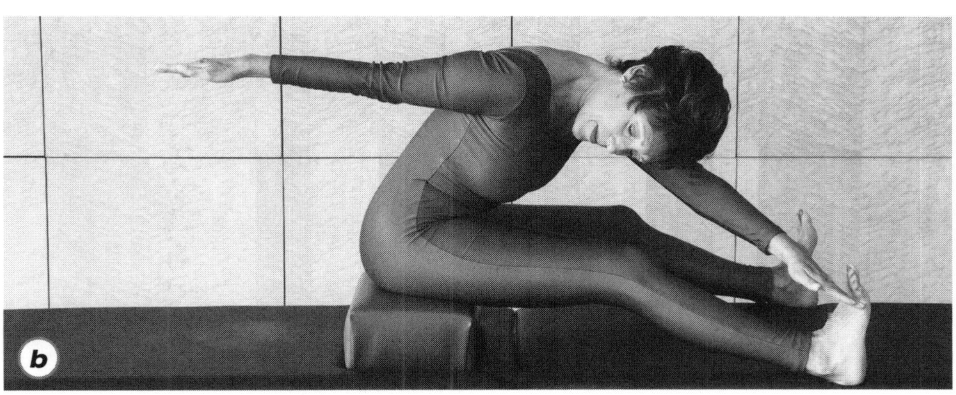

b

(continued)

- **Hip:** Keep the knees slightly bent and soft.
  - Inhale to prepare. Exhale, draw the abdominals in and up, and twist from the waist toward the right while drawing the left hip back in opposition. Hold for 2 counts.
  - Inhale and rotate back to the center, sitting tall.
  - Exhale and twist from the waist toward the left while drawing the right hip back in opposition. Hold for 2 counts.
  - Repeat 5 times in each direction.
  - Perform the twist portion of the exercise only for the first 3 months postop.

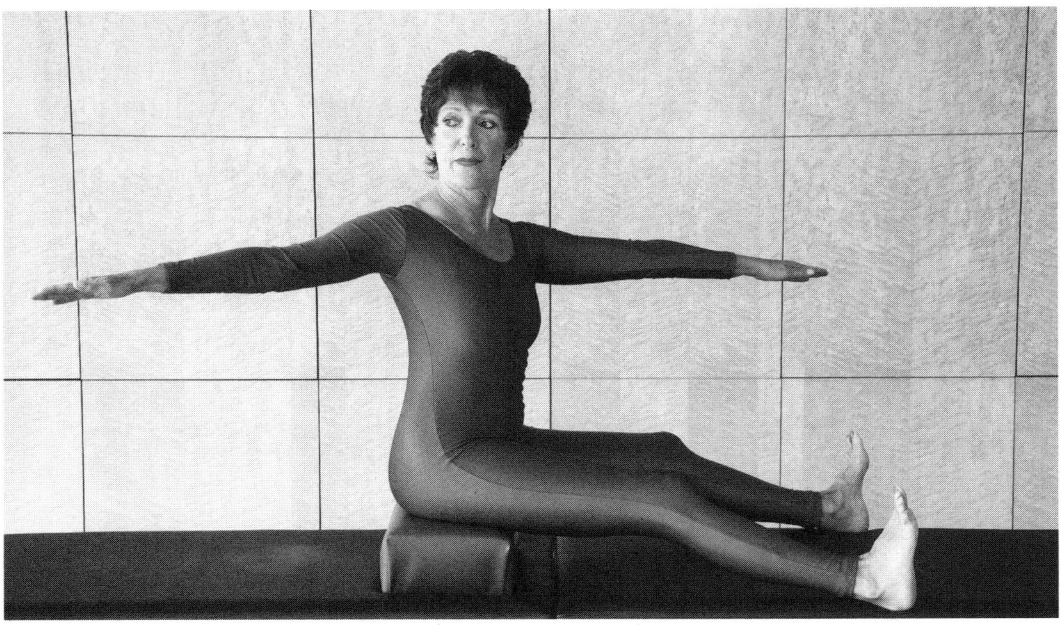

Look for . . . Encourage

- Thinking of the spine stretch forward exercise when reaching to the outside little toe with the palm facing the floor
- Reaching up and over toward the little toe
- Taking the ear to the knee and listening to the knee
- Shoulders gliding toward the hip as if suspenders were hooked to the bottom tips of the shoulder blades and attached to the hips
- Abdominals drawing deeply into the spine
- Sitting tall as if against a wall and maintaining a neutral spine

Be aware of . . . Prevent

- Feet rolling in or out when reaching to the little toe
- Folding from the hip to create the movement
- Loss of shoulder alignment

Primary Muscles Activated

Abdominals, biceps, triceps, shoulder complex, multifidi, rotators, iliopsoas, rectus femoris, pectineus, gracilis, sartorius, adductor longus, adductor brevis, vastus medialis, vastus intermedius, vastus lateralis, tensor fasciae latae, tibialis anterior, hamstrings are stretched (biceps femoris, semitendinosus, semimembranosus)

Swan Prep

Timeline: 6 weeks to 3 months postop
Appropriate for: knee and hip
Location: a raised mat, hip height

Instructions

- Lie prone (facedown) on the mat. Make a pillow with the hands and place them under the forehead *(a)*.
- Place the feet hip-distance apart, keep the legs parallel, and feel the shoulders gliding toward the hips.
- Feel the tops of the toes, deepen the pubic bone toward the mat, and slightly engage the gluteus muscles and hamstrings.
- Draw the abdominals in and up; feel as though you could shoot air between the mat and the belly button.
- Inhale and begin to lift the head and chest away from the hands and mat. Hold for 2 counts, exhale, and lengthen back down to mat *(b)*.
- Repeat 3 to 5 times.

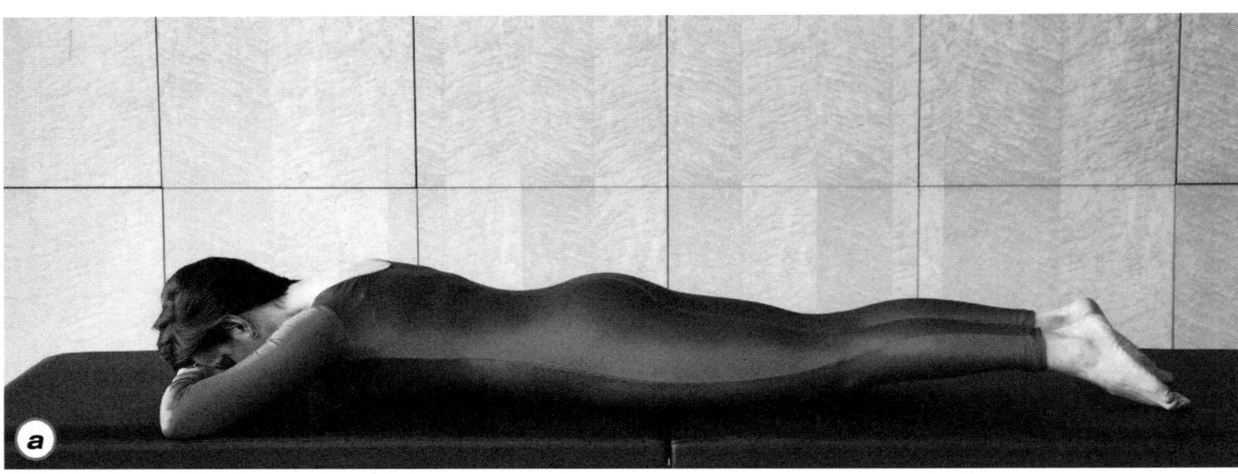
a

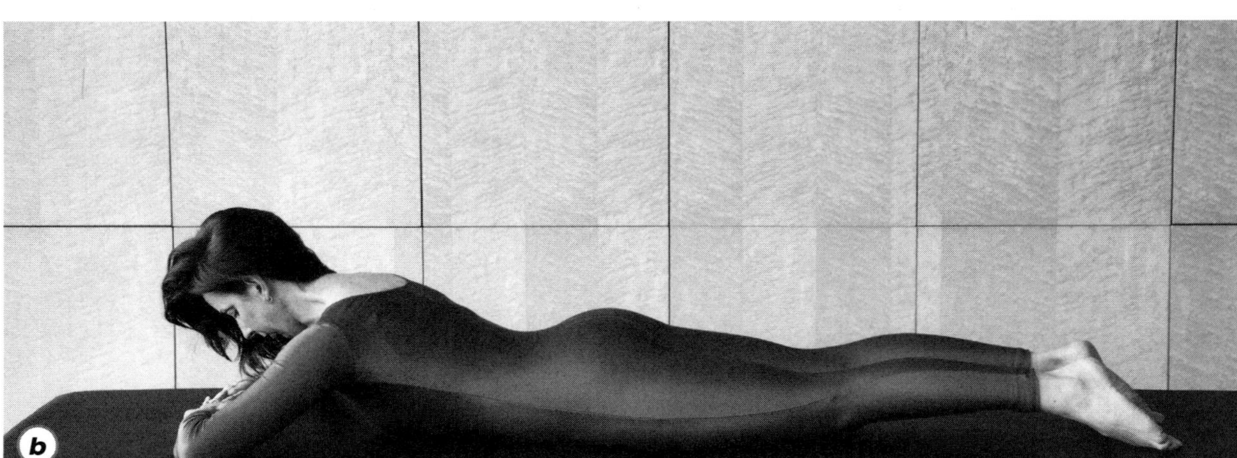
b

Options

1. Fold a towel into quarters and place it under the abdominals and hips.

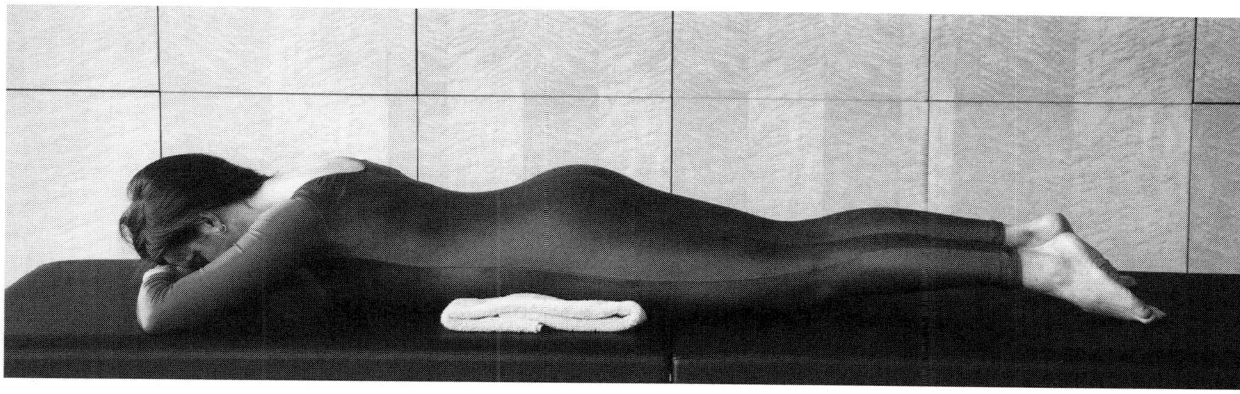

2. Fold a towel into quarters and place it under the abdominals and hips and place another folded towel under the knees.

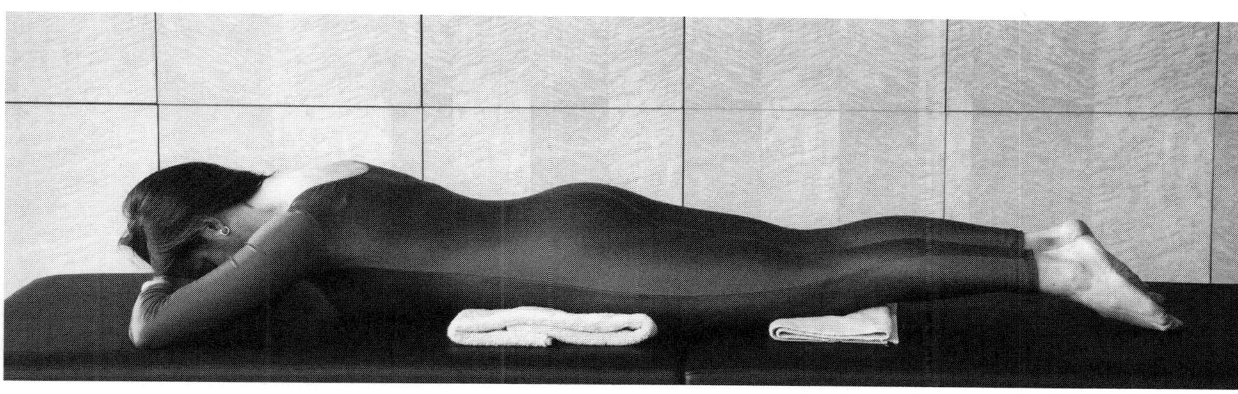

3. Lie prone (facedown) on the mat. Place the forehead on the mat and rest the arms by and slightly under the sides of the body with the palms facing up. Place the feet hip-distance apart, keep the legs parallel, and feel the shoulders gliding down the back side. Draw the abdominals in and up; feel as though you could shoot air between the mat and the belly button. Inhale and begin to lift the head and then the chest away from the mat. Hold for 2 counts, exhale, and lengthen back down to mat.

(continued)

Look for . . . Encourage

- The head following the alignment of the spine
- The shoulders gliding toward the hip points as the body lengthens up
- Navel snapped to spine

Be aware of . . . Prevent

Hyperextension of the lumbar spine

Primary Muscles Activated

Abdominals, splenius capitis, splenius cervicis, transversospinalis group, erector spinae group, quadratus lumborum (assists), intertransversarii, interspinalis, latissimus dorsi, gluteus maximus, gluteus medius (posterior portion), adductor magnus (ischiocondylar portion), biceps femoris, semitendinosus, semimembranosus, rectus femoris, vastus medius, vastus intermedius, vastus lateralis, tensor fasciae latae, tibialis posterior, gastrocnemius, soleus, plantaris

Single-Leg Kick

Timeline: 6 weeks to 3 months postop

Appropriate for: knee and hip

Location: a raised mat, hip height

Instructions

- Lie prone and prop the upper body on the forearms with the elbows in line with the shoulders. Make fists with the hands and face the palms toward each other. Extend the legs all the way onto the mat, positioning them hip-distance apart.
- Lift the head, chest, and rib cage off the mat as one unit. The head and neck should act as an extension of the spine. Keep the upper body lifted away from the mat.
- Feel the forearms pressing into the mat and hugging to the midline as if you were holding a magic circle. Feel as if you were pulling yourself through the window of your arms (press, hug, and pull).
- Keep this stable position as you perform the movement.
- Rest the tops of the toes on the mat, draw the abdominals in and up toward the spine, and engage the gluteus muscles, keeping the pubic bone guided toward the mat, hip bones on the mat.
- Bend the right knee and kick, kick the right heel in toward the buttocks; lengthen the right leg down to the mat; and then kick, kick the left heel in toward the buttocks; lengthen the left leg down to the mat. Make the movement slow and controlled, and work one leg at a time. Maintain a normal breath throughout the sets. (Action: kick, kick and lengthen leg to mat.)
- **Knee:** Bend the knee only 5 to 8 inches (13-20 centimeters). Keep the movement slow and controlled. *Do not* pulse *(a)*.

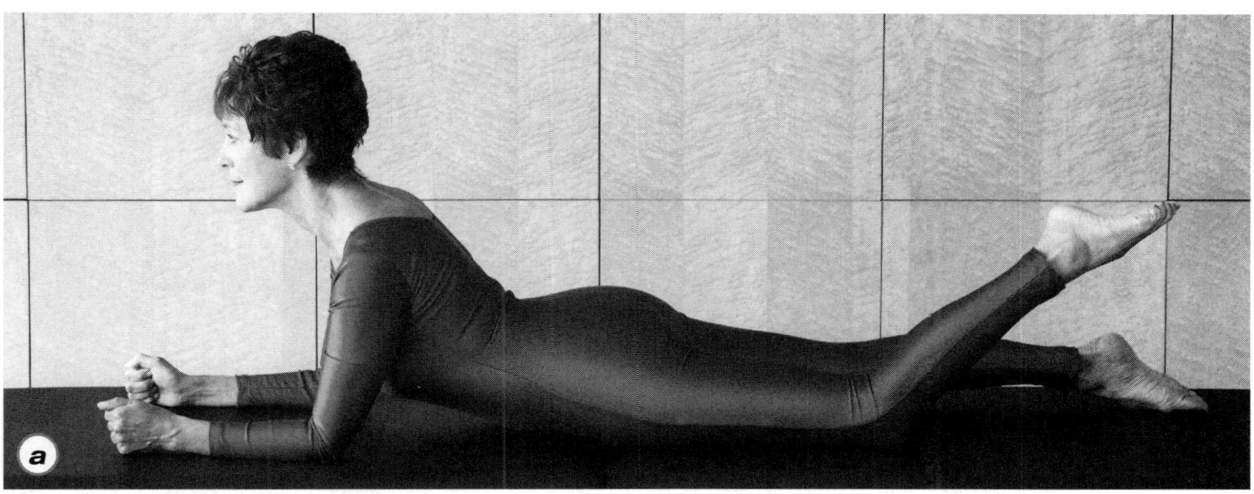

(continued)

- **Hip:** Bend the knee toward the buttocks as far as possible without experiencing discomfort *(b)*.
- Repeat 6 times on each leg.

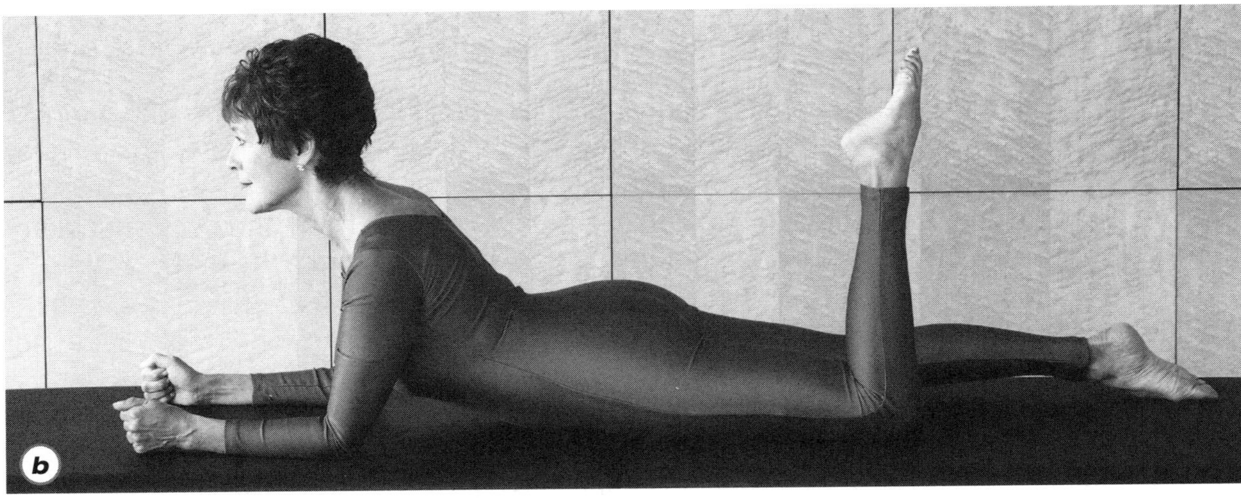

b

Options

1. Lower the torso all the way down onto the mat and make a pillow with the hands. Place the forehead on the pillow. Lengthen both legs out onto the mat, positioning them hip-distance apart. Draw the abdominals in and up. Bend the right knee toward the buttocks. Kick, kick the heel in toward the buttocks; lengthen the right leg down toward the mat; kick, kick the left heel in toward the buttocks and lengthen the left leg down toward the mat. Make the movement slow and controlled, and work one leg at a time. Maintain a normal breath throughout the sets. If you do this modification for the knee version, *do not* pulse.

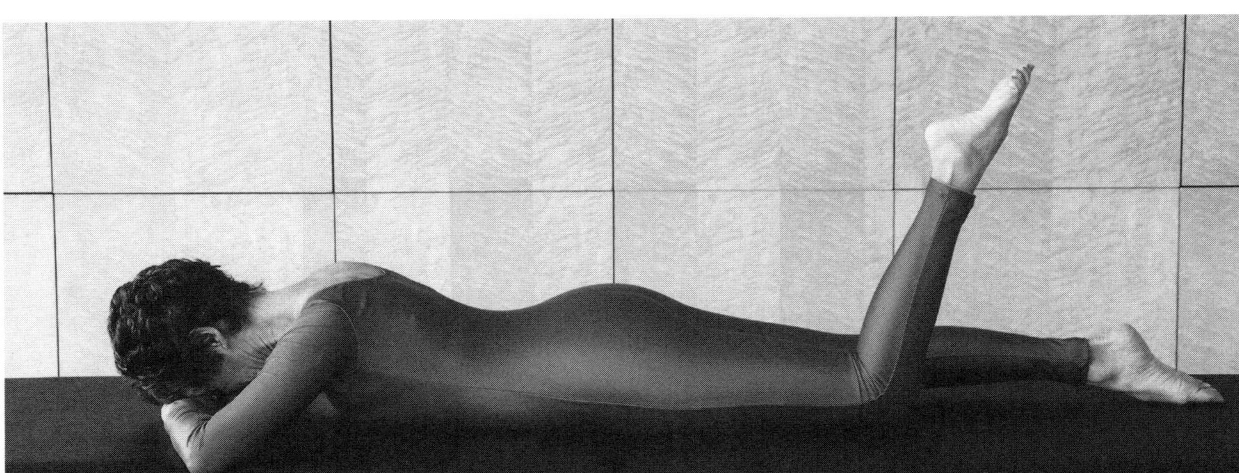

2. Place a towel under the torso for comfort as needed for either the hip *(a)* or the knee *(b)* version of the exercise.

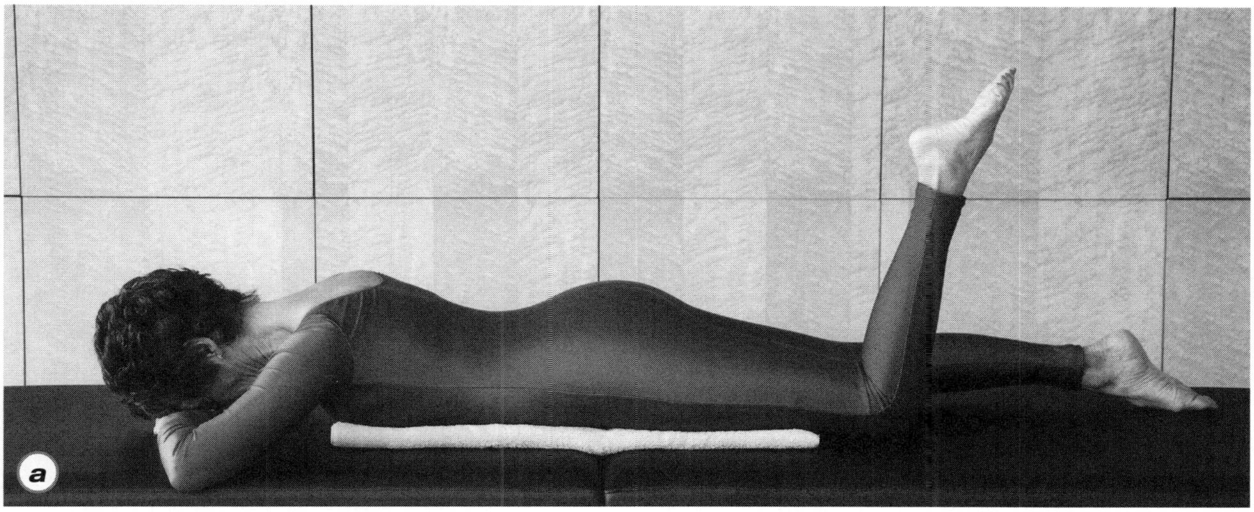

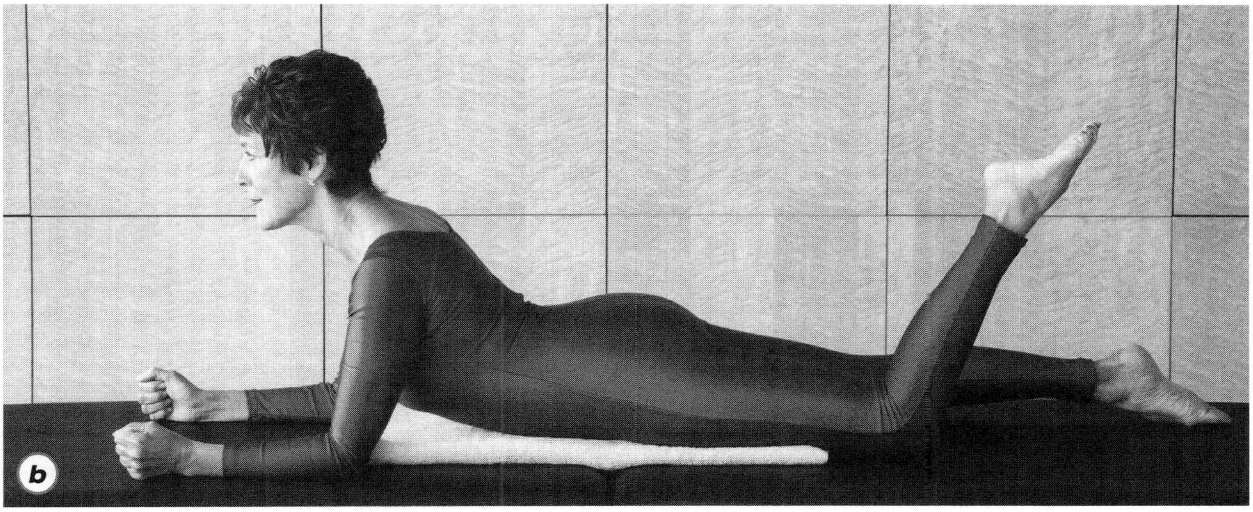

(continued)

Single-Leg Kick *(continued)*

Look for . . . Encourage

- The chest lifted away from the mat and the forearms
- The shoulders gliding toward the hips as if suspenders were hooked to the bottom tips of the shoulder blades and attached to the hips
- Movement without pain in the knee and hip
- Abdominals lifted in and up and away from the mat
- Hips stable on the mat during the movement of the legs

Be aware of . . . Prevent

- Hyperextension of the lumbar spine
- Sinking between the shoulder blades
- Loss of core control
- Torso swaying side to side with the movement

Primary Muscles Activated

Abdominals, triceps, biceps, shoulder complex, splenius capitis, splenius cervicis, transversospinalis group, erector spinae group, quadratus lumborum (assists), intertransversarii, interspinalis, latissimus dorsi, gluteus maximus, gluteus medius (posterior portion), adductor magnus (ischiocondylar part), biceps femoris, semimembranosus, semitendinosus, gracilis, gastrocnemius, sartorius, popliteus, plantaris, rectus femoris, vastus medialis, vastus intermedius, vastus lateralis, tibialis posterior, soleus

Shoulder Bridge (Modified)

Timeline: 6 weeks to 3 months postop
Appropriate for: knee and hip
Location: a raised mat, hip height

Instructions

- Lie supine on the mat with the knees bent into a mountain shape and the feet placed on a small barrel. Position the feet hip-distance apart, the arms long by the sides of the body or out in a slight V, and the palms face down on the mat.
- Place a small, soft ball between the knees. Hug the legs toward the ball. Make sure the toes, heels, knees, and hips are in alignment.
- Inhale to prepare. Exhale and press the feet down on the barrel and curl the tailbone toward the nose. Roll up one vertebra at a time to the waist only *(a)*.

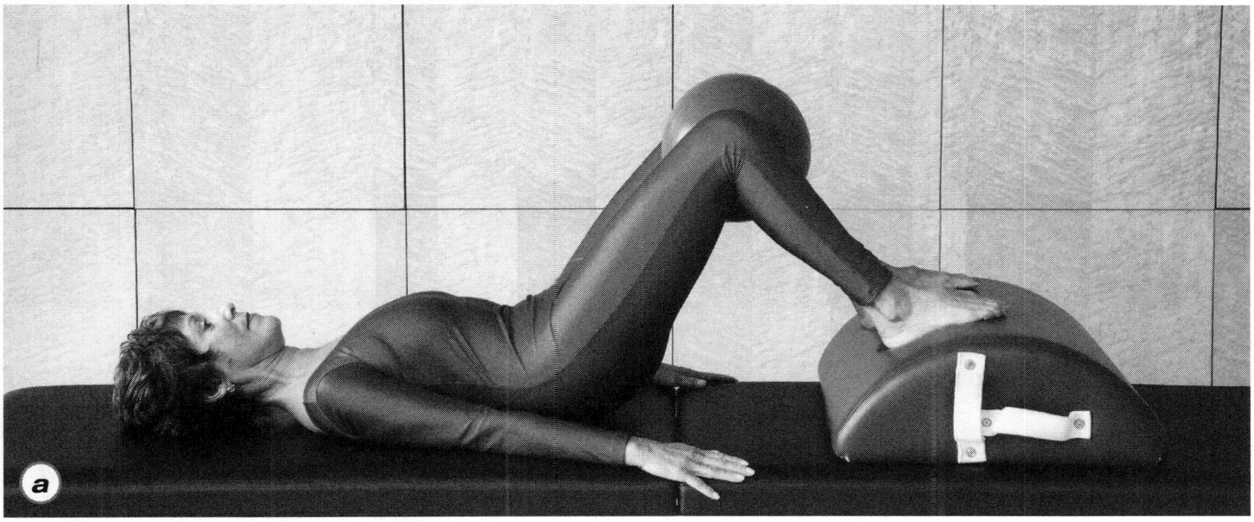
a

(continued)

Shoulder Bridge (Modified) *(continued)*

- Inhale to prepare. Exhale and roll back down to the starting position. Slowly roll up and down.
- Repeat 3 times.
- Next roll up to the shoulder blades and roll back down one vertebra at a time. Slowly roll up and down *(b)*.
- As you are rolling down, think of drawing the tailbone to the heels to deepen the articulation of the spine back down to the mat.
- When not using a barrel, place the heels about 3 inches (8 centimeters) in front of the knees on the mat as tolerated *(c)*.

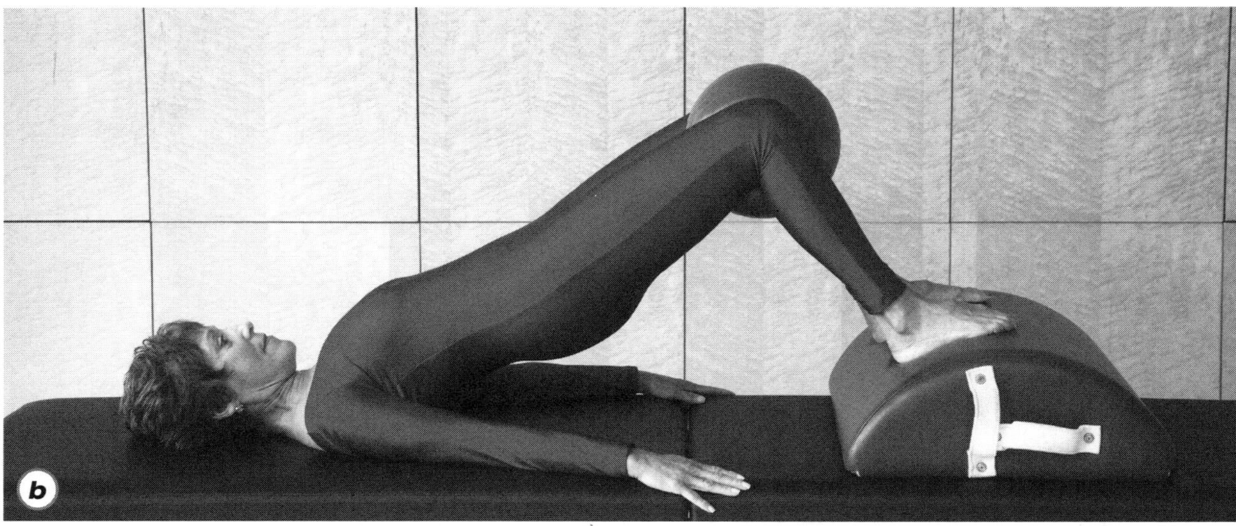
b

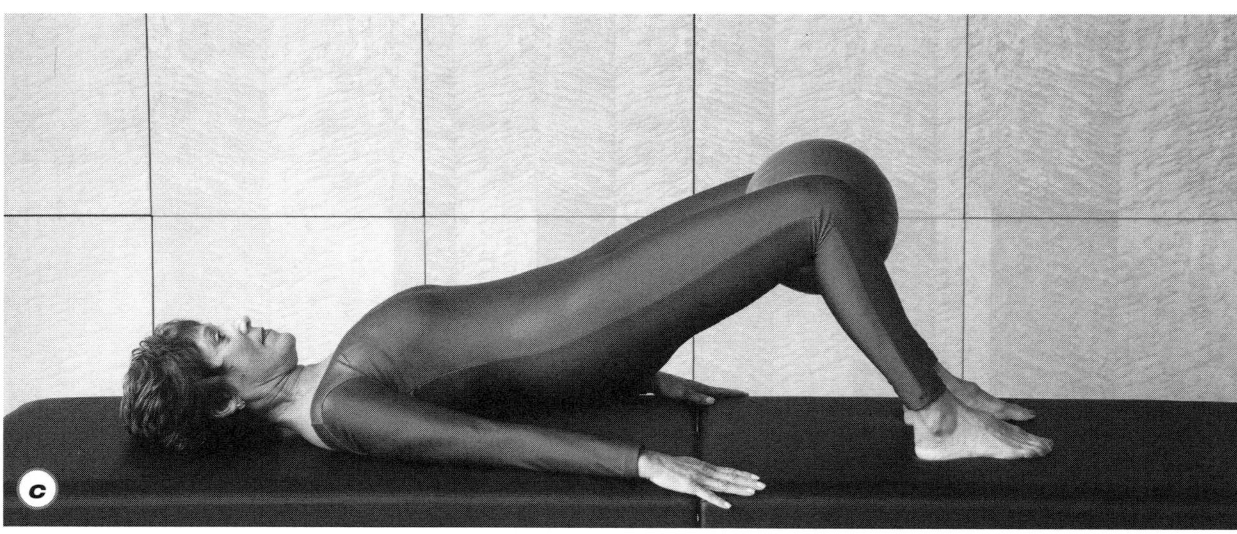
c

Option

Use a large box or two sturdy pillows with *(a)* or without *(b)* the use of a small, soft ball to perform the movement. Keep legs hip-distance apart.

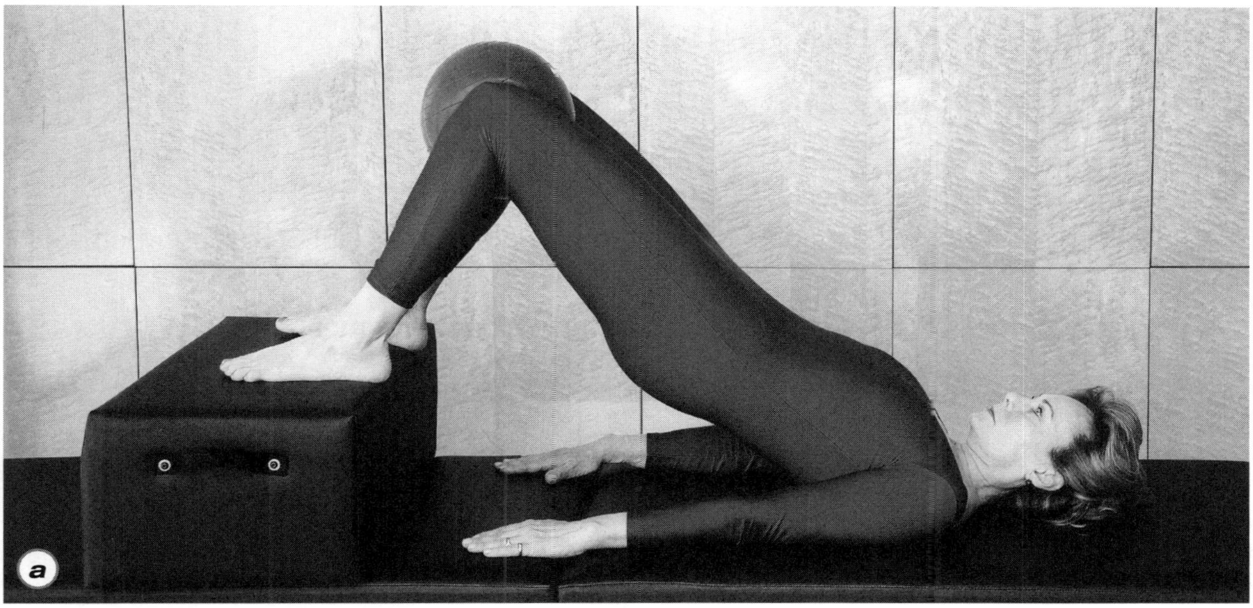

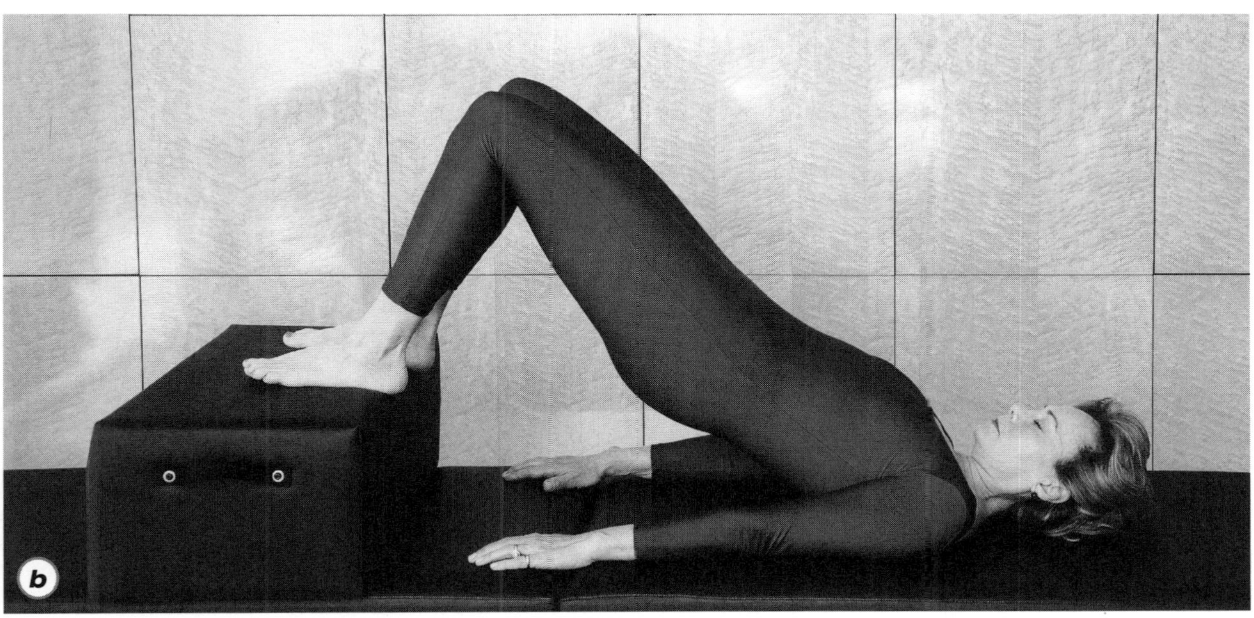

(continued)

Shoulder Bridge (Modified) *(continued)*

Look for . . . Encourage

- The abdominals drawing in and up
- Articulation of the vertebrae as if they were a string of pearls being laid out on the mat one pearl at a time
- Rolling up to one long line between the shoulder blades and the knees
- Hips steady and parallel throughout the movement

Be aware of . . . Prevent

- Hyperextension of the lumbar spine
- Cramping in the hamstrings (to avoid cramping, reduce the ROM or rest between sets)
- Pelvic instability and tilting
- Over-recruitment of the gluteus muscles to perform the movement

Primary Muscles Activated

Abdominals, rectus femoris, sartorius, pectineus, iliopsoas, gluteus maximus, gluteus medius (posterior portion), biceps femoris, semitendinosus, semimembranosus, tensor fasciae latae, adductor magnus, adductor longus, adductor brevis, gracilis, popliteus, plantaris, gastrocnemius

Teaser Prep 1

Timeline: 6 weeks to 3 months postop
Appropriate for: knee and hip
Location: a raised mat, hip height

Instructions

- Lie supine on the mat with the knees slightly bent into a mountain shape. Place a small, soft ball between the knees and lengthen the arms to the ceiling with the palms facing the thighs and the shoulders away from the ears *(a)*.
- Inhale to prepare. Curl the head, neck, and shoulders off the mat; bring the chin toward the chest; exhale; lower the arms parallel to the thighs; and slowly roll up. Scoop the navel to the spine and draw the abdominals in and up. Lengthen the arms up on a diagonal *(b)*.

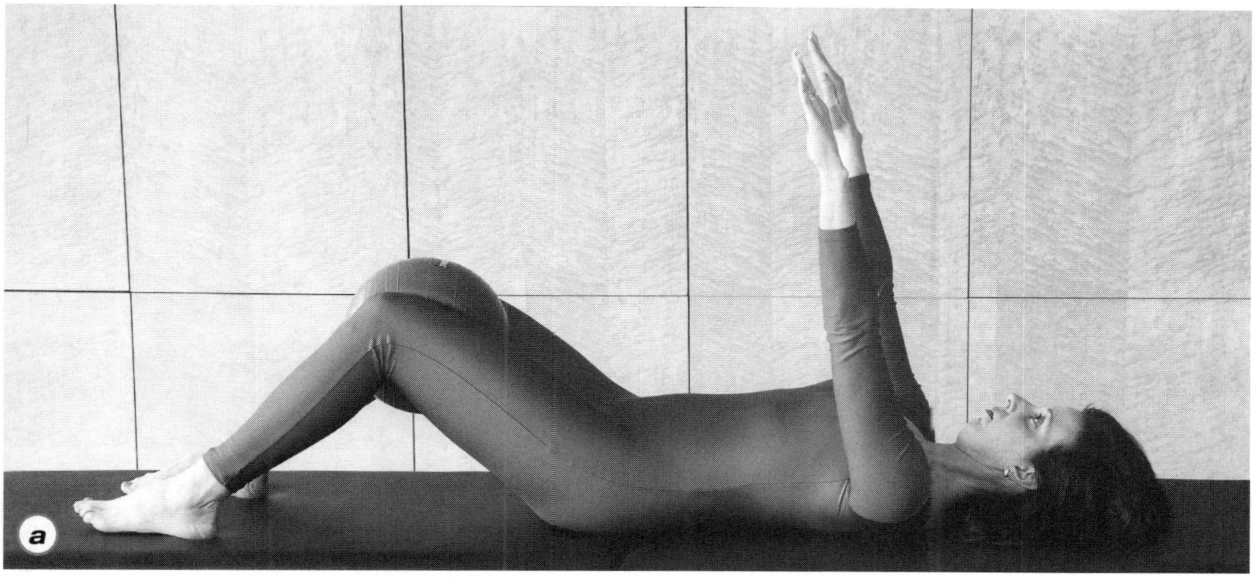

a

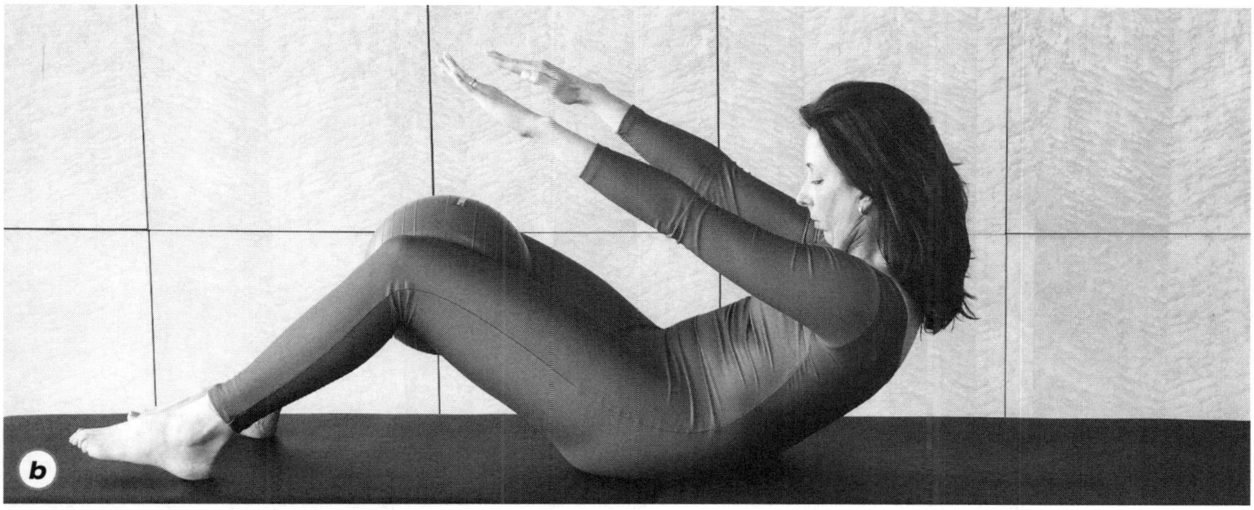

b

(continued)

Teaser Prep 1 *(continued)*

- **Knee:** Keep the knees soft and parallel with a small, soft ball. Hold for a count of 5 *(c)*.
- **Hip:** For up to 3 months, roll up to keep 90° to 100° of flexion as the upper body reaches into the teaser position. Hold for a count of 5 *(d)*.
- Exhale and slowly roll down to the mat. Resist through the abdominals and hug the ball to the midline of the body.
- Repeat 3 times.
- Challenge: Roll down and up to a count of 8.

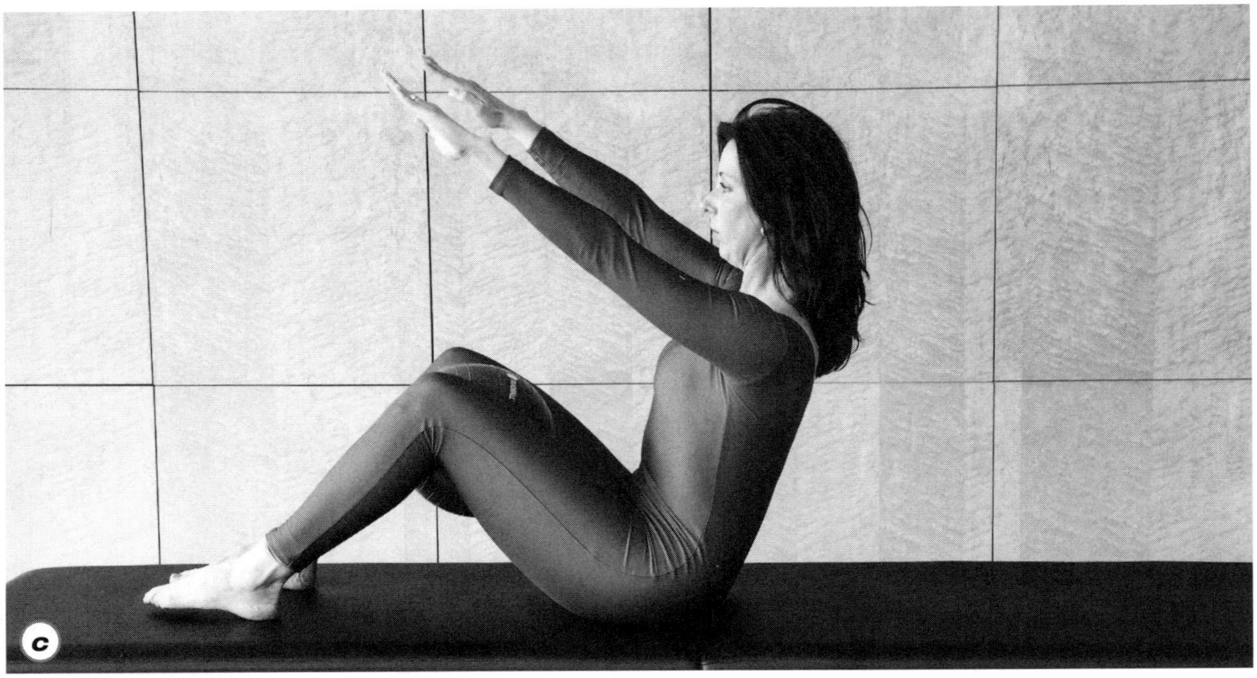

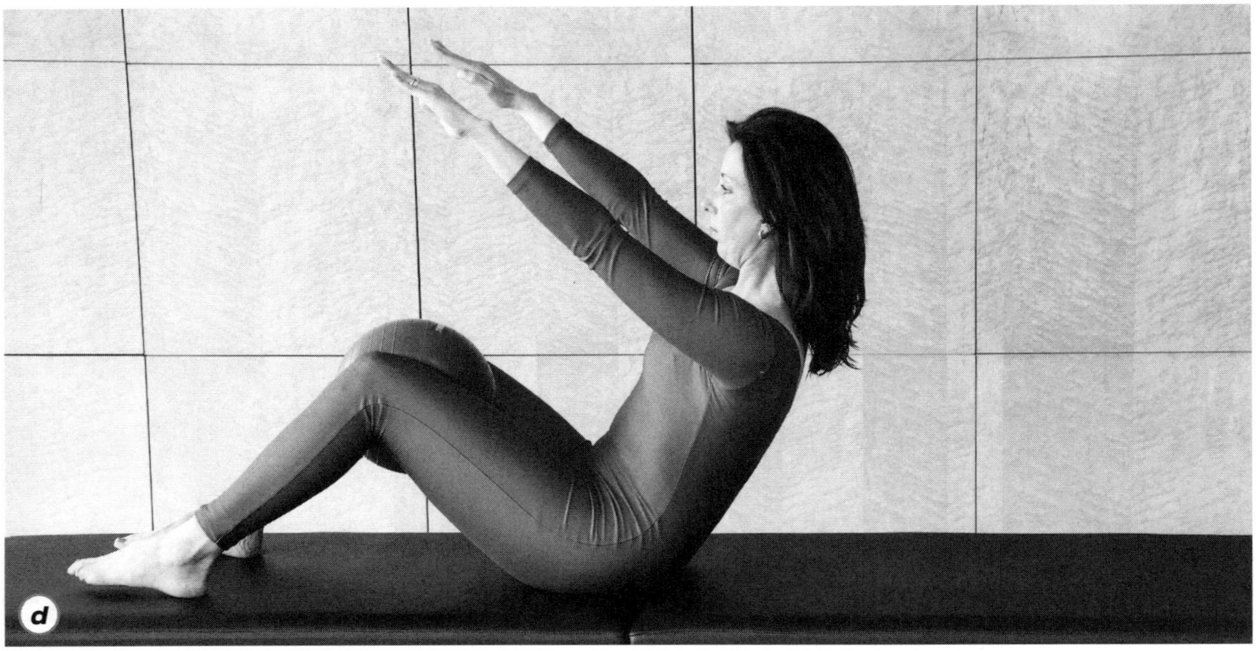

Option

Use the hands to walk up the sides of the legs in order to assist with the slow and controlled articulation of the spine into the teaser position.

Look for . . . Encourage

- Shoulders gliding toward the hips as if suspenders were hooked to the bottom tips of the shoulder blades and attached to the hips
- Abdominals drawn in and up
- Even articulation of the spine
- Gaze following the movement
- Moving as if a set of helium balloons were lifting the torso up to the teaser position
- Rolling up to the point where there is control without forceful momentum

Be aware of . . . Prevent

- Excessive momentum into the teaser position
- Loss of core control
- Loss of shoulder alignment

Primary Muscles Activated

Abdominals, biceps, shoulder complex, rectus femoris, sartorius, pectineus, iliopsoas, adductor magnus, adductor longus, adductor brevis, gracilis, biceps femoris, semitendinosus, semimembranosus, tensor fasciae latae, gastrocnemius, popliteus, plantaris

Teaser Prep 2

Timeline: 6 weeks to 3 months postop

Appropriate for: knee and hip

Location: a raised mat, hip height

Instructions

- Lie supine on the mat with the left knee slightly bent into a mountain shape and the right leg extended along the inside of the thigh and knee of the left leg, toe pointed toward the opposite wall on a diagonal. Lengthen the arms to the ceiling, with the palms facing the thighs and the shoulders away from the ears *(a)*.
- Inhale to prepare. Curl the head, neck, and shoulder off the mat; bring the chin toward the chest; exhale; lower the arms parallel to the thighs; and slowly roll up. Scoop the navel to the spine, drawing the abdominals in and up. Lengthen the arms up on a diagonal *(b)*.

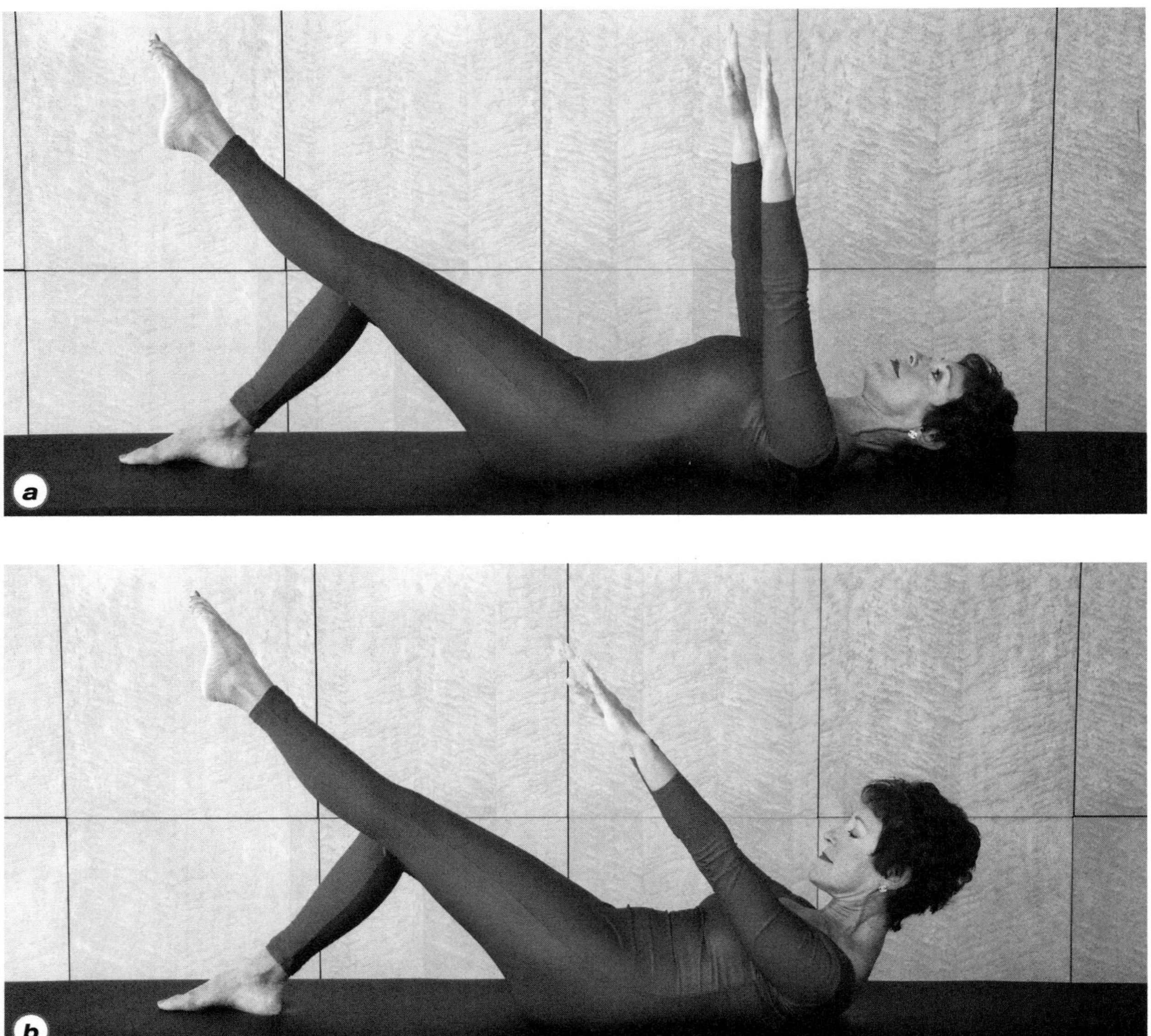

- Roll up and maintain a C-curve in the lower spine with a proud chest.
- Hold for a count of 5.
- Exhale and slowly roll down to the mat, resisting through the abdominals and articulating the spine vertebra by vertebra to the mat.
- **Knee:** Keep the knees soft and the legs parallel, hugging to the midline as tolerated *(c)*. Place a thick pad between the knees as needed.
- **Hip:** For up to 3 months, keep a small mountain shape in the leg in order to keep 90° to 100° of flexion as the upper body reaches into the teaser position *(d)*.
- Repeat for 3 times.
- Challenge: Roll up and down to a count of 8.

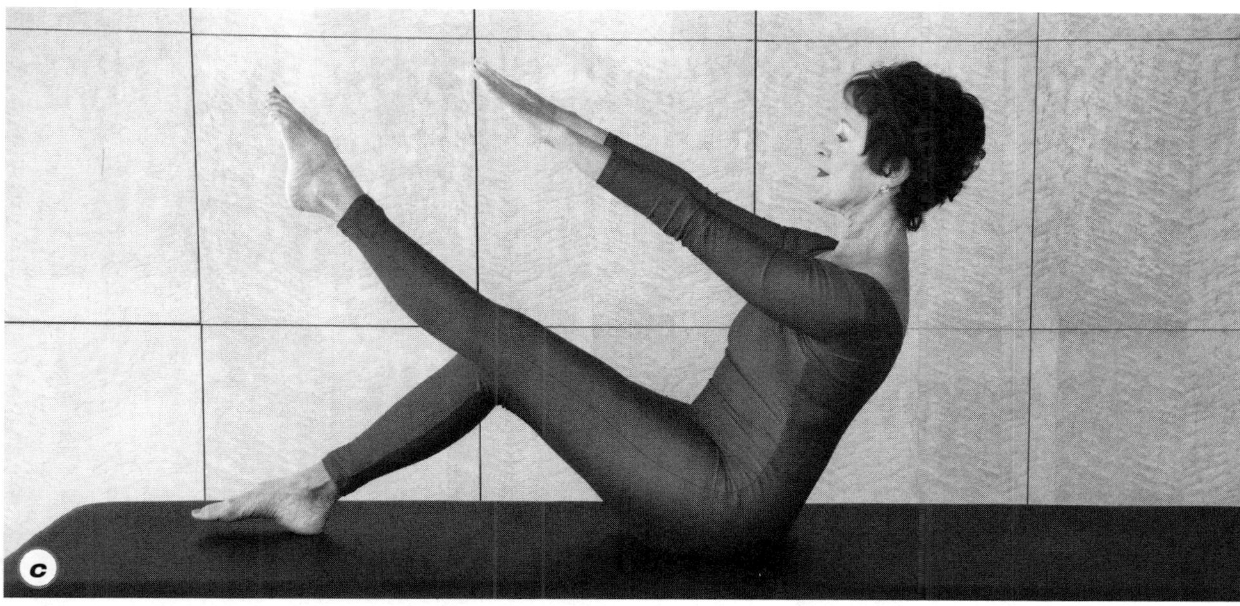

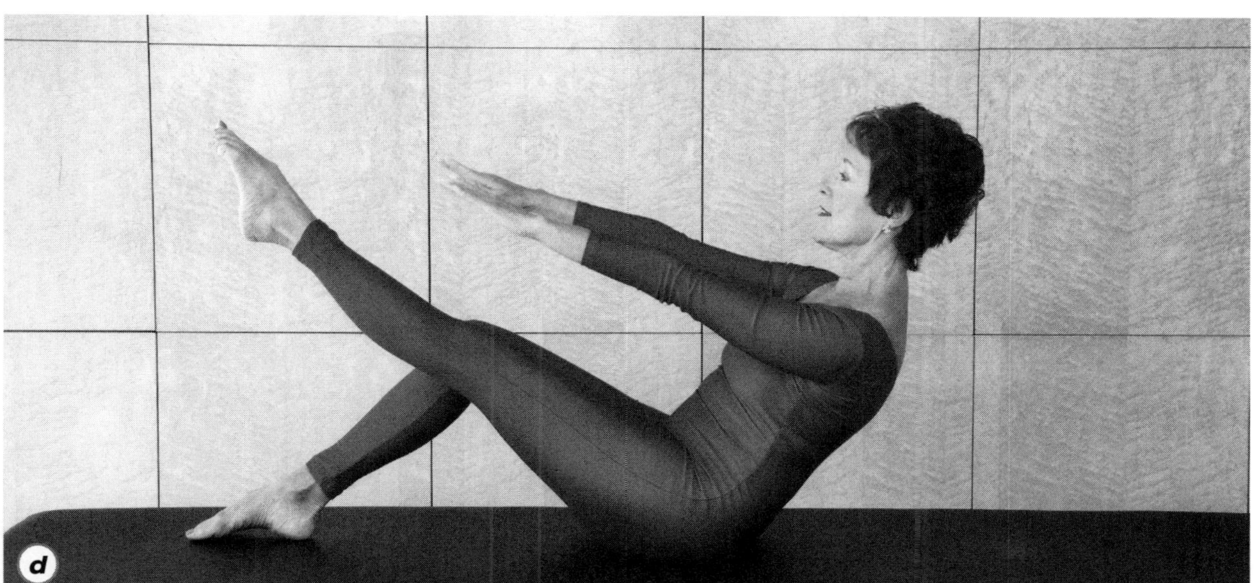

(continued)

Options

1. Walk the hands up the sides of the legs to articulate the spine into the teaser position.

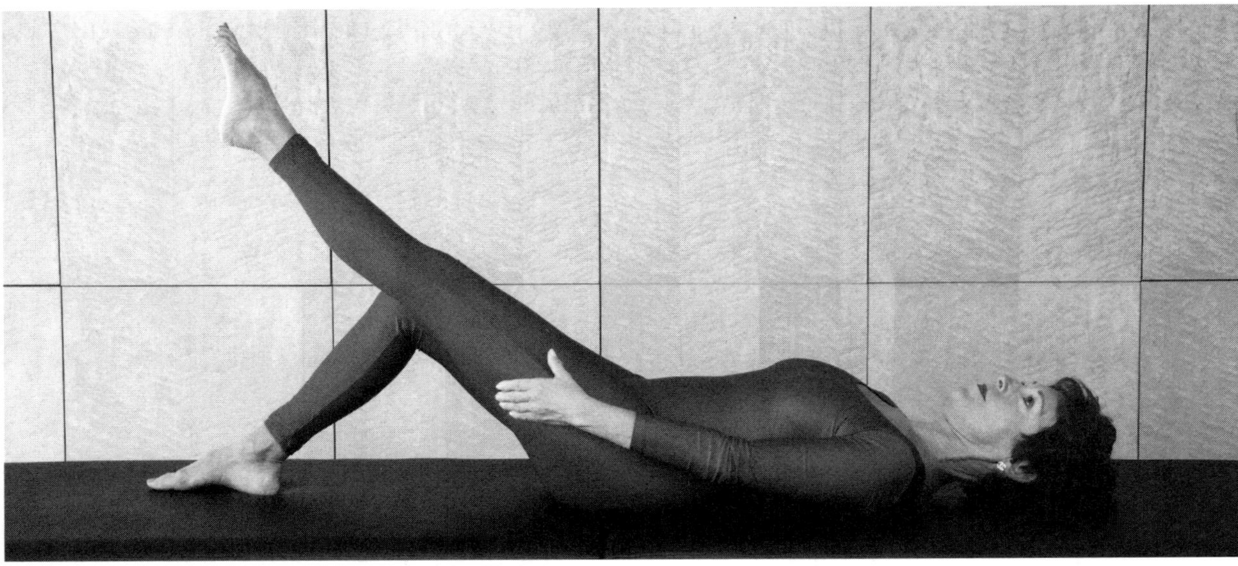

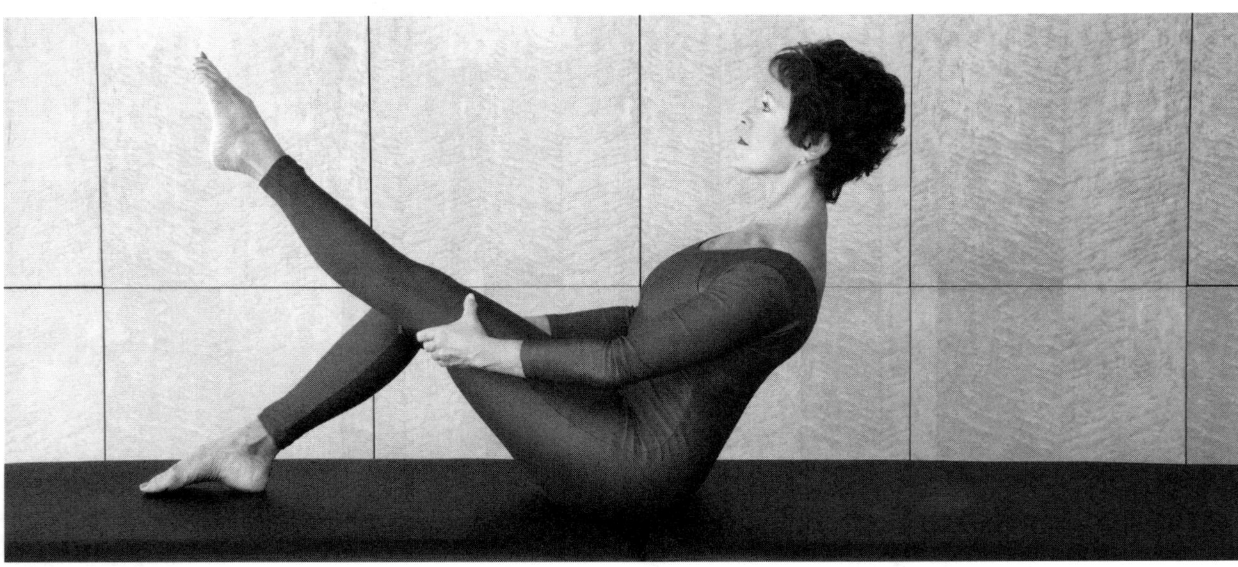

2. Place a long exercise band wide across the bottom of the foot that is extended. Choke up on the band to begin the teaser. The tension of the band will ease as you roll up, so walk the hands up the band as you roll up into the teaser position.

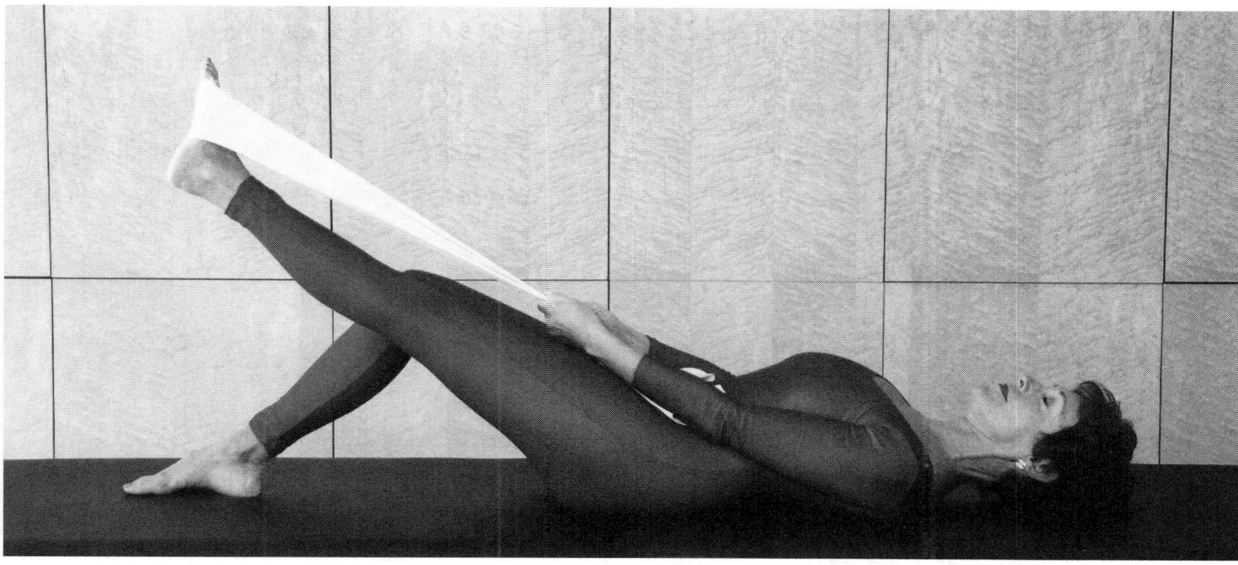

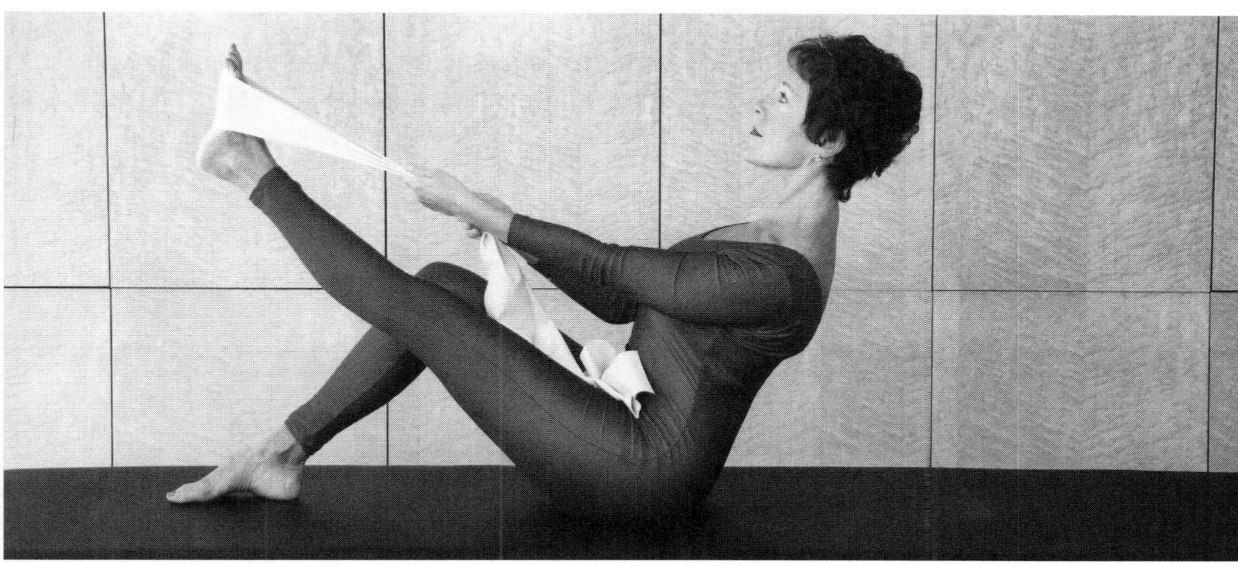

(continued)

Look for . . . Encourage

- Shoulders gliding toward the hips as if suspenders were hooked to the bottom tips of the shoulder blades and attached to the hips
- Abdominals drawn in and up
- Even articulation of the spine
- Gaze following the movement
- Moving as if a set of helium balloons were lifting the torso up to the teaser position
- Rolling up to the point where there is control without forceful momentum

Be aware of . . . Prevent

- Excessive momentum
- Loss of core control
- Uneven articulation of the spine up to the teaser and down to the mat
- Loss of shoulder alignment

Primary Muscles Activated

Abdominals, biceps, shoulder complex, rectus femoris, sartorius, pectineus, iliopsoas, adductor longus, adductor brevis, gracilis, biceps femoris, semitendinosus, semimembranosus, tensor fasciae latae, gastrocnemius, popliteus, plantaris, vastus lateralis, vastus medialis, tibialis posterior, soleus

Side Stretch

Timeline: 6 weeks to 3 months postop

Appropriate for: knee and hip

Location: a raised mat, hip height

Instructions

- Sit tall on the side of the table with the feet on a box or the floor so that the hips stay slightly higher than the knees.
- Position the legs hip-distance apart and keep them parallel.
- Place a small, soft ball between the legs and hug it toward the midline of the body. Keep the head and shoulders and hips in alignment.
- Extend the arms out to the sides of the body at shoulder height as if you were reaching out to touch the side walls *(a)*.

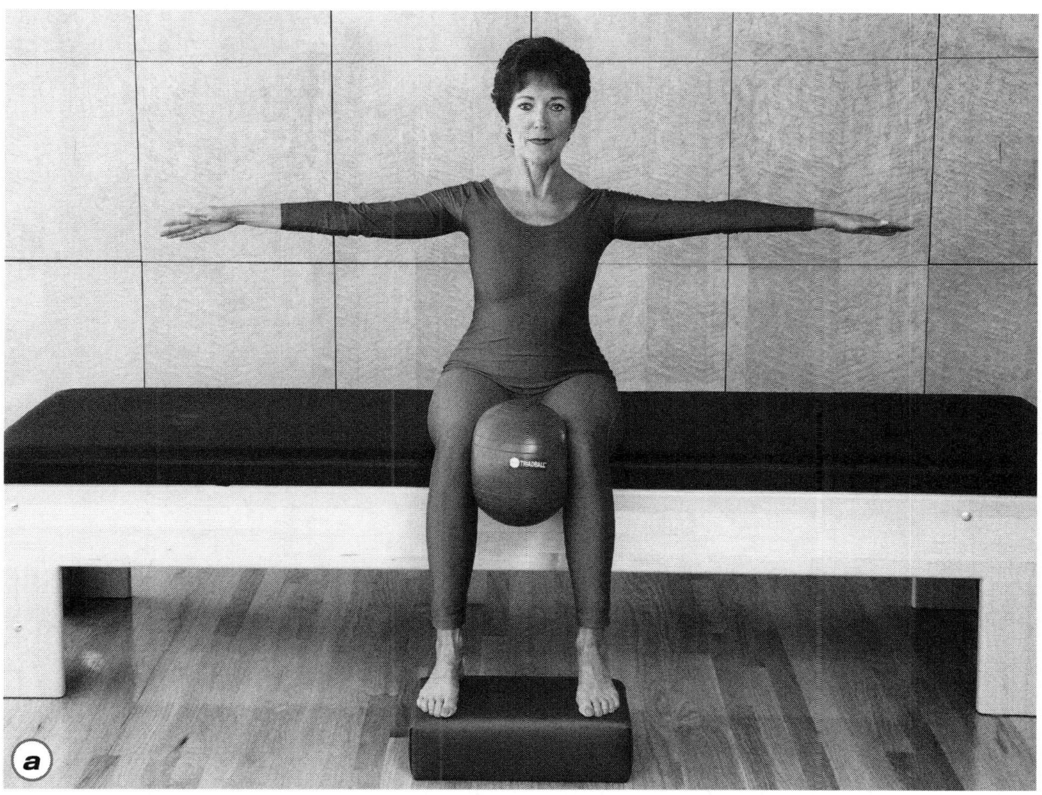
a

(continued)

Side Stretch *(continued)*

- Bring the right arm up next to the ear, with the right palm facing the head. Extend the left arm to the mat and rest the left palm on the mat *(b)*.
- Inhale to prepare. Exhale and begin to bring the right arm up and over as the left hand keeps reaching for the mat *(c)*.

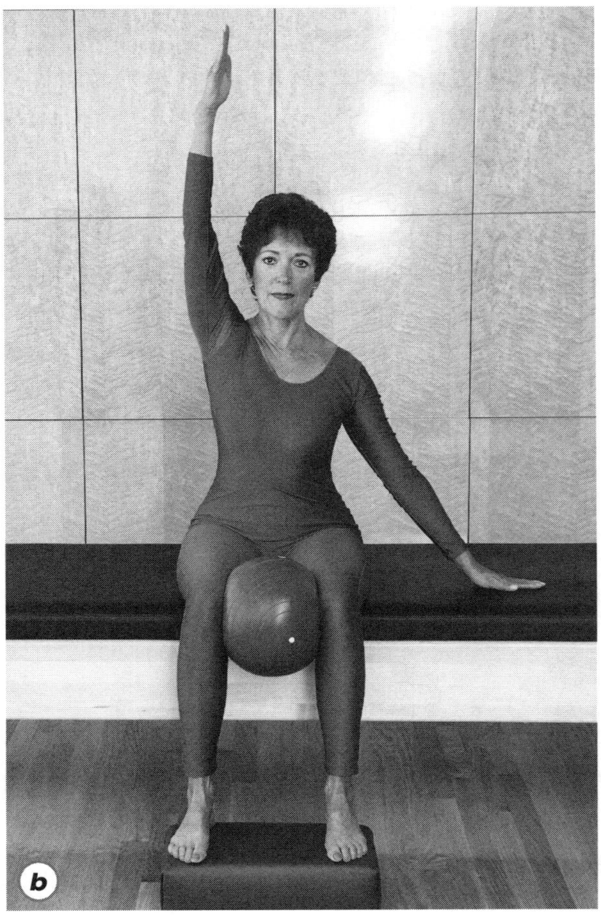

b

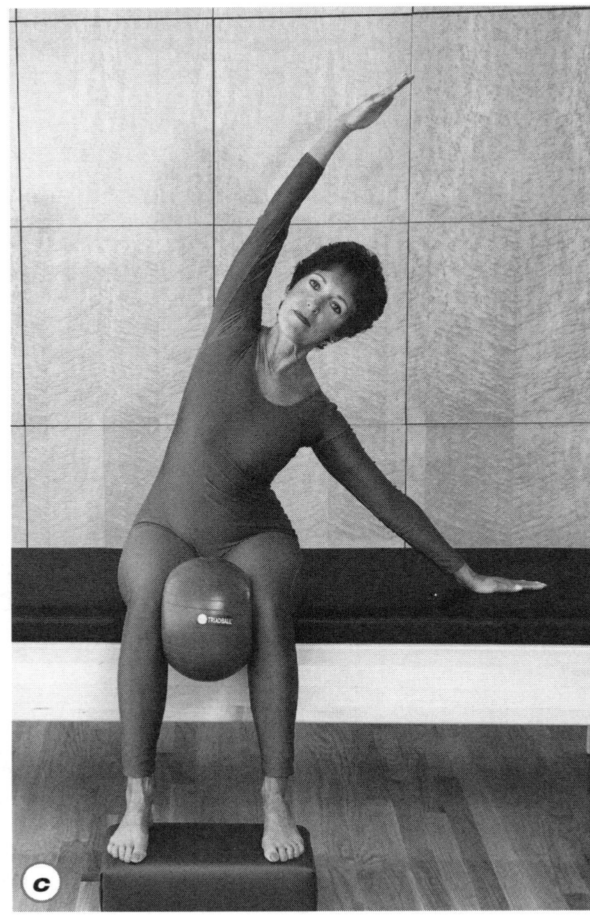

c

- Bend the left arm as needed or allow the arm to slide along the mat as the right arm reaches up and over toward the left, creating the side stretch on the right side of the body.
- Hold for a count of 5, and then slowly return back to the starting position *(a)*.
  - Keep the right shoulder blade flowing toward the right hip even though you are extending the arm up and over on a diagonal line.
  - Imagine that there is a cactus on the mat and that you are rounding up and over the cactus.
  - Keep the right hip glued to the mat during the entire movement.
- Breathe into the right ribs when leading back to the starting position.
- Repeat 3 times. Reverse and stretch the left side.

Look for . . . Encourage

- Shoulders gliding toward the hips
- Hip deepening to the mat during the lateral flexion up and over to the opposite side
- Gazing straight ahead
- Creating a long arc
- Thinking of arching up and over the rainbow

Be aware of . . . Prevent

- Bending the arm that is extending up and over
- Leading back with the arm instead of the lateral spine
- Loss of alignment during the bend to the side
- Loss of abdominal engagement with the movement

Primary Muscles Activated

Abdominals, shoulder complex, quadratus lumborum, erector spinae group, intertransversarii, latissimus dorsi, adductor magnus, adductor longus, adductor brevis, gracilis, pectineus

chapter 5

Pilates Mat Exercises for Three to Six Months and Six Months and Beyond Postoperative

This chapter describes and illustrates the classical Pilates mat exercises with fewer modifications but in keeping with the specified ROM guidelines for clients with hip or knee arthroplasty. The exercises in this chapter match the second and third columns in tables 3.2 and 3.3 (see p. 31).

Clients who have been practicing Pilates regularly for 3 months should be able to understand and demonstrate core control and stability. In addition, after 3 months postop, the ROM guidelines decrease, allowing for increased flexion and internal and external rotation, especially for the hips. Please refer to the ROM guidelines in chapter 3 (see pp. 32-36). Over the next 9 months, the client works toward the ideal expression of the Pilates movements. However, clients who are just starting Pilates exercises must first start with the pre-Pilates movements and any optional movements within the 6 weeks to 3 months postop category. Demonstrating movement with core control and stability and disassociation at the joints is important before moving into a postop timeline that the client may be at but is not ready for. For the client with a bilateral joint replacement and sometimes for a client with a syndrome, it may be important to continue to perform the movements on a raised mat that is at hip height. See page 38 in chapter 3 for further guidelines on where to perform the Pilates exercises. Clients with a unilateral joint replacement should be able to perform the mat exercises on a floor mat by the end of 3 months.

When working with a client with a syndrome, select movements with modifications that allow the client to move without pain and gradually build the core and muscle strength of the joints and improve ROM. Start slowly and reduce the modifications as the client builds core strength and stability.

In many of the exercises you will see the use of a small, soft ball approximately 8 to 10 inches (20-25 centimeters) in diameter. For the purposes of this book, the Triadball was used in the various exercises and options. The ball should not be fully inflated. It should be firm enough to support the body yet pliable enough to hold and squeeze. When the ball is used under the head and neck, the shoulders will be slightly off the mat and the eye line will be at a 45° angle. Make sure the weight of the head is resting on the ball. There should be no tension in the neck (Fritzke and Voogt 2009).

Each exercise presented in this chapter shows the setup and action of the movement with several options. The instructions also include what to look for and encourage and what to be aware of and prevent. The primary muscles of the movement are listed, with emphasis on the muscles that are activated or stabilized from the pelvis, hip, and knee.

All exercises should be performed under the guidance of a qualified Pilates instructor and with referral from the operative physician. The client's needs, restrictions, and ROM recommendations should be specified by the physician and followed accordingly. These guidelines may vary from the protocols that follow, and the protocols should be modified based on the individual's needs and the surgeon's preferences.

Hundred

Timeline: 3 to 6 months postop

Appropriate for: knee and hip

Location: a floor mat or a raised mat as needed; a raised mat for a bilateral knee or hip replacement as needed

Instructions

- Lie supine on the mat with the arms long by the sides of the body, the legs in tabletop position, and a small, soft ball between the knees. Lightly hug the ball to the midline of the body.
- Curl the head, neck, and shoulders up off the mat. Look toward the thighs.
- Draw the abdominals in and up.
- Lift the arms straight up in line with the abdominals.
- Inhale and vigorously pump the arms for 5 counts and exhale and pump the arms for 5 counts. With the exhale, scoop deeper into the abdominals.
- Repeat for 5 to 10 breaths.

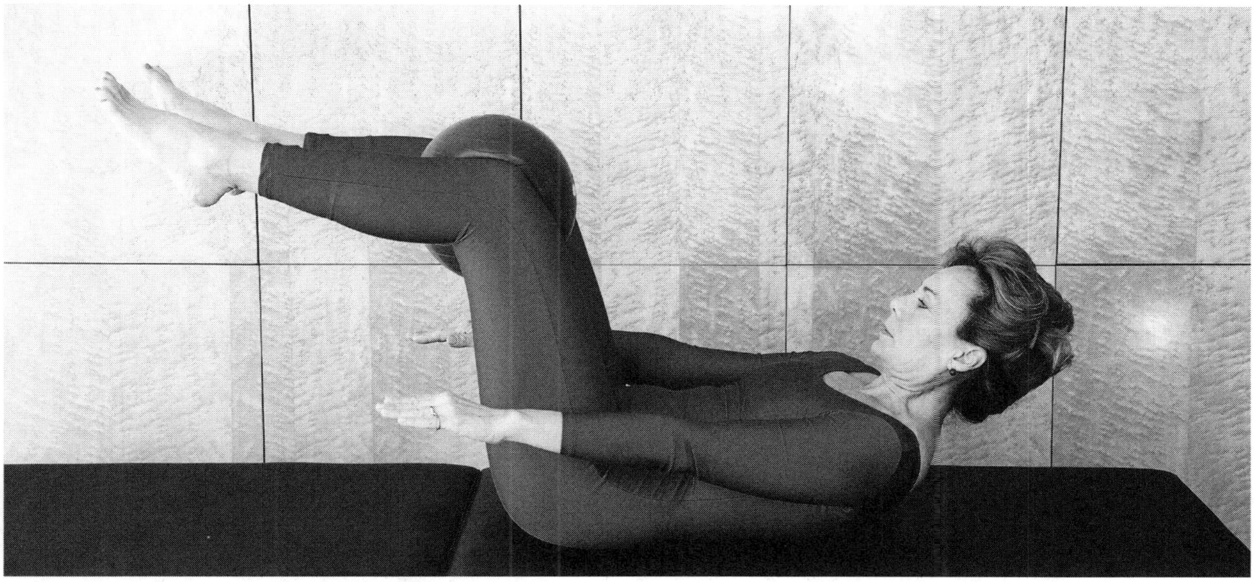

(continued)

Hundred *(continued)*

Option

Place a soft ball 8 to 10 inches (20-25 centimeters) in diameter under the head and neck; see page 134 for instructions for placement.

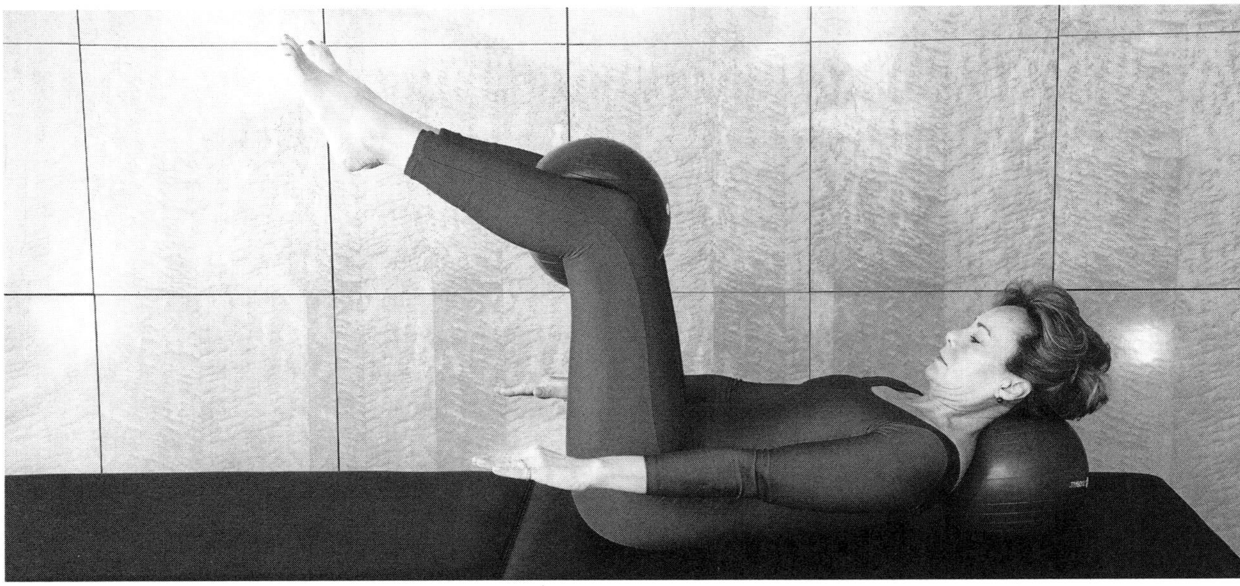

Look for . . . Encourage

- Shoulders gliding toward the hips as if suspenders were hooked to the bottom tips of the shoulder blades and attached to the hips
- Abdominals drawn in and up
- The tailbone long on the mat, maintaining neutral spine
- Pumping straight arms in line with the hands as if splashing into water against resistance
- Open collarbones, as if taffy were stretched across the shoulders
- Chin toward the chest and rounded up to the bottom tips of the shoulder blades with the space the size of a tangerine between the chin and the chest
- Eyes gazing at the thighs

Be aware of . . . Prevent

- Pumping the hands up and down
- Arching the low back (lumbar spine) and losing the neutral spine
- Bulging abdominals

HUNDRED

Timeline: 6 months postop and beyond
Appropriate for: knee and hip
Location: a floor mat or a raised mat as needed

Instructions

- Lie supine on the mat with the arms long by the sides of the body and the legs in tabletop position.
- Curl the head, neck, and shoulders up off the mat, looking toward the thighs.
- Extend the legs toward the ceiling to 90° of flexion or out to a 45° angle with or without a small, soft ball between the knees. Point the toes.
- Draw the abdominals in and up.
- Lift the arms straight up in line with the abdominals.
- Inhale and vigorously pump the arms for 5 counts and exhale and pump the arms for 5 counts. With the exhale, scoop deeper into the abdominals.
- Repeat for 10 breaths.
- **Hip:** Placing the legs in a longer and lower position increases the stress on the hip flexors. Keep the legs slightly bent or in a tabletop position to lessen the stress and prevent overuse of the hip flexors. In addition, place a small, soft ball between the knees, shins, or ankles to further engage the adductors, decrease overuse of the hip flexors, and increase connection to the core.

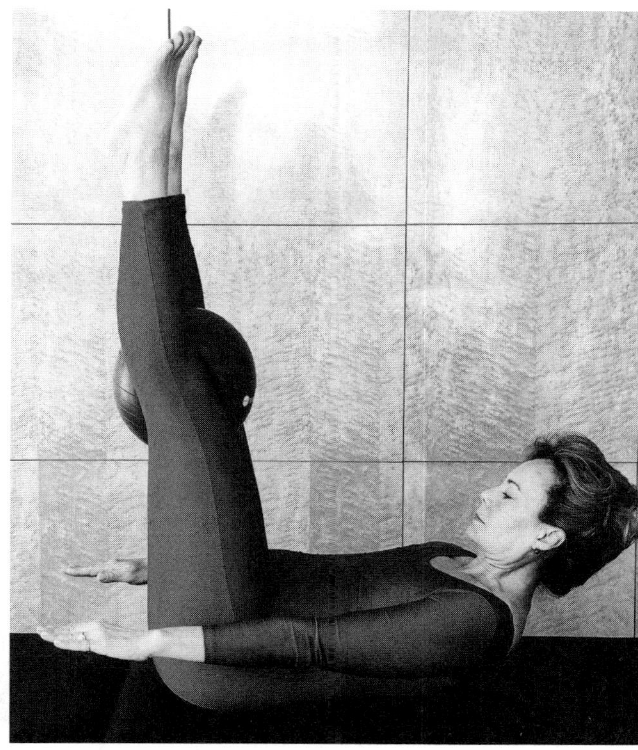

(continued)

Hundred *(continued)*

Options

1. Place a small, soft ball between the knees or ankles. Lightly hug the ball to the midline of the body.

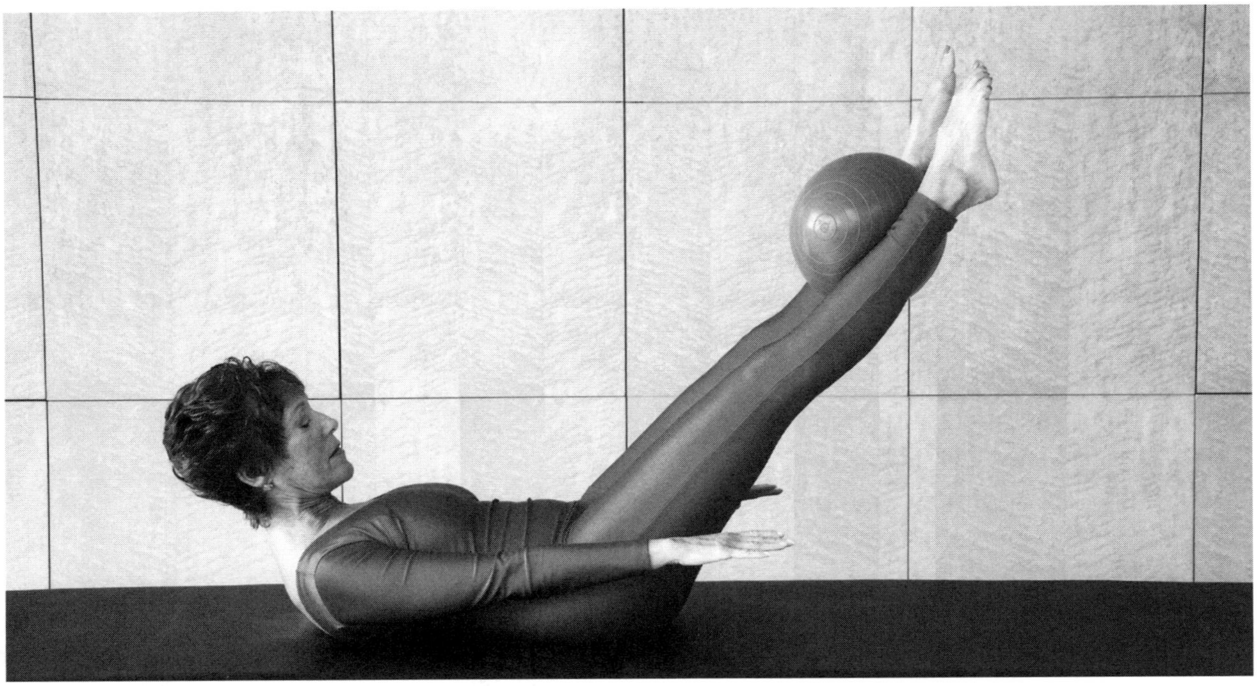

2. Bend the knees slightly with or without a cushion between the knees.

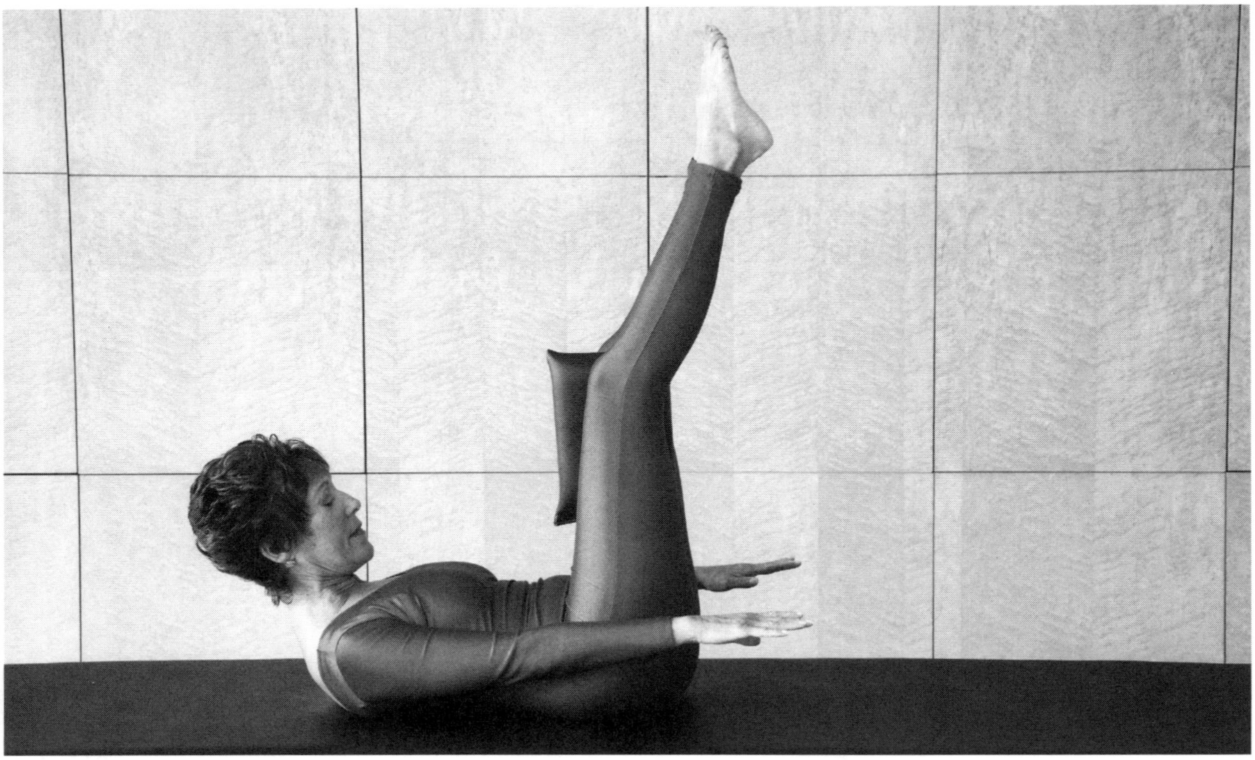

3. Extend the legs out to 45° from the floor only if the core is stable and engaged. Keep a neutral spine. You should feel no gripping or discomfort in the hip flexors.

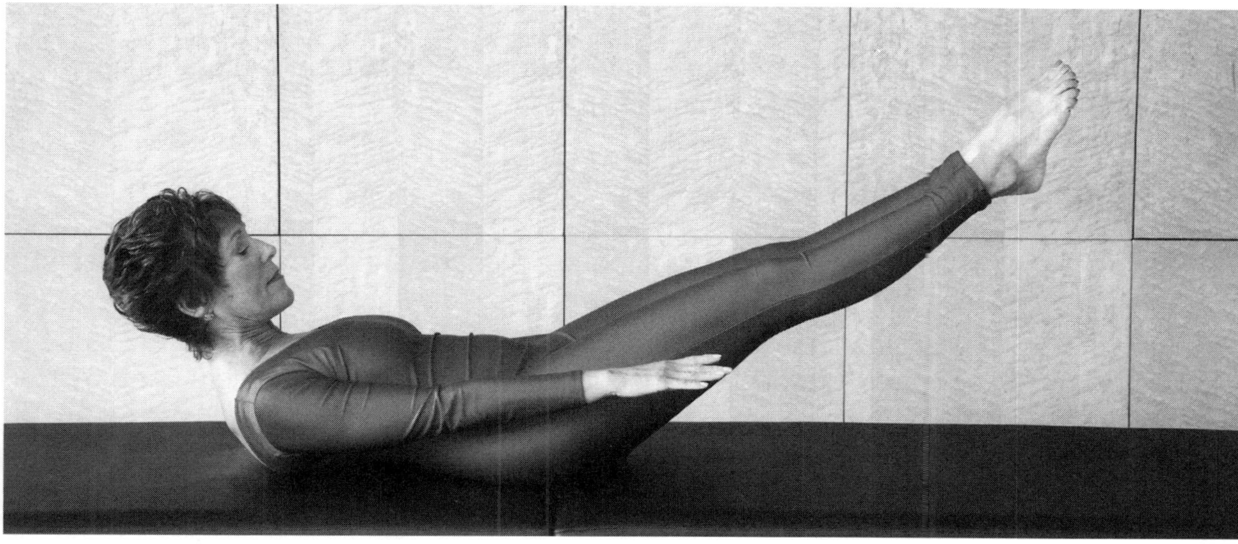

Look for . . . Encourage

- Shoulders gliding toward the hips as if suspenders were hooked to the bottom tips of the shoulder blades and attached to the hips
- Abdominals drawn in and up
- The tailbone long on the mat and the spine neutral
- Pumping straight arms in line with the hands as if splashing into water against resistance
- Open collarbones as if taffy were stretched across the shoulders
- Chin toward the chest and rounded up to the bottom tips of the shoulder blades
- Eyes gazing at the thighs

Be aware of . . . Prevent

- Pumping the hands up and down
- Arching the low back (lumbar spine) and losing a neutral spine
- Bulging abdominals

Primary Muscles Activated

The primary muscles activated depend on the chosen option. The primary muscles include the following: Abdominals, anterior scalene, sternocleidomastoid, biceps, triceps, deltoids, shoulder complex, iliopsoas, rectus femoris, sartorius, pectineus, adductor magnus, adductor longus, adductor brevis, gracilis, vastus medialis, vastus intermedius, vastus lateralis, biceps femoris, semimembranosus, semitendinosus, popliteus, gastrocnemius, tensor fasciae latae, plantaris, tibialis posterior, soleus

Half Roll-Down and Half Roll-Up

Timeline: 3 to 6 months and 6 months and beyond postop

Appropriate for: knee and hip

Location: a floor mat or a raised mat as needed; a raised mat for a bilateral knee or hip replacement as needed for up to 6 months postop

Instructions for Half Roll-Down

- Sit on the mat with the knees bent into a mountain shape and a small, soft ball placed between the knees with the hands under the thighs, holding with a light touch.
- Bring the chin toward the chest, look toward the thighs, and inhale to prepare. Exhale and roll off the sit bones, drawing the abdominals in deeply, and forming a C-curve in the lower spine *(a)*.
- Continue to exhale and roll down to the length of the arms, hugging the ball between the knees *(b)*.

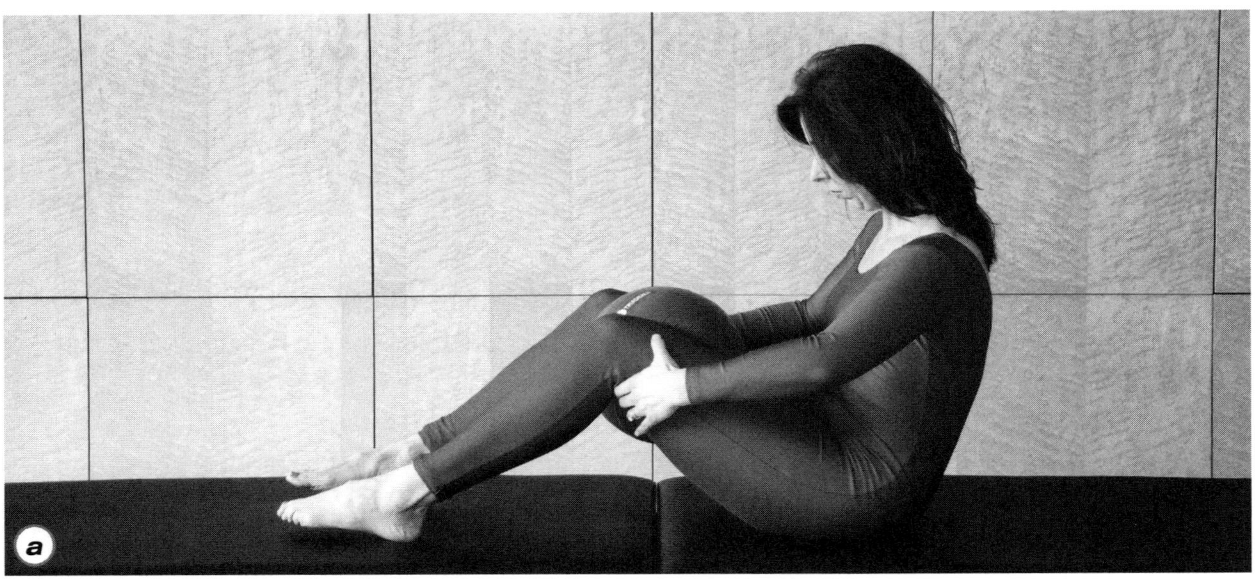

a

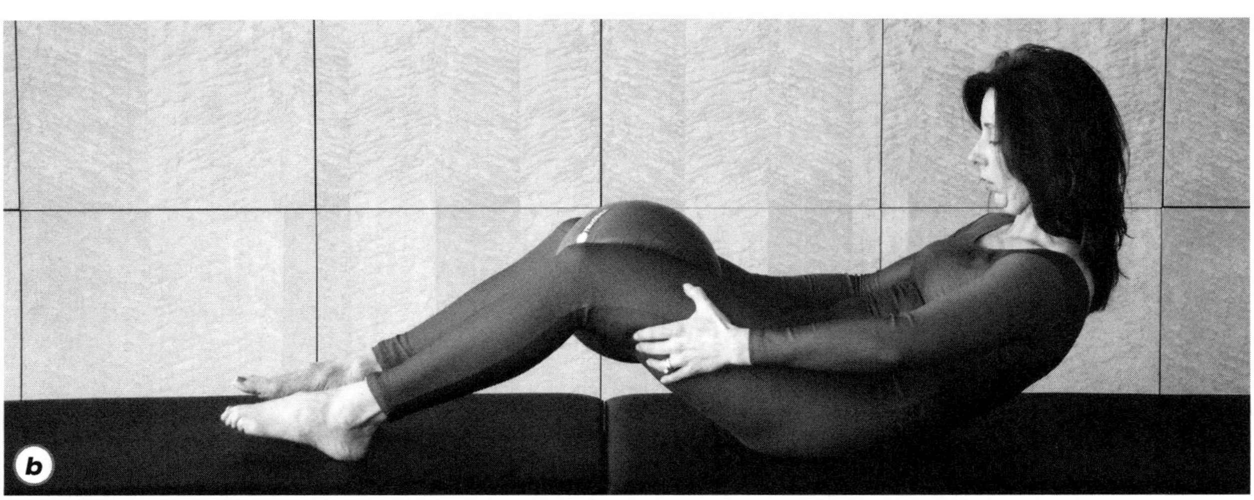

b

- Inhale to prepare. Exhale and round back up. Maintain the flexion of the spine as you round back up to the start.
- **Hip:** Keep 110° of hip flexion for up to 6 months, and do not exceed 115° of hip flexion for 6 months and beyond.
- **Knee and hip:** Roll down to the length of the arms only if you can maintain control of the movement by not lifting the legs or losing the articulation of the spine.
- Repeat 5 to 10 times. Keep the rhythm slow and controlled.
- Note: As you roll down and back up it may be necessary to tuck the feet under a support strap to provide stability in order to perform the move correctly.

Instructions for Half Roll-Up

- Sit on the mat with the knees bent into a mountain shape and a small, soft ball placed between the knees and the hands under the thighs, holding with a light touch *(a)*.
- Bring the chin toward the chest, look down toward the abdominals, and inhale to prepare. Exhale and roll off the sit bones, scooping the navel to the spine, drawing the abdominals in deeply, and forming a C-curve in the lower spine *(b)*.

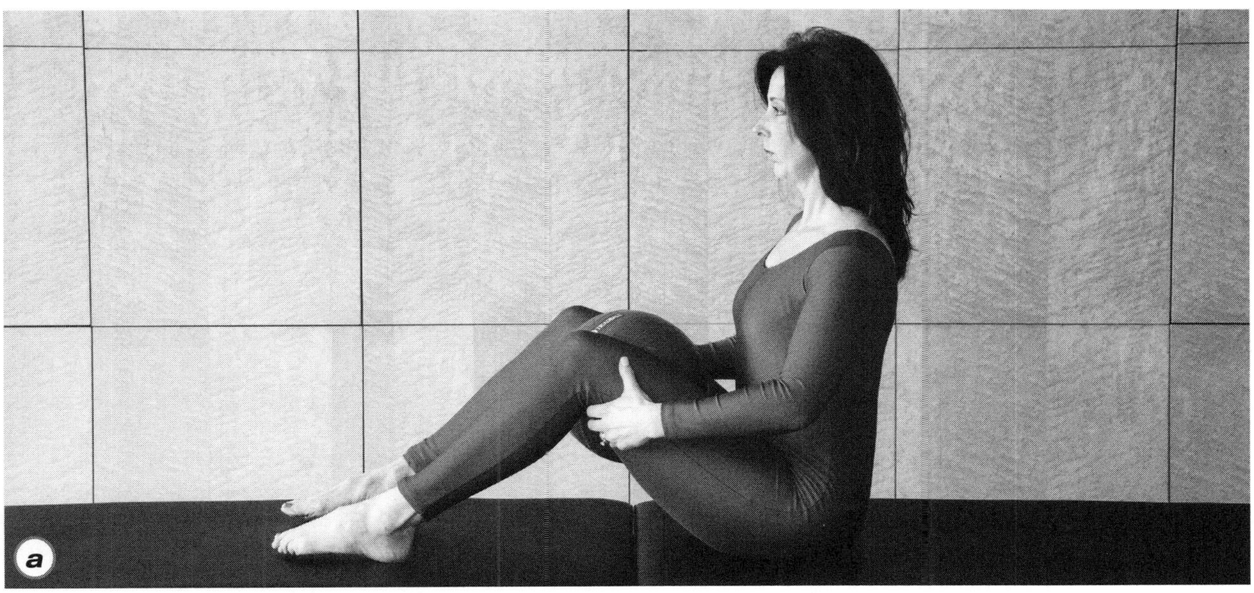

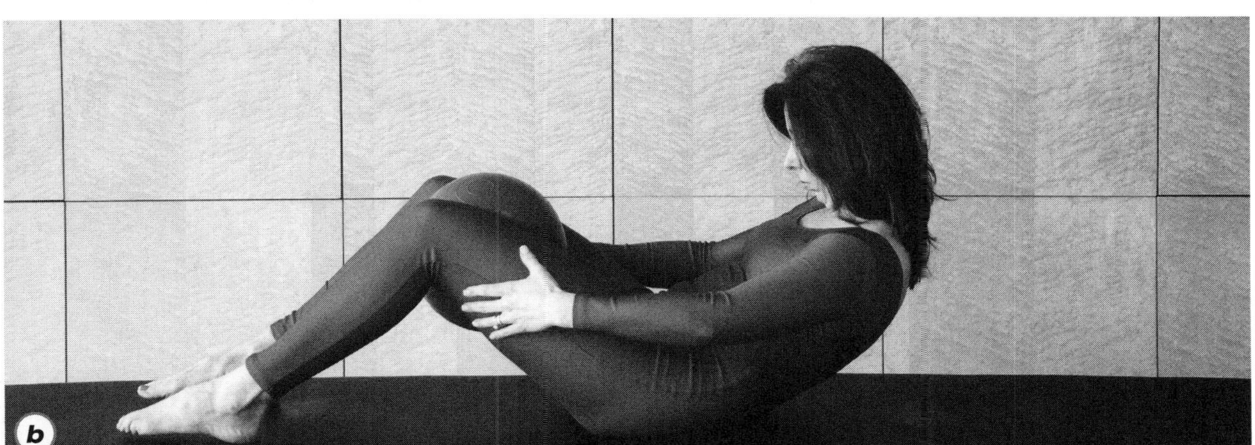

(continued)

- Continue to exhale and roll all the way down to the mat, articulating each vertebra into the mat as if you were imprinting the spine into a bed of wet sand *(c)*.

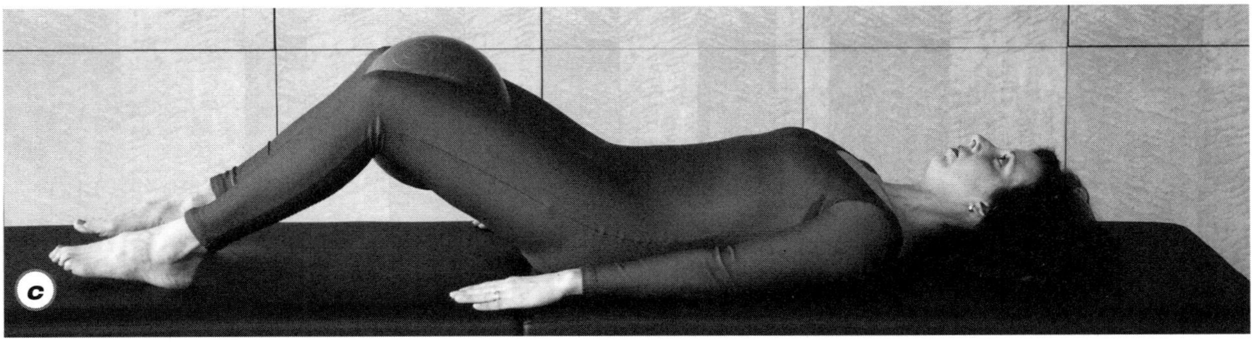

- Inhale to prepare. Exhale and bring the chin toward the chest. Place the hands back under the thighs and use them as needed to roll up one vertebra at a time to the start position. Maintain the flexion in the spine as you round back up to the start.
- **Hip:** Keep 110° of hip flexion for up to 6 months, and do not exceed 115° of hip flexion for 6 months and beyond.
- Keep the knees in a flexed position as tolerated, hugging the ball to the midline of the body.
- Repeat 5 to 10 times. Keep the rhythm slow and controlled.
- Note: As you roll down and back up it may be necessary to tuck the feet under a strap to provide stability in order to perform the move.

Look for . . . Encourage

- Articulation of each vertebra down to the mat as if each piece of the spine were being imprinted into a bed of wet sand
- A deep scoop in the abdominals
- Shoulders gliding toward the hips as if suspenders were hooked to the bottom tips of the shoulder blades and attached to the hips
- Hugging the legs toward the midline of the body

Be aware of . . . Prevent

- Gripping in the hip flexors
- Rolling down or up in segments of the spine

Primary Muscles Activated

Abdominals, iliopsoas, rectus femoris, sartorius, pectineus, gracilis, adductor magnus, adductor longus, adductor brevis, biceps femoris, semitendinosus, semimembranosus, tensor fasciae latae, gastrocnemius, popliteus, plantaris

Roll-Up

Timeline: 3 to 6 months postop

Appropriate for: knee and hip

Location: a floor mat or a raised mat as needed; a raised mat for a bilateral knee or hip replacement as needed

Instructions

- Lie supine on the mat with the arms extended to the ceiling, shoulder-width apart, and the palms facing away or slightly turned in and facing each other. Root the shoulder blades into the mat and away from the ears. Extend the legs long on the mat, hip-distance apart, with a small, soft ball between the ankles and the knees slightly bent. Hug the ball to the midline of the body *(a)*.

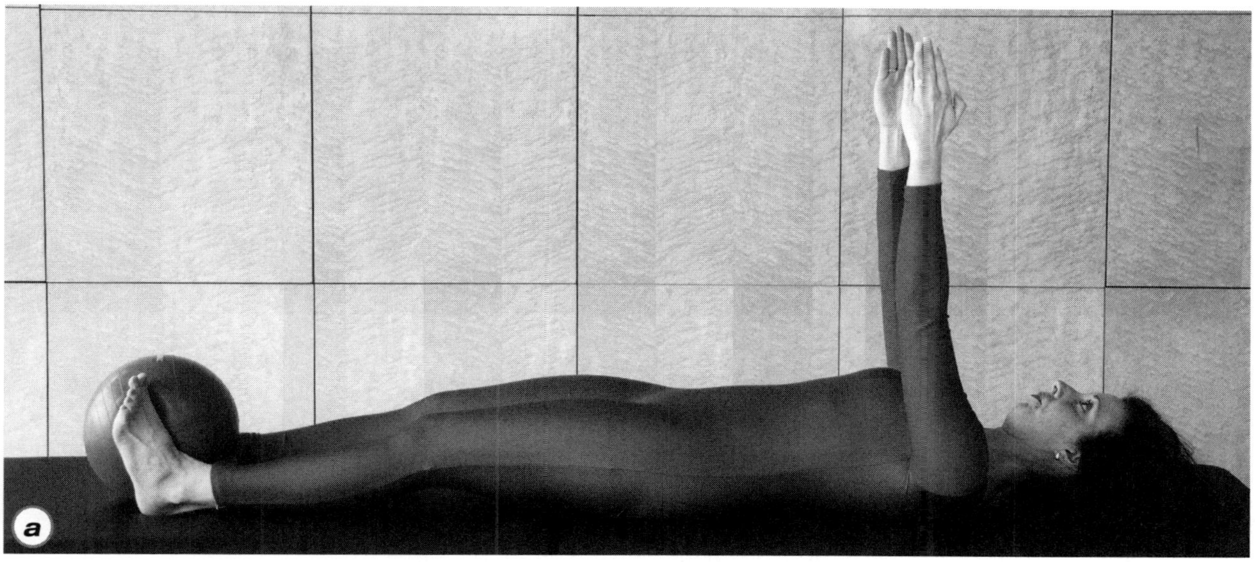
a

(continued)

- Inhale to prepare. Exhale and begin to lower the arms parallel to the legs while curling the head, neck, and shoulders off the mat. Look toward the feet.
- **Knee:** Scoop the navel to the spine, drawing the abdominals in and up, and round up and over, reaching long toward the feet with a deep scoop in the abdominals. Maintain slightly bent knees.
- **Hip:** Scoop the navel to spine, drawing the abdominals in and up, and round up and over, keeping 110° of hip flexion with a deep scoop in the abdominals *(b).*

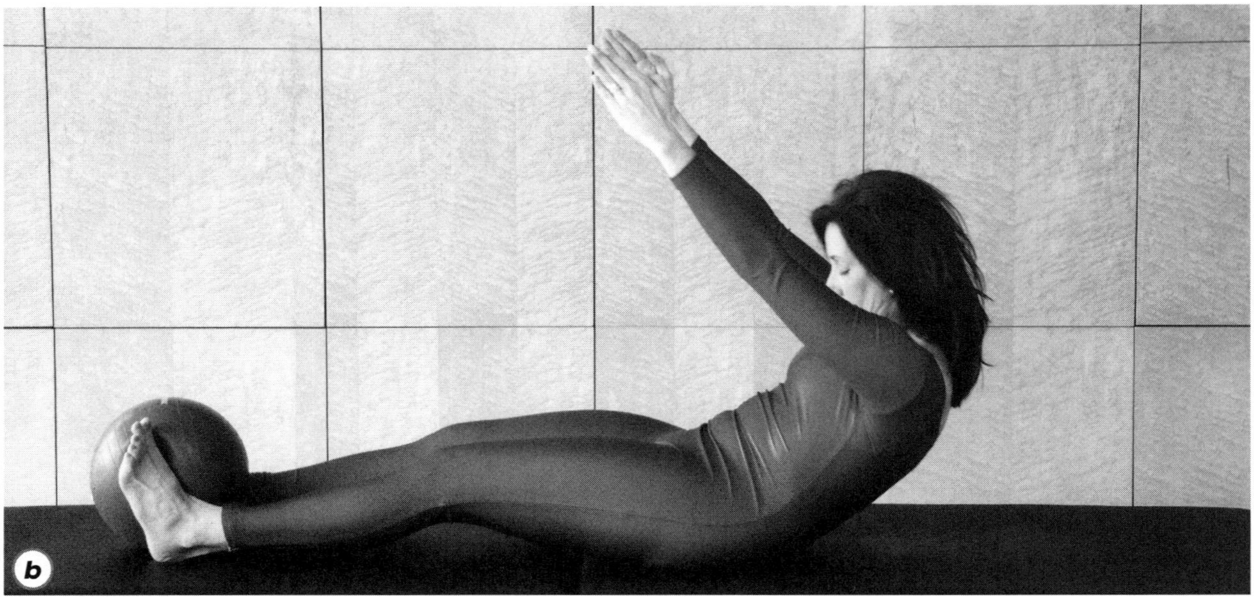
b

- Lengthen the arms long toward the feet in opposition to the navel, which is pulled deeply in toward the spine *(c)*.
- Inhale and then exhale and roll back down to the mat one vertebra at a time. Try to find each vertebra as you roll down to the mat.
- Repeat 5 to 10 times. Roll up and down with a slow rhythm.

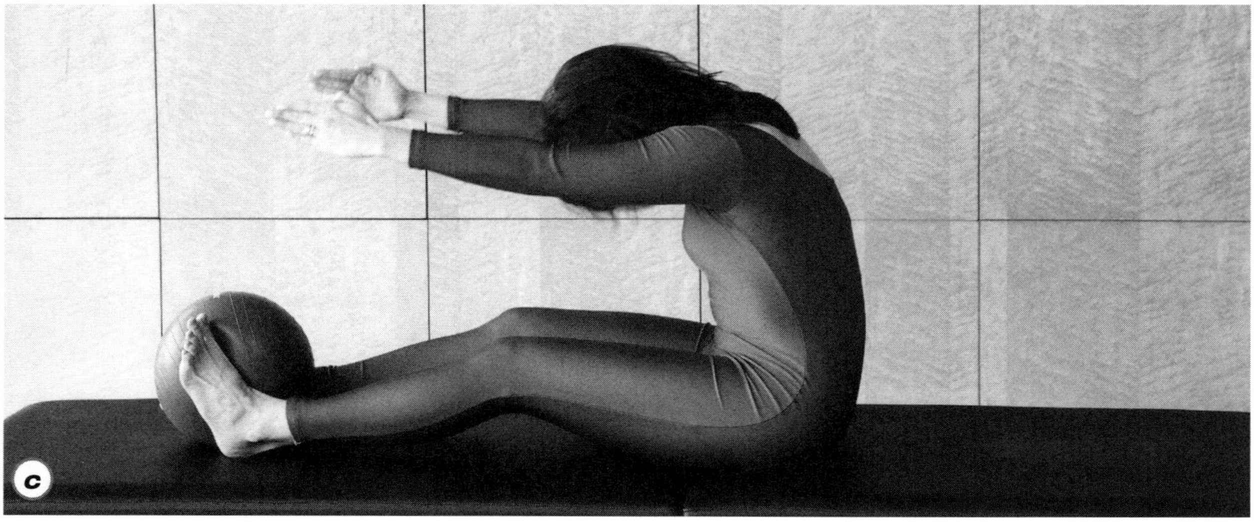
c

Options

1. Place a rolled-up towel or pillow under the knees with the feet flexed or relaxed as needed. Snugly hold a small, soft ball in the hands while rolling up.

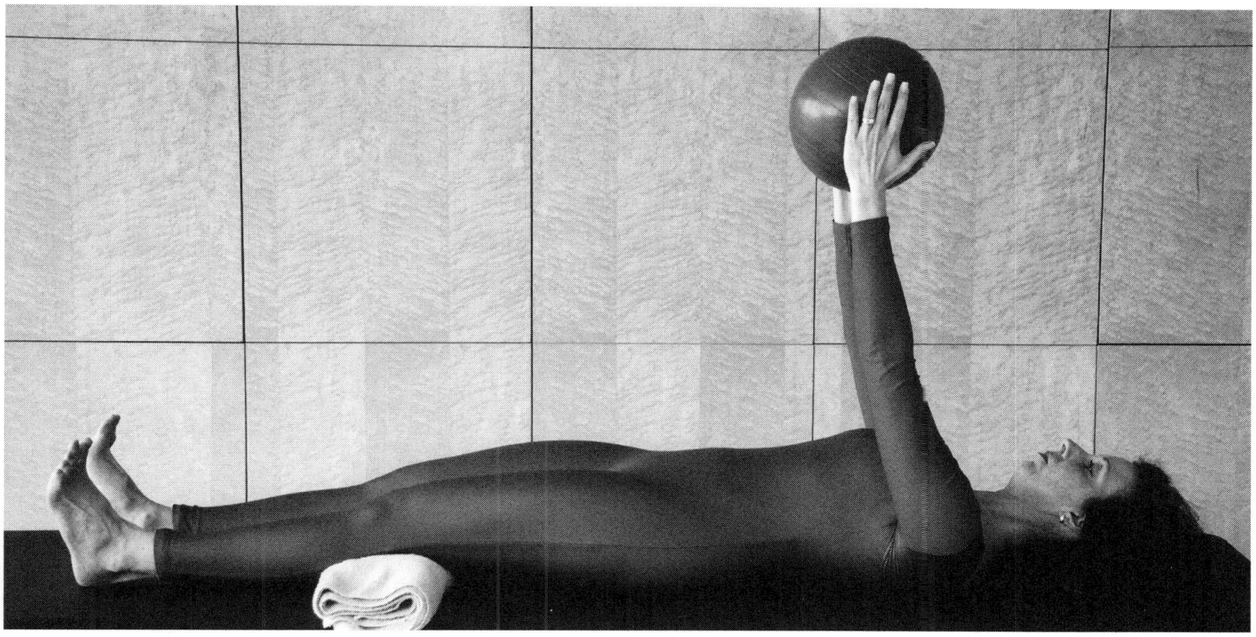

2. Place a thick pad or a small, soft ball between the knees.

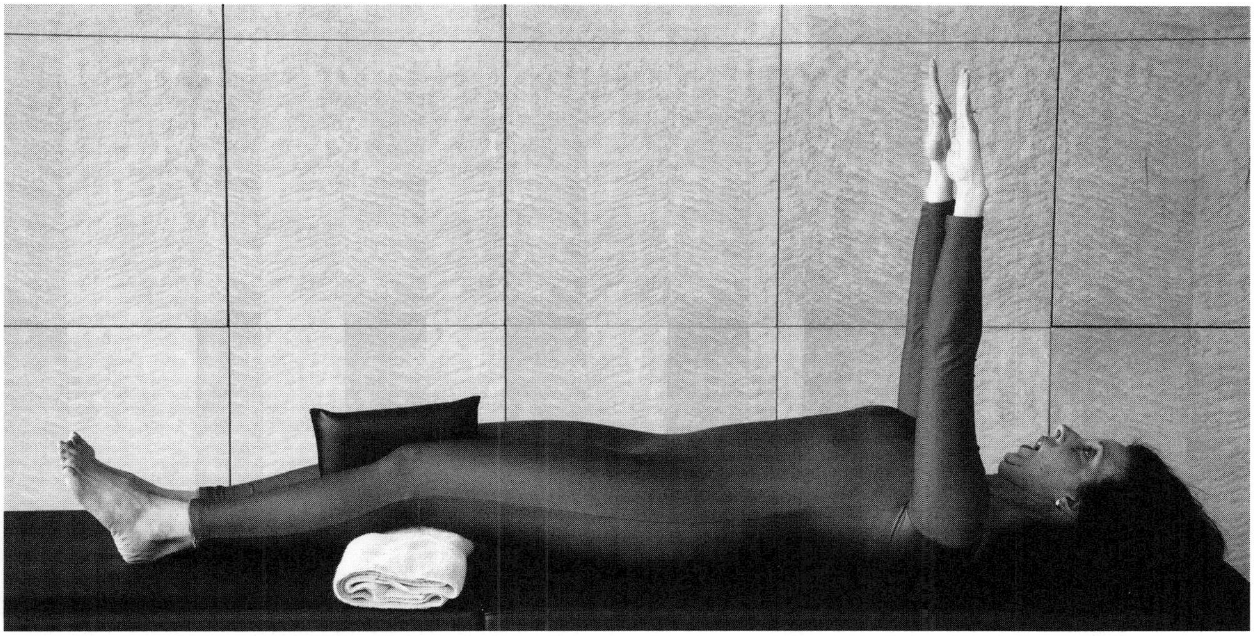

(continued)

Look for . . . Encourage

- Articulation of each vertebra down to the mat as if each piece of the spine were being imprinted into a bed of wet sand
- A deep scoop in the abdominals
- Shoulders gliding toward the hips as if suspenders were hooked to the bottom tips of the shoulder blades and attached to the hips
- Hugging the legs toward the midline of the body

Be aware of . . . Prevent

- Gripping in the hip flexors
- Rolling down or up in segments of the spine
- Hinging from the hips, folding the chest onto the thighs

ROLL-UP

Timeline: 6 months postop and beyond

Appropriate for: knee and hip

Location: a floor mat or a raised mat as needed

Instructions

- Lie supine on the mat with the arms extended to the ceiling, shoulder-width apart, and the palms facing away. The shoulders are gliding toward the hip points, the legs are long on the mat and hugging toward the midline, and the feet are flexed *(a)*.
- Inhale to prepare. Exhale and curl the head and shoulders off the mat. Look toward the feet. Lower the arms parallel to the legs.
- **Knee:** Scoop the navel to the spine, drawing the abdominals in and up, and round up and over, reaching long toward the feet with a deep scoop in the abdominals.
- **Hip:** Scoop the navel to the spine, drawing the abdominals in and up, and round up and over. Do not exceed 115° of hip flexion with a deep scoop in the abdominals *(b)*.
- Lengthen the arms long toward the feet in opposition to the navel, which is pulled deeply in toward the spine *(c)*.
- Inhale and then exhale and roll back down to the mat one vertebra at a time. Try to find each vertebra as you roll down to the mat.
- Repeat 10 times. Roll up and down with a slow rhythm for the first 4 repeats and then increase the flow.

(continued)

Roll-Up *(continued)*

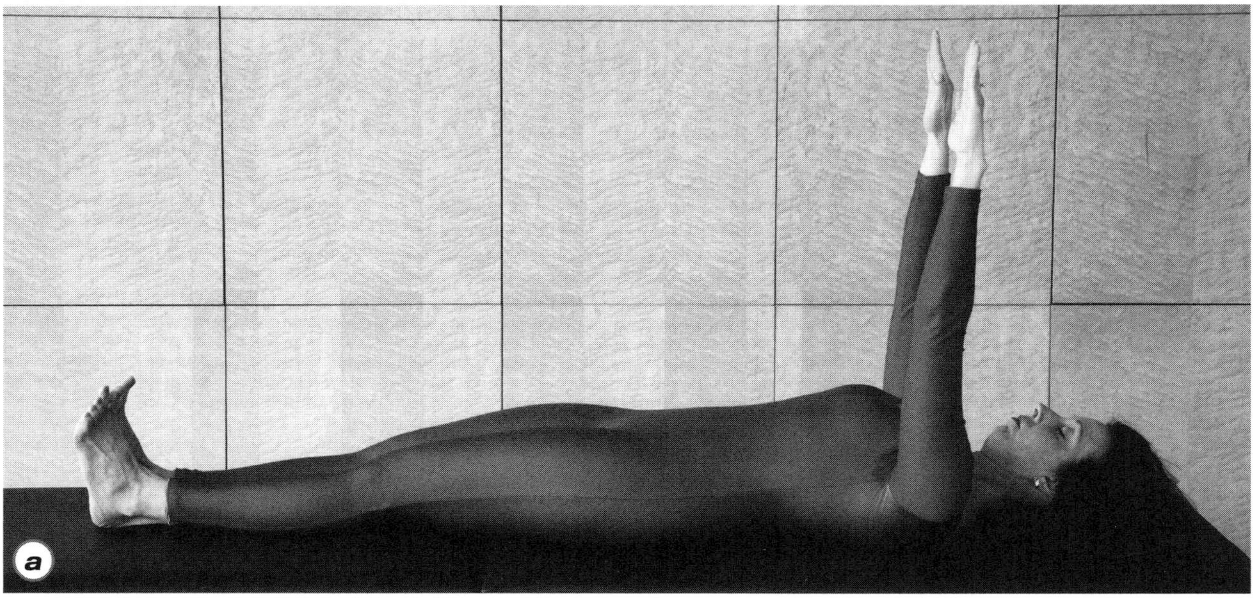

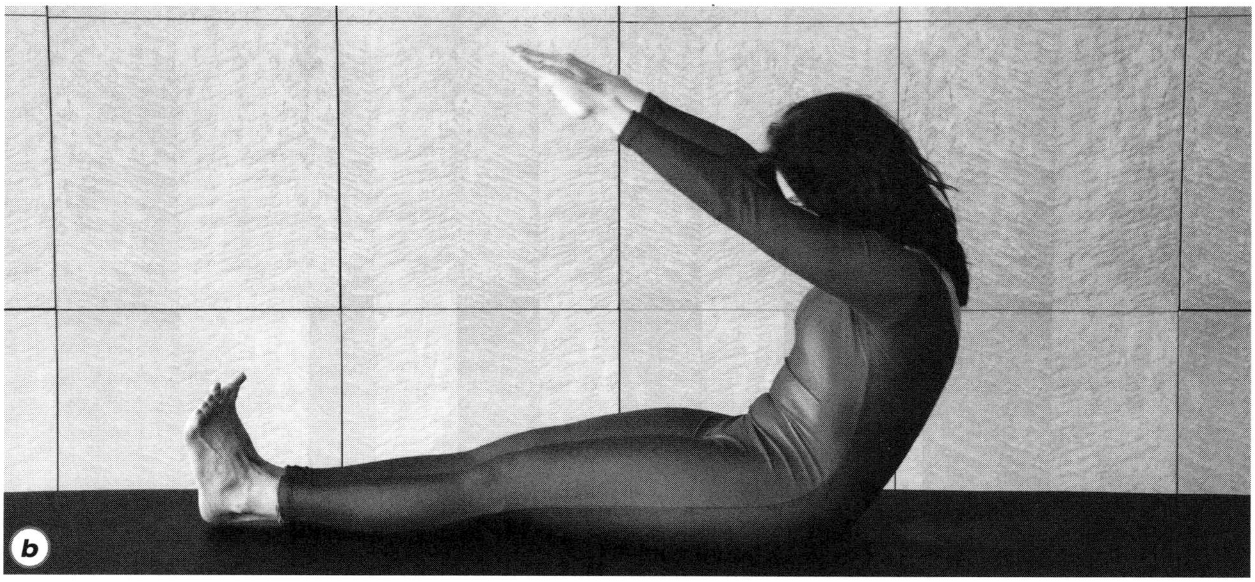

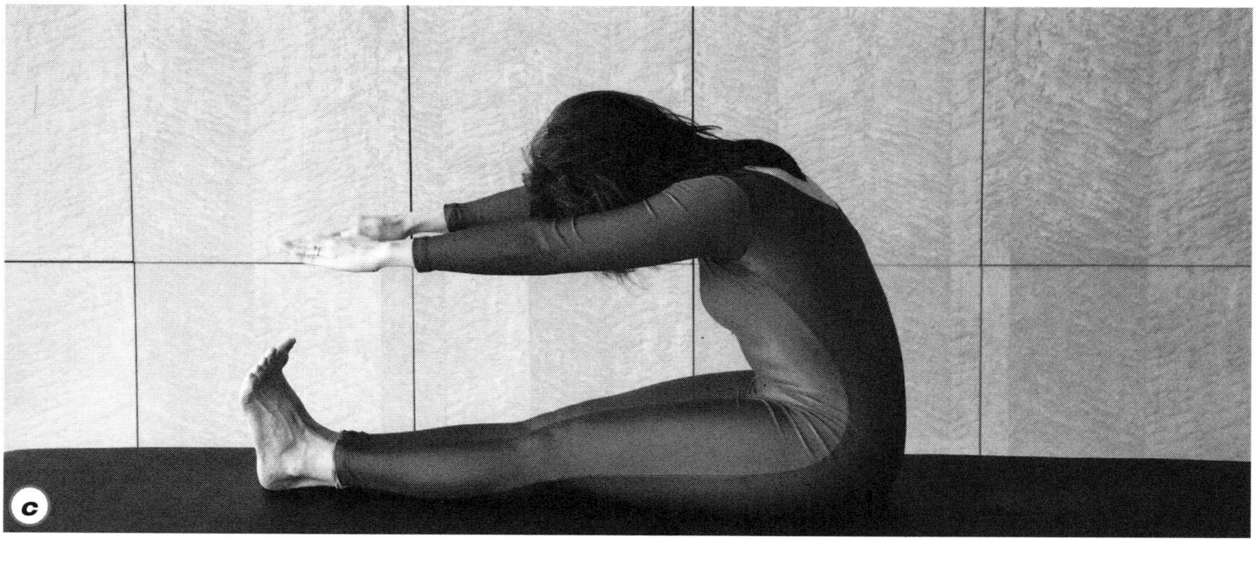

Look for . . . Encourage

- Articulation of each vertebra down to the mat as if each piece of the spine were being imprinted into a bed of wet sand
- A deep scoop in the abdominals
- Shoulders gliding toward the hips as if suspenders were hooked to the bottom tips of the shoulder blades and attached to the hips
- Hugging the legs toward the midline of the body

Be aware of . . . Prevent

- Gripping in the hip flexors
- Rolling down or up in segments of the spine
- Hinging from the hips, folding the chest onto the thighs

Primary Muscles Activated

Abdominals, biceps, triceps, deltoids, shoulder complex, iliopsoas, rectus femoris, sartorius, pectineus, gracilis, adductor magnus, adductor longus, adductor brevis, biceps femoris, semitendinosus, semimembranosus, gluteus maximus, gluteus medius (posterior portion), tensor fasciae latae, gastrocnemius, popliteus, plantaris, vastus medialis, vastus intermedius, vastus lateralis, tibialis anterior

Single-Leg Circle

Timeline: 3 to 6 months postop

Appropriate for: knee and hip

Location: a floor mat or a raised mat as needed; a raised mat for a bilateral knee or hip replacement as needed

Instructions

- Lie supine on the mat with the head resting on a small pad as needed. Extend the left leg out onto the mat and hug the leg toward the midline of the body with a rolled-up towel under the knee as needed.
- Extend the right leg to 90° of flexion without *(a)* or with *(b)* a slight bend in the knee. Keep the leg parallel, point the toes toward the ceiling, and keep the arms long by the sides of the body.
- Draw the abdominals in and up, stabilizing the core.
- **Knee:** Inhale to prepare. Exhale and circle the right leg across the midline toward the left hip and down and around to the width of the right shoulder; stop at the top. Slightly bend your right knee as needed. Make small circles the size of a basketball. A cue for the movement is deep cross, shallow out, stop at the top.
- **Hip:** Inhale to prepare. Exhale and circle the right leg across the midline, moving no more than 20° across the midline, and around to the width of the right shoulder; stop at the top. Make small circles the size of a basketball.
- Circle 5 times and then reverse the direction and circle 5 times. Change legs and repeat.
- Keep the hips planted on the mat with the movement.

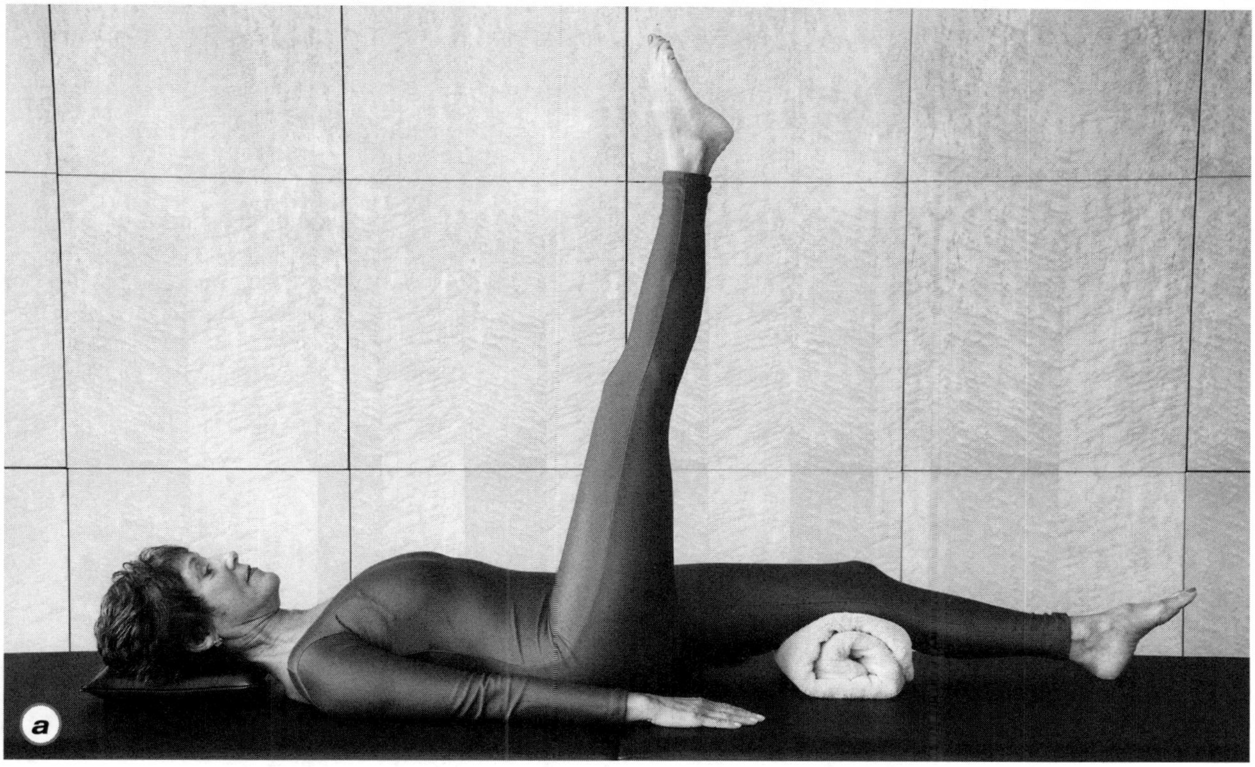

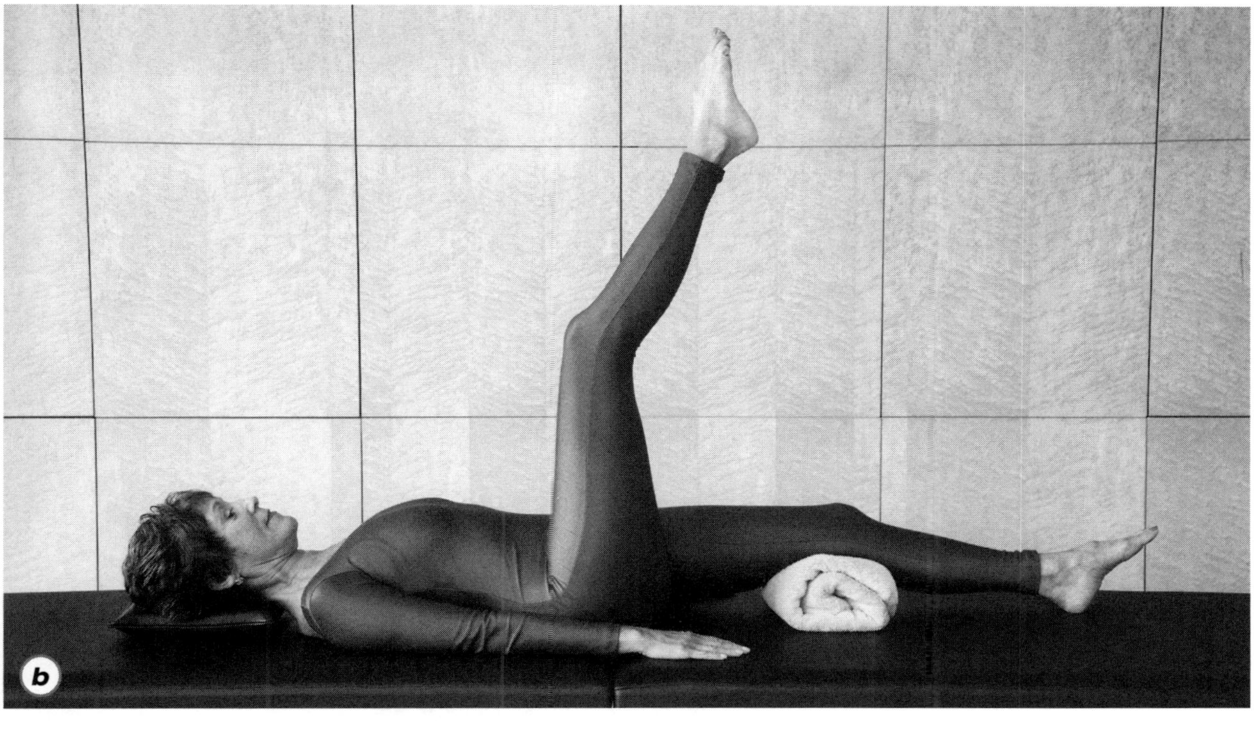

(continued)

Single-Leg Circle *(continued)*

Options

1. Place a small, soft ball under the thigh of the extended leg. The working leg is straight to the ceiling at 90° of flexion with or without a slight bend in the knee as needed.

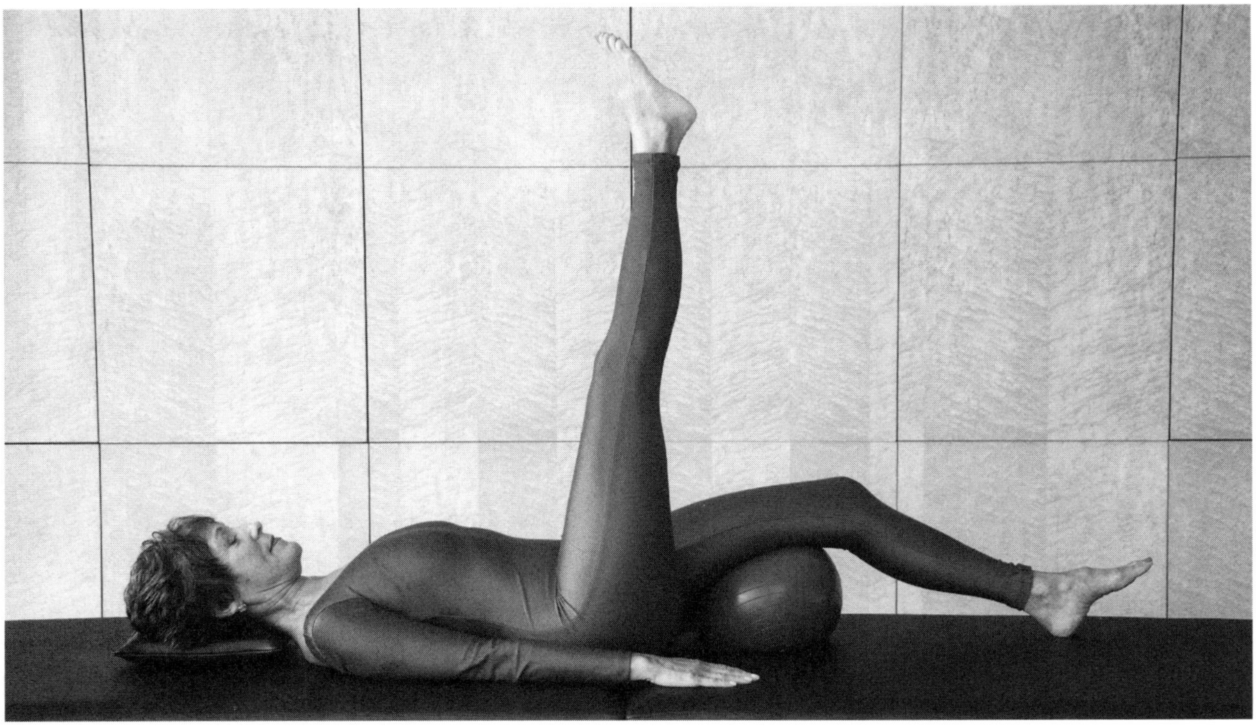

2. Bend the knee of the extended leg and keep the working leg straight at 90° of flexion with or without a slight bend in the knee.

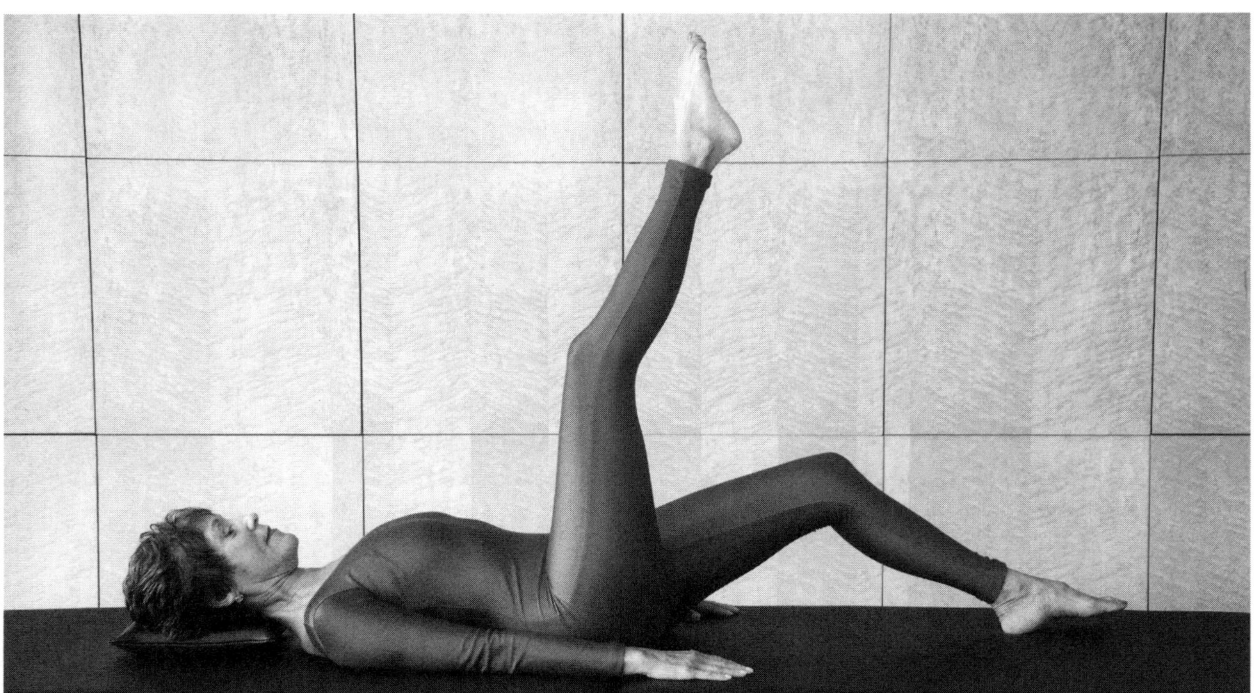

Look for . . . Encourage

- Working leg engaged hip to toe
- Shoulders gliding toward the hips as if suspenders were hooked to the bottom tips of the shoulder blades and attached to the hips
- Stable core and torso and leg working with precision and control
- Open collarbones as if taffy were strung across the shoulders
- Arms long on the mat
- Disassociation of the head of the femur from the acetabulum (stable pelvis with a flowing movement of the working leg)

Be aware of . . . Prevent

- Arching the lower lumbar region away from the mat, losing the neutral spine
- Movement of the hips and pelvis

(continued)

SINGLE-LEG CIRCLE

Timeline: 6 months and beyond postop
Appropriate for: knee and hip
Location: a floor mat or a raised mat as needed

Instructions

- Lie supine on the mat with the left leg extended out onto the mat and hugging toward the midline of the body; bend the knee as needed.
- Extend the right leg to 90° of flexion. The arms are long by the sides of the body. Keep the raised leg parallel to itself and toes pointed.
- Draw the abdominals in and up to stabilize the torso.
- **Knee and hip:** Inhale to prepare. Exhale and circle the right leg across the midline toward the width of the left hip and down and around to the width of the right shoulder. Stop at the top. The size of the circle depends on keeping the hips stable and the abdominals engaged. The flow is deep cross, shallow out, stop at the top.
- Circle 5 to 8 times in each direction and then change legs.
- Keep the hips planted on the mat.
- Bend knees of both legs as needed.

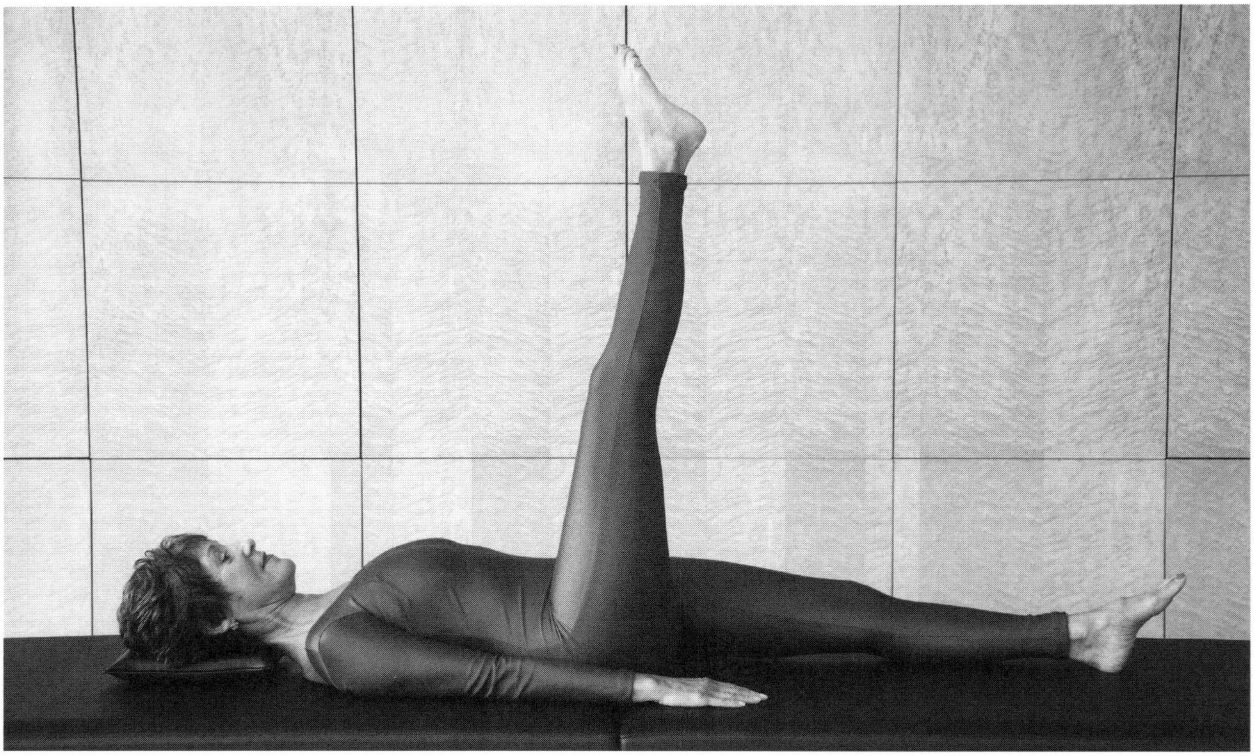

Look for . . . Encourage

- Working leg engaged hip to toe
- Shoulders gliding toward the hips as if suspenders were hooked to the bottom tips of the shoulder blades and attached to the hips
- Stable core and torso and leg working with precision and control
- Open collarbones as if taffy were strung across the shoulders
- Arms long on the mat
- Disassociation of the head of the femur from the acetabulum (stable the pelvis with a flowing movement of the working leg)

Be aware of . . . Prevent

- Arching the lower lumbar region away from the mat, losing the neutral spine
- Movement of the hips and pelvis

Primary Muscles Activated

Abdominals, rectus femoris, vastus medialis, vastus intermedius, vastus lateralis, sartorius, pectineus, iliopsoas, gluteus maximus, gluteus medius, gluteus minimus, tensor fasciae latae, adductor magnus, adductor longus, adductor brevis, gracilis, sartorius, tibialis posterior, gastrocnemius, soleus, plantaris, hamstrings are stretched (biceps femoris, semitendinosus, semimembranosus)

Rolling Like a Ball

Restrictions: not applicable for the hip at 3 to 6 months postop; instead, perform the half roll-down on page 140

Timeline: 3 to 6 months postop

Appropriate for: knee

Location: a floor mat or a raised mat as needed; a raised mat for a bilateral knee or hip replacement as needed

Instructions

- Sit tall, place the hands under the thighs close to the knees, position the legs in parallel with a small, soft ball between the knees, and squeeze the ball, hugging the legs to the midline of the body.
- Keep the heels drawing in toward the buttocks and bring the chin toward the chest, keeping a small space between the chin and the chest, looking down toward the abdominals,
- Draw the navel to the spine with the abdominals in and up.
- Roll slightly off the sit bones, lifting the heels off the mat, and balance.
- Inhale; leading with the lower back, rock back toward the bottom tips of the shoulder blades.
- Exhale, draw deep into the abdominals, and rock back up and balance.
- Repeat 6 to 8 times.

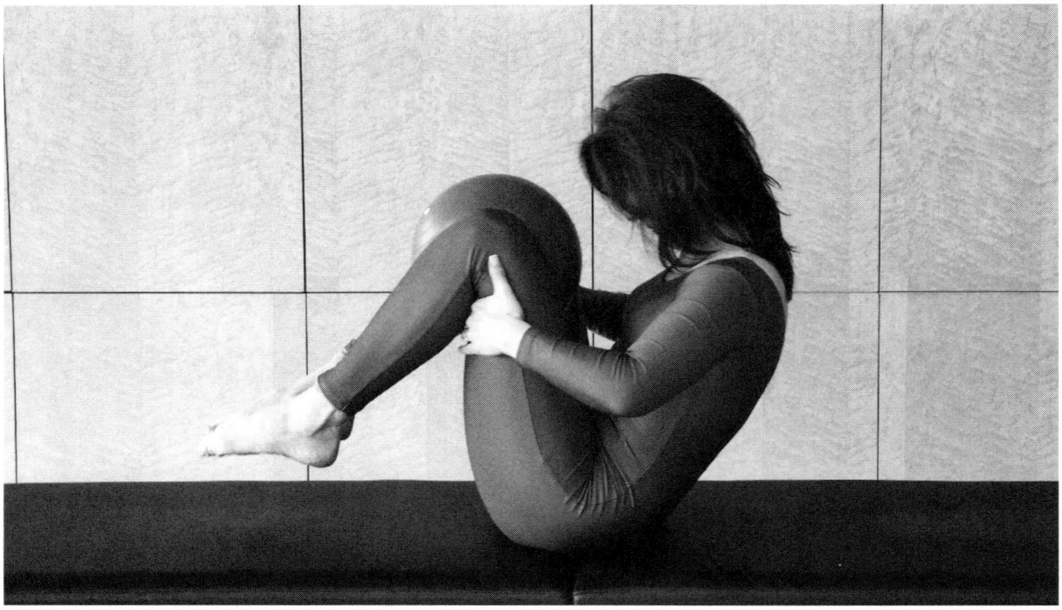

Look for . . . Encourage

- Moving as one unit, no seesaw action with the legs and torso
- Shoulders gliding toward the hips as if suspenders were hooked to the bottom tips of the shoulder blades and attached to the hips
- The core, not momentum, creates the roll
- The lower back and not the head is leading
- Moving as if the spine were a wheel, rolling and massaging the spine
- Thinking of the resistance of a stretched rubber band to help create a stable torso during the roll, pressing the thighs into the hands, and drawing back into the core
- Shoulders gliding away from the ears

Be aware of . . . Prevent

- Rolling too far back to the neck
- Flaring the shins away from the torso with the movement
- Using momentum to create the roll

(continued)

ROLLING LIKE A BALL

Timeline: 6 months and beyond
Appropriate for: knee and hip
Location: a floor mat or a raised mat as needed

Instructions

- **Knee:** Position the hands on the fronts of the calves or on the ankles with the heels together and the toes apart. Place a rolled-up towel under the crease of the knees as needed. Bring the chin toward the chest and keep a small space between the chin and the chest. Look down toward the abdominals. Draw the abdominals in and up. Roll slightly back, lift the heels off the mat, and balance.
- Inhale and rock back toward the tips of the shoulder blades.
- Exhale, rock back up, and balance.

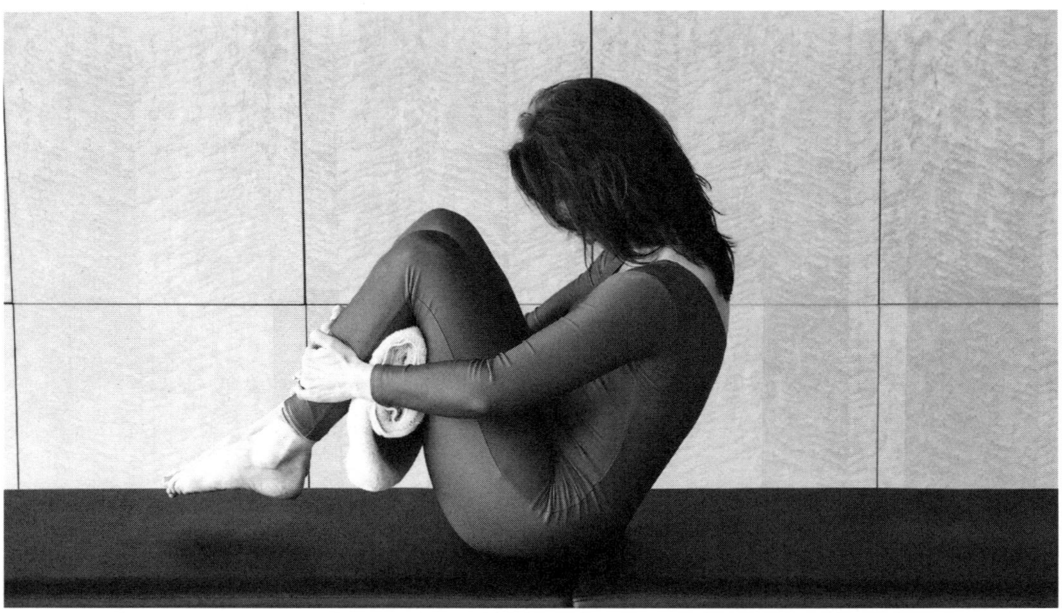

- **Hip:** Sit slightly off the sit bones with the hands under the thighs close to the knees. Maintain a maximum of 115° of hip flexion. Use a small ball between the knees to keep the legs open and parallel with a connection to the midline of the body. Keep the knees at least hip-distance apart. Bring the chin toward the chest and keep a small space between the chin and the chest. Look down toward the abdominals. Draw the abdominals in and up. Roll slightly back and lift the heels off the mat and balance.
- Inhale and rock back toward the tips of the shoulder blades.
- Exhale, rock back up, and balance.

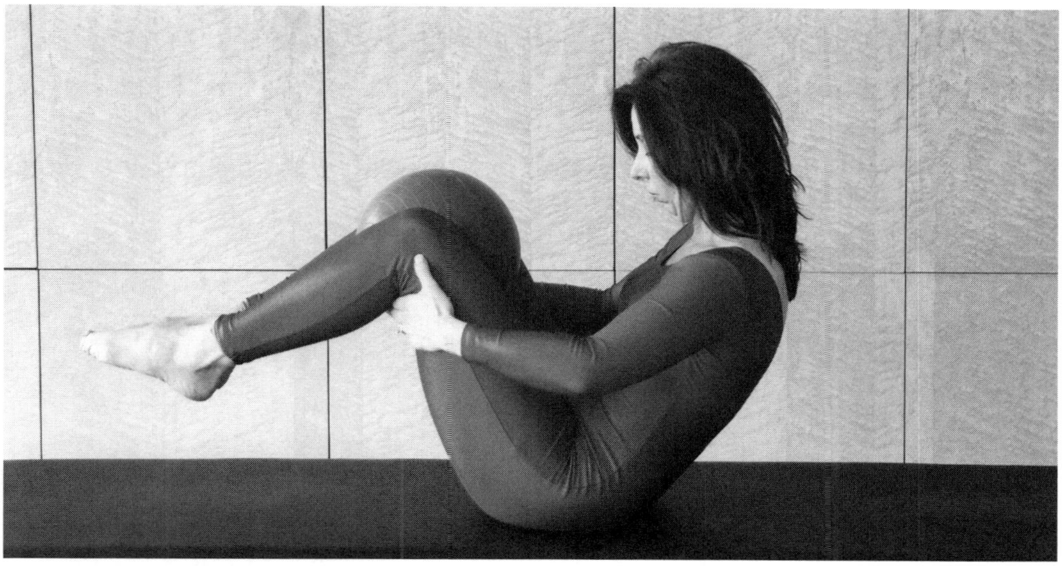

Look for . . . Encourage

- Moving as one unit, no seesaw action with the legs and torso
- Shoulders gliding toward the hips as if suspenders were hooked to the bottom tips of the shoulder blades and attached to the hips
- The energy of the heels flowing in toward the sit bones
- Using the core, not momentum, to create the roll
- Leading with the lower back, not the head
- Moving as if the spine were a wheel, rolling and massaging the spine
- Thinking of the resistance of a stretched rubber band to help create a stable torso during the roll, pressing the thighs into the hands, and drawing back into the core

Be aware of . . . Prevent

- Rolling too far back to the neck
- Flaring the shins away from the torso with the movement
- Using momentum to create the roll

Primary Muscles Activated

Abdominals, rectus femoris, sartorius, pectineus, iliopsoas, biceps femoris, semitendinosus, semimembranosus, tensor fasciae latae, adductor magnus, adductor longus, adductor brevis, gracilis, gastrocnemius, popliteus, plantaris

Single-Leg Stretch

Timeline: 3 to 6 months and 6 months and beyond postop

Appropriate for: knee and hip

Location: a floor mat or raised mat as needed; a raised mat for a bilateral knee or hip replacement as needed for up to 6 months postop

Instructions

- Lie supine on the mat, with the knees bent into tabletop position.
- Move the outside hand toward the ankle and the inside hand to the inside aspect of the knee.
- Curl the head, neck, and shoulders off the mat up to the bottom tips of the shoulder blades. Look toward the thighs.
- **Knee:** Lengthen the left leg out to 45° from the mat and bring the right knee in toward the chest as tolerated, keeping the tailbone long on the mat. Scoop the navel to the spine and switch legs. Bend the left knee as tolerated and lengthen the right leg to 45° *(a)*.

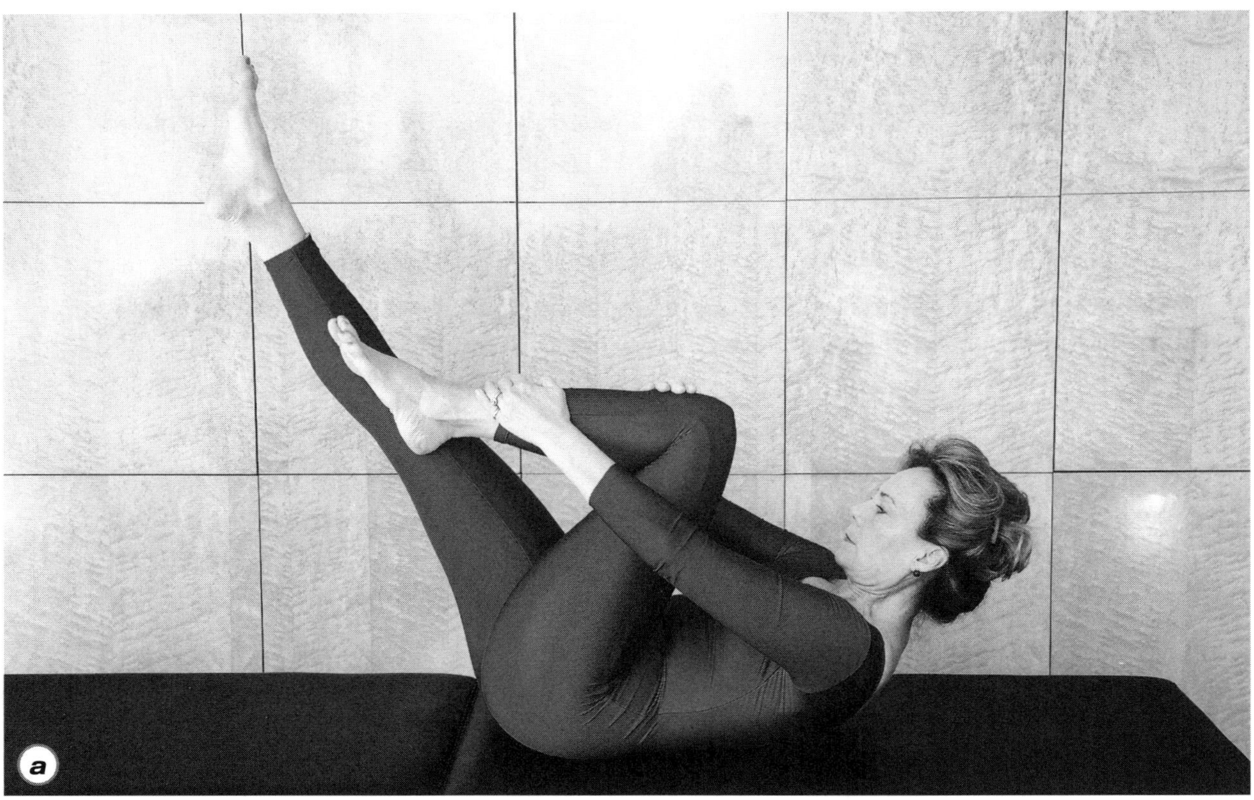

- **Hip:** Lengthen the left leg to 45° from the mat and bring the right knee in toward the chest. Maintain up to 110° of hip flexion for up to 6 months (as shown here) and up to 115° of hip flexion for 6 months and beyond. Scoop the navel to the spine and switch legs. Bend the left knee and lengthen the right leg to 45° *(b)*.
- Inhale for two leg movements and exhale for two leg movements.
- Repeat 8 times per leg.

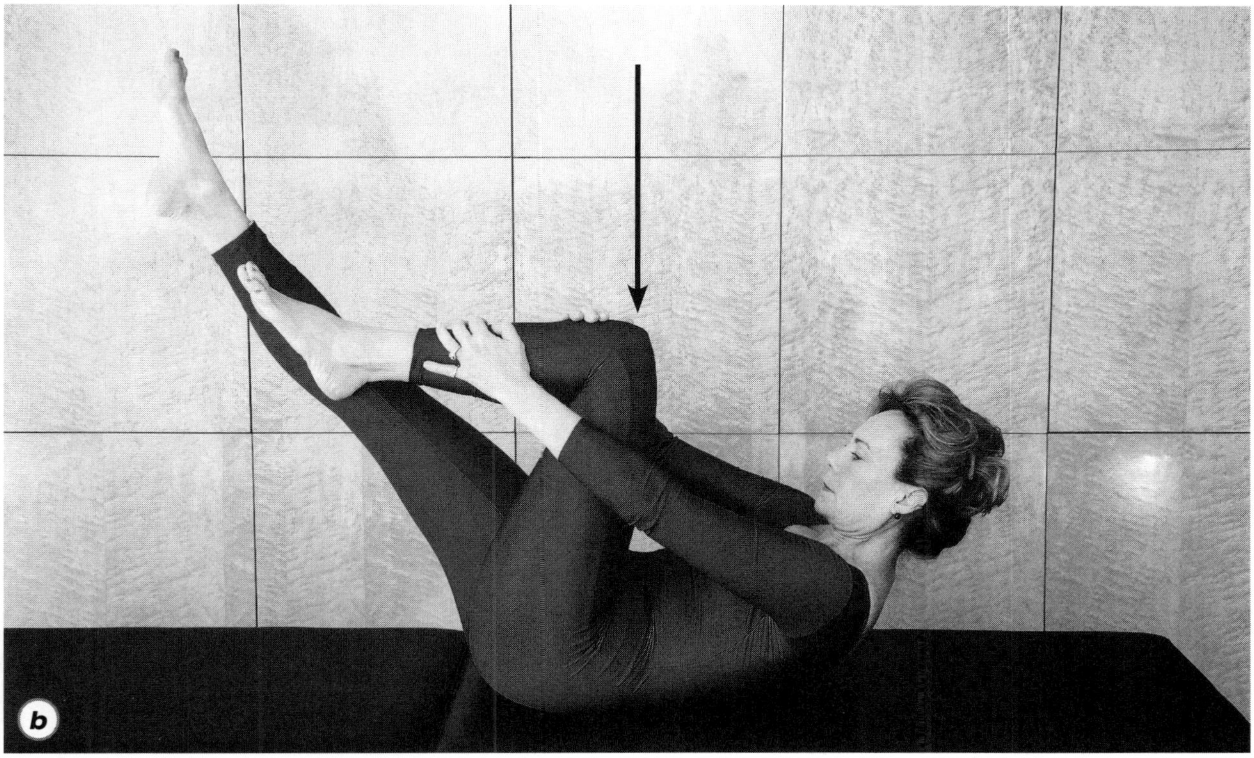

(continued)

Option

Place a small, soft ball 8 to 10 inches (20-25 centimeters) in diameter under the head and neck; see page 134 for instructions for placement.

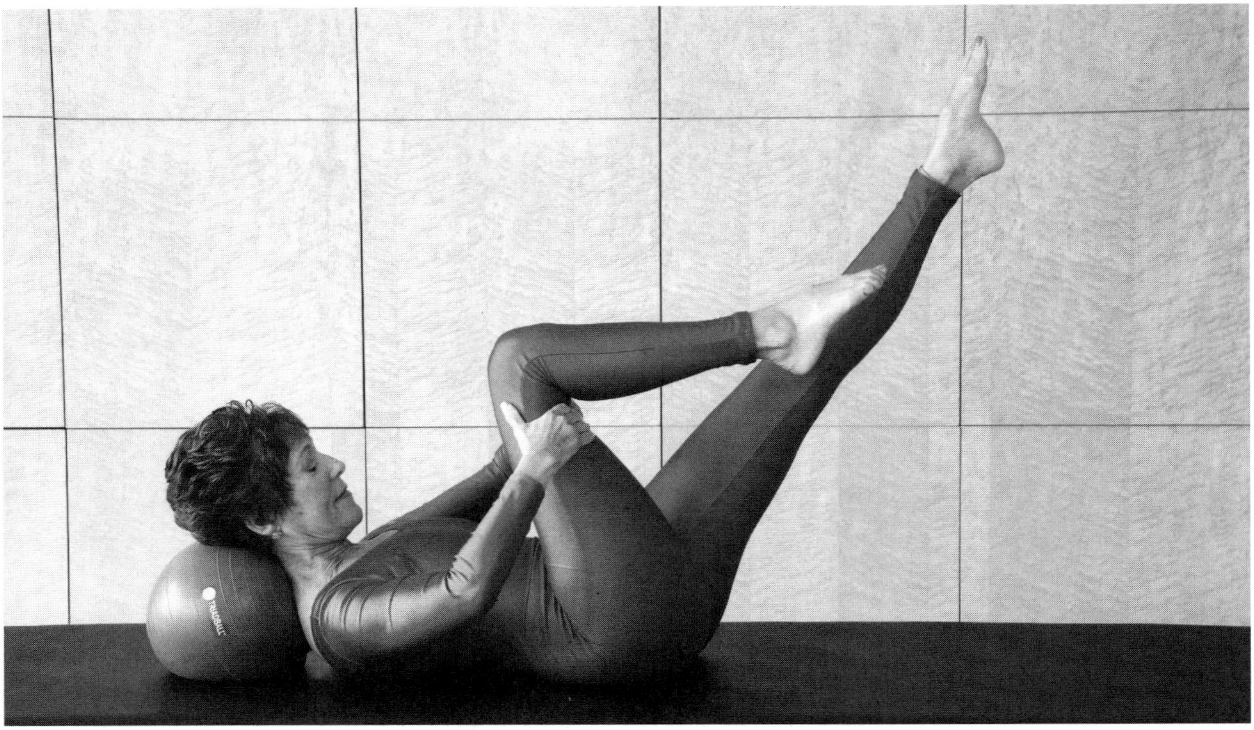

Look for . . . Encourage

- Precision and control as the legs are switched
- The tailbone long on the mat, keeping neutral spine
- The shoulder blades gliding toward the tailbone as if suspenders were attached to the bottom tips of the shoulder blades and attached to the hips
- Abdominals drawn in and up
- Stable pelvis

Be aware of . . . Prevent

- Tension in the head, neck, and shoulders
- Arching (hyperextension) of the lumbar spine
- Loss of core control

Primary Muscles Activated

Abdominals, biceps, triceps, deltoids, anterior scalene, sternocleidomastoid, rectus femoris, vastus medialis, vastus intermedius, vastus lateralis, sartorius, pectineus, iliopsoas, biceps femoris, semitendinosus, semimembranosus, tensor fasciae latae, adductor longus, adductor brevis, gracilis, popliteus, gastrocnemius, plantaris

Double-Leg Stretch

Timeline: 3 to 6 months postop

Appropriate for: knee and hip

Location: a floor mat or a raised mat as needed; a raised mat for a bilateral knee or hip replacement as needed

Instructions

- **Knee:** Lie supine on the mat, with the knees bent in toward the chest as tolerated. Place the hands on the shins and place a pad or small ball between the knees. Hug the legs to the midline of the body and keep the tailbone down on the mat.
- **Hip:** Lie supine on the mat with the legs bent in toward the chest to maintain up to 110° of hip flexion. Place the hands on the shins and place a pad or small, soft ball between the knees. Hug the legs to the midline of the body and keep the tailbone down on the mat.
- Curl the head, neck, and shoulders off the mat up to the bottom tips of the shoulder blades. Look toward the thighs *(a)*.
- Draw the abdominals in and up.
- Inhale and simultaneously lengthen both legs up to 90° or out to 65° from the floor and extend the arms toward the ears *(b)*.
- Exhale and circle the arms out and around as you bring the knees in toward the chest as tolerated, keeping 110° of flexion for the hips, with the tailbone long on the mat. Place the hands back on the shins *(c)*.
- Keep the low back and ribs glued to the mat and the abdominals scooped in and up as you extend the arms and legs away from the core of the body.
- As the arms extend back toward the ears, think about rounding up further toward the abdominals.
- Repeat 8 times.

(continued)

Double-Leg Stretch *(continued)*

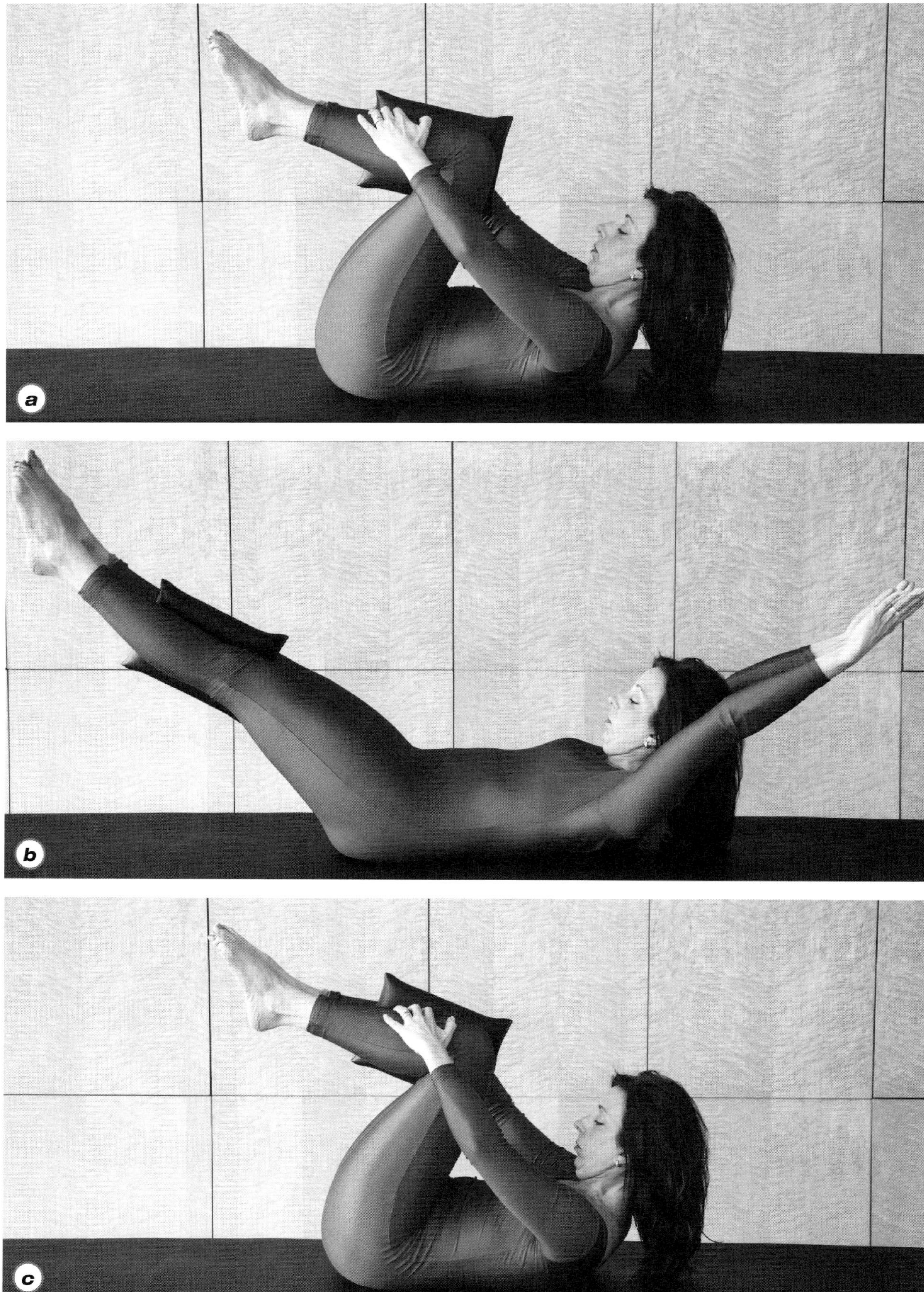

Options

1. Support the head, neck, and shoulders by placing a ball 8 to 10 inches (20-25 centimeters) in diameter under the head and neck; see page 134 for instructions for placement.

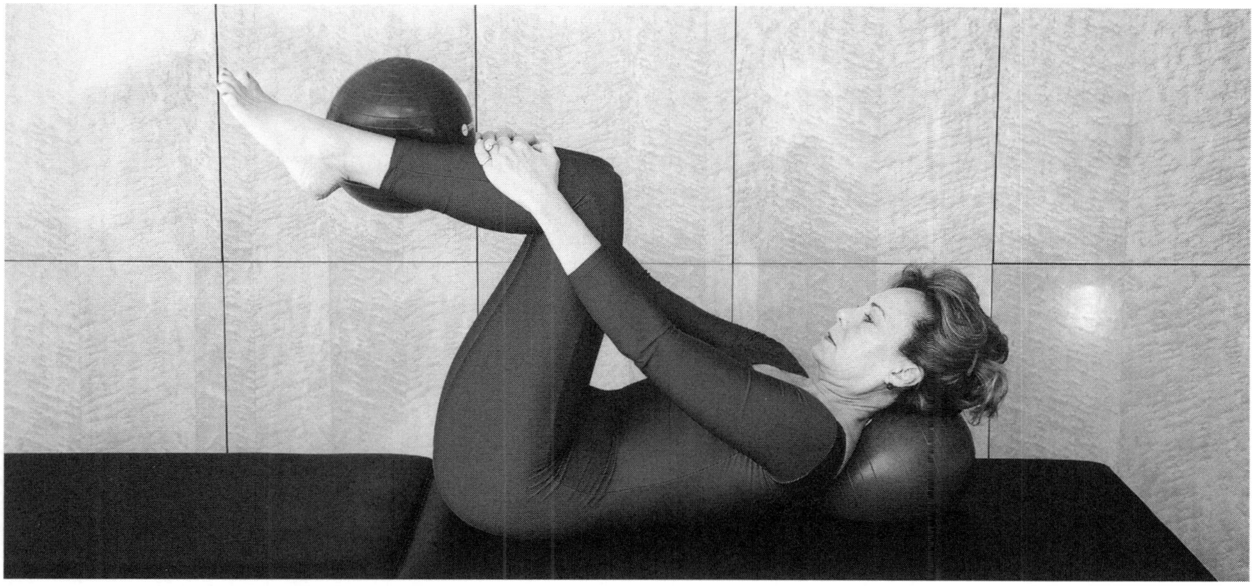

2. Keep the legs in tabletop position and perform only the arm portion of exercise.
3. Use a large exercise ball, 22 to 26 inches (55-66 centimeters) in diameter. Place the legs in tabletop position with the heels resting on top of the ball. Inhale and simultaneously extend the arms back toward the ears. Use the legs to roll the ball out, keeping the heels in place. Exhale and roll the ball back to the starting position with the feet on the ball as you circle the arms around to the shins.

Look for . . . Encourage

- Precision of movement
- Shoulders gliding toward the hips as if suspenders were hooked to the bottom tips of the shoulder blades and attached to the hips
- Tailbone long on the mat
- Abdominals drawn in and up

Be aware of . . . Prevent

- Tension in the head, neck, and shoulders
- Lowering the head back toward the mat when the arms extend back in line with the ears
- Arching (hyperextension) of the lumbar spine
- Shoulders elevated toward the ears

(continued)

DOUBLE-LEG STRETCH

Timeline: 6 months postop and beyond
Appropriate for: knee and hip
Location: a floor mat or a raised mat as needed

Instructions

- **Knee:** Lie supine on the mat with the knees bent in toward the chest, the hands on the shins, the legs hugged to the midline of the body, and the tailbone down on the mat.
- **Hip:** Lie supine on the mat with the knees bent in toward the chest to maintain up to 115° of hip flexion. Place the hands on the shins and hug the legs to the midline of the body. Keep the tailbone long on the mat.
- Curl the head, neck, and shoulders off the mat up to the bottom tips of the shoulder blades. Look toward the thighs.
- Draw the abdominals in and up.
- Inhale and simultaneously lengthen both legs out to 45° from the mat and extend the arms toward the ears.
- Exhale and circle the arms out and around as you bring the knees in toward the chest as tolerated, keeping 115° of flexion for the hips (as shown here), with the tailbone long on the mat. Place the hands back on the shins.
- Keep the low back and ribs glued to the mat and the abdominals drawn deeply in and up as you extend the arms and legs away from the core of the body.
- As the arms extend back toward the ears, think about rounding up further toward the abdominals.
- Keep the legs parallel and hugging the midline of the body.
- Repeat 8 to 10 times.

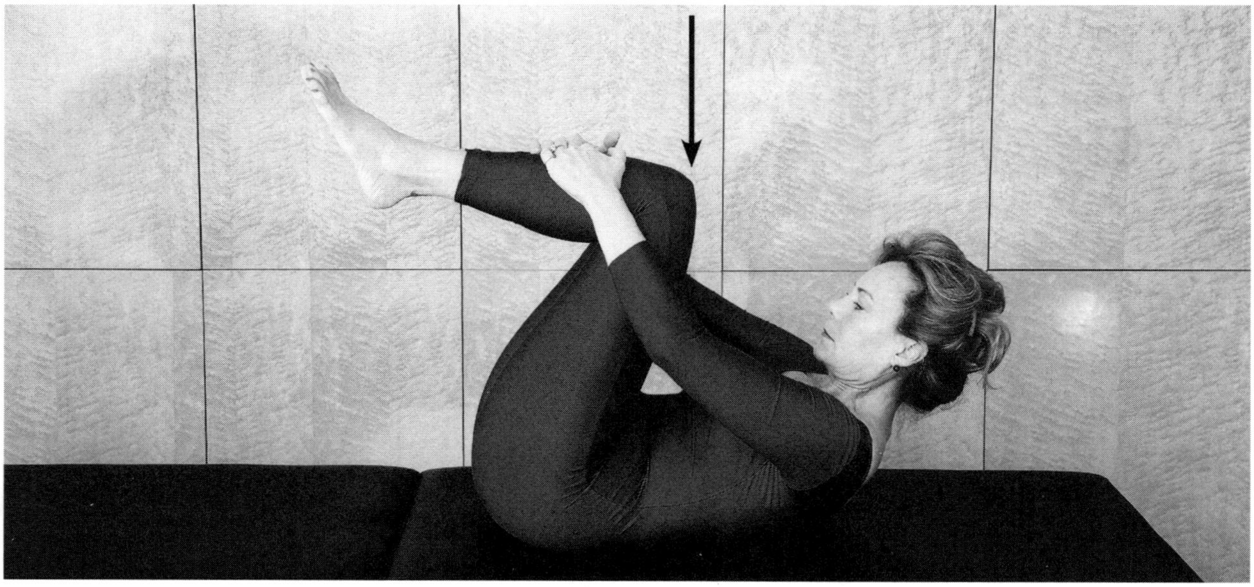

Option

Continue to use a pad between the thighs or a small ball between the knees as needed. Placing a small, soft ball between the knees and ankles further engages the adductors, decreases overuse of the hip flexors, and increases connection to the core.

Look for . . . Encourage

- Precision of movement
- Shoulders gliding toward the tailbone as if suspenders were attached to the bottom tips of the shoulder blades and stretching to the hip pockets
- Tailbone long on the mat
- Thinking about rounding up further toward the abdominals as the arms extend back toward the ears
- Abdominals drawn in and up

Be aware of . . . Prevent

- Tension in the head and shoulders
- Lowering of the head back toward the mat when the arms extend back in line with the ears
- Arching (hyperextension) of the lumbar spine

Primary Muscles Activated

Abdominals, biceps, deltoids, shoulder complex, scalene, sternocleidomastoid, rectus femoris, sartorius, adductor magnus, adductor longus, adductor brevis, pectineus, gracilis, iliopsoas, biceps femoris, semitendinosus, semimembranosus, tensor fasciae latae, gastrocnemius, popliteus, plantaris, vastus medialis, vastus intermedius, vastus lateralis

Single Straight-Leg Stretch and Scissors

Timeline: 3 to 6 months and 6 months and beyond postop

Appropriate for: knee and hip

Location: a floor mat or a raised mat as needed; a raised mat for a bilateral knee or hip replacement as needed up to 6 months postop

Instructions

- Lie supine on the mat and place the legs in tabletop position.
- Curl the head, neck, and shoulders off the mat up to the bottom tips of the shoulder blades. Look toward the thighs and stay in the deep scoop to complete the repetitions of the exercise.
- **Knee:** Extend both legs to the ceiling. Walk the hands up to the right calf. Keeping the knees soft, scissor the left leg to 45° with toes pointed. Draw the abdominals in and up. Pull the right leg in toward the chest with a gentle double pulse and then switch legs and double pulse the left leg while the right leg reaches out to 45°. Keep the legs long with either a small bend in the knee *(a)* or soft knees *(b)*.

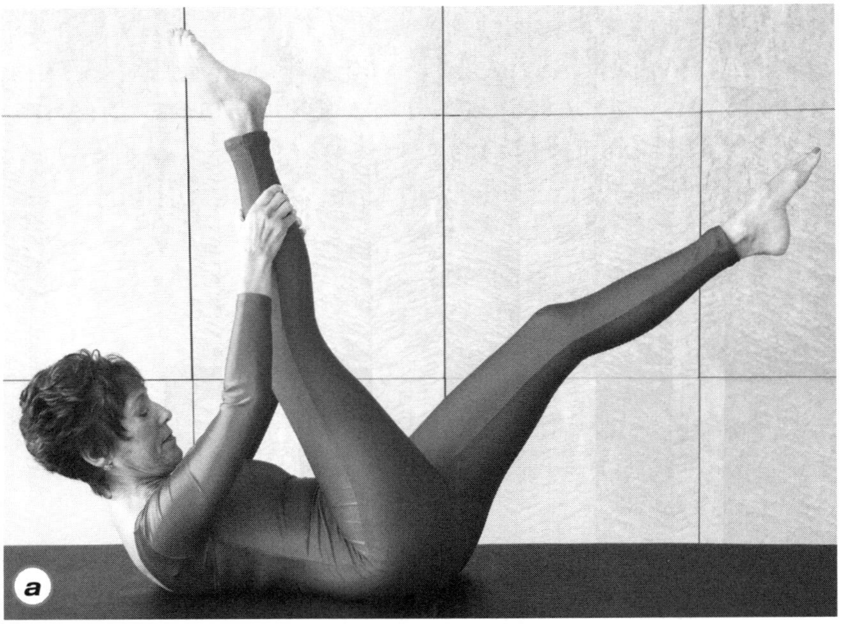

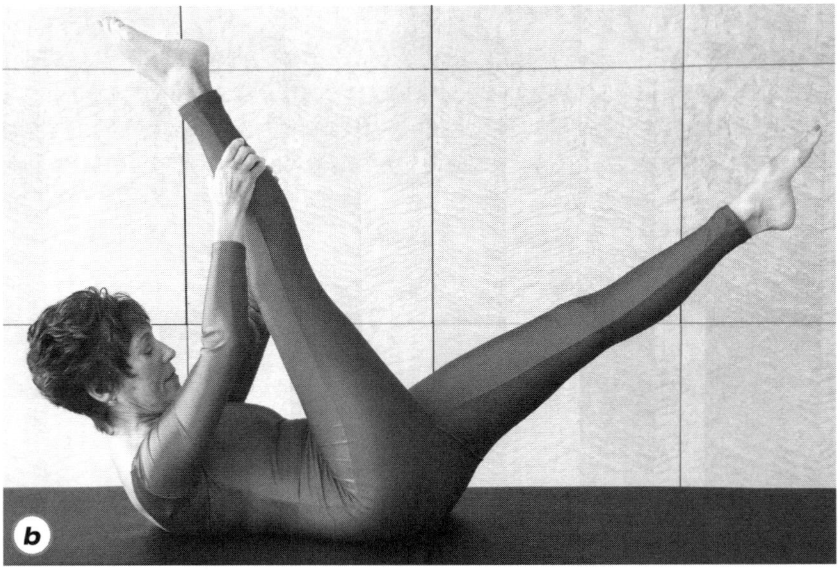

- **Hip:** Extend both legs to the ceiling. Walk the hands up to the right calf. Keeping the knees soft, scissor the left leg to 45° with toes pointed. Draw the abdominals in and up. Pull the right leg in toward the chest with a gentle double pulse, keeping 110° of hip flexion for up to 6 months (as shown in *c*), and no more than 115° of hip flexion for 6 months and beyond, while the left leg reaches out to 45°. Switch legs and double pulse the left leg while the right leg reaches out to 45°.
- Scoop deep into the abdominals with each action of the leg.
- Inhale for two leg movements and exhale for two leg movements.
- Repeat 8 times per leg.

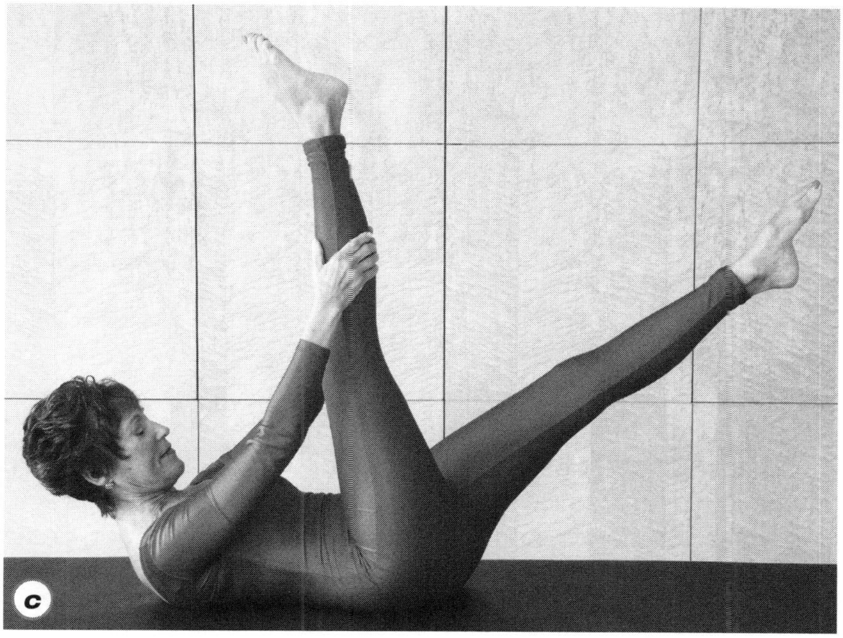

(continued)

Single Straight-Leg Stretch and Scissors *(continued)*

Option

For an additional challenge, place the arms long on the mat, palms down, and perform the scissors.

Look for . . . Encourage

- Shoulders gliding toward the tailbone as if suspenders were hooked to the bottom tips of the shoulder blades and attached to the hips
- Open collarbones
- Abdominals drawing in and up
- Legs long with a small bend in the knees, especially if the hamstrings are tight
- Tailbone long on the mat

Be aware of . . . Prevent

- Tension in the head, neck, and shoulders
- Arching (hyperextension) of the lumbar spine

Primary Muscles Activated

Abdominals, biceps, deltoids, triceps, anterior scalene, sternocleidomastoid, iliopsoas, rectus femoris, sartorius, adductor longus, adductor brevis, pectineus, tensor fasciae latae, gracilis, vastus medialis, vastus lateralis, vastus intermedius, hamstrings are stretched (biceps femoris, semimembranosus, semitendinosus), tibialis posterior, gastrocnemius, plantaris, soleus

Double Straight-Leg Stretch (Lower Lift)

Timeline: 3 to 6 months and 6 months and beyond postop

Appropriate for: knee and hip

Location: a floor mat or a raised mat as needed; a raised mat for a bilateral knee or hip replacement as needed for up to 6 months postop

Instructions

- Lie supine on the mat with the legs in tabletop position. Layer the hands and place them behind the head at the base of the skull with the elbows wide and the thumbs running down the sides of the neck.
- Curl the head, neck, and shoulders off the mat up to the bottom tips of the shoulder blades. Look toward the thighs. Deeply scoop the navel to the spine, drawing the abdominals in and up.
- Extend the legs to 90° with the tailbone long on the mat *(a)*.

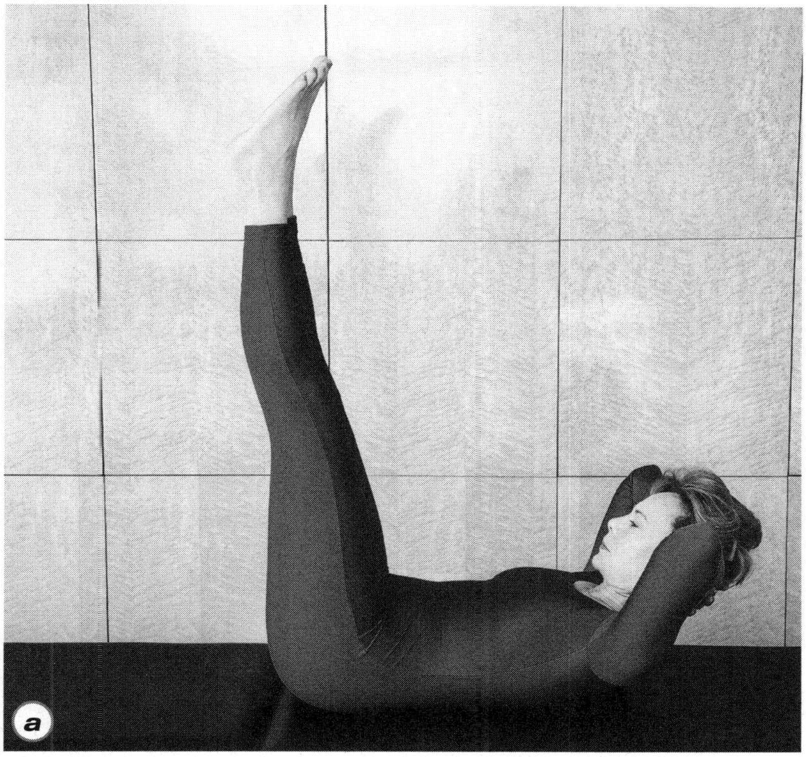

- Inhale and slowly lower the legs 5 to 7 inches (13-18 centimeters) for the count of 3 *(b)*, and then exhale and bring the legs back to 90° on the count of 1.
- Change flow: lower on the count of 1 and lift on the count of 3 back to 90°.
- **Knees and hips:** Keep the legs parallel and hugging the midline of the body and the knees soft with or without a pad or ball between the knees or between the ankles.
- Repeat 8 times.

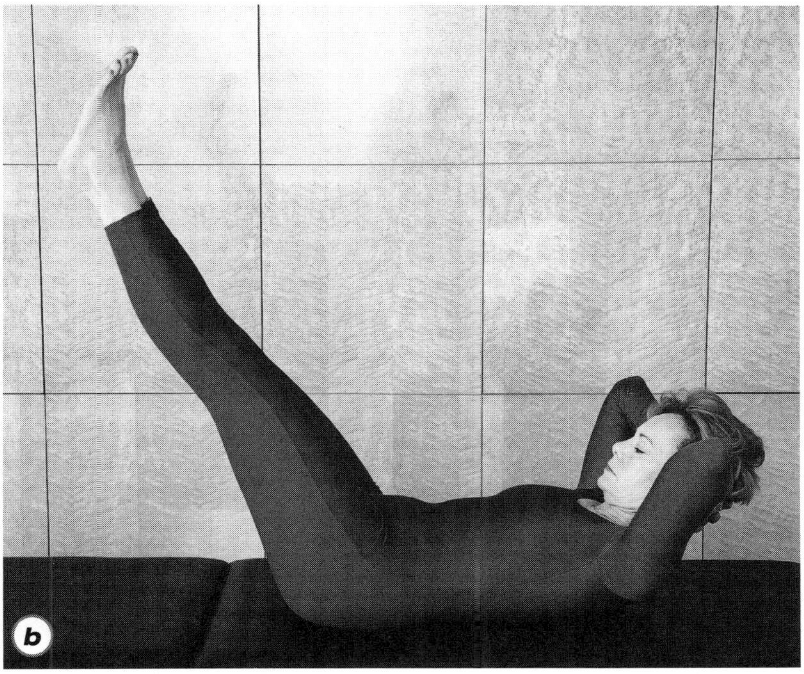

(continued)

Double Straight-Leg Stretch (Lower Lift) *(continued)*

Options

1. Place an exercise band wide around the bottom of the feet with the legs parallel. Hold the exercise band in both hands with light tension. The upper arm to elbow should rest on the mat. Place a small, soft ball behind the head, neck, and shoulders and perform the lower lift. (See p. 134 for the placement of the ball.)

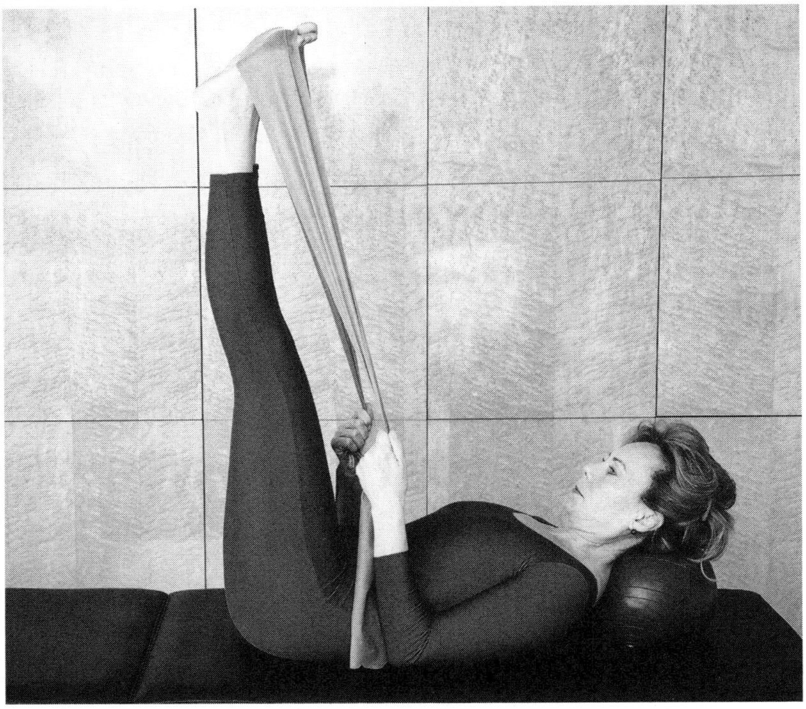

2. Place a small, soft ball behind the head, neck, and shoulders with the hands in a diamond shape under the tailbone. Keep the elbows wide and on the mat. If desired, place a second small ball between the shins and ankles, keeping the knees slightly flexed.

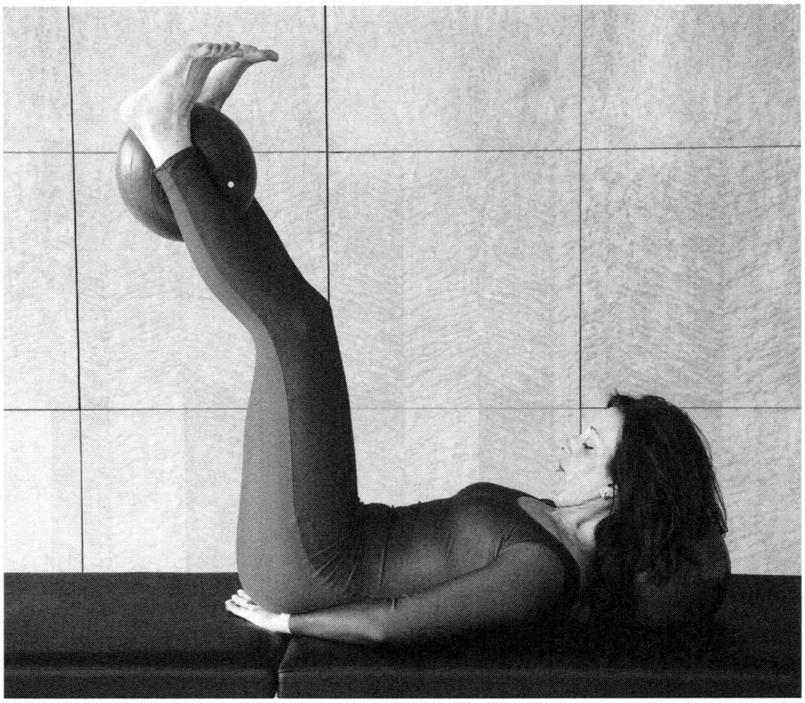

3. Using a small ball between the legs further engages the adductors, decreases overuse of the hip flexors, and increases connection to the core.

Look for . . . Encourage

- Tailbone long on the mat
- Shoulders gliding toward the tailbone as if suspenders were hooked to the bottom tips of the shoulder blades and attached to the hips
- Abdominals drawn in and up
- Collarbones open
- Low back on the mat and the abdominals scooped deeply in and up during the lower lift

Be aware of . . . Prevent

- Tension in the head and neck
- Arching (hyperextension) of the lumbar spine when the legs lower

Primary Muscles Activated

Abdominals, anterior scalene, sternocleidomastoid, iliopsoas, rectus femoris, sartorius, adductor magnus, adductor longus, adductor brevis, pectineus, gracilis, vastus medialis, vastus intermedius, vastus lateralis, tensor fasciae latae, hamstrings are stretched (biceps femoris, semitendinosus, semimembranosus)

Crisscross

Timeline: 3 to 6 months and 6 months and beyond postop

Appropriate for: knee and hip

Location: a floor mat or a raised mat as needed; a raised mat for a bilateral knee or hip replacement as needed for up to 6 months postop

Instructions

- Lie supine on the mat with the legs in tabletop position.
- Place the head and shoulders on the mat with the hands layered and placed behind the head with the thumbs running down the sides of the neck. The elbows are slightly off the mat.
- Inhale to prepare. Exhale and curl the head, neck, and shoulders off the mat. Gaze at the thighs.
- Extend the left leg out to 45° and bring the right knee in toward the chest.
- Inhale to prepare. Exhale and twist the torso from the waist to the right (left shoulder to right hip). Gaze diagonally forward and draw the abdominals in and up.
- Hold for 3 counts.
- Inhale center (stay rounded up), and exhale and twist to the left as you simultaneously change legs (right leg extends, left knee comes in toward the chest).
- Hold for 3 counts.
- Repeat 6 to 8 sets.
- **Hip:** Keep 110° of hip flexion for up to 6 months and then work toward 115° of hip flexion as tolerated. Maintain a neutral spine.
- Try to stay curled up to the bottom tips of the shoulder blades for all sets.
- Play with rhythm and flow as tolerated.

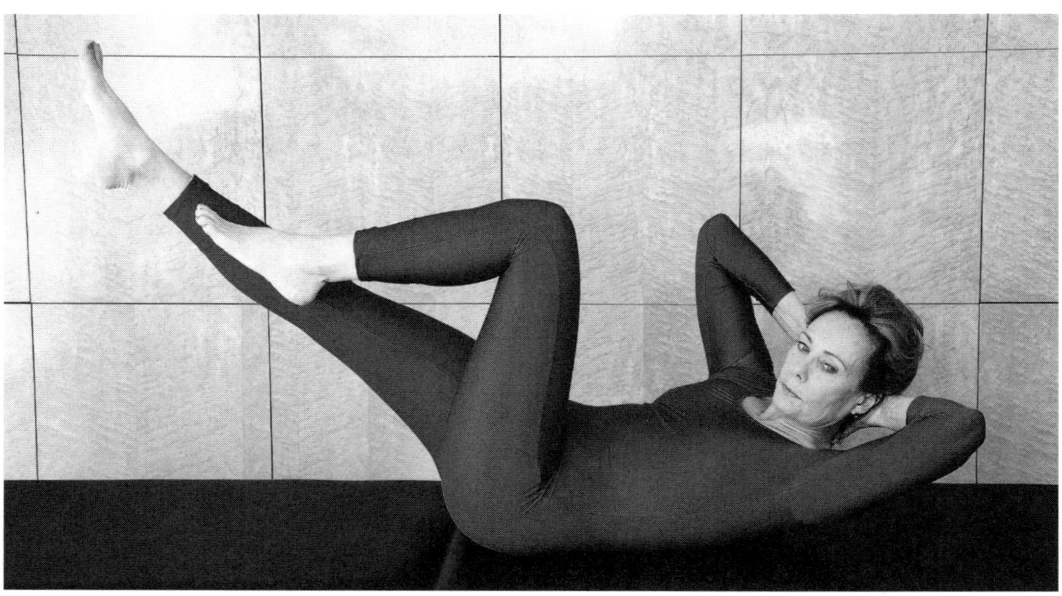

Option

Use a soft ball between the knees.

- Lie supine on the mat with the legs in tabletop position and a small, soft ball between the knees.
- Place the head and shoulders on the mat. Layer the hands and place them behind the head with the thumbs running down the sides of the neck.
- Inhale to prepare. Exhale and curl the head, neck, and shoulders off the mat. Gaze at the thighs.
- Extend the right leg to the ceiling, twist the torso from the waist to the left (right shoulder to left hip), gaze diagonally forward, and draw the abdominals in and up.
- Hold for 3 counts.
- Inhale, center, and exhale to switch sides. Simultaneously extend the left leg to the ceiling and twist to the right (left shoulder to right hip).
- Hold for 3 counts.
- Repeat 6 to 8 sets.

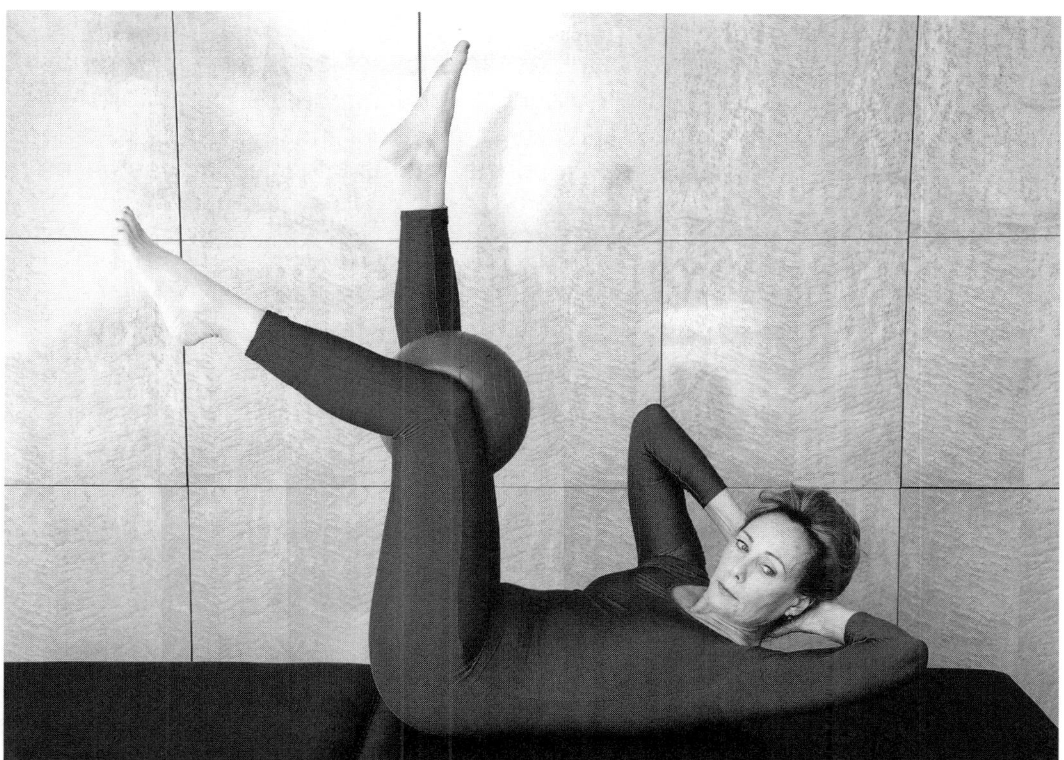

(continued)

Look for . . . Encourage

- Stable pelvis on the mat during the twist from the waist, no excess movement of the hips when the legs switch
- Twisting from the waist, bringing the obliques toward the opposite hip
- Elbows wide and stable with the twist
- Lifting up to the bottom tips of the shoulder blades
- Over time, extending legs out to 45° with movement

Be aware of . . . Prevent

- Tension in the head, neck, and shoulders
- Folding the elbow in toward the opposite hip
- Twisting only the elbows and shoulders
- Loss of shoulder alignment

Primary Muscles Activated

Abdominals, biceps, deltoids, shoulder complex, anterior scalene, sternocleidomastoid, iliopsoas, rectus femoris, sartorius, adductor magnus, adductor longus, adductor brevis, pectineus, gracilis, biceps femoris, semitendinosus, semimembranosus, tensor fasciae latae, gastrocnemius, popliteus, plantaris, vastus medialis, vastus intermedius, vastus lateralis

Spine Stretch Forward

Timeline: 3 to 6 months and 6 months and beyond postop

Appropriate for: knee and hip

Location: a floor mat or a raised mat as needed; a raised mat for a bilateral knee or hip replacement as needed for up to 6 months postop

Instructions

- Sit tall on the mat with a folded towel under the buttocks and a rolled-up towel under the knees as needed. Extend the legs, keeping them hip-distance apart, and flex the feet.
- Position the arms at shoulder width and shoulder height, keeping them long and parallel to the legs *(a)*.

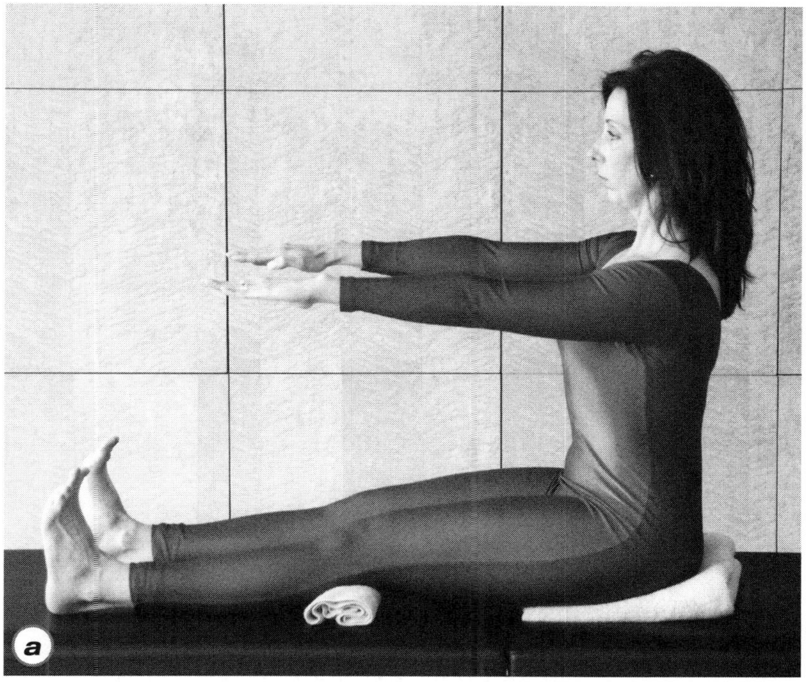

- Sit tall as if you were sitting up against a wall. Inhale and lift the abdominals in and up. Exhale and round up and over an imaginary large beach ball, creating a large C-curve in the middle of the spine; draw the abdominals in even deeper and keep the shoulder blades gliding toward the hip points *(b)*.

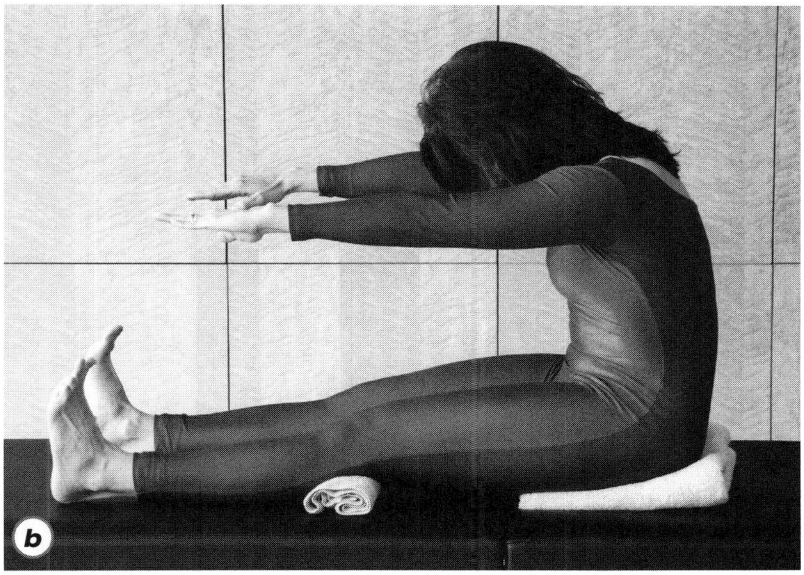

(continued)

Spine Stretch Forward *(continued)*

- Allow the belly button to flow back toward the spine in opposition to the hands reaching for the opposite wall.
- Inhale and begin to roll the spine up slowly back to the tall starting position.
- Repeat 5 to 7 times.

Option

Perform the exercise while seated against a wall.

Look for . . . Encourage

- Shoulders gliding toward the hip points
- Thinking of lifting up and over a big beach ball
- Waistband flowing in toward the spine
- Feeling as though the ribs are being drawn to the hips during the lift up and over
- Sitting tall as if a string were attached to the crown of the head and extended to the ceiling to start the movement

Be aware of . . . Prevent

- Rounding from the upper back
- Gripping in the hip flexors
- Shoulders reaching for the opposite wall

Primary Muscles Activated

Abdominals, biceps, triceps, shoulder complex, iliopsoas, rectus femoris, pectineus, gracilis, sartorius, adductor longus, adductor brevis, vastus medialis, vastus intermedius, vastus lateralis, tensor fasciae latae, tibialis anterior, hamstrings are stretched (biceps femoris, semitendinosus, semimembranosus)

Open-Leg Rocker

Restriction: not applicable for knee and hip at 3 to 6 months postop; perform the half roll-down on page 140

Timeline: 6 months and beyond postop

Appropriate for: knee and hip

Location: a floor mat or a raised table as needed

Instructions

- Sit tall with the legs bent into a mountain shape. Place a small, soft ball between the knees.
- Place the hands under the thighs near the knees.
- Draw the abdominals in and up, creating a deep scoop in the abdominals.
- Roll back off the sit bones a few inches and lift the heels and then the toes. Pick the legs up to the tabletop position to prepare for the movement. Hold this pose and balance, maintaining a deep scoop in the abdominals and a proud chest. Gaze forward.
- Inhale to prepare. Exhale and bring the chin toward the chest, drawing the abdominals in and up and rock back toward the bottom tips of the shoulder blades, leading with the lower spine.
- Exhale and rock back up to a proud chest and a big scoop in the abdominals and balance in this pose.
- Repeat 6 to 8 times.
- **Hip:** Maintain up to a maximum of 115° of hip flexion.

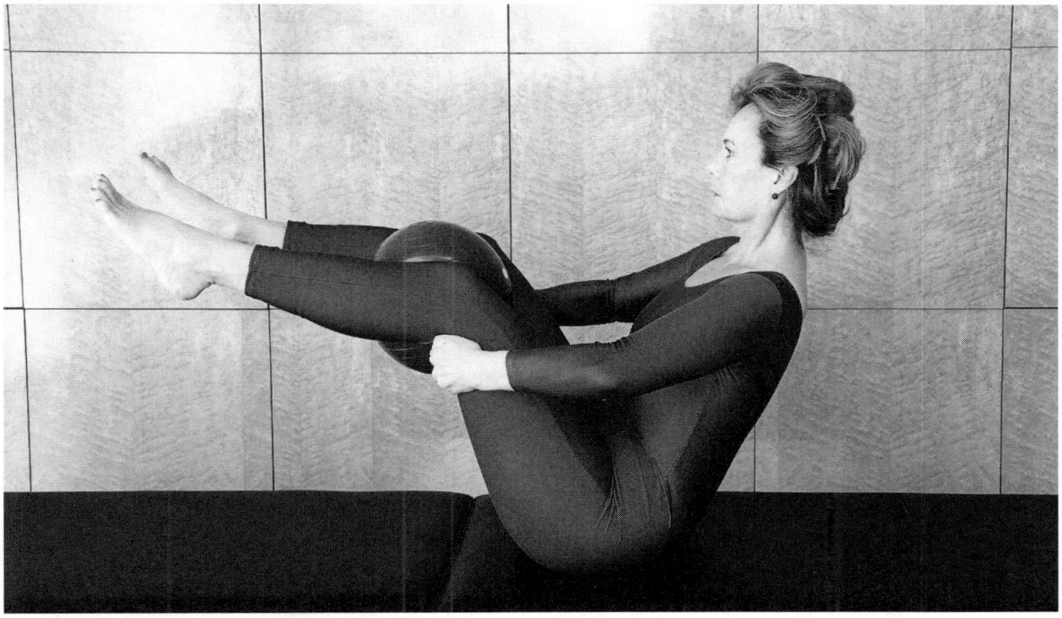

(continued)

Options

1. **Knee:** Move the hands up toward the outsides of the calves. Keep the legs in tabletop position or extend them out on a diagonal and balance. Keep the hands in position throughout the movement. Use a ball or thick pad as needed between the knees.

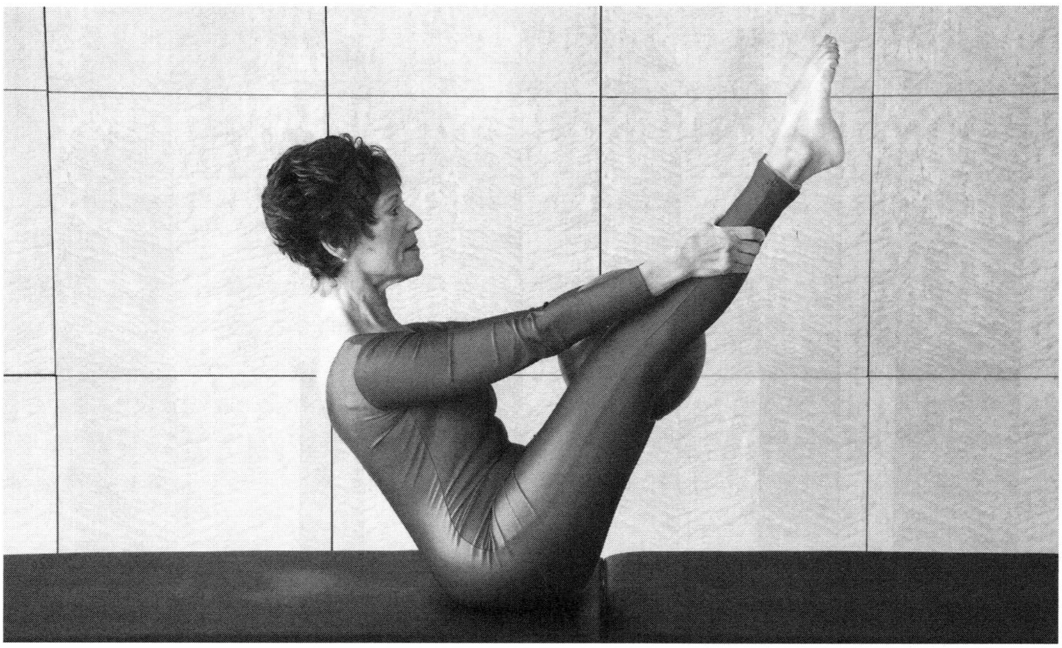

2. **Hip:** Keep the hands near the knees to maintain up to 115° of hip flexion. Extend the legs out on a diagonal with soft knees. Use a ball between the knees or ankles if desired.

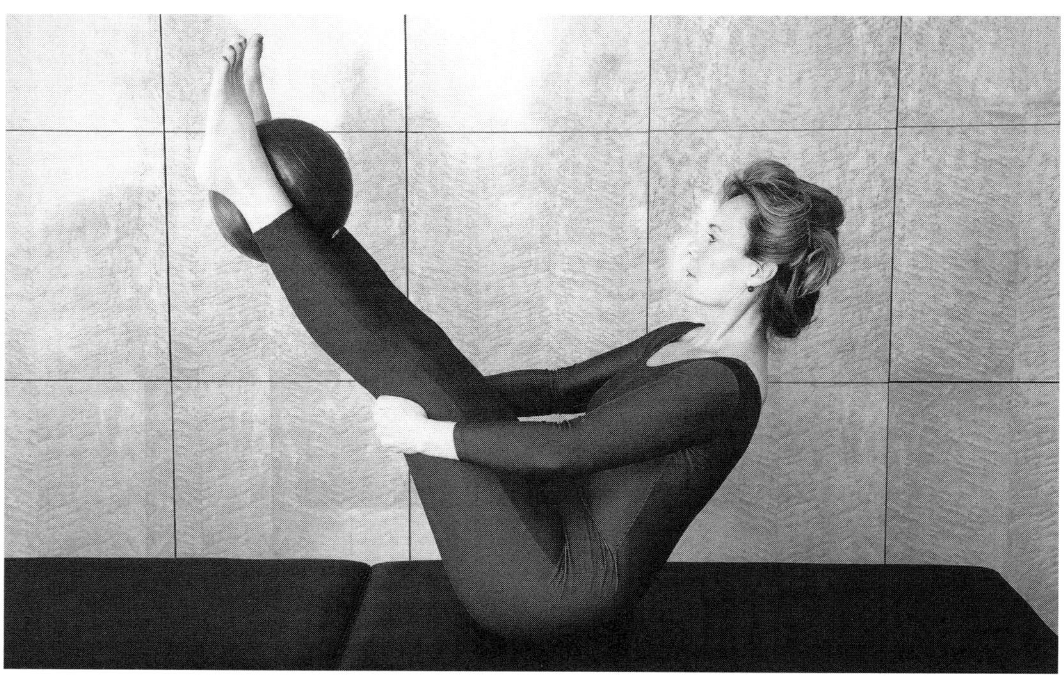

3. Without a ball:
   - Sit tall with the legs slightly bent on the mat. Place the hands under the thighs.
   - Draw the abdominals in and up and roll back off the sit bones, creating a deep scoop in the abdominals and a C-curve in the lower spine.
   - Pick the right leg up into the tabletop position. Follow with the left leg.
   - Keep the legs hip-distance apart and hold the position with a deep scoop in the abdominals and a proud chest. Gaze forward.
   - If desired, extend the right leg out on a diagonal and follow with the left leg. Hold the hands under the thighs or up on the calves. Keep the hands stable on the legs throughout the movement.
   - Inhale and bring the chin to the chest. Exhale and rock back, leading with the lower spine to the bottom tips of the shoulder blades.
   - Exhale and roll back up to a proud chest and a deep scoop in the abdominals.

Look for . . . Encourage

- Moving as one unit—no seesaw with the legs and torso
- Shoulders gliding toward the hip points
- Leading with the lower back, not the head
- Thinking of massaging the spine
- Thinking of the abdominals as a sling through which the body is rolling back and up
- Keeping the hands in the starting position throughout the movement
- If the arms are extended to the calves, keeping the arms straight throughout the movement

Be aware of . . . Prevent

- Rolling too far back to the neck
- Leading the movement with the head and not the lower back
- Loss of core stability

Primary Muscles Activated

The primary muscles activated depend on the chosen option. The primary muscles include the following: Abdominals, shoulder complex, rectus femoris, sartorius, pectineus, iliopsoas, gracilis, biceps femoris, tensor fasciae latae, adductor magnus, adductor longus, adductor brevis, semimembranosus, semitendinosus, gastrocnemius, popliteus, plantaris, vastus lateralis, vastus medialis, vastus intermedius

Corkscrew

Timeline: 3 to 6 months postop

Appropriate for: knee and hip

Location: a floor mat or a raised table as needed; a raised mat for a bilateral knee or hip replacement as needed for up to 6 months postop

Instructions

- Lie supine on the mat with the arms long by the sides of the body and the palms down on the mat.
- Bring one leg at a time into a tabletop position. Exhale and extend both legs to the ceiling, with slightly flexed knees hugging to the midline with or without a small, soft ball between the knees or ankles. Point the toes toward the ceiling. Keep the tailbone long on the mat.
- Prepare to make small circles on the ceiling with both legs moving as one unit.
- Visualize a clock on the ceiling. Inhale to prepare; circle the legs as one unit to 3 o'clock, 6 o'clock, 9 o'clock, and then back to 12 o'clock; pause at the top and reverse. Exhale while circling the legs, drawing the abdominals in and up.
- Inhale to prepare and exhale to 9 o'clock, 6 o'clock, 3 o'clock, and then back to 12 o'clock.
- Keep the circle the size of a large clock on the ceiling.
- Repeat 5 times in each direction.

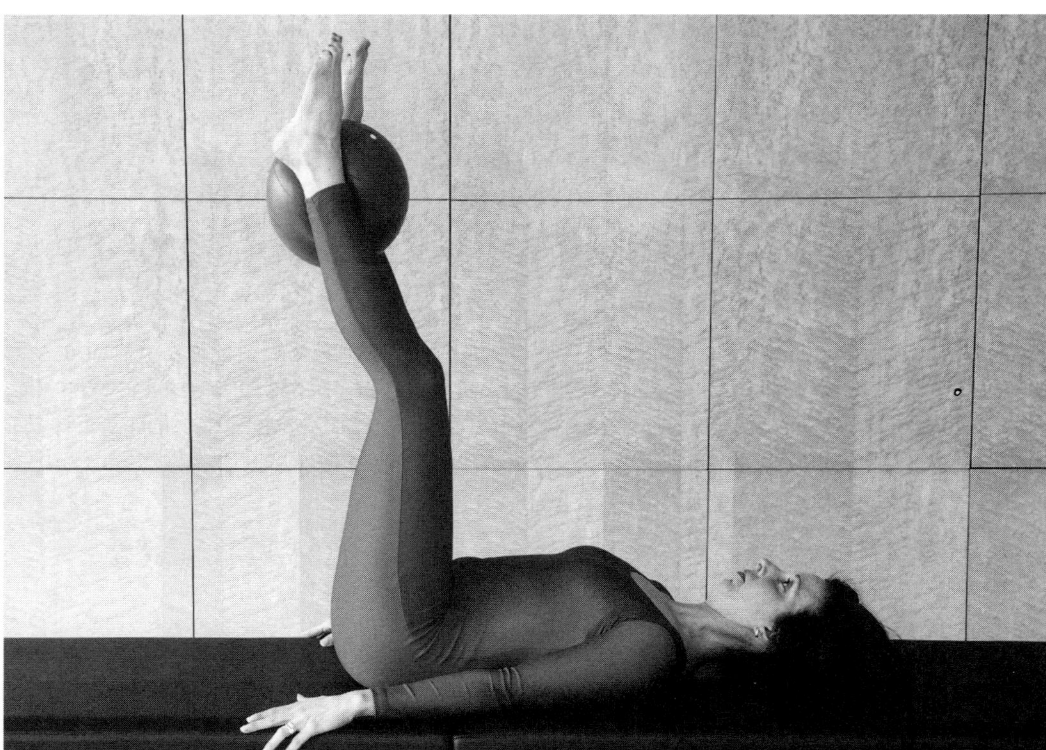

Options

1. **Knee:** Place a small pad between the knees as needed.

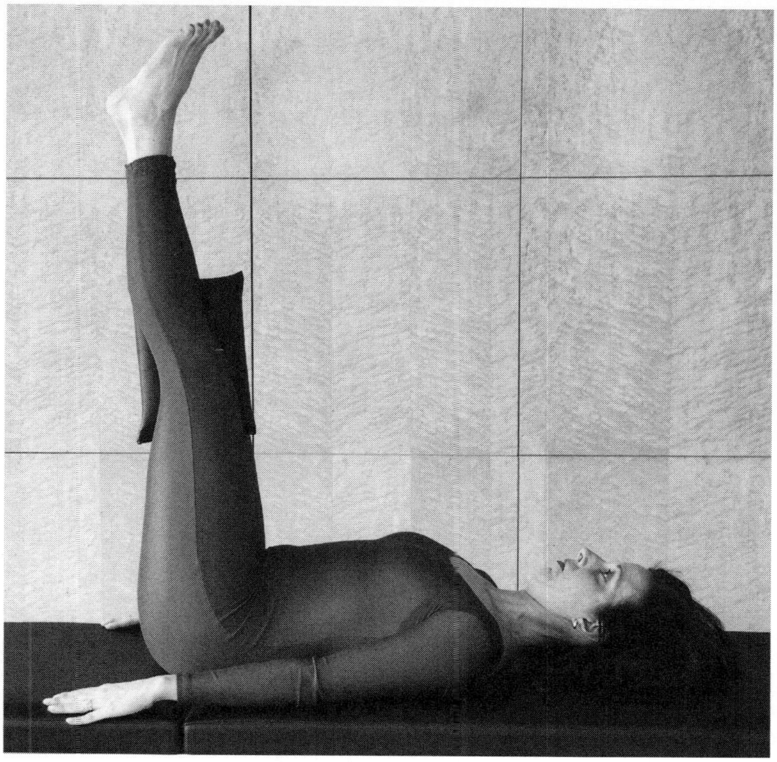

2. **Knee and hip:** Place an exercise band wide around the bottoms of the feet (ball of foot to arch) with the legs in parallel. Lightly grasp the exercise band in each hand and rest the elbows and upper forearm on the mat. Let the legs and abdominals work together to make the circle. Keep the arms and hands fixed with the movement of the legs. Perform the corkscrew.

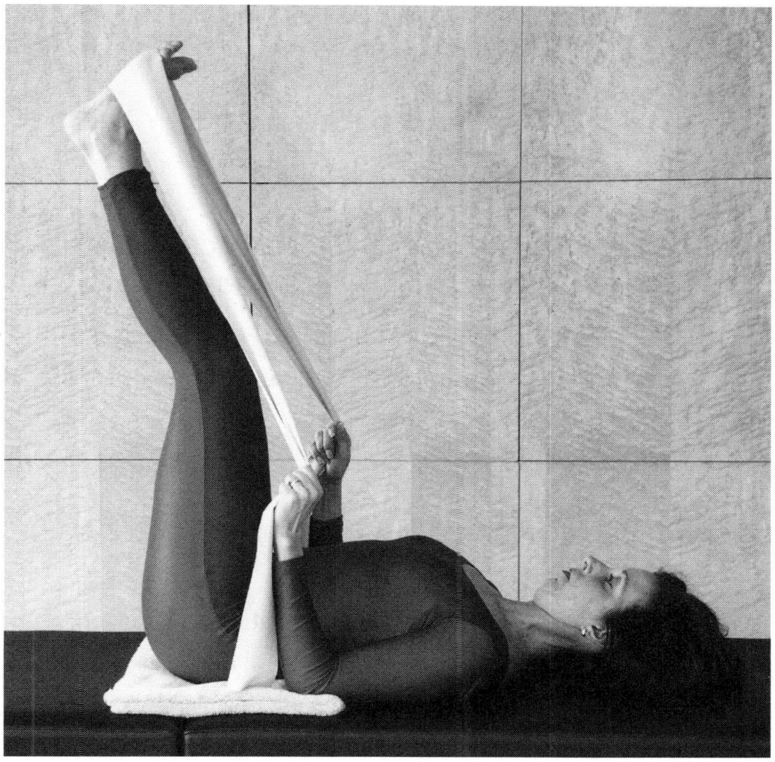

(continued)

Corkscrew *(continued)*

3. Place the hands in a diamond shape under the tailbone. Keep the elbows wide and on the mat. Perform the corkscrew.

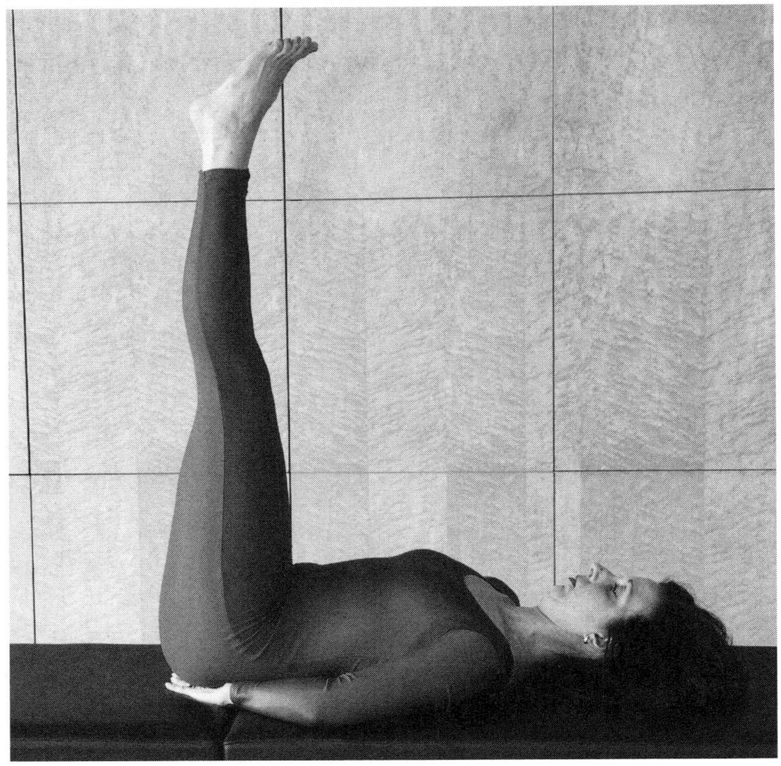

4. **Hip:** Place a small, soft pad or towel under the hip and tailbone to use as a cushion.

Look for . . . Encourage

- Torso and hips stable on the mat, collarbones open, and shoulders away from the ears and gliding toward the hip points
- The back ribs on the mat and the abdominals scooped deeply in and up
- Thinking of the ball of the femur gliding around within the hip socket to make the circle
- Open collar bones with shoulders gliding toward the hip points
- Think of both legs as one unit with the movement

Be aware of . . . Prevent

- Arching the lumbar spine when moving the leg
- Loss of core control
- Rocking the pelvis side to side with the movement

CORKSCREW

Timeline: 6 months and beyond postop
Appropriate for: knee and hip
Location: a floor mat or a raised table as needed

Instructions

- Lie supine on the mat with the arms long by the sides of the body and the palms down on the mat.
- Bring one leg at a time into a tabletop position. Exhale and extend both legs to the ceiling, hugging them together and keeping them parallel. Point the toes to the ceiling. Keep the tailbone long on the mat and the legs at 90°. Use a pad between the knees as needed.
- Prepare to make circles on the ceiling with both legs moving as one unit.
- Visualize a clock on the ceiling. Inhale to prepare; circle the legs as one unit to 3 o'clock, 6 o'clock, 9 o'clock, and then back to 12 o'clock; pause at the top and reverse. Exhale during the circling of the legs, drawing the abdominals in and up.
- Next, add a small lift of the coccyx and the sacrum (1-3 inches [3-8 centimeters] as tolerated) straight up off the mat toward the ceiling with the circling of the legs.
- Inhale to prepare; circle the legs to 3 o'clock, 6 o'clock, 9 o'clock, and then up to 12 o'clock and exhale; lift straight up away from the mat.
- To incorporate the lift, exhale, press the full arm into the mat, create a deep scoop in the abdominals, and lift straight up.
- Repeat 5 times in each direction.
- To advance the movement, make the circle larger by sending the legs out toward a 45° angle all around the circle as tolerated. Keep the hips on the mat and a deep scoop into the abdominals with the circling of the legs.

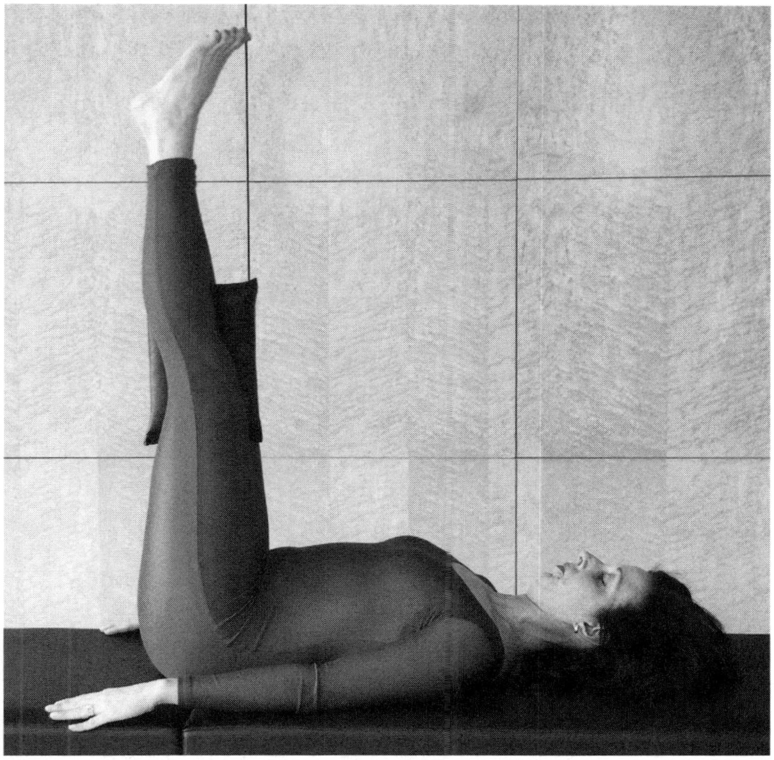

(continued)

Corkscrew *(continued)*

Look for . . . Encourage

- Torso and hips stable on the mat, collarbones open, and shoulders away from the ears and gliding toward the hip points
- Flat palms on the mat
- The back ribs on the mat and the abdominals scooped deeply in and up
- Thinking of the ball of the femur gliding around within the hip socket to make the circle
- Lifting straight up
- Think of both legs as one unit with the movement

Be aware of . . . Prevent

- Arching the lumbar spine when moving the legs
- Folding the legs in toward the chest during the lift
- Claw hands with the movement
- Loss of core control

Primary Muscles Activated

Abdominals, rectus femoris, sartorius, pectineus, iliopsoas, gluteus maximus, gluteus medius, gluteus minimus, tensor fasciae latae, adductor magnus, adductor longus, adductor brevis, gracilis, vastus medialis, vastus intermedius, vastus lateralis, gastrocnemius, soleus, tibialis posterior, plantaris, hamstrings are stretched (biceps femoris, semitendinosus, semimembranosus)

Saw

Timeline: 3 to 6 months and 6 months and beyond postop

Appropriate for: knee and hip

Location: a floor mat or a raised mat as needed; a raised mat for a bilateral knee or hip replacement as needed for up to 6 months postop

Instructions

- Sit tall with the legs extended out to each corner of the mat. The arms are perpendicular to the sides of the body and slightly below shoulder height. The feet are flexed.
- **Knee:**
  - Keep the knees slightly bent and soft.
  - Inhale and twist from the waist to the left.
  - Exhale, bring the chin to the chest, and reach up and over toward the left little toe with the right hand, pinky finger toward pinky toe. The left arm reaches back in opposition.
  - Draw the abdominals in and up while drawing the opposite hip back in opposition.
  - Inhale, roll up in the twist to an upright position, and rotate the spine back to center.
  - Reverse directions and repeat 5 sets.

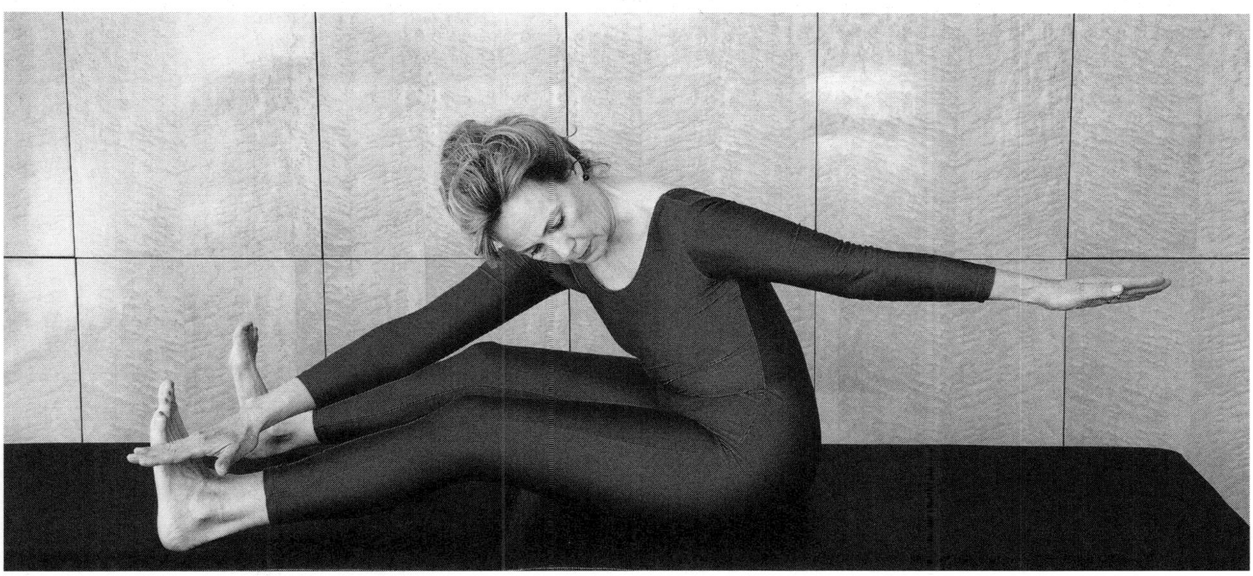

(continued)

- **Hip:**
  - Inhale and twist from the waist to the left.
  - Exhale, bring the chin to the chest, and round up and over toward the left foot, keeping 110° of hip flexion for up to 6 months postop and up to 115° of hip flexion after 6 months postop as shown here. The left arm reaches back in opposition.
  - Draw the abdominals in and up while drawing the opposite hip back in opposition.
  - Inhale, roll the spine to an upright position, and then rotate the spine back to center.
  - Reverse directions and repeat 5 sets.

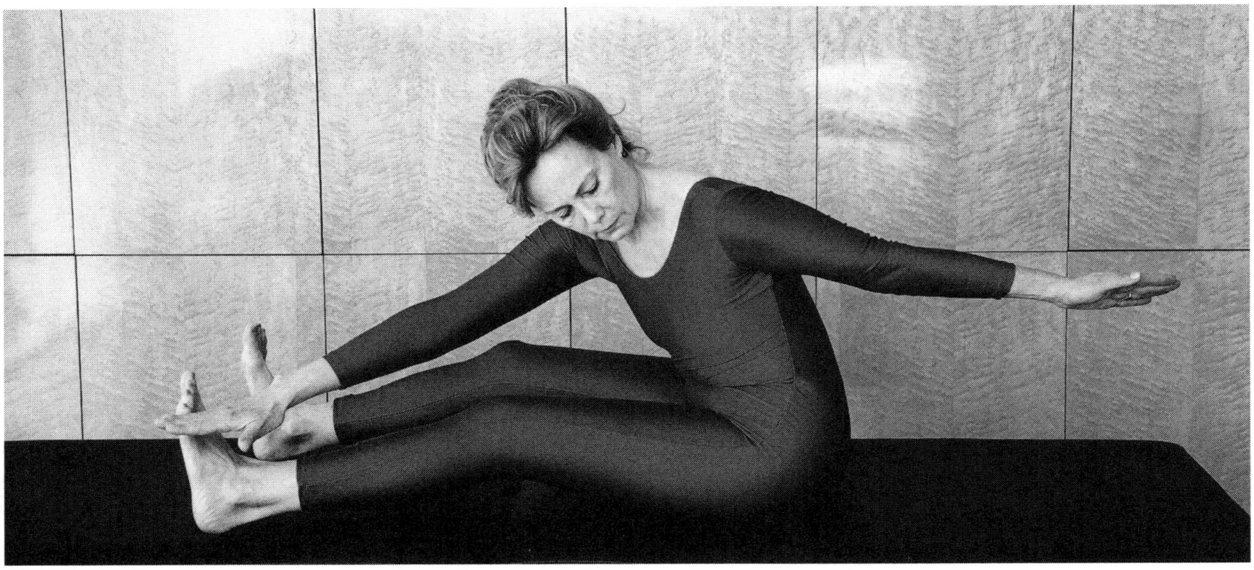

Options

1. Place a rolled-up towel under knees.

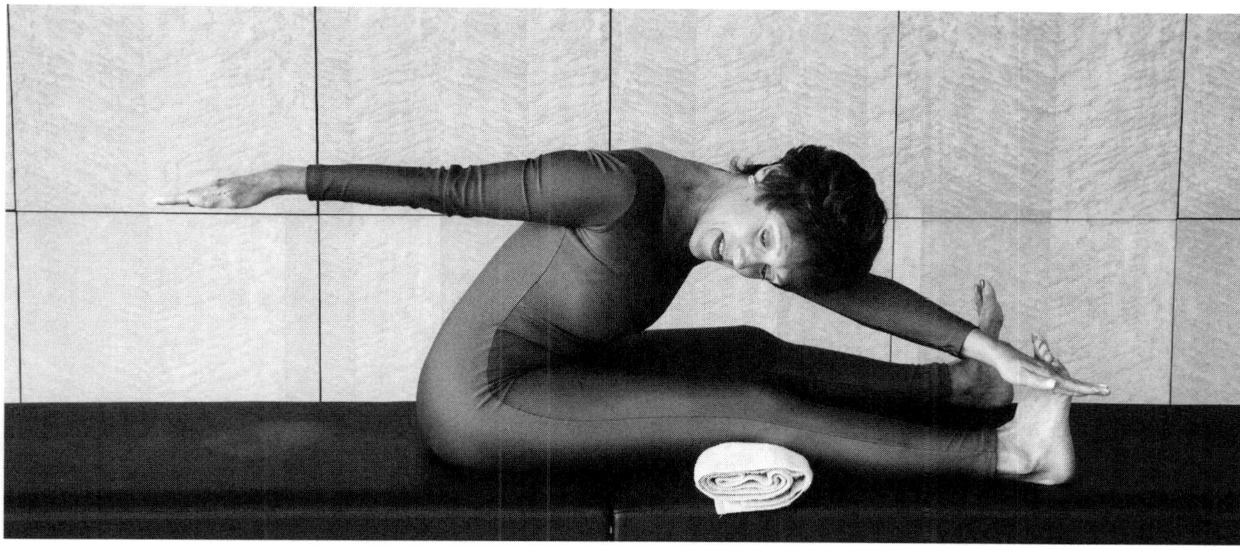

2. Use an exercise band to increase the resistance and guide the movement.

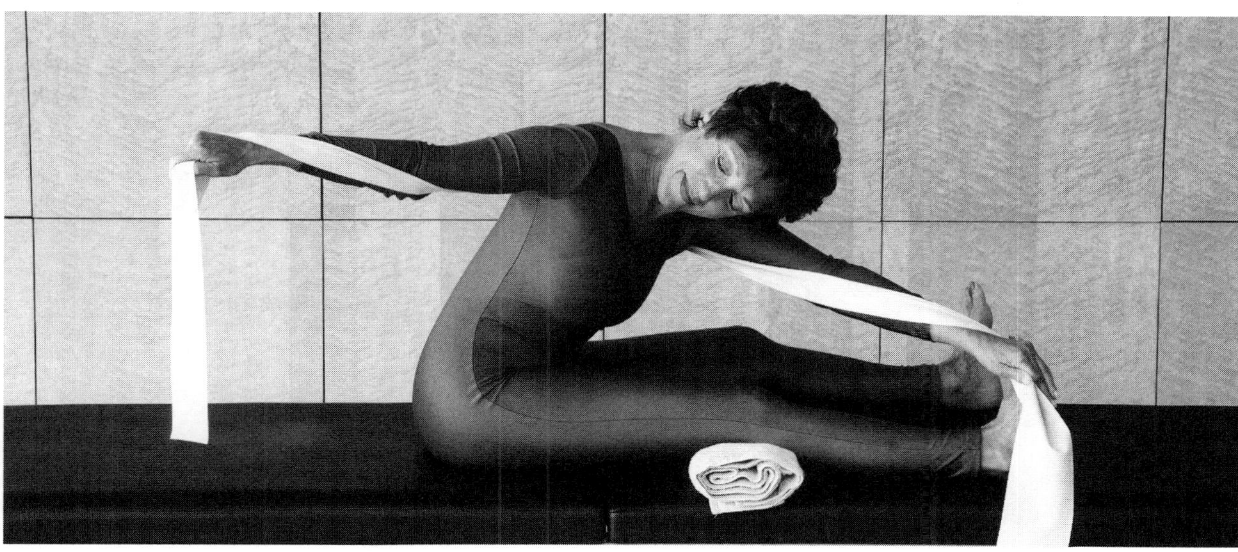

3. Place a folded towel under the buttocks as needed.
4. Sit on a small raised box such as a moon box to raise the pelvis from the mat. This is very helpful when the hamstrings are shortened and tight.

(continued)

Look for . . . Encourage

- Thinking of the spine stretch forward exercise when reaching to the outside little toe with the palm facing the floor
- Thinking of reaching up and over toward the little toe
- Shoulders gliding toward the hips as if suspenders were hooked to the bottom tips of the shoulder blades and attached to the hips
- Abdominals drawn in deeply to the spine
- Sitting tall as if against a wall
- Stable pelvis

Be aware of . . . Prevent

- Feet rolling in or out when reaching to the little toe
- Folding from the hip to create the movement
- Loss of core control
- Stable pelvis

Primary Muscles Activated

Abdominals, biceps, triceps, shoulder complex, multifidi, rotators, iliopsoas, rectus femoris, pectineus, gracilis, sartorius, adductor longus, adductor brevis, vastus medialis, vastus intermedius, vastus lateralis, tensor fasciae latae, tibialis anterior, hamstrings are stretched (biceps femoris, semitendinosus, semimembranosus)

Swan Prep

Timeline: 3 to 6 months postop

Appropriate for: knee and hip

Location: a floor mat or a raised mat as needed; a raised mat for a bilateral knee or hip replacement as needed for up to 6 months postop

Instructions

- Lie prone on the mat, make a pillow with the hands, and place the forehead onto the tops of the hands *(a)*.
- Keep the feet hip-distance apart, the legs parallel, and the shoulders gliding toward the hips.
- Feel the tops of the toes, deepen the pubic bone toward the mat, and slightly engage the gluteus muscles and hamstrings.
- Draw the abdominals in and up; feel as though you could shoot air between the mat and the belly button.
- Inhale and begin to lift the head, neck, and chest, with the hands glued to the forehead, as one unit from the mat *(b)*. Hold for 2 counts, exhale, and lengthen back down to the mat.
- Keep the head in line with the spine.
- Repeat 3 to 5 times.

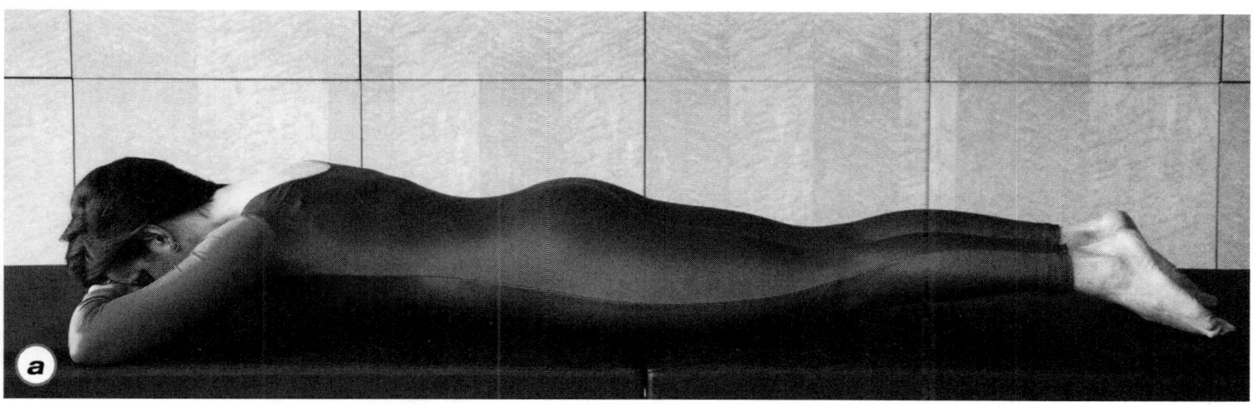

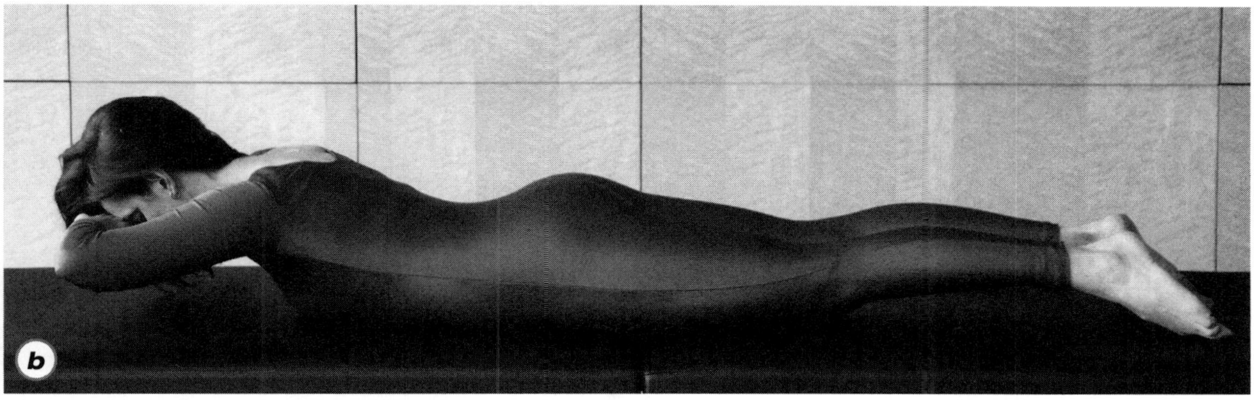

(continued)

Option

To increase the degree of difficulty, try the following:

- Inhale and begin to lift the head, chest, and arms as one unit away from the mat.
- Exhale and lengthen both arms, palms down, out to the side as if to touch the walls.
- Inhale and return the hands to a pillow under the head.
- Exhale and lengthen back down to the mat.

Look for . . . Encourage

- The head follows the alignment of the spine
- The shoulders glide toward the hip points as the upper body lengthens up
- Abdominals are drawn in and up, feeling the waistband snapping to the spine

Be aware of . . . Prevent

- Hyperextension of the lumbar spine
- Head lower than the rest of the spine with the movement
- Loss of core control

Primary Muscles Activated

Abdominals, splenius capitis, splenius cervicis, transversospinalis group, erector spinae group, quadratus lumborum (assists), intertransversarii, interspinalis, latissimus dorsi, gluteus maximus, gluteus medius (posterior portion), adductor magnus (ischiocondylar portion), biceps femoris, semitendinosus, semimembranosus, rectus femoris, vastus medius, vastus intermedius, vastus lateralis, tensor fasciae latae, tibialis posterior, gastrocnemius, plantaris, soleus

Swan

Restrictions: not applicable for knee and hip at 3 to 6 months postop; perform the swan prep on page 191

Timeline: 6 months and beyond postop

Appropriate for: knee and hip

Location: a floor mat or a raised table as needed

Instructions

- Lie prone on the mat and place the hands with the fingers open wide a few inches (centimeters) in front of the shoulders. Hold the elbows up off the mat and in by the sides of the rib cage *(a)*.

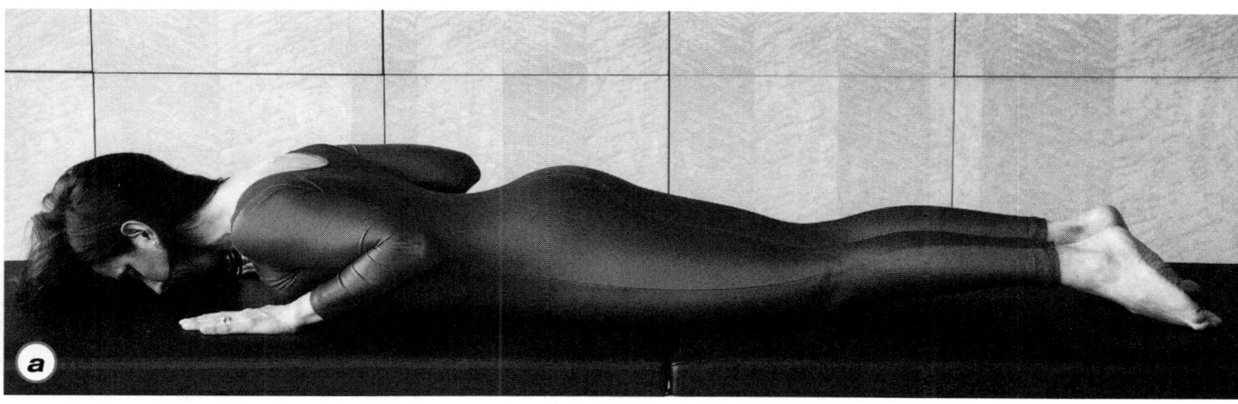

- Keep the shoulders away from the ears and gliding toward the hips.
- With the feet about 6 inches (15 centimeters) apart and the legs parallel, feel the tops of the toes, deepen the pubic bone toward the mat, and slightly engage the gluteus muscles and hamstrings.

(continued)

Swan *(continued)*

- Draw the abdominals in and up; feel as though you could shoot air between the mat and the belly button.
- Inhale and lift the head, neck, and chest away from the mat. Press into the hands and continue to lift up as high as you can, keeping the shoulders away from the ears and the abdominals in and up *(b)*. Hold for 3 counts and then exhale and lengthen back down to the mat rib by rib.
- Repeat 3 to 5 times.

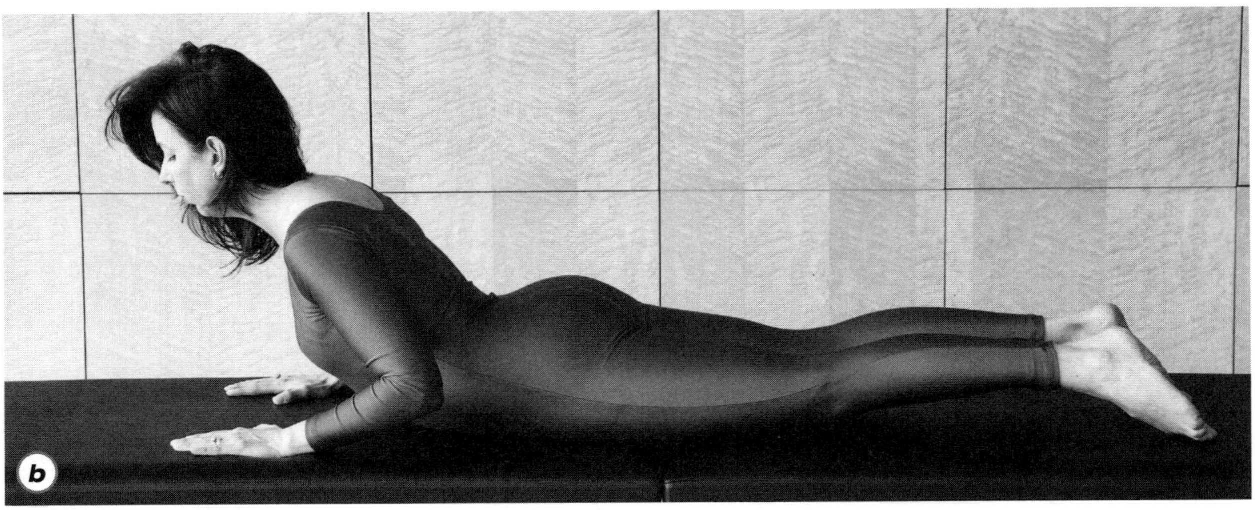

Options

1. Reverse the breath. Exhale to lengthen up and inhale to return.
2. Start with the forearms on the mat. Move hands closer toward the face to place the forearms and then lift into extension.

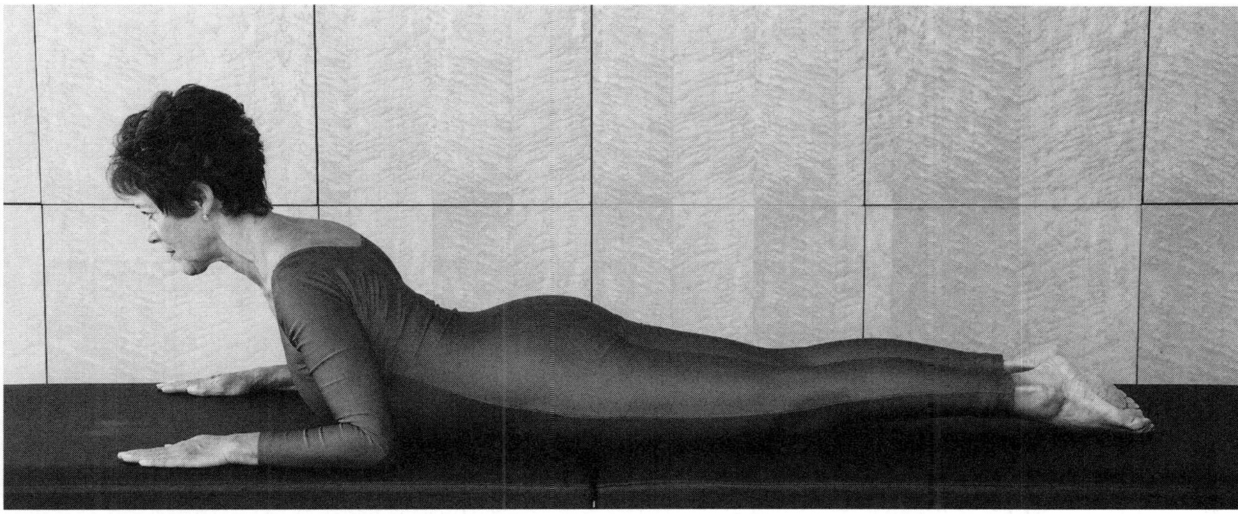

Look for . . . Encourage

- The head following the alignment of the spine
- The shoulders gliding toward the hip points as the upper body lengthens up
- Lengthening away from the mat only to the point that the shoulders remain gliding toward the hip points and the abdominals remain engaged
- Even articulation of the spine into extension

Be aware of...Prevent

- Hyperextension of the lumbar spine
- Head lower than the rest of the spine during the movement
- Loss of core control

Primary Muscles Activated

Abdominals, splenius capitis, splenius cervicis, transversospinalis group, erector spinae group, quadratus lumborum (assists), intertransversarii, interspinalis, latissimus dorsi, gluteus maximus, gluteus medius (posterior portion), adductor magnus (ischiocondylar portion), biceps femoris, semitendinosus, semimembranosus, rectus femoris, vastus medius, vastus intermedius, vastus lateralis, tensor fasciae latae, tibialis posterior, gastrocnemius, plantaris, soleus

Single-Leg Kick

Timeline: 3 to 6 months and 6 months and beyond postop

Appropriate for: knee and hip

Location: a floor mat or a raised mat as needed; a raised mat for a bilateral knee or hip replacement as needed for up to 6 months postop

Instructions

- Lie prone and prop up on the forearms with the elbows under the shoulders. Make a fist with the hands and face the palms toward each other. Extend the legs all the way onto the mat and keep them hip-distance apart.
- Lift the head, chest, and rib cage away from the floor as one unit. The head and neck are an extension of the spine. Keep the upper body lifted from the floor.
- Feel the forearms press into the mat and hug the midline as if you were holding a magic circle. Feel as though you are pulling yourself through the window of your arms (press, hug, and pull).
- Keep this stable position as you perform the movement.
- Place the tops of the toes on the mat, draw the abdominals in and up toward the spine, and engage the gluteus muscles, keeping the hips on the mat.
- Lift both legs a few inches off the mat and hold. Bend the right knee and kick the heel toward the buttocks.
- Kick, kick the right heel in toward the buttocks and lengthen the right leg back down and hover it over the mat while you kick, kick the left heel.
- Smoothly flow from one leg to the next.
- Maintain normal breathing throughout the set.
- **Knee:** Bend the knee toward the buttocks with control. Use a slower pace. Keep working to increase flexion, and add a double pulse as tolerated.
- Repeat 8 times per leg.

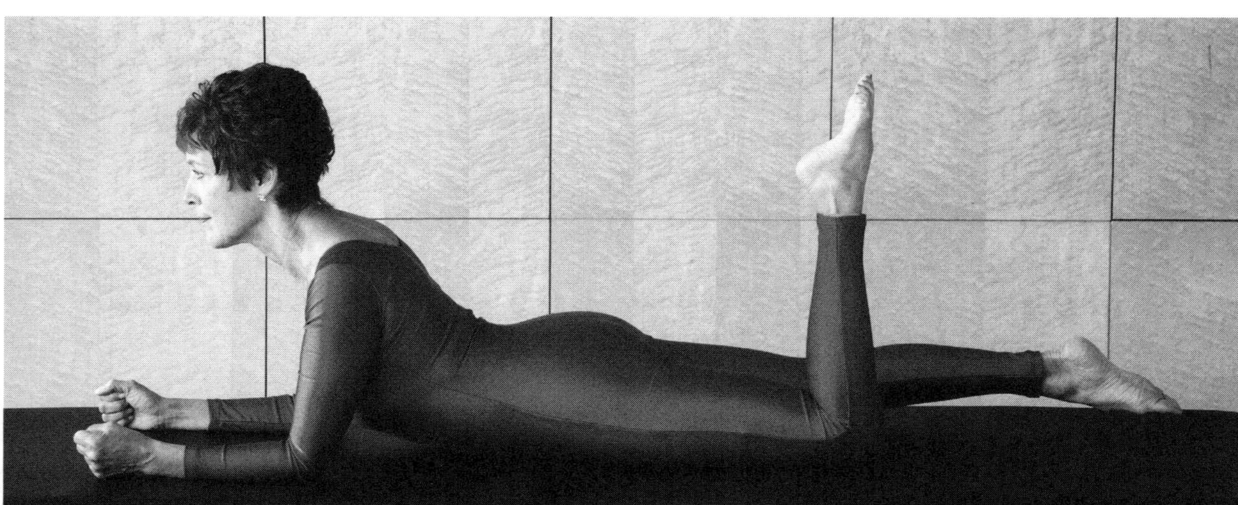

Option

Continue with the 6 weeks to 3 month postop version (see p. 113) as needed, especially for bilateral knee and hip replacement.

Look for . . . Encourage

- Chest lifted away from the mat and forearms
- Shoulders gliding toward the hips as if suspenders were hooked to the bottom tips of the shoulder blades and attached to the hips
- Movement without pain in the knee and hip
- Abdominals lifted in and up and away from the mat
- Hips stable on the mat with the movement of the legs

Be aware of . . . Prevent

- Hyperextension of the lumbar spine
- Sinking between the shoulder blades
- Loss of core control
- Torso swaying side to side with the movement

Primary Muscles Activated

Abdominals, triceps, biceps, shoulder complex, splenius capitis, splenius cervicis, transversospinalis group, erector spinae group, quadratus lumborum (assists), intertransversarii, interspinalis, latissimus dorsi, gluteus maximus, gluteus medius (posterior portion), adductor magnus (ischiocondylar part), biceps femoris, semimembranosus, semitendinosus, gracilis, gastrocnemius, sartorius, popliteus, plantaris, rectus femoris, vastus medialis, vastus intermedius, vastus lateralis, tibialis posterior, soleus

Double-Leg Kick

Timeline: 3 to 6 months and 6 months and beyond postop

Appropriate for: knee and hip

Location: a floor mat or a raised mat as needed; a raised mat for a bilateral knee or hip replacement as needed for up to 6 months postop

Instructions

- Lie prone on the mat with the face turned toward the left and the right cheek on the mat. Extend the legs all the way onto the mat, keeping them hip-distance apart.
- Clasp the hands together and place them on the back (hand over hand). Move the hands up as high as you can with the elbows reaching toward the floor *(a)*.
- Rest the tops of the toes on the mat, draw the abdominals in and up, and engage the gluteus muscles, keeping the hips on the mat.
- Exhale and bend both knees, bringing the heels to the buttocks. Pulse 1, 2, 3. Inhale and extend both legs back onto the mat. Lift the head, neck, shoulders, and chest away from the mat as the arms extend, hovering away from the back toward the feet *(b)*. Follow the alignment of the spine with the head.

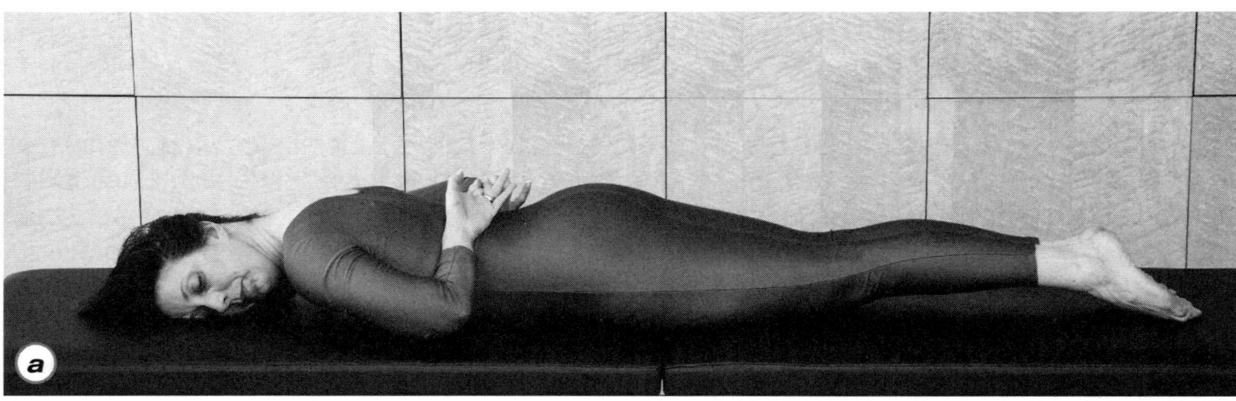

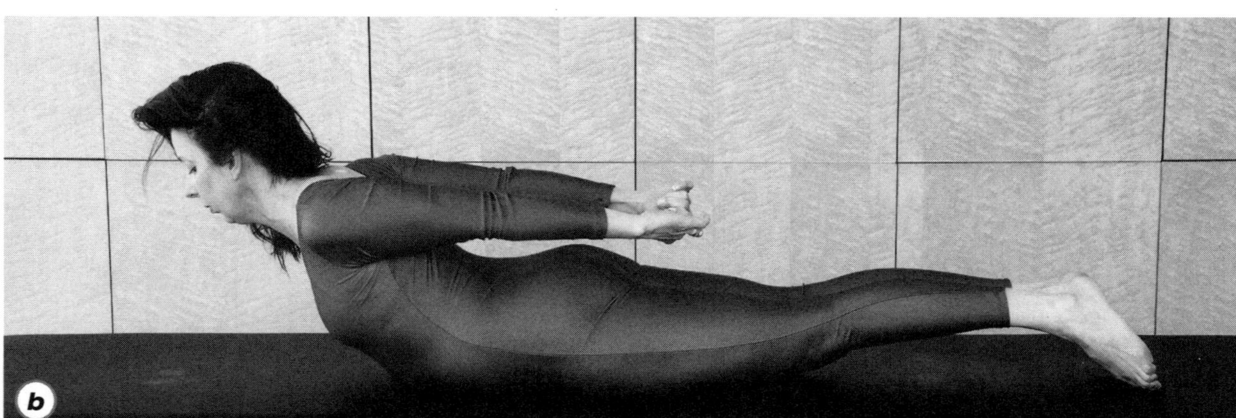

- Draw the shoulder blades away from the ears as you extend the spine.
- Exhale and lower the upper body back to the starting position. Turn the head to the opposite side.
- **Knee:** Bend the knees toward the buttocks with control (use a slower pace). Keep working to increase flexion, and add the pulse as tolerated. Move without pain.
- **Hip:** Bend the knees toward the hips as tolerated.
- Repeat 6 to 8 times.

Option

This option may be necessary for bilateral hip or knee replacements:

- Make a pillow with the hands and place the forehead facedown on the hands.
- Exhale and bend both legs. Bring the heels to the buttocks and pulse 1, 2, 3.
- Inhale and extend both legs back to the mat while drawing the abdominals in and up. Keep the head, neck, and shoulders on the mat.
- Place a towel under the hips and lower abdominals.

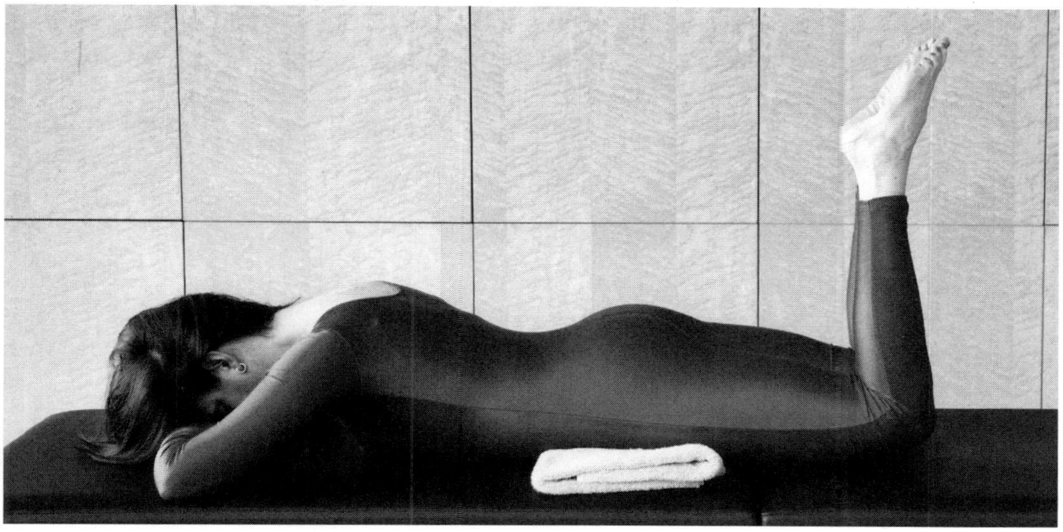

(continued)

Look for . . . Encourage

- Hip points on the mat with the movement of the legs
- The shoulders gliding toward the hips as if suspenders were hooked to the bottom tips of the shoulder blades and attached to the hips
- Abdominals drawn in deep at all times
- Movement without pain

Be aware of . . . Prevent

- Hyperextension of the lumbar spine
- Hyperextension of the neck
- Loss of core control

Primary Muscles Activated

Abdominals, triceps, biceps, shoulder complex, splenius capitis, splenius cervicis, transversospinalis group, erector spinae group, quadratus lumborum (assists), intertransversarii, interspinalis, latissimus dorsi, gluteus maximus, biceps femoris, semimembranosus, semitendinosus, gracilis, gastrocnemius, sartorius, popliteus, plantaris, rectus femoris, vastus medialis, vastus intermedius, vastus lateralis, tibialis posterior, soleus

Spine Twist

Timeline: 3 to 6 months and 6 months and beyond postop

Appropriate for: knee and hip

Location: a floor mat or a raised mat as needed; a raised mat for a bilateral knee or hip replacement as needed for up to 6 months postop

Instructions

- Sit tall with the legs lengthened out on the mat and the feet flexed. Place a rolled-up towel under the knees and a small, soft ball between the ankles. Keep the legs hip-distance apart. Hug the ball to the midline of the body.
- Think of a rod holding you up tall and a string running from the crown of your head to the ceiling.
- Keep the arms perpendicular to the sides of the body and lengthened out slightly below shoulder height. Reach out as if to touch the walls.
- Inhale to prepare. Exhale and rotate from the waist, twisting to the right. Let the head and neck continue the rotation. Look over the fingers. Sit tall as you twist, drawing the abdominals in deeply as if you were wringing all the air out of the lungs.
- Hold the position for a count of 2.
- Inhale and return to the center.
- Exhale and twist to the left from the waist. Maintain a tall back, and hold for a count of 2.
- As you twist to one direction, draw the opposite hip back in opposition to the twist and keep it stable on the mat.
- **Knee and hip:** Sit up on a moon box or folded towel or blanket as needed. Place a rolled-up towel or ball under the knees as needed.
- Repeat 4 times in each direction.

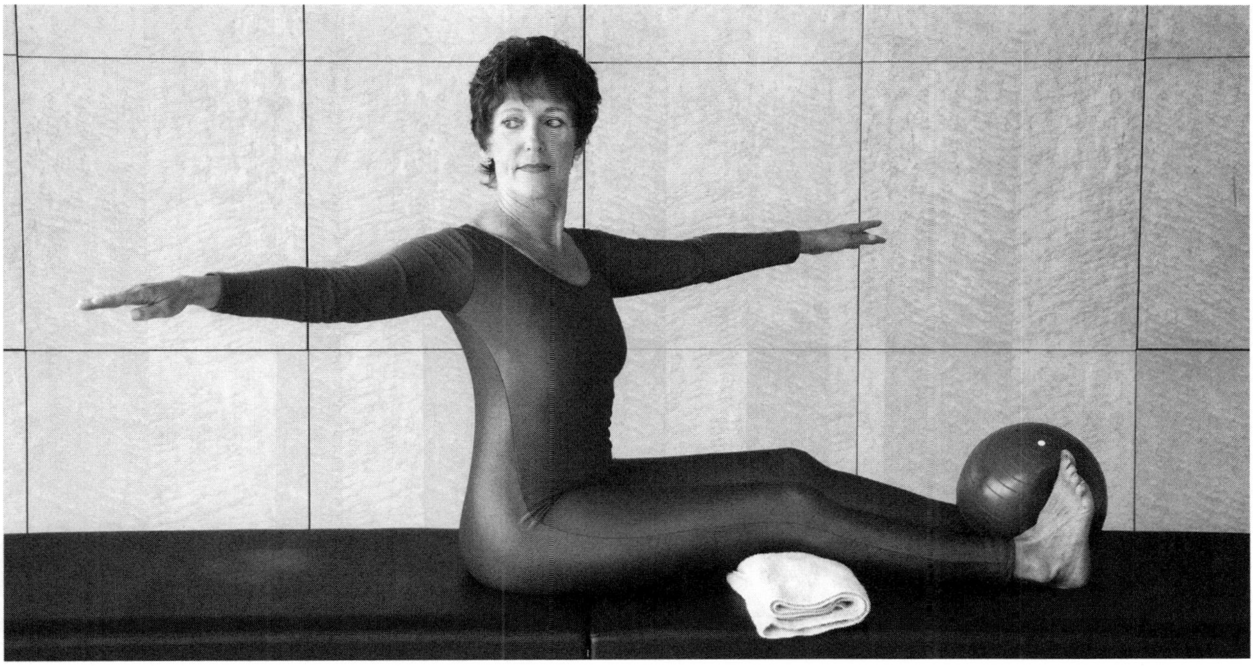

(continued)

Options

1. Sit tall on a moon box with a small, soft ball under the knees.

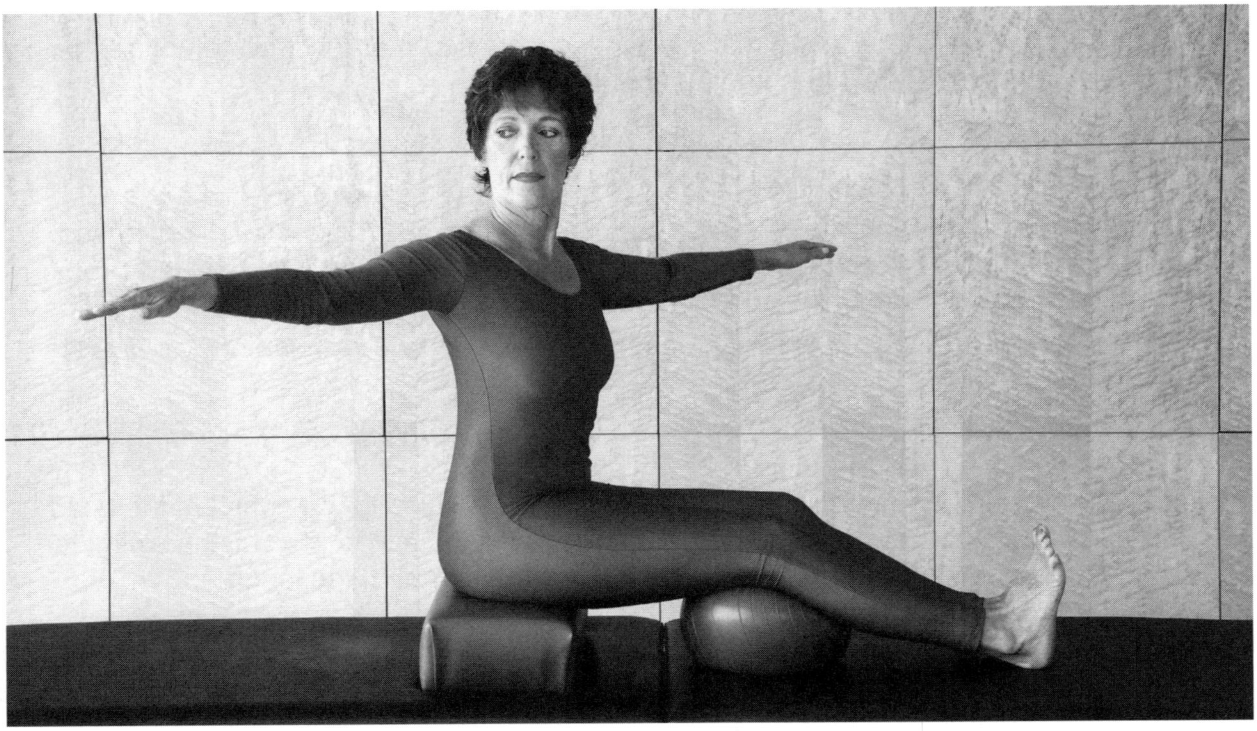

2. Sit tall with a small, soft ball under the knees.

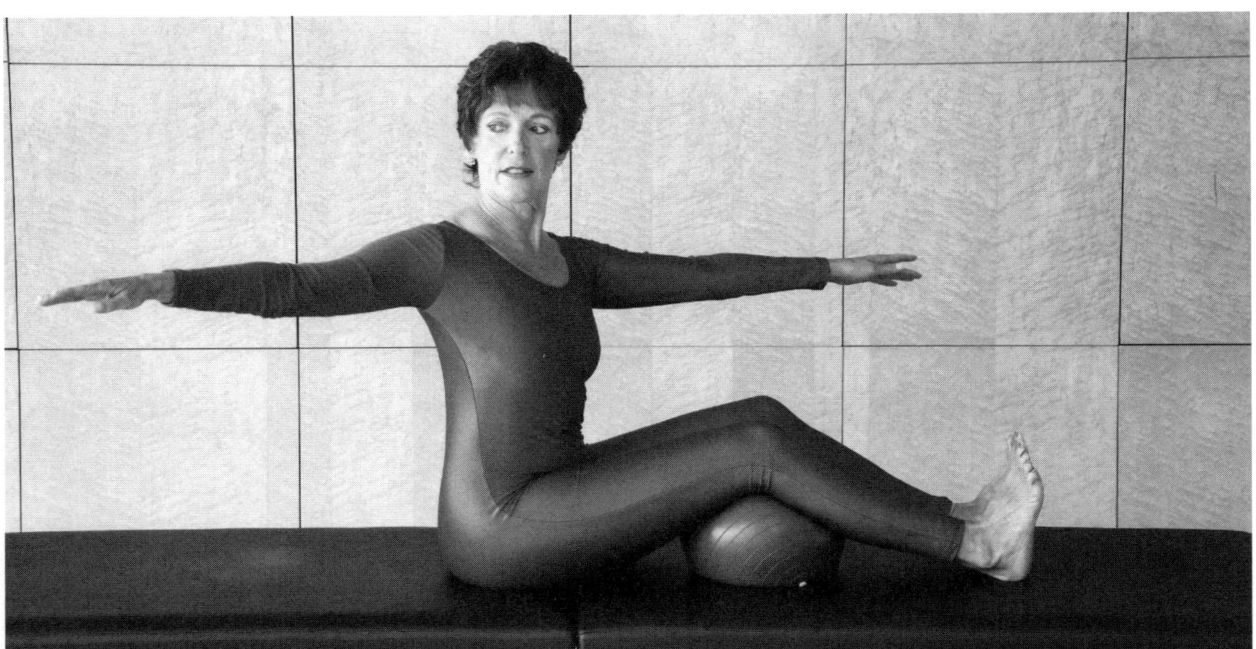

Look for . . . Encourage

- The shoulders gliding down the back
- Twisting only to the point that shoulder alignment is maintained
- The head following in the twist and looking out over the hand
- The abdominals drawn in deeply
- Feeling as if the twist were wringing all of the water out of a sponge
- Sitting tall like a tree reaching to the clouds
- Stable pelvis

Be aware of . . . Prevent

- Feet rolling in, out, or apart when twisting
- Shoulders lifting with the twist
- Hips shifting when twisting

Primary Muscles Activated

Abdominals, biceps, triceps, shoulder complex, multifidi, rotators, iliopsoas, rectus femoris, pectineus, gracilis, sartorius, adductor longus, adductor brevis, adductor magnus, vastus medialis, vastus intermedius, vastus lateralis, tensor fasciae latae, tibialis anterior, hamstrings are stretched (biceps femoris, semitendinosus, semimembranosus)

Neck Pull (Modified)

Timeline: 3 to 6 months postop

Appropriate for: knee and hip

Location: a raised mat for a bilateral knee or hip replacement as needed for up to 6 months postop

Instructions

- Sit tall with the knees slightly bent and the legs extended hip-distance apart on the mat. Flex the feet. Place a small, soft ball between the ankles or shins. Lightly hug the ball to the midline of the body. Place a rolled-up towel under the knees as needed. Place the hands on each side of thighs *(a)*.
- Inhale to prepare. Exhale and bring the chin toward the chest (keeping the space of a tangerine between the chin and chest). Draw the abdominals in and up, leading with the lower back. Roll off the sit bones toward the mat and slowly roll down one vertebra at a time all the way to the mat *(b)*.

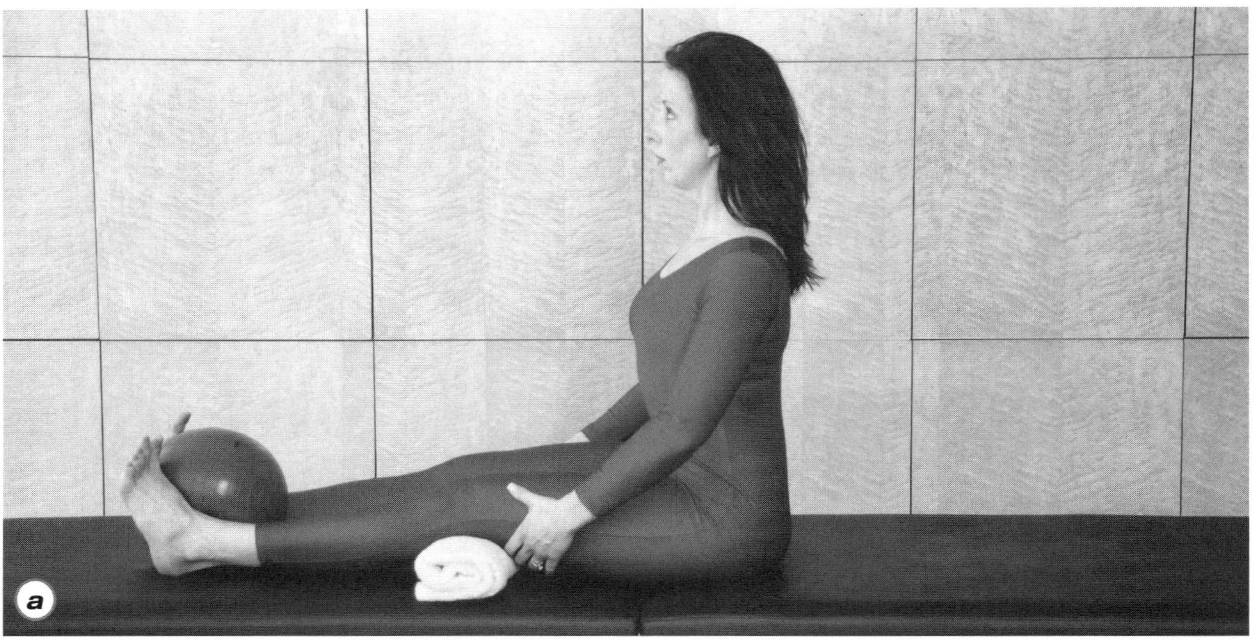

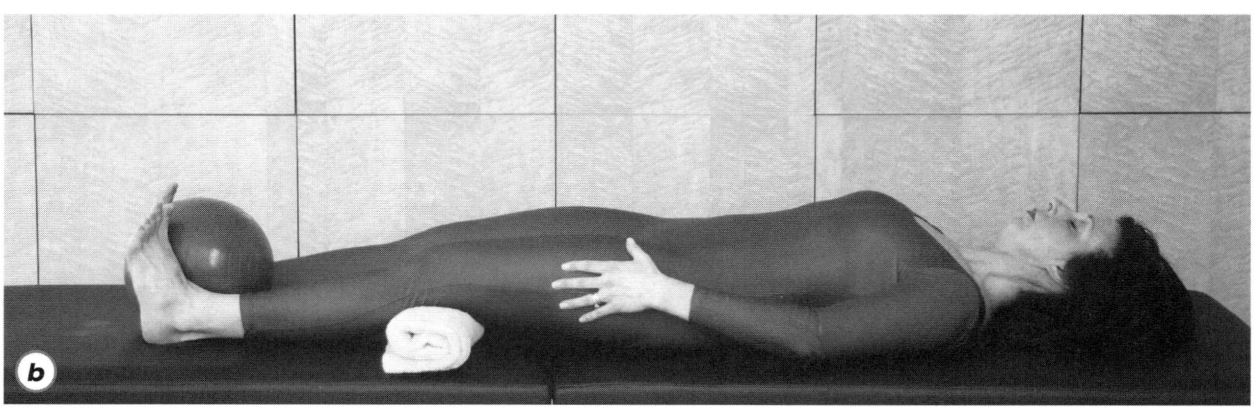

- Keep the hands on the thighs next to the hips. Inhale to prepare. Exhale and curl the head and shoulders off the mat. Looking toward the feet, draw the abdominals in deeply as you round all the way over to kiss your knees.
- Inhale and roll up one vertebra at a time, sitting tall.
- **Knee:** Slightly flex the knees or bend the knees as needed.
- **Hip:** Roll back up and over to no more than 110° of hip flexion, as shown here *(c)*. Place a small towel or pad under the buttocks and low back for comfort as needed. Keep the knees soft.
- When rolling down to the mat, think of rolling toward the sacrum, waist, ribs, upper back, shoulders, and then head. Lower down in opposition to the heels. Reach through the heels to create opposition and resistance.
- Repeat 5 to 10 times.

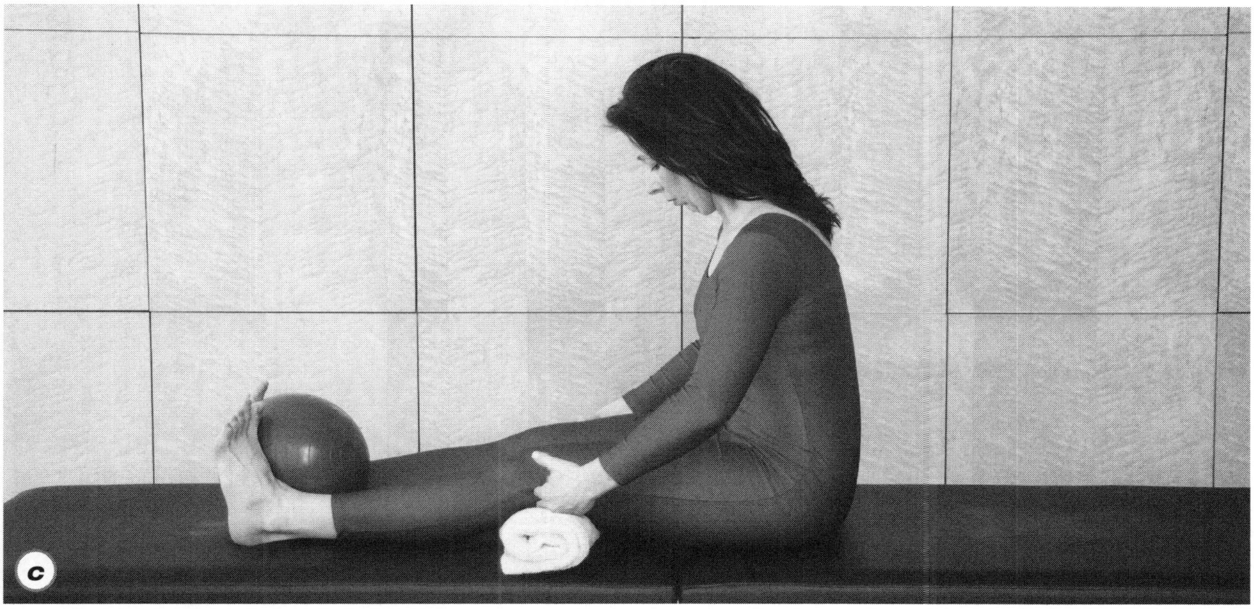

(continued)

Neck Pull (Modified) *(continued)*

Options

1. Place a towel under the hips for comfort.
2. Use two soft balls 9 inches (23 centimeters) in diameter; place one between the ankles and one between the knees. Gently squeeze to increase the engagement of the adductors.

Look for . . . Encourage

- The shoulders gliding toward the hips as if suspenders were hooked to the bottom tips of the shoulder blades and attached to the hips
- Even articulation of the spine
- Abdominals drawn in and up

Be aware of . . . Prevent

- Rolling the legs in and turning the toes in instead of pointing them to the ceiling
- Using momentum and lifting the legs to roll up
- Loss of core control
- Hyperextension of the knees
- Loss of shoulder alignment

Primary Muscles Activated

Abdominals, biceps, deltoid, shoulder complex, back extensors, iliopsoas, rectus femoris, gluteus medius, gluteus maximus, sartorius, pectineus, gracilis, adductor magnus, adductor longus, adductor brevis, biceps femoris, semitendinosus, semimembranosus, vastus medialis, vastus intermedius, vastus lateralis, tensor fasciae latae, tibialis anterior

Neck Pull

Restrictions: not applicable for knee and hip at 3 to 6 months postop; perform the modified neck pull on page 204

Timeline: 6 months and beyond postop

Appropriate for: knee and hip

Location: a floor mat or a raised table as needed

Instructions

- Sit tall with the legs extended hip-distance apart and the feet flexed with or without a small, soft ball between the ankles or shins. Use a rolled-up towel under knees as needed.
- Clasp one hand on top of the other and place the hands behind the head at the base of the skull with the thumbs running down the sides of the neck *(a)*.
- Inhale to prepare. Exhale, keep the chin to the chest (separated by the space of a tangerine), and draw the abdominals in and up. Leading with the lower back, roll off the sit bones and slowly roll down one vertebra at a time to the mat *(b)*.
- Keep the hands behind the head with the elbows in peripheral vision or pointed to the ceiling. Inhale to prepare. Exhale and curl the head and shoulders off the mat, looking toward the feet. Draw the abdominals in deeply as you roll back up, rounding over as if to kiss the knees *(c)*.
- Inhale and roll up one vertebra at a time to sitting tall *(d)*.
- **Knee:** Slightly flex the knees as needed. Place a rolled-up towel under the knees as needed. Prevent hyperextension of the knees when you roll down to the mat.
- **Hip:** Roll up and over to keep up to 115° of hip flexion *(c)*. Keep the knees soft.
- Repeat 5 to 10 times.
- When rolling down to the mat, think of rolling toward the sacrum, waist, ribs, upper back, shoulders, and then head. Lower down in opposition to the heels. Reach through the heels to create opposition and resistance.
- Note: The neck pull is a strong intermediate exercise and requires concentration and good core control to perform the movement without lifting the legs and overengaging the hip flexors. You should be able to perform the modified neck pull with good core control before the full version is initiated.

(continued)

Neck Pull *(continued)*

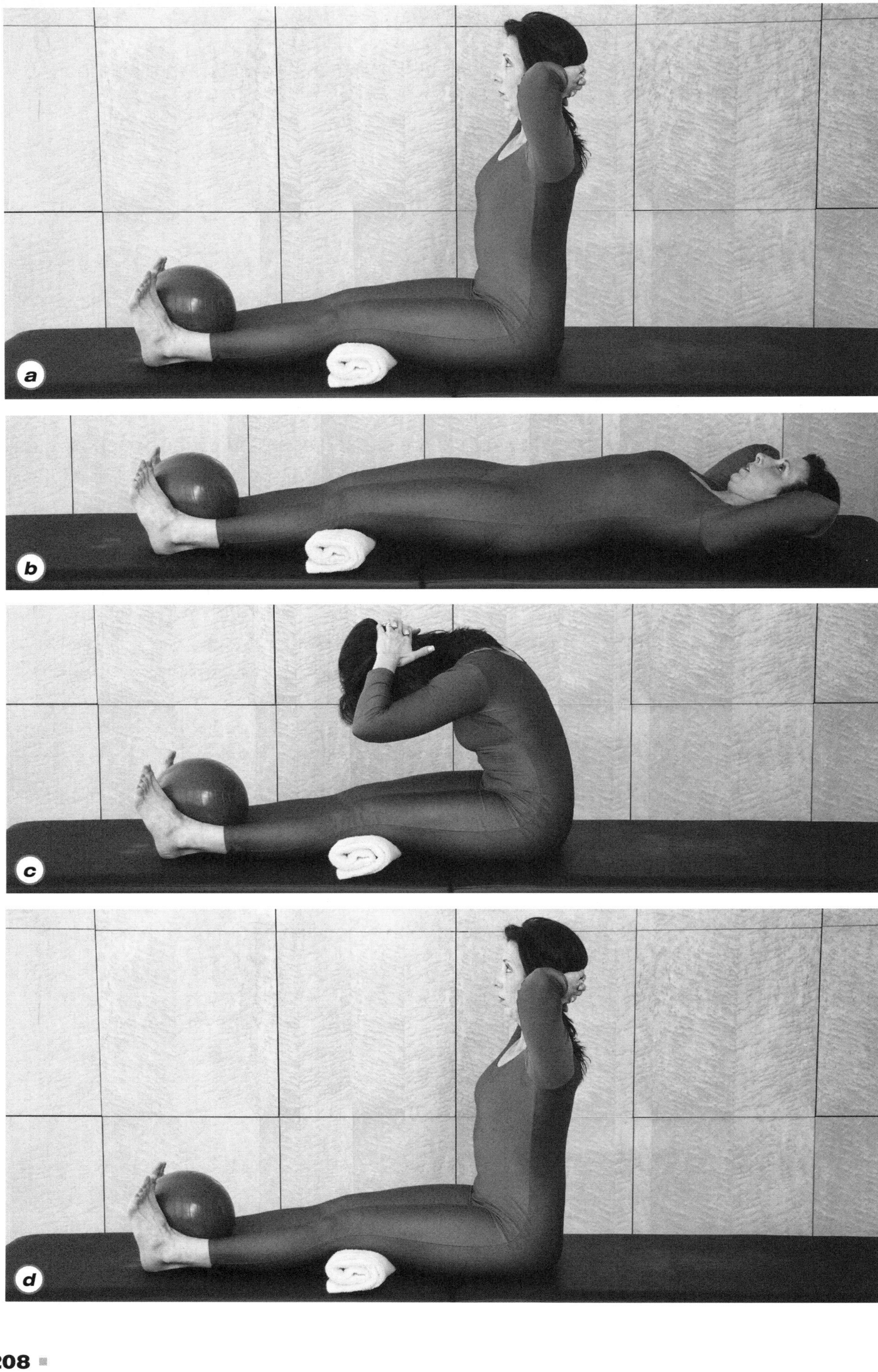

Options

1. Begin with a straight back *(a)*. Inhale, hinge back with a flat back a few inches, and then exhale *(b)*. With the chin to the chest, scoop the abdominals in and up and roll down to the mat one vertebra at a time. Inhale to prepare. Exhale and curl the head and shoulders off the mat, looking toward the feet. Draw the abdominals in deeply as you roll back up, rounding over as if to kiss the knees.
2. Place a small, soft ball between the knees and gently squeeze to increase the engagement of the adductors.

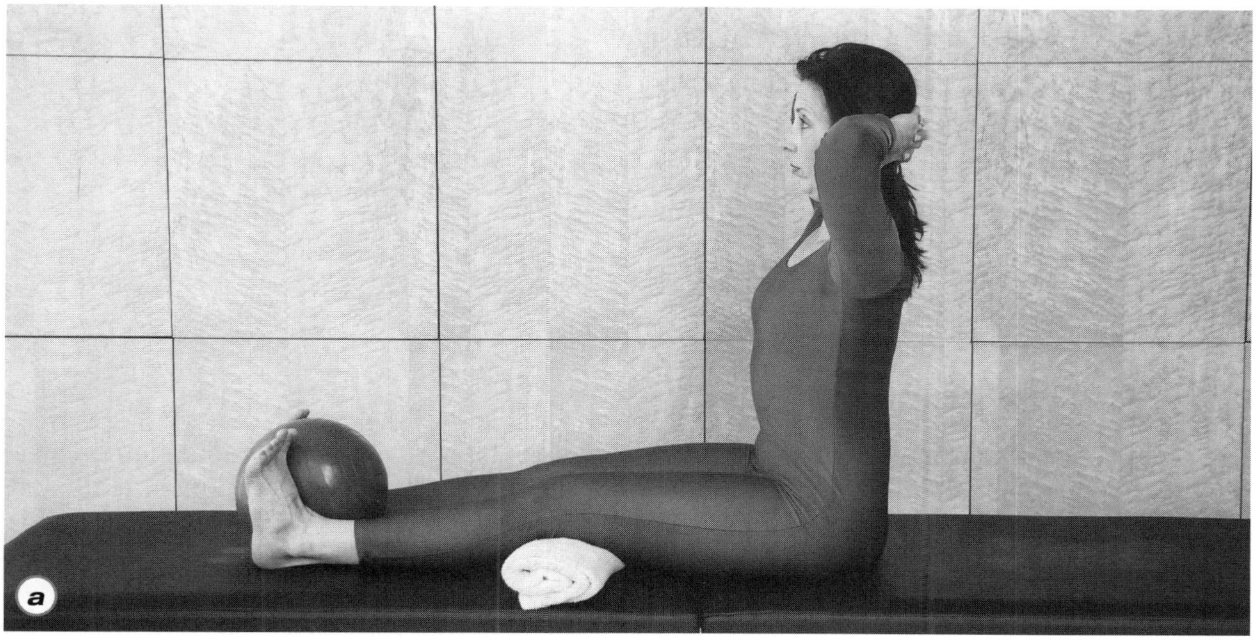

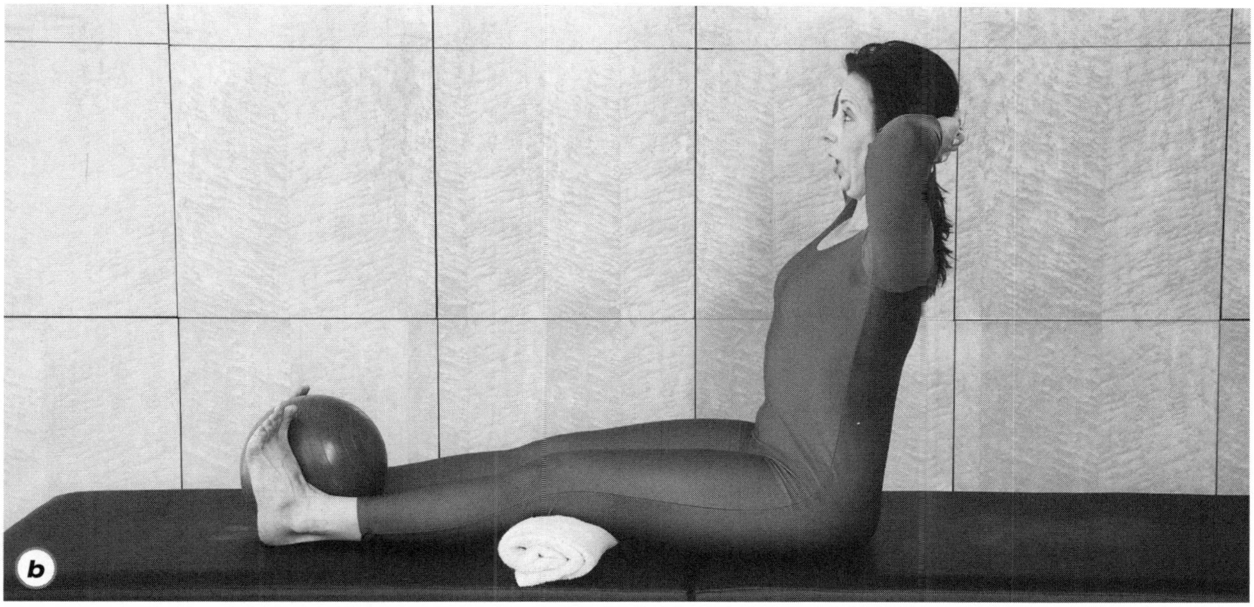

(continued)

Neck Pull *(continued)*

Look for . . . Encourage

- The shoulders gliding toward the hips as if suspenders were hooked to the bottom tips of the shoulder blades and attached to the hips
- Even articulation of the spine
- Abdominals drawn in and up
- Toes pointed to the ceiling, heels to the wall

Be aware of . . . Prevent

- Rolling the legs in and turning the toes in
- Using momentum and lifting the legs to roll up
- Loss of core control
- Hyperextension of the spine when performing the flat-back version
- Hyperextension of the knees
- Pulling on the neck
- Loss of shoulder alignment

Primary Muscles Activated

Abdominals, biceps, deltoid, shoulder complex, back extensors, iliopsoas, rectus femoris, gluteus medius, gluteus maximus, sartorius, pectineus, gracilis, adductor magnus, adductor longus, adductor brevis, biceps femoris, semitendinosus, semimembranosus, vastus medialis, vastus intermedius, vastus lateralis, tensor fasciae latae, tibialis anterior

Shoulder Bridge

Timeline: 3 to 6 months and 6 months and beyond postop

Appropriate for: knee and hip

Location: a floor mat or a raised mat as needed; a raised mat for a bilateral knee or hip replacement as needed for up to 6 months postop

Instructions

- Lie supine on the mat with the knees bent. Ideally, the heels are lying under the bent knees and the feet are hip-distance apart with or without a smal , soft ball between the knees. Position the arms long by the sides or out in a slight V, with the palms down on the mat.
- Make sure the toes, heels, knees, and hips are in alignment.
- Inhale to prepare. Exhale and press the feet into the mat and curl the tailbone toward the nose. Roll up one vertebra at a time to the shoulder blades.
- Inhale to prepare. Exhale and roll back down to the starting position. Slowly roll up and down.
- As you are rolling down, think of drawing the tailbone to the heels to deepen the articulation of the spine on the mat. Bridging challenges the pelvis to maintain stability throughout the movement.
- **Knee and hip:** Move the feet away from the bent knees as needed in order to move into the bridge position without stressing the knees or hips. Keep the knees hip-distance apart.
- Repeat 3 times.
- Additional action: While in the bridge position, lift and lower the bridge 3 to 4 inches (8-10 centimeters). Inhale to lower a little and exhale to lift back up, repeat 8 times, and then lower all the way down. Repeat the set.

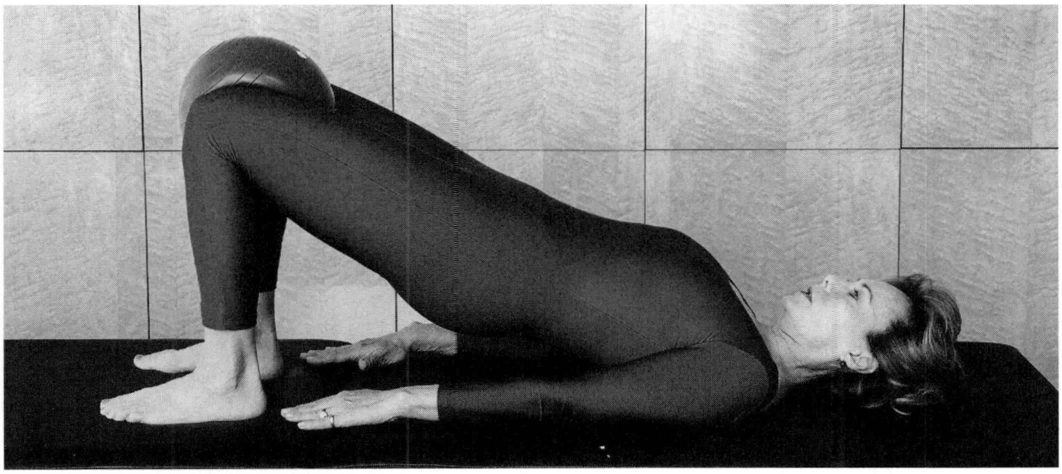

(continued)

Options

1. To increase the difficulty, roll up into the bridge position and hold. Lift the right leg up to a tabletop position, hold for a count of 5, lower the right leg down, and then switch legs. Repeat 3 times on each side.

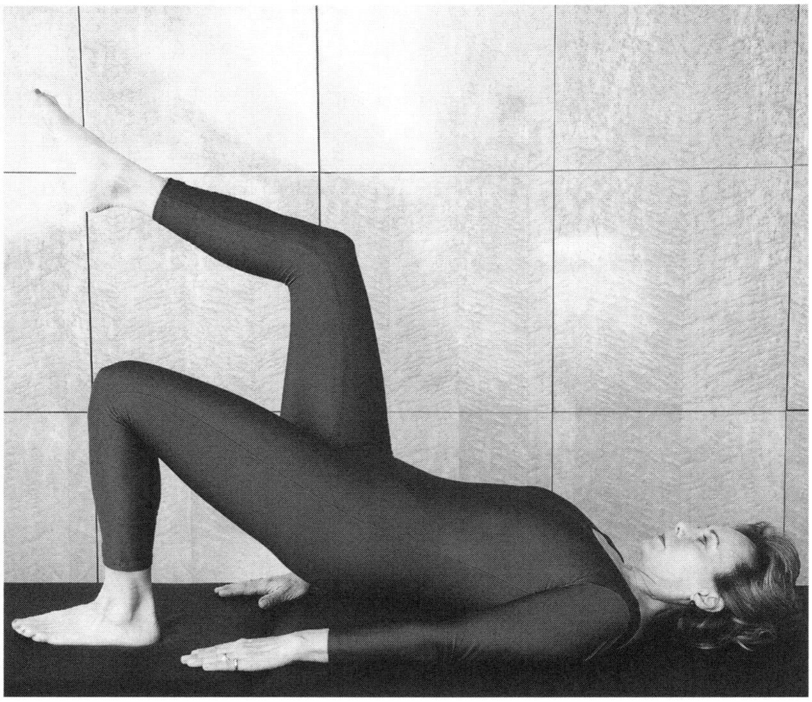

2. Roll up into the bridge position and hold. Lift the right leg up and point the toe to the ceiling. Keeping the pelvis steady, hold for a count of 5, bend the knee and lower the leg down, place the foot on the mat, and then switch legs. Repeat 2 times on each leg. Roll down in between sets as needed.

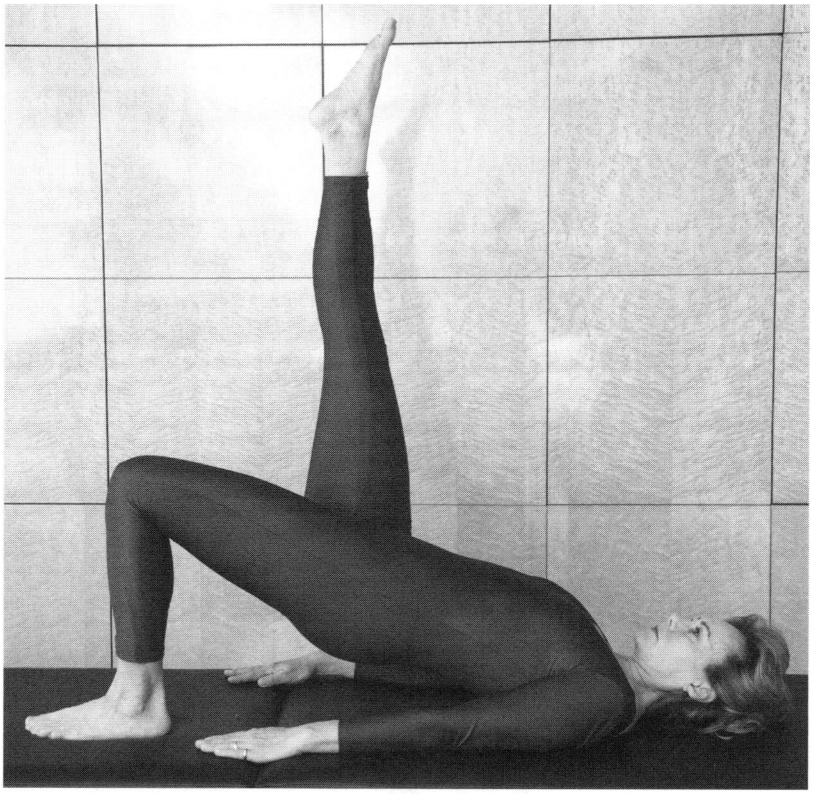

3. Place a Pilates ring in the hands and lift the arms to the ceiling with a light squeeze to the midline of the body. Roll up to the bridge position. Pulse the ring for 8 counts and then slowly roll down with the arms still reaching to the ceiling.

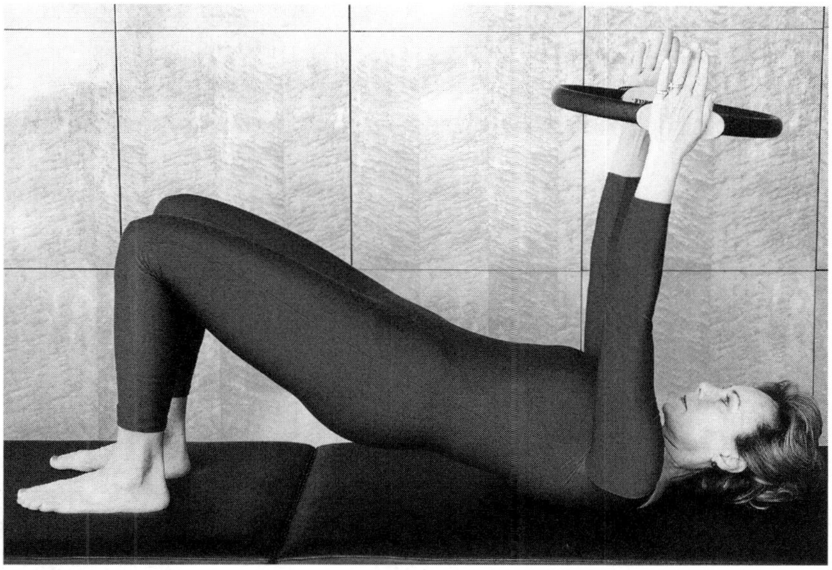

4. Roll up into the bridge position with a Pilates ring in the hands pointing to the ceiling. Lift one leg to the ceiling, keeping pelvis steady. Pulse the ring 8 counts, lower the leg, place the foot on the mat, and roll slowly down on the mat. Repeat 2 times on each leg.

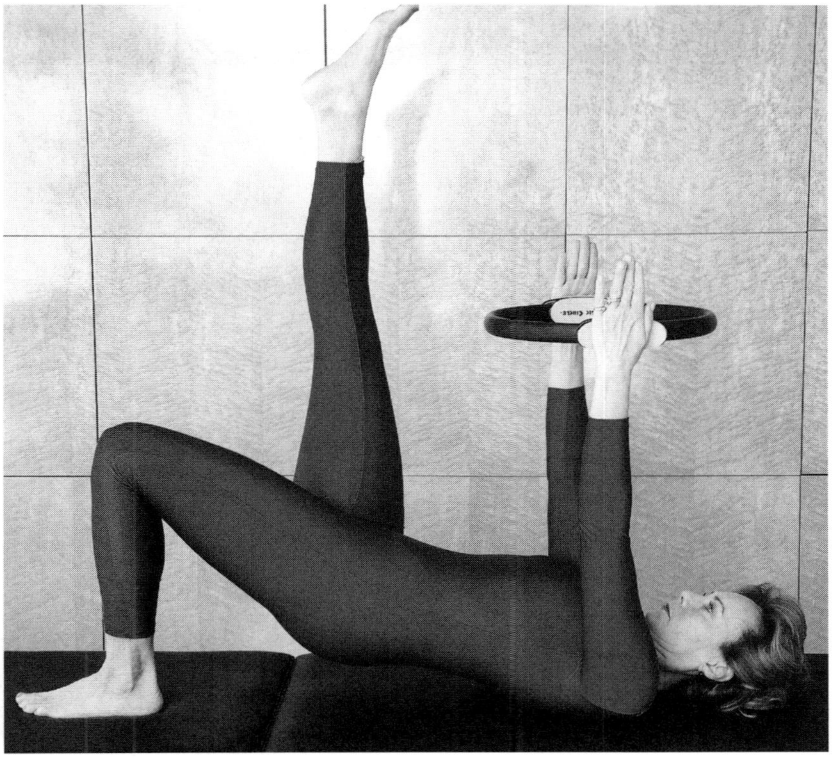

(continued)

Shoulder Bridge *(continued)*

5. Perform the shoulder bridge by placing the feet and shins a few inches (centimeters) apart on a large exercise ball *(a)*. If desired, place a second small ball between the ankles and hug the ball to the midline of the body *(b)*. Roll up into the bridge position, hold for 5 counts, and slowly roll down one vertebra at a time.

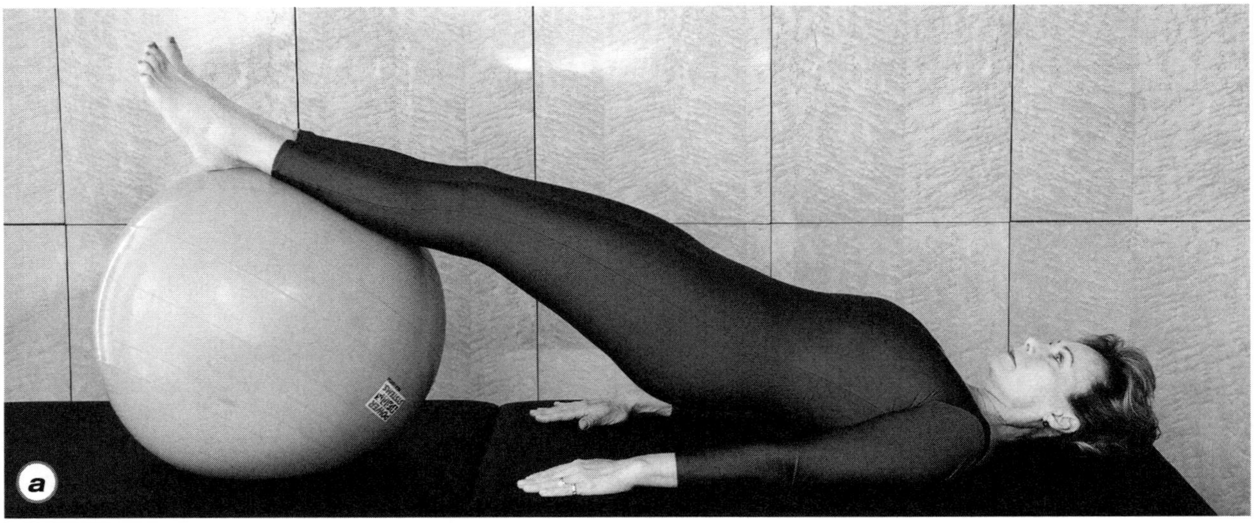
a

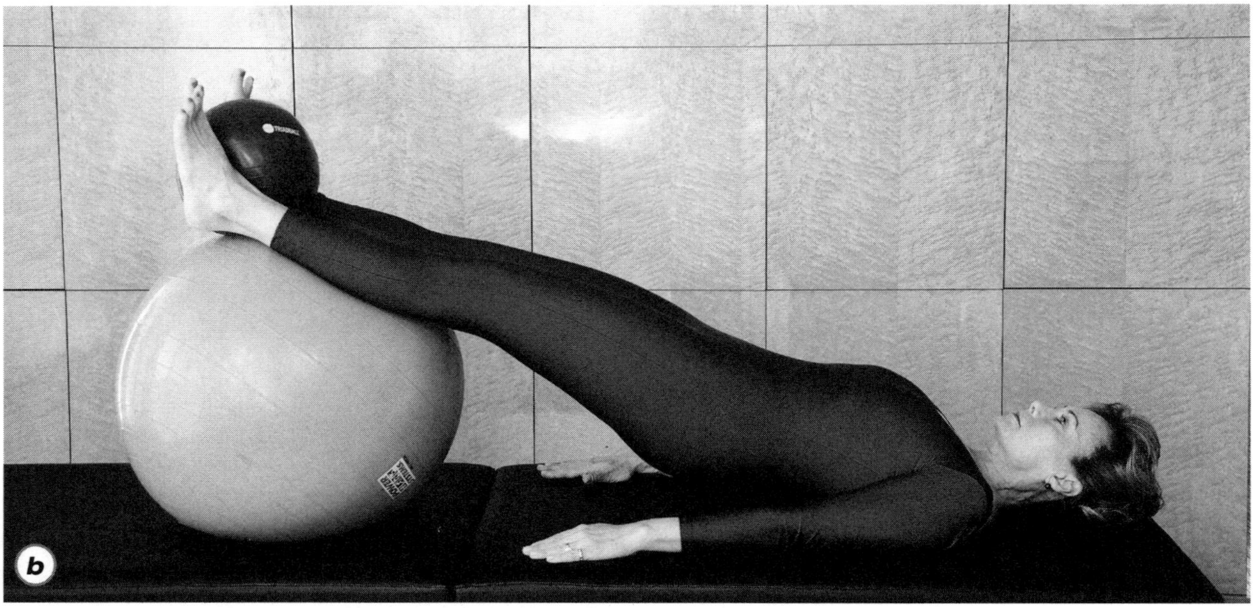
b

6. Tie an exercise band around the legs, keeping the legs hip-distance apart. Roll up into the bridge position. Engage the abductors and press out on the band without rolling the feet out. The exercise band has to be snug enough to create enough tension to perform the movement. Press in and out 8 times. Roll down to the mat. Repeat the set 3 times.

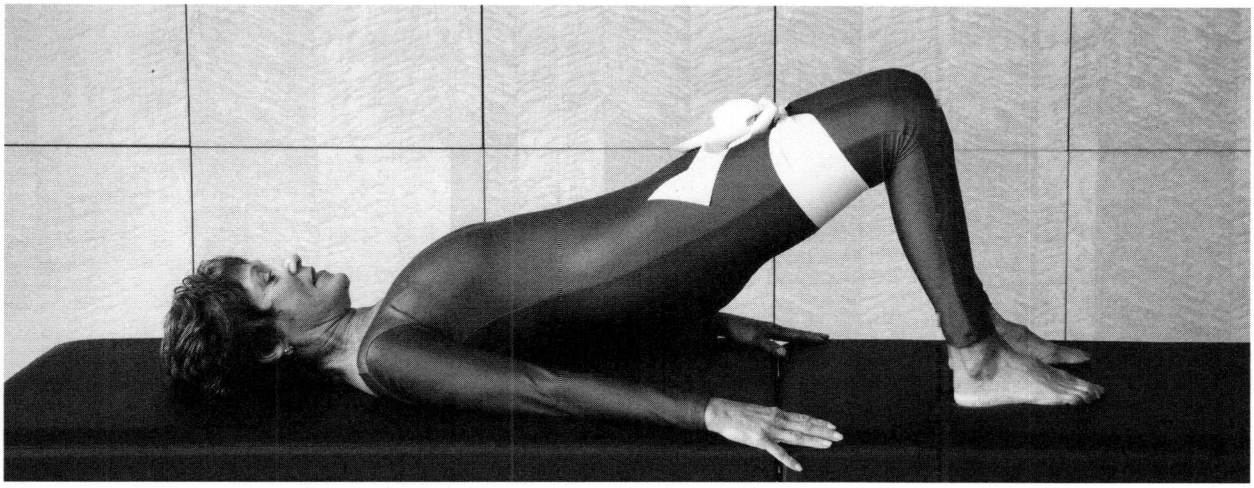

7. Roll up into the bridge position. Keep the pelvis very steady as you lift the right foot 1 inch (2.5 centimeters) off the mat. Hold for 2 counts and then switch sides. Lift the left foot and hold for 2 counts. Repeat 3 to 5 times per leg and then slowly roll down to the mat.

(continued)

Look for . . . Encourage

- The abdominals drawing in and up
- Articulation of the vertebrae as if they were a string of pearls being laid out on the table one pearl at a time
- Rolling up to one long line between the shoulder blades and the knees
- Pelvic stability with the movements
- Open collar bones and shoulders away from ears

Be aware of . . . Prevent

- Hyperextension of the lumbar spine
- Cramping in the hamstrings—reduce the ROM or rest between sets
- Pelvic instability and tilting, especially with unilateral heel or leg lifts
- Excessive recruitment of the gluteus muscles and hamstrings
- Tension in the neck and shoulders
- Loss of shoulder alignment

Primary Muscles Activated

The primary muscles activated depend on the chosen option. The primary muscles include the following: Abdominals, rectus femoris, sartorius, pectineus, iliopsoas, gluteus maximus, gluteus medius, biceps femoris, semitendinosus, semimembranosus, tensor fasciae latae, adductor magnus, adductor longus, adductor brevis, gracilis, popliteus, plantaris, gastrocnemius, vastus lateralis, vastus medialis, vastus intermedius, gluteus minimus, tibialis anterior, tibialis posterior, soleus

Teaser Prep 1

Timeline: 3 to 6 months and 6 months and beyond postop

Appropriate for: knee and hip

Location: a floor mat or a raised mat as needed; a raised mat for a bilateral knee or hip replacement as needed for up to 6 months postop

Instructions

- Lie supine on the mat with the knees slightly bent into a mountain shape. Place a small, soft ball between the knees, lengthen the arms to the ceiling with the palms facing the thighs, and draw the shoulders away from the ears *(a)*.
- Inhale to prepare; curl the head, neck, and shoulders off the mat, bringing the chin toward the chest. Exhale and lower the arms parallel to the thighs and slowly roll up, scooping the navel to the spine and drawing the abdominals in and up. Lengthen the arms up on a diagonal *(b)*.

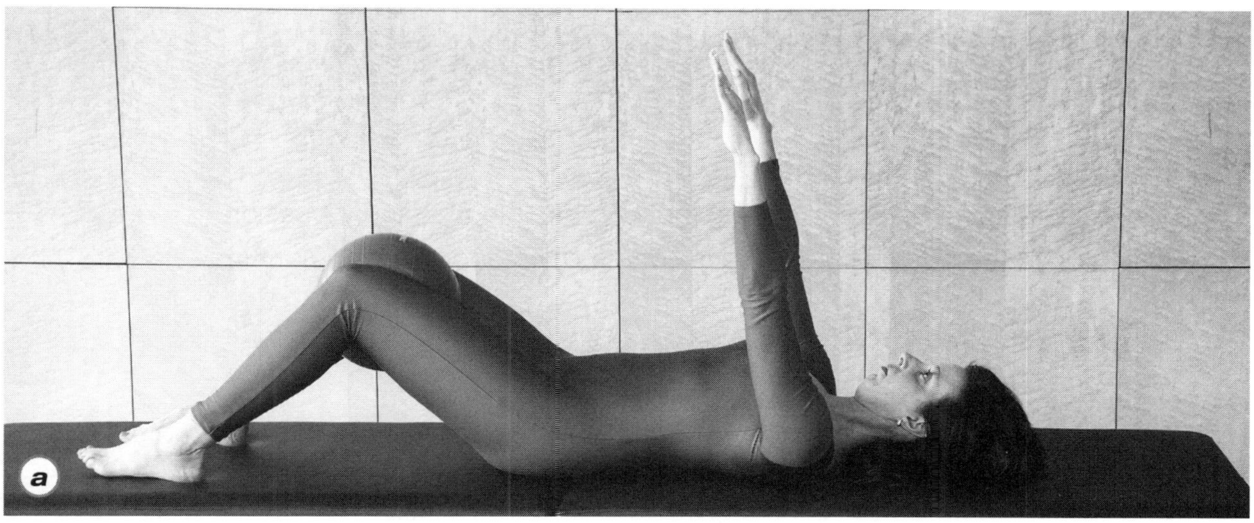

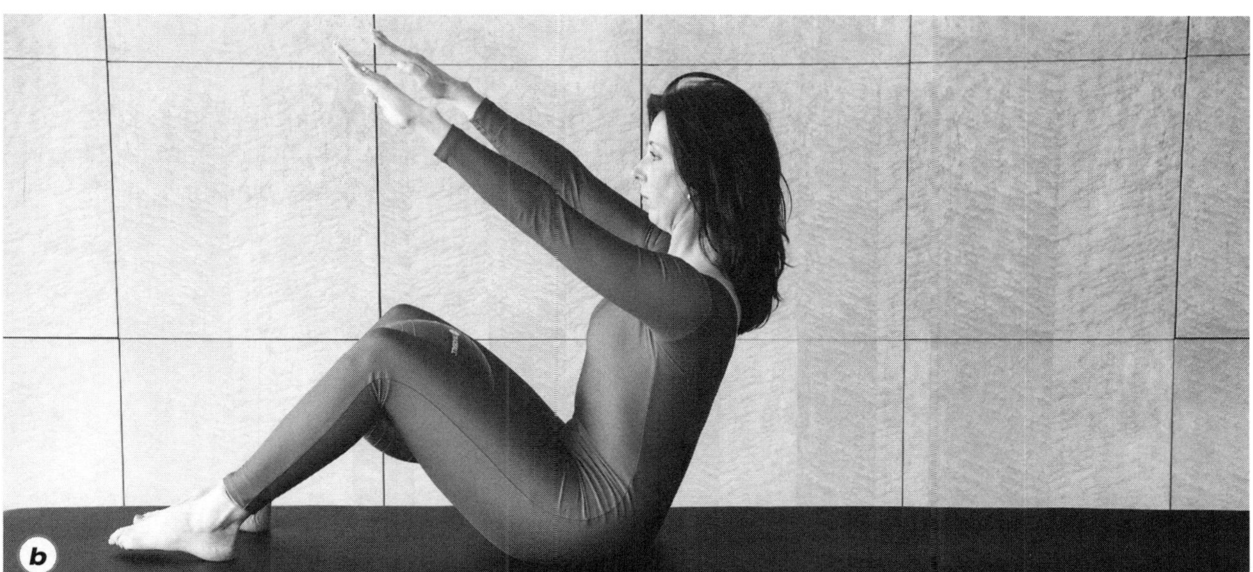

(continued)

- Hold for a count of 5.
- Exhale and slowly roll down to the mat, resisting through the abdominals and hugging the ball to the midline of the body.
- **Knee:** Keep the knees soft.
- **Hip:** Roll up to keep 110° of hip flexion for up to 6 months postop and 115° of hip flexion for 6 months and beyond postop as the upper body reaches into the teaser position.
- Repeat 3 times.
- Challenge: Roll down and up to a count of 8.

Option

Use the hands to walk up the sides of the legs to assist with the articulation of the spine into the teaser position. Keep the movement slow and controlled.

Look for . . . Encourage

- Shoulders gliding toward the hips as if suspenders were hooked to the bottom tips of the shoulder blades and attached to the hips
- Abdominals drawn in and up
- Even articulation of the spine
- Gaze following the movement
- Thinking of helium balloons floating the torso up into the teaser position
- Rolling up to the point where there is control without forceful momentum

Be aware of . . . Prevent

- Excessive momentum into the teaser
- Loss of core control
- Loss of shoulder alignment

Primary Muscles Activated

Abdominals, biceps, shoulder complex, rectus femoris, sartorius, pectineus, iliopsoas, adductor magnus, adductor longus, adductor brevis, gracilis, biceps femoris, semitendinosus, semimembranosus, tensor fasciae latae, gastrocnemius, popliteus, plantaris

Teaser Prep 2

Timeline: 3 to 6 months and 6 months and beyond postop

Appropriate for: knee and hip

Location: a floor mat or a raised mat as needed; a raised mat for a bilateral knee or hip replacement as needed for up to 6 months postop

Instructions

- Lie supine on the mat with the right knee slightly bent into a mountain shape and the left leg extended along the inside of the thigh and knee of the right leg. Point the toe toward the opposite wall on a diagonal. Lengthen the arms to the ceiling with the palms facing the thighs and the shoulders away from the ears *(a)*.
- Inhale to prepare; curl the head, neck, and shoulders off the mat, bringing the chin toward the chest. Exhale and lower the arms parallel to the thighs. Slowly roll up, scooping the navel to the spine and drawing the abdominals in and up. Lengthen the arms up on a diagonal.
- Roll up and maintain a C-curve in the lower spine with a proud chest *(b)*.

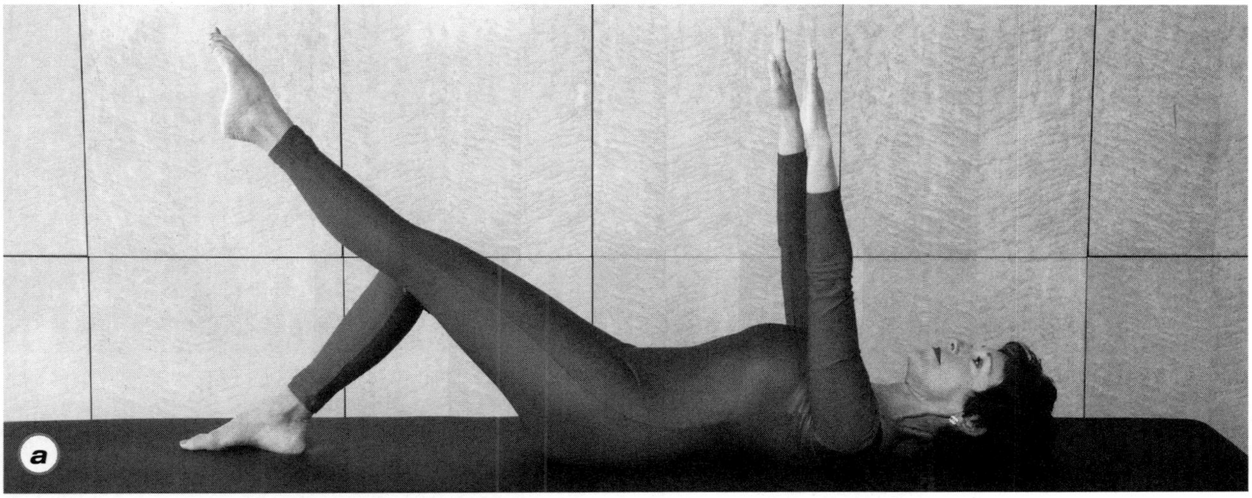

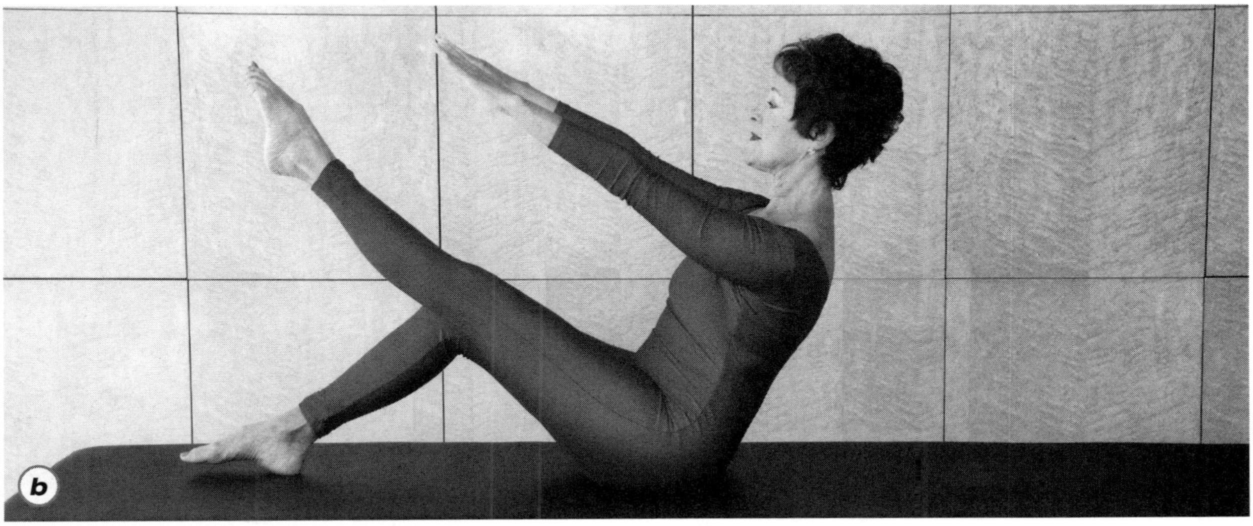

(continued)

Teaser Prep 2 *(continued)*

- Hold for a count of 5.
- Exhale and slowly roll down to the mat, resisting through the abdominals and articulating the spine vertebra by vertebra.
- **Knee:** Keep the knees soft.
- **Hip:** Roll up to keep 110° of hip flexion for up to 6 months postop and 115° of hip flexion for 6 months and beyond postop as the upper body reaches into the teaser position.
- Repeat 3 times.
- Challenge: Roll up and down to a count of 8.

Options

1. Use the hands to walk up the sides of the legs to articulate into the teaser position.

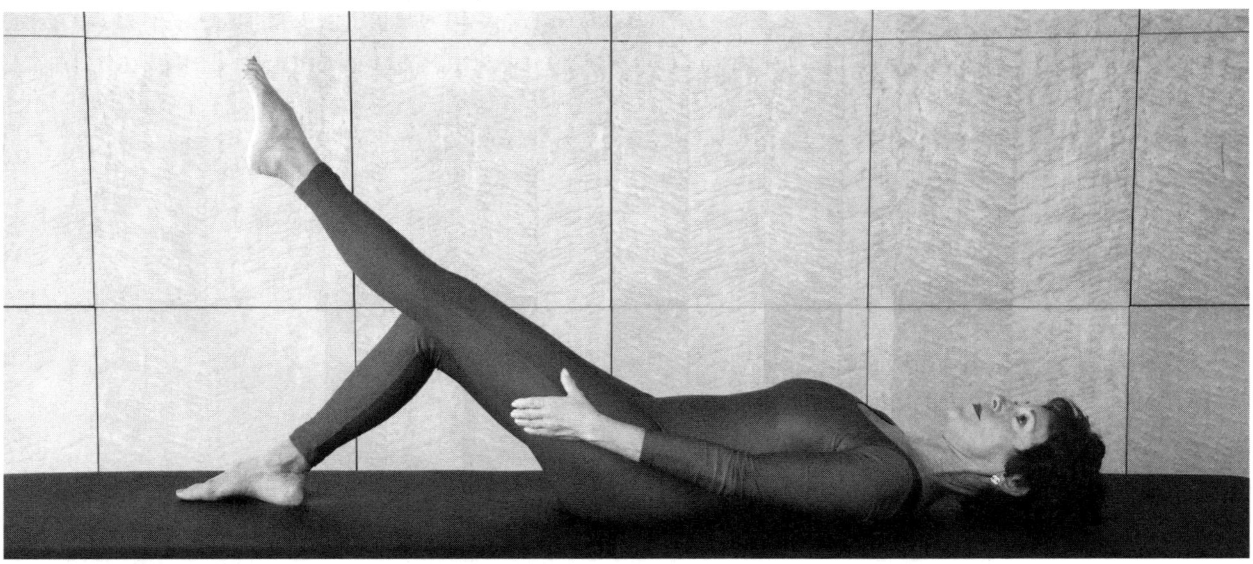

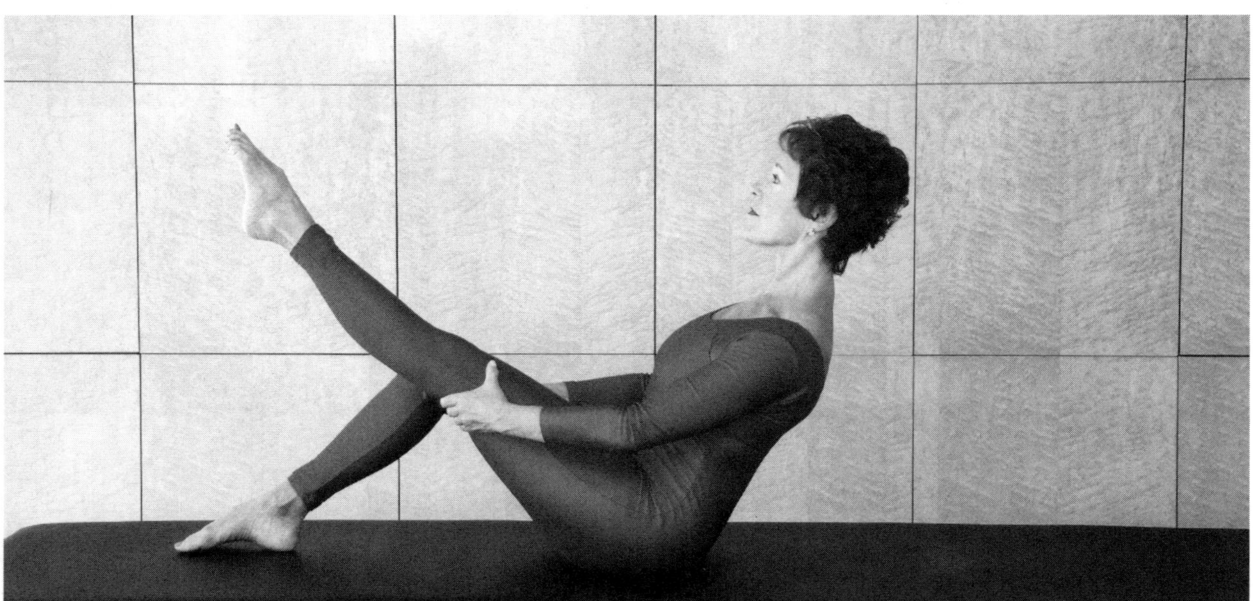

2. Use a long exercise band placed wide across the bottom of the foot that is extended. Choke up on the band to begin the teaser. The tension of the band will reduce as you roll up, so walk the hands up the band as you roll up to the teaser position.

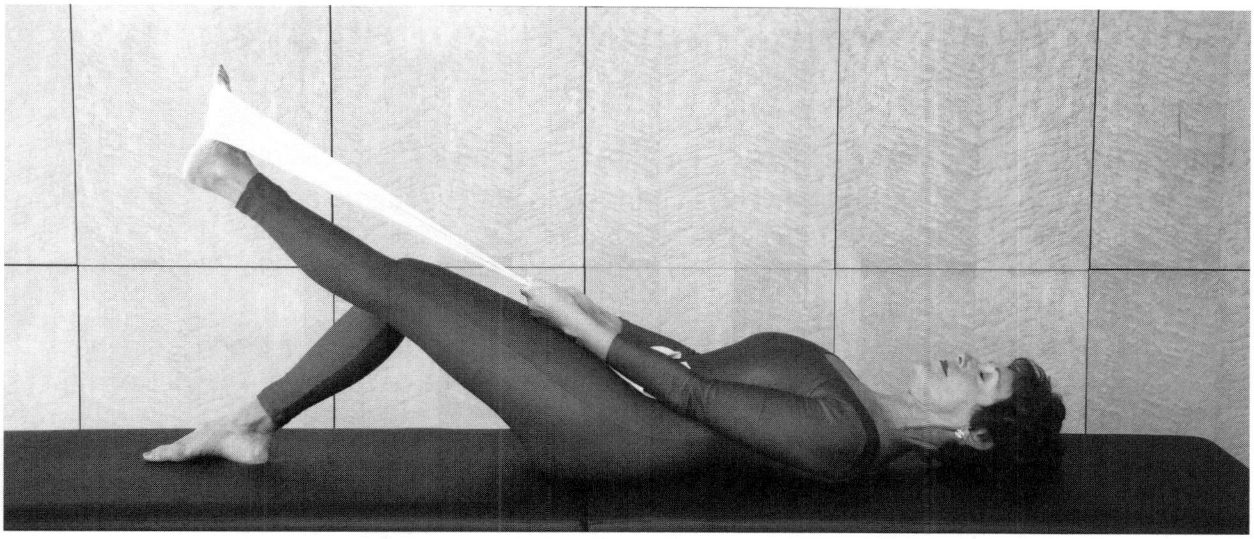

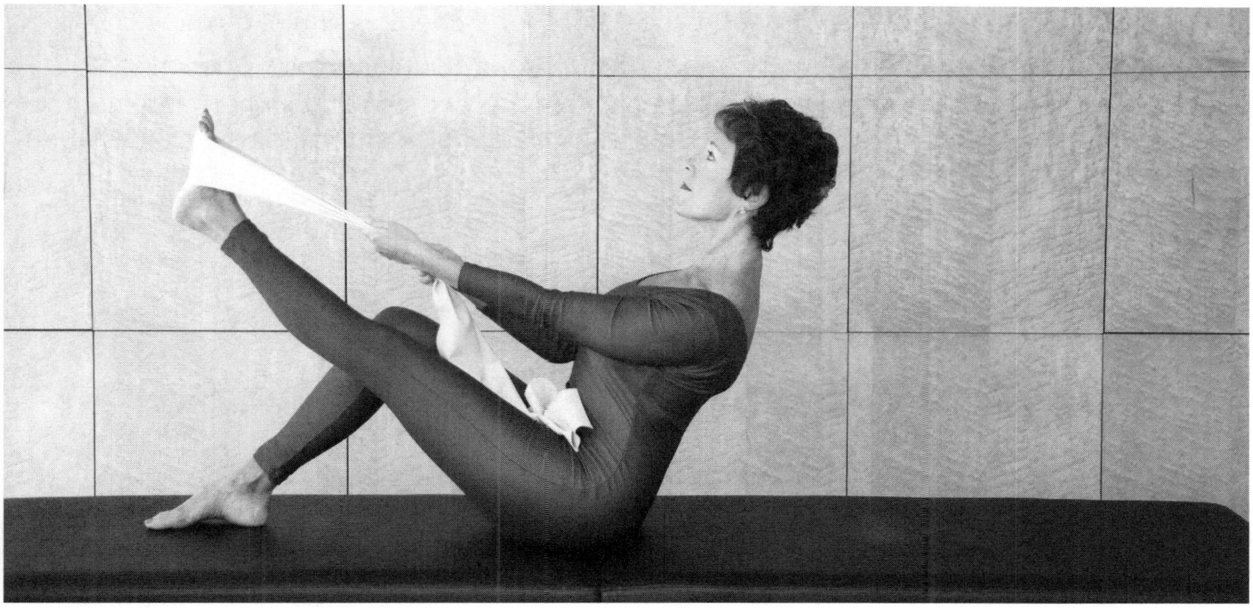

(continued)

Look for . . . Encourage

- Shoulders gliding toward the hips as if suspenders were hooked to the bottom tips of the shoulder blades and attached to the hips
- Abdominals drawn in and up
- Even articulation of the spine
- Gaze following the movement
- Thinking of helium balloons floating the torso up to the teaser position
- Rolling up to the point where there is control without forceful momentum

Be aware of . . . Prevent

- Excessive momentum
- Loss of core control
- Uneven articulation of the spine up to teaser and down to the mat
- Loss of shoulder alignment

Primary Muscles Activated

Abdominals, biceps, shoulder complex, rectus femoris, sartorius, pectineus, iliopsoas, adductor longus, adductor brevis, gracilis, biceps femoris, semitendinosus, semimembranosus, tensor fasciae latae, gastrocnemius, popliteus, plantaris, vastus medialis, vastus lateralis, vastus medialis, tibialis posterior, soleus

Teaser 1

Timeline: 3 to 6 months and 6 months and beyond postop

Appropriate for: knee and hip

Location: a floor mat or a raised mat as needed; a raised mat for a bilateral knee or hip replacement as needed for up to 6 months postop

Instructions

- Lie supine on the mat with the legs bent into a tabletop position with or without a small, soft ball between the knees. Lengthen the arms toward the ceiling with the palms facing the thighs and the shoulders away from ears *(a)*.
- Hug the ball or legs to the midline. Inhale to prepare and curl the head, neck, and shoulders off the mat. Exhale, draw the abdominals deeply in and up, and roll up vertebra by vertebra on a diagonal with the arms reaching up on a high diagonal.
- As you roll up, hug the ball to the midline and press your thighs forward as you roll your upper body up off the mat.
- Roll up and maintain a C-curve in the lower spine with a proud chest *(b)*.
- Hold for a count of 5.
- Exhale and slowly roll down vertebra by vertebra, resisting through the abdominals.
- Challenge: Roll down to a count of 6 to 8.
- **Knee:** Keep the legs parallel and the knees soft and hugging the ball.

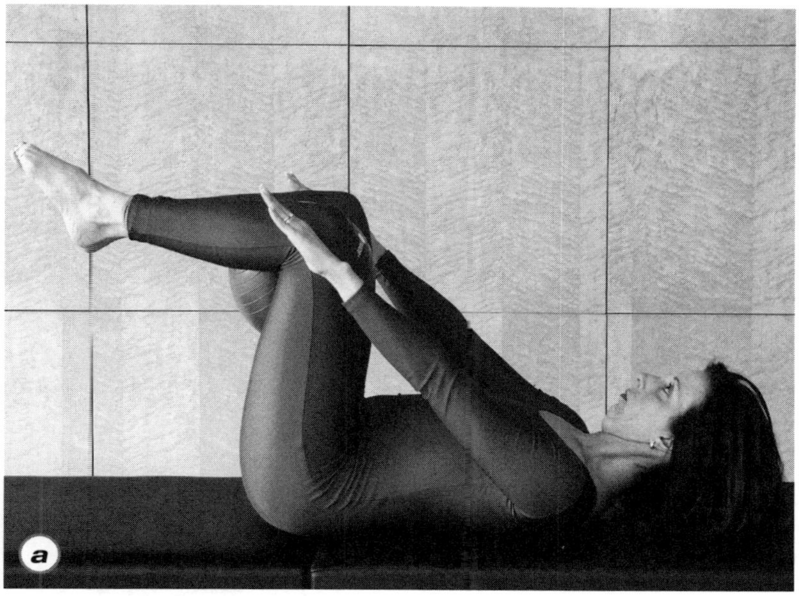
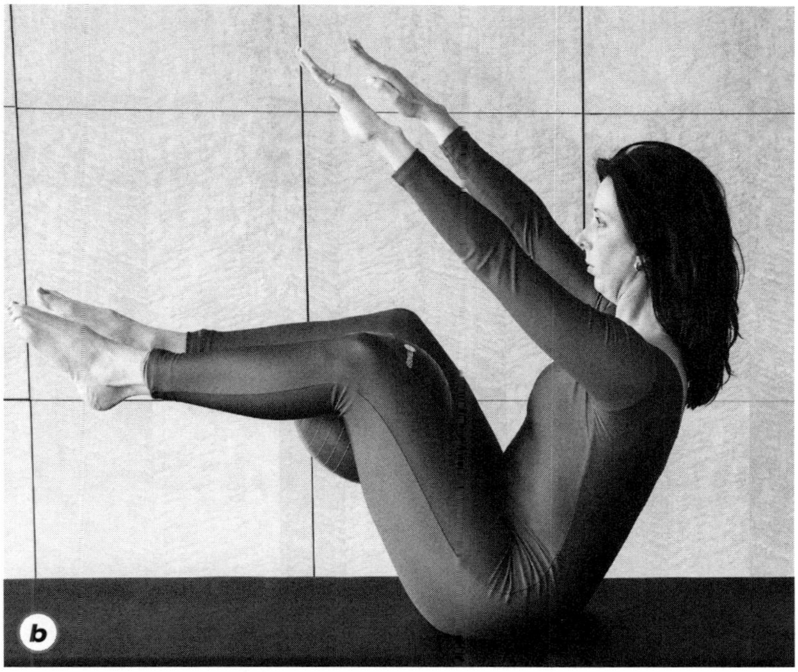

(continued)

Teaser 1 *(continued)*

- **Hip:** Roll up to keep 110° of hip flexion for up to 6 months postop *(c)* and 115° of hip flexion for 6 months and beyond postop *(d)* as the upper body rolls up into the teaser position.
- Repeat 3 times.

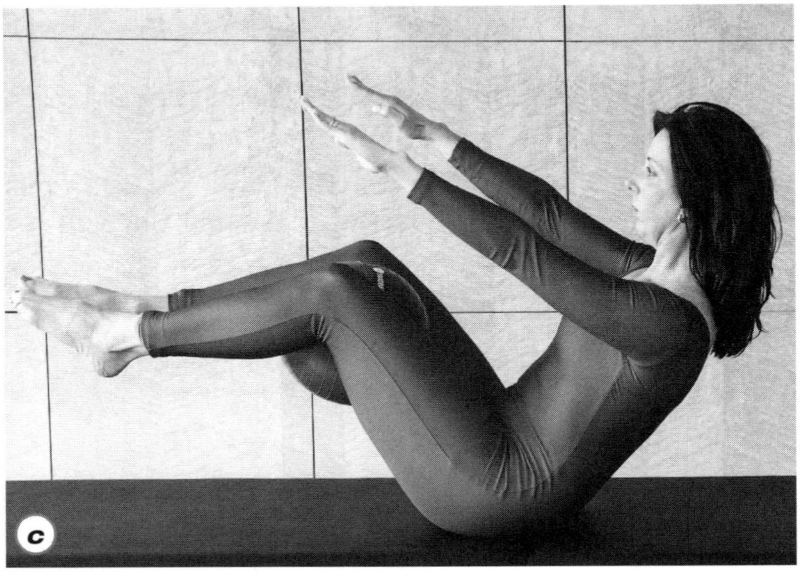

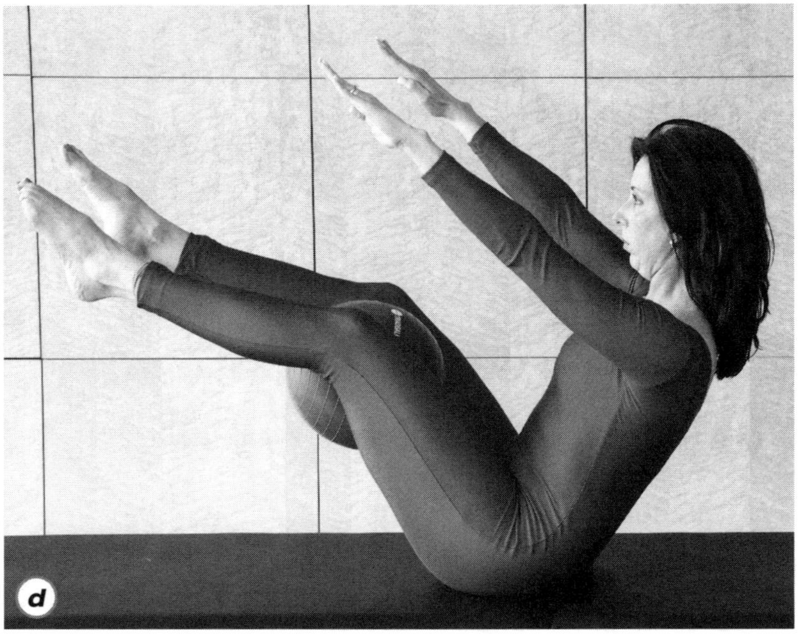

Look for . . . Encourage

- Shoulders gliding toward the hips as if suspenders were hooked to the bottom tips of the shoulder blades and attached to the hips
- Abdominals drawn in with the exhale on the roll up into the teaser
- Even articulation of the spine
- Gaze following the movement
- Thinking of helium balloons floating the torso up to the teaser position
- Rolling up to the point where there is control without forceful momentum

Be aware of . . . Prevent

- Excessive momentum
- Loss of core control
- Loss of shoulder alignment

Primary Muscles Activated

Abdominals, biceps, shoulder complex, rectus femoris, sartorius, pectineus, iliopsoas, adductor longus, adductor magnus, adductor brevis, gracilis, biceps femoris, semitendinosus, semimembranosus, tensor fasciae latae, gastrocnemius, popliteus, plantaris

Teaser 2

Timeline: 3 to 6 months and 6 months and beyond postop

Appropriate for: knee and hip

Location: a floor mat or a raised mat as needed; a raised mat for a bilateral knee or hip replacement as needed for up to 6 months postop

Instructions

- Lie supine on the mat with the legs extended to the ceiling or out to a 45° angle. Lengthen the arms toward the ceiling, with the palms facing the thighs, and point the fingers to the ceiling *(a)*.
- Inhale to prepare and curl the head, neck, and shoulders off the mat. Exhale, draw the abdominals deeply in and up, and roll the spine up vertebra by vertebra on a diagonal with the arms parallel to the thighs.
- As you roll up, hug the ball to the midline and press your thighs forward as you roll your upper body up off the mat.
- Roll up and maintain a C-curve in the lower spine with a proud chest *(b)*.
- Hold for a count of 5.
- Exhale and slowly roll down vertebra by vertebra, resisting through the abdominals.
- Challenge: Roll down to a count of 6 to 8.
- **Knee:** Keep the legs parallel with the knees soft or slightly bent.

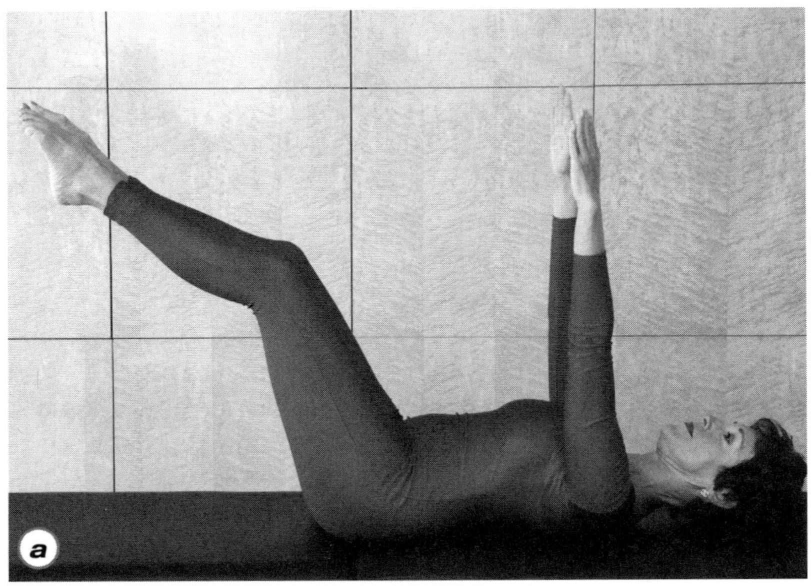

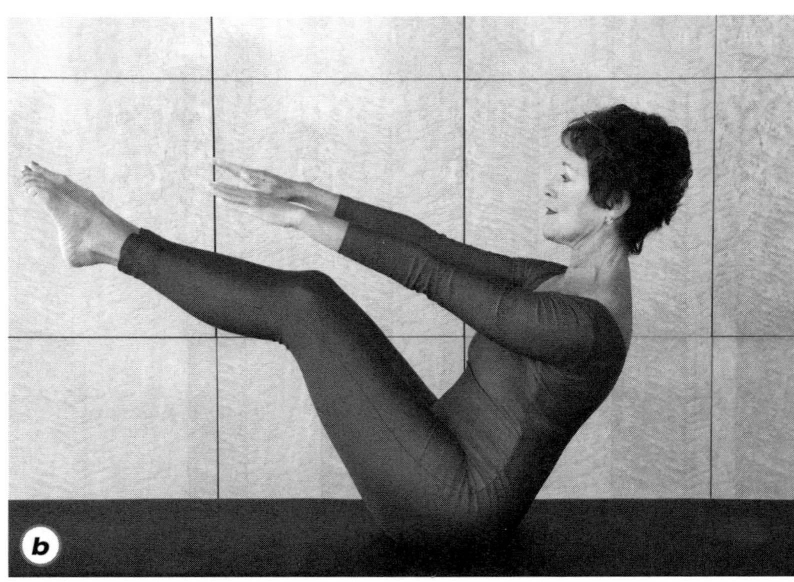

- **Hip:** Roll up to keep 110° of hip flexion for up to 6 months postop and 115° of hip flexion for 6 months and beyond postop as the upper body reaches to the teaser position *(c-d)*. Bend the knees as needed to avoid straining the hip flexors.
- Repeat 3 times.

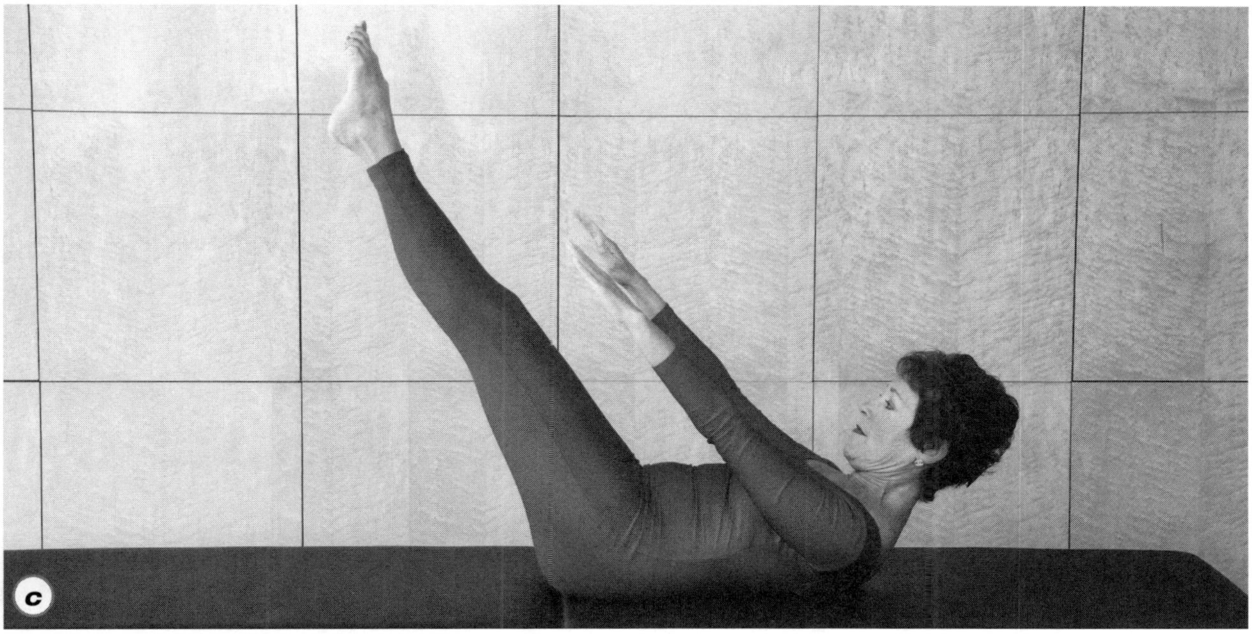

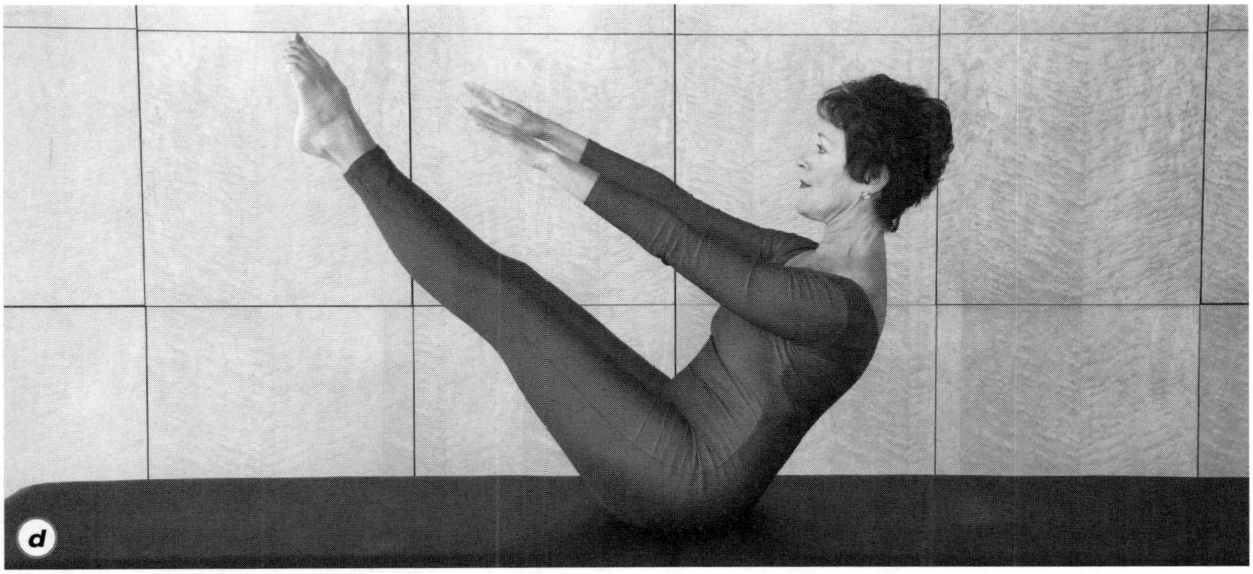

(continued)

Teaser 2 *(continued)*

Options

1. Place a long, lightweight exercise band around the base of the feet when performing the teaser 1 and 2 as needed until you can successfully engage the core and incrementally roll the spine up and down vertebra by vertebra, resisting through the abdominals.

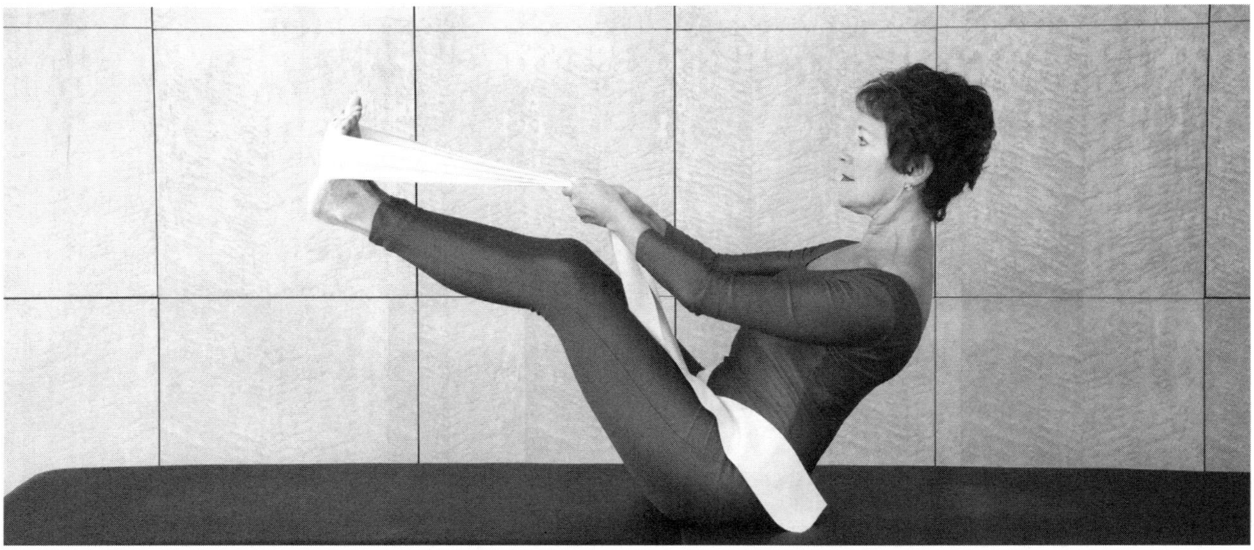

2. Place the feet on a large exercise ball to roll up to the teaser position.

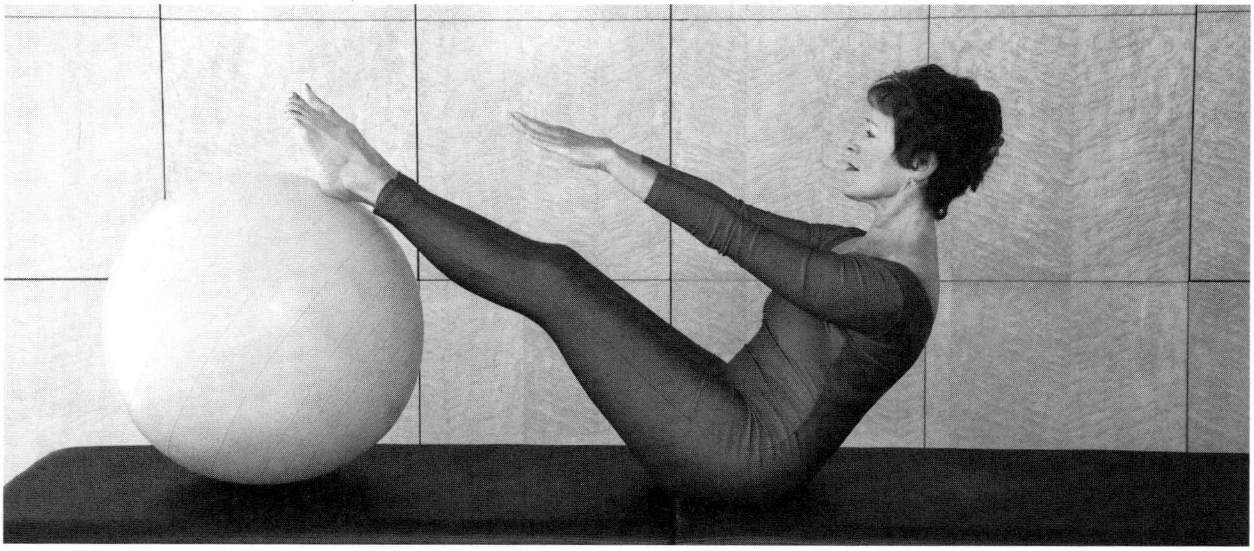

3. Use the hands to walk up the outsides of the legs to assist with moving into the teaser position.

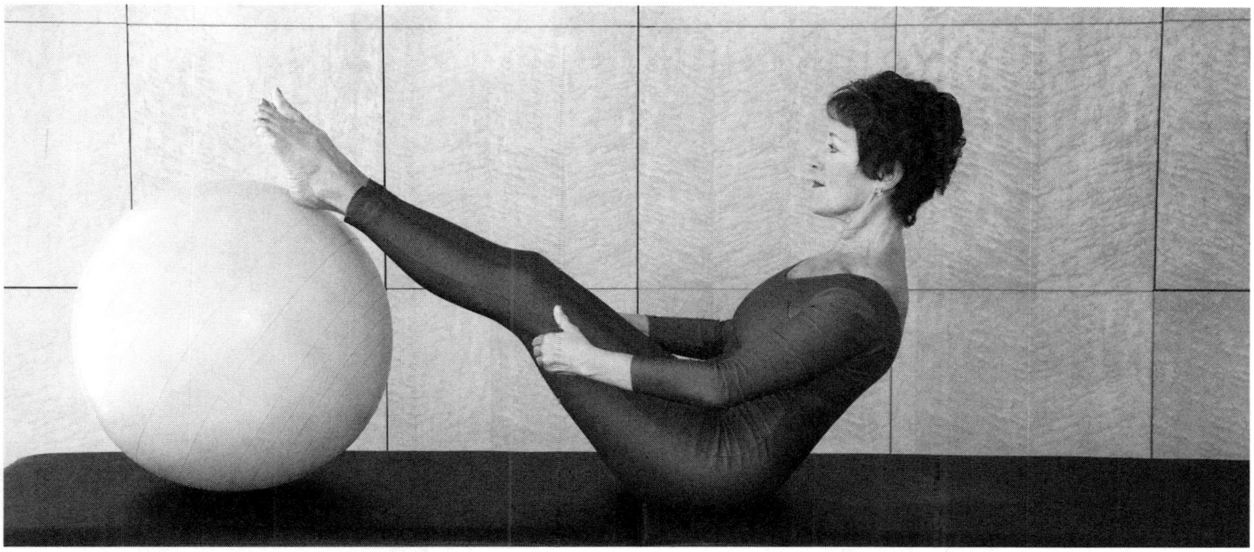

4. Use the exercise band and place a pad between the knees.

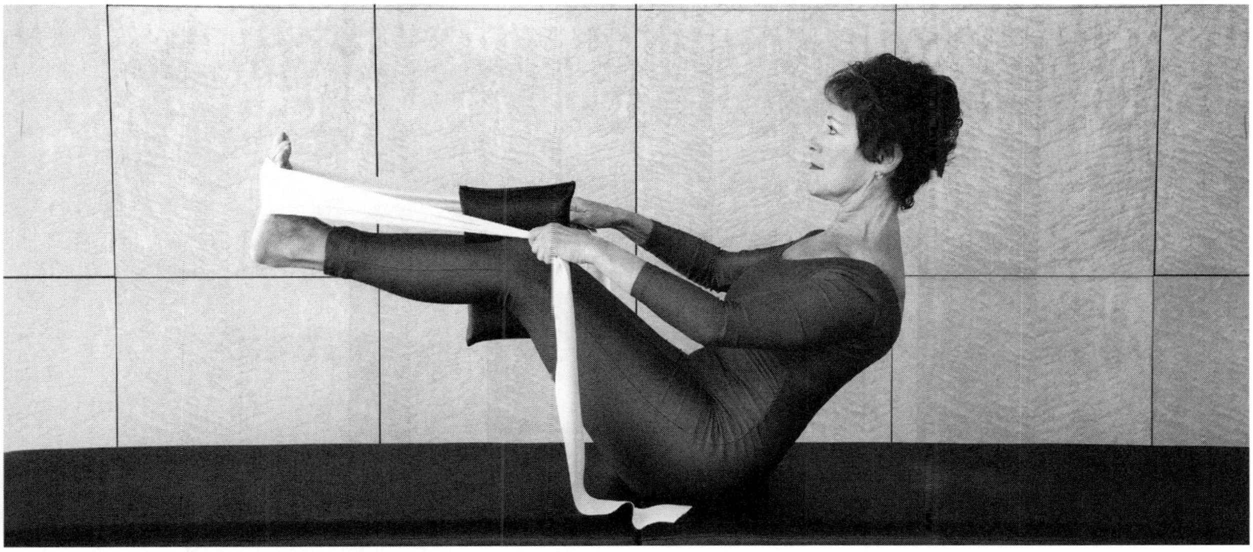

(continued)

Look for . . . Encourage

- Shoulders gliding toward the hips as if suspenders were hooked to the bottom tips of the shoulder blades and attached to the hips
- Abdominals drawn in with the exhale when rolling up into the teaser
- Even articulation of the spine
- Gaze following the movement
- Thinking of helium balloons floating the torso up to the teaser position
- Bent knees to avoid straining the hip flexors
- Rolling up to the point where there is control without forceful momentum

Be aware of . . . Prevent

- Excessive momentum
- Loss of core control
- Loss of shoulder alignment
- Gripping in the hip flexors

Primary Muscles Activated

The primary muscles activated depend on the chosen option: Abdominals, biceps, shoulder complex, rectus femoris, sartorius, pectineus, iliopsoas, adductor longus, adductor magnus, adductor brevis, gracilis, biceps femoris, semitendinosus, semimembranosus, tensor fasciae latae, gastrocnemius, popliteus, plantaris, vastus medialis, vastus intermedius, vastus lateralis, tibialis posterior, tibialis anterior, soleus

Teaser 3

Restrictions: not applicable for knee or hip at 3 to 6 months postop
Timeline: 6 months and beyond postop
Appropriate for: knee and hip
Location: a floor mat or a raised table as needed

Instructions

- Lie supine with the legs extended out on the mat and hugging to the midline of the body. Extend the arms back in line with the ears and turn the palms away from the face *(a)*.
- Inhale and bring the arms above the chest while curling the head, neck, and shoulders off the mat.
- Exhale, deeply engage the abdominals, and roll up to the lower thoracic area, keeping the waist flowing toward the spine. Pick the legs up and continue to roll up to a high diagonal *(b)*.

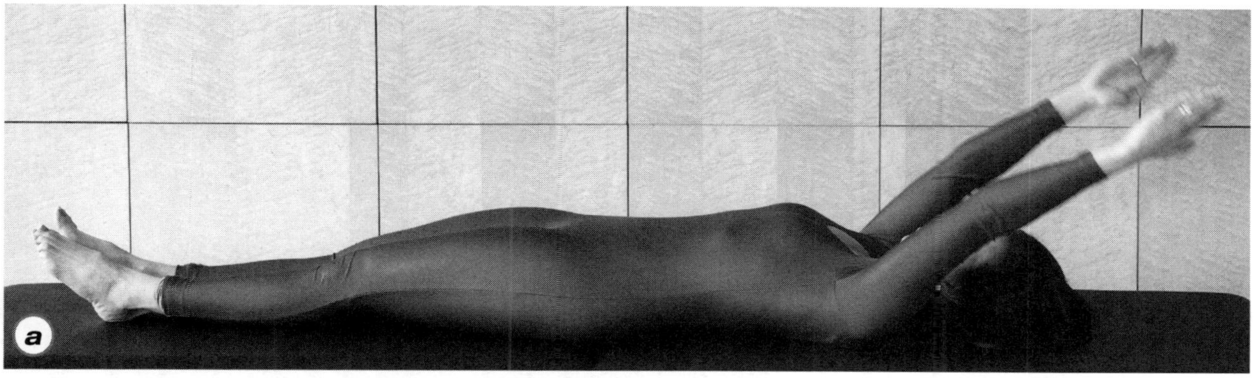

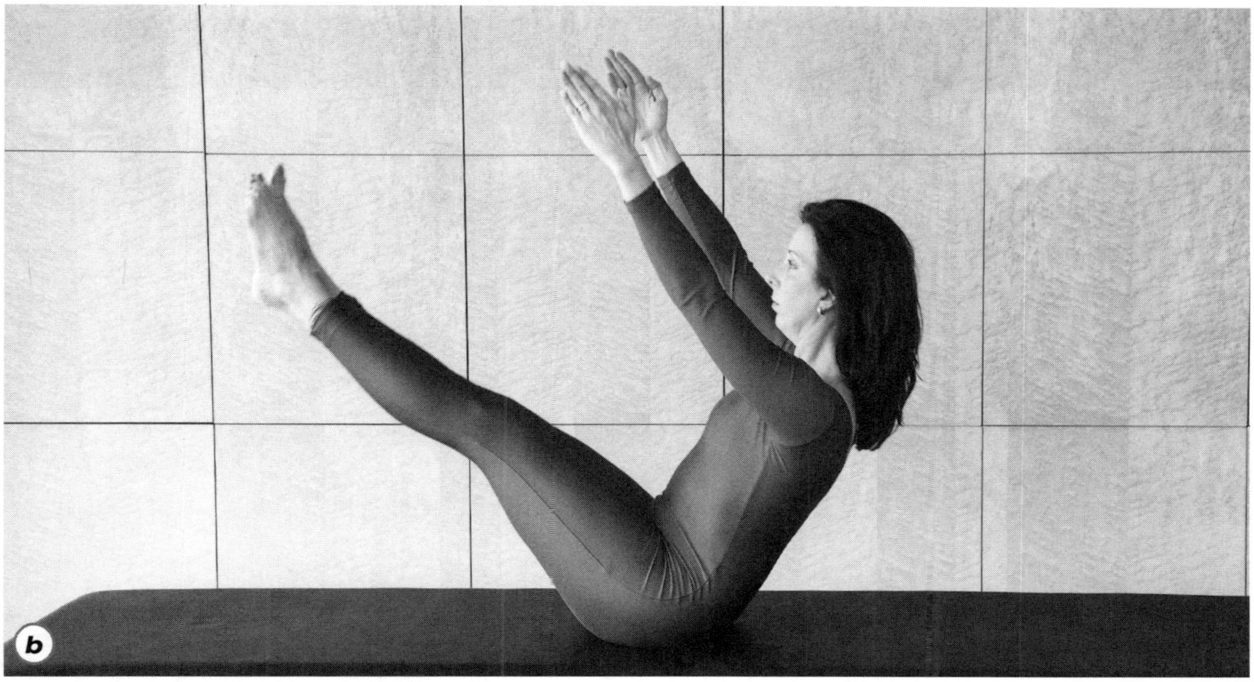

(continued)

Teaser 3 *(continued)*

- Hold for a count of 5.
- Exhale and, leading with the lower back, roll back down to the starting position vertebra by vertebra.
- The feet and head should arrive on the mat at the same time.
- **Knee:** Keep the knees soft but the legs extended as tolerated.
- **Hip:** Roll up to keep 115° of hip flexion and keep the knees soft.
- Repeat 3 times.

Options

1. Hold a ring or ball between the legs or in the hands.

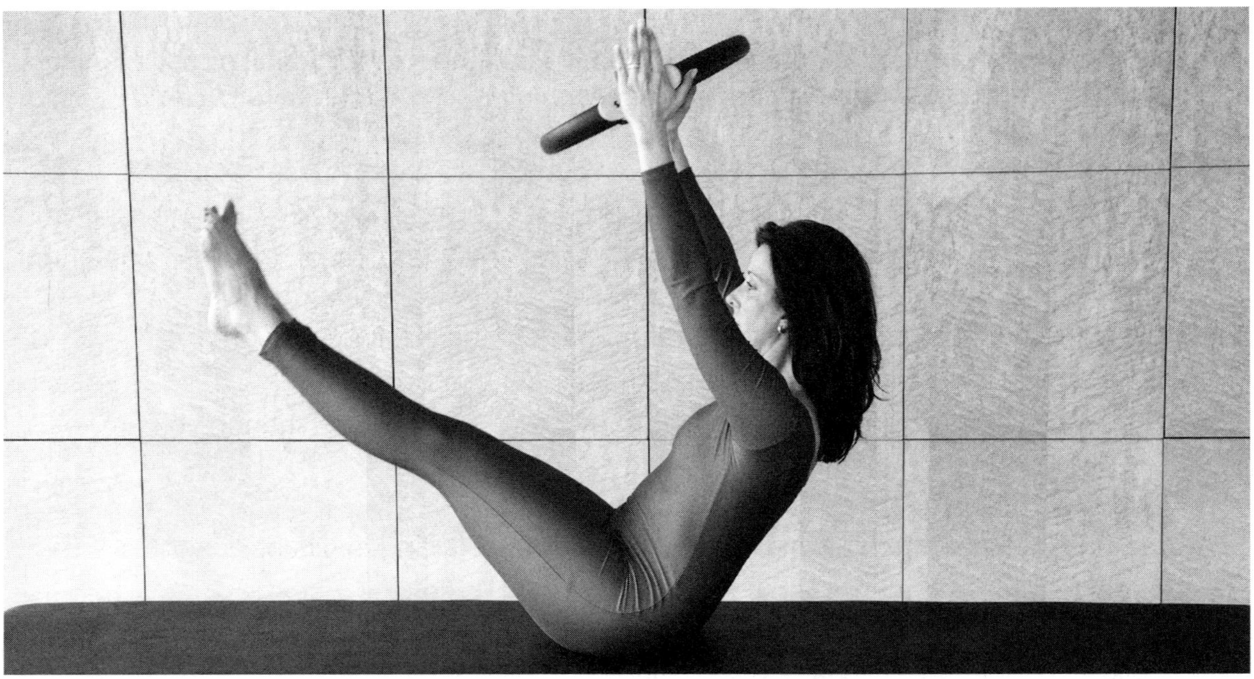

2. Hold an exercise band in the hands, keeping an even tension on the band.

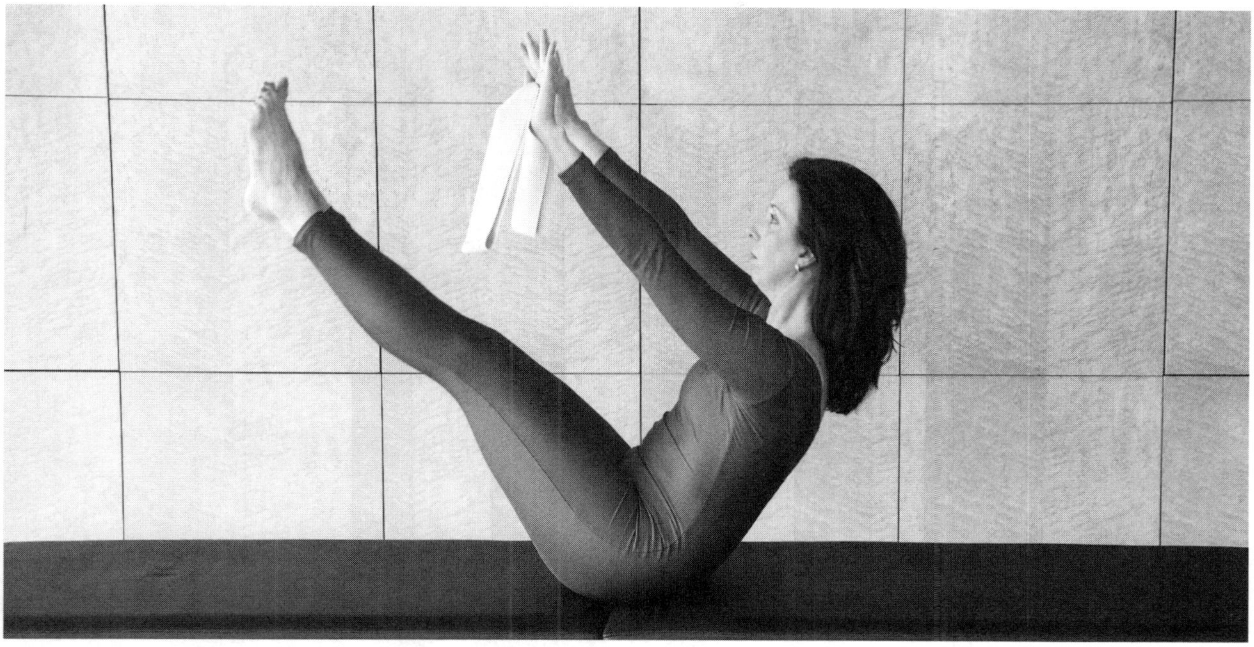

Look for . . . Encourage

- Shoulders gliding toward the hips as if suspenders were hooked to the bottom tips of the shoulder blades and attached to the hips
- Abdominals drawn in with the exhale when rolling up into the teaser
- Even articulation of the spine
- Gaze following the movement
- Thinking of helium balloons floating the torso up to the teaser position
- Bent knees as needed to avoid straining the hip flexors

Be aware of . . . Prevent

- Excessive momentum
- Loss of core control
- Stress and strain on the hip flexors
- Loss of shoulder alignment
- Gripping the hip flexors
- Rib cage lifted away from the mat when arms are extended back in line with the ears

Primary Muscles Activated

Abdominals, biceps, shoulder complex, rectus femoris, sartorius, pectineus, iliopsoas, adductor longus, adductor magnus, adductor brevis, gracilis, biceps femoris, semitendinosus, semimembranosus, gluteus maximus, gluteus medius (posterior portion), tensor fasciae latae, vastus medialis, vastus intermedius, vastus lateralis, back extensors, tibialis posterior, soleus, gastrocnemius, plantaris

Cancan (Modified)

Restrictions: not applicable for hip at 3 to 6 months postop

Timeline: 3 to 6 months and 6 months and beyond postop

Appropriate for: knee

Timeline: 6 months and beyond postop

Appropriate for: hip

Location: a floor mat or a raised mat as needed; a raised mat for a bilateral knee or hip replacement as needed for up to 6 months postop

Instructions

- Sit tall with the legs together. Lean back and place the forearms on the mat with the palms down and the fingers pointing toward the hips or lightly to the sides of the buttocks.
- Bend the knees into a mountain shape, hugging the legs together. Use a small, soft ball or pad between the knees as needed. Lift the heels with the toes slightly touching the floor *(a)*.

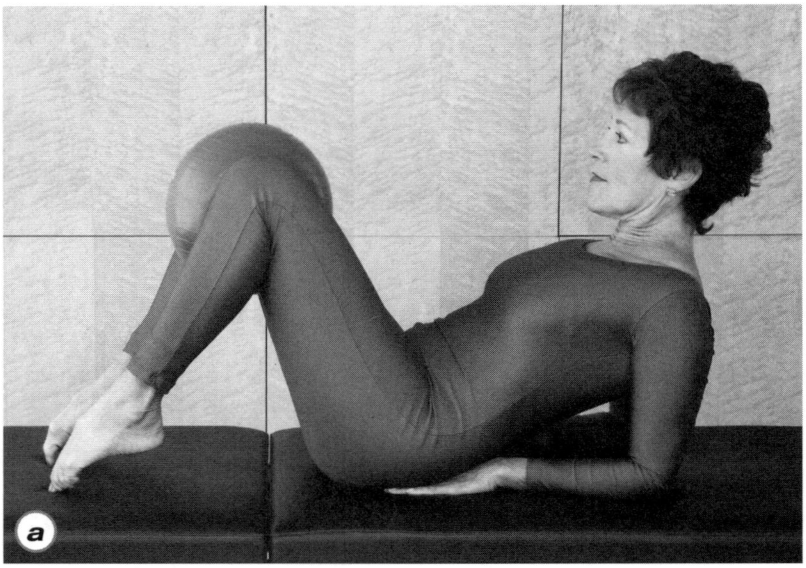

- Lift the chest away from the forearms. Maintain a neutral spine with the chest lifted. Gaze forward, lengthen the shoulder blades toward the hips, and keep the collarbones open.
- Inhale to prepare. Exhale and rotate the knees as one unit to the right, rolling toward the outside of the little toe *(b)*. Rotate back to the center and

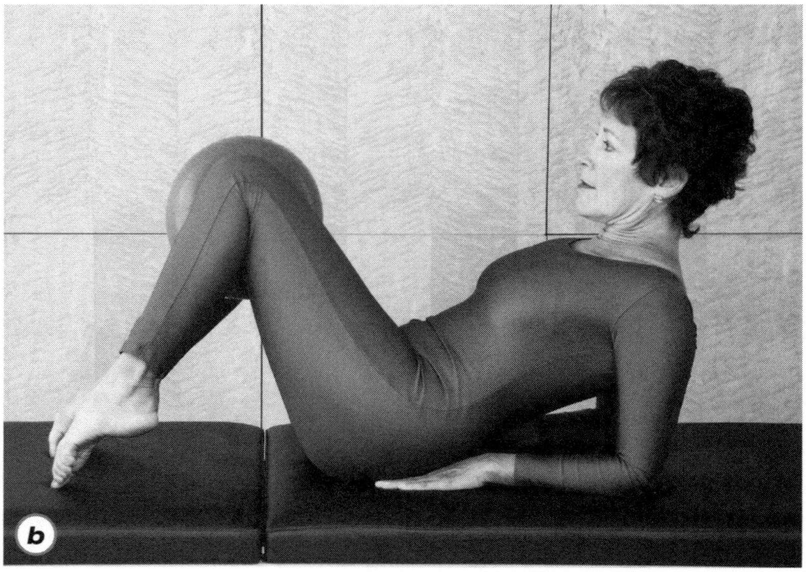

then rotate to the left *(c)*. Rotate back to the center and then rotate to the right.

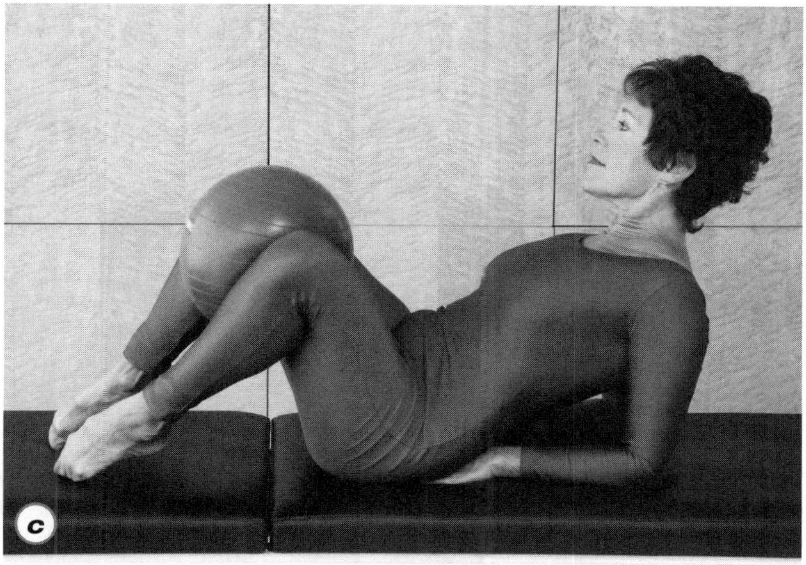

- Exhale, drawing the abdominals in and up, and lift the legs to the ceiling on the diagonal from the right rotation *(d)*.
- Bend the knees back into the right rotation and then rotate to the left, then to the right, and then to the left. Exhale and extend the legs toward the ceiling on the diagonal.
- Keep the torso square and stable. Think of pulling the opposite hip back toward the mat when you extend the legs on a diagonal toward the ceiling.
- The flow is center, right, center, left, center, right, extend, bend, center, left, center, right, center, left, extend, bend, center.
- **Hip:** Maintain the flexion precautions of 115° of hip flexion for 6 months and beyond postop.
- Repeat 5 times in each direction.

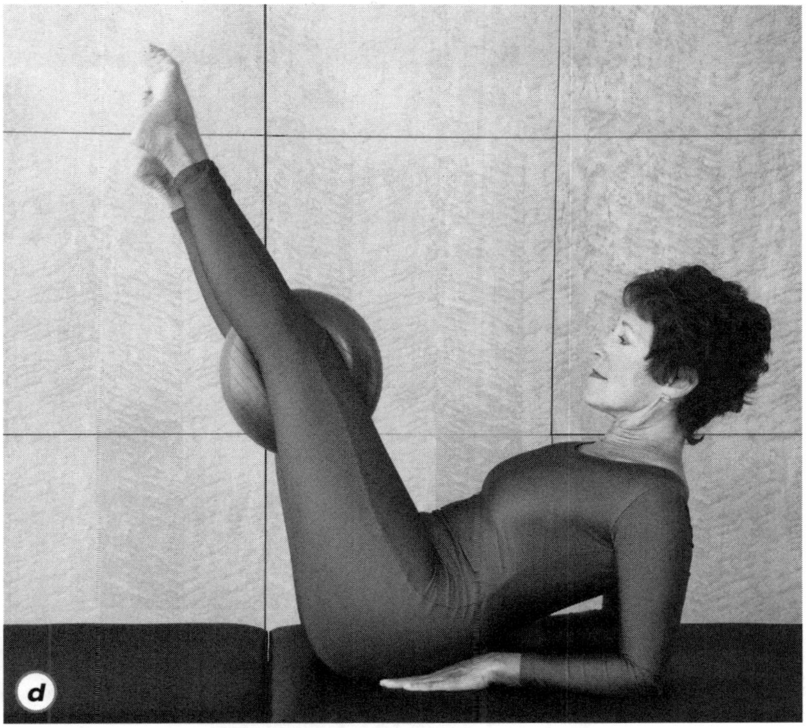

(continued)

Cancan (Modified) *(continued)*

Options

1. Keep the arms by the sides of the body.
- Lie supine on the mat with the arms by the sides and bend the knees into mountain shape.
- Lift the heels and lightly touch the floor with the toes *(a)*.
- Rotate right *(b)*, then left *(c)*, then right, and extend the legs to the ceiling on a diagonal *(d)*.
- Keep the torso square and stable on the mat and maintain a neutral spine.

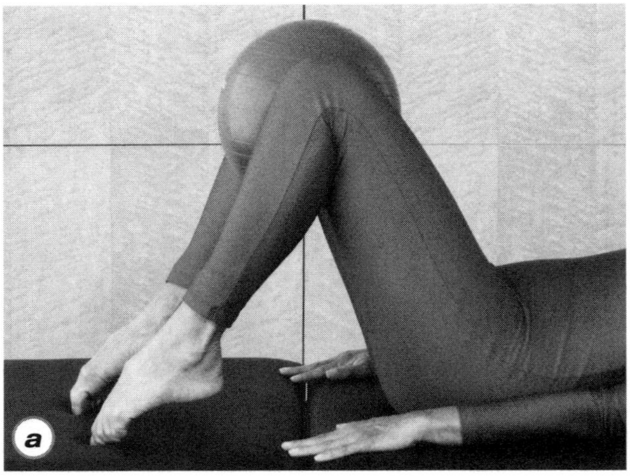

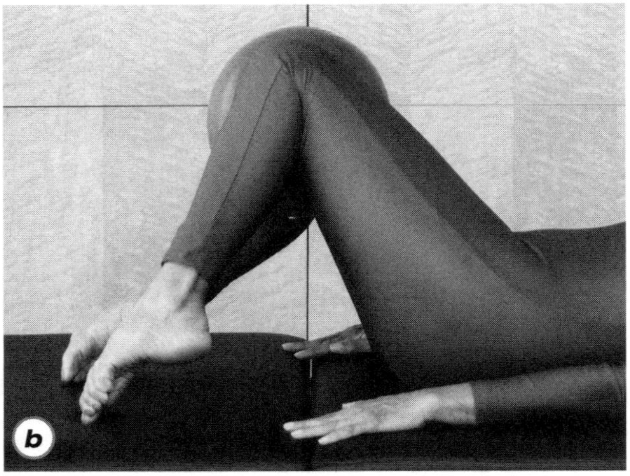

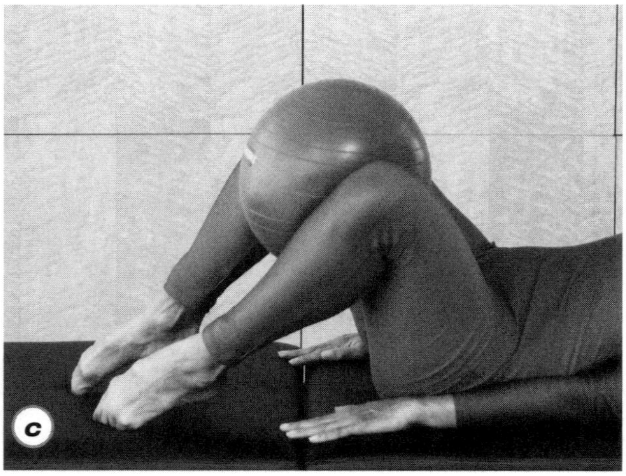

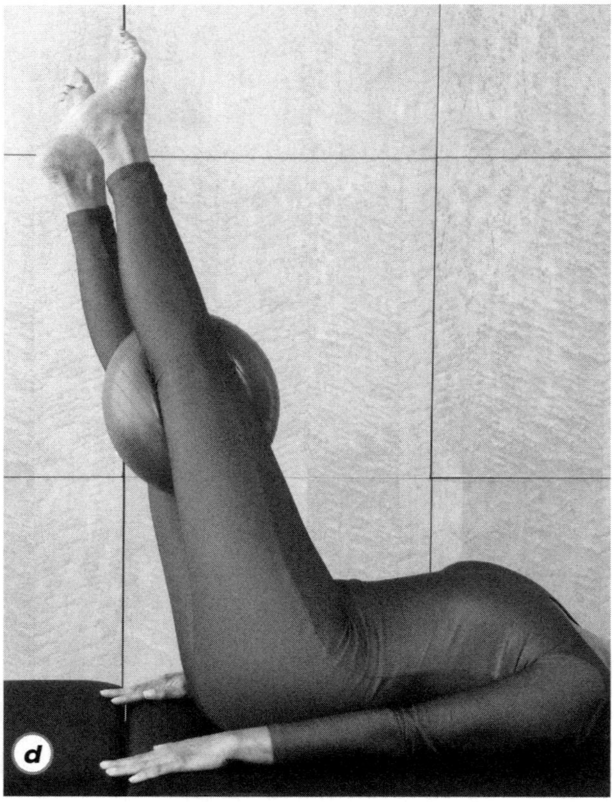

2. Perform a knee-only option for 6 months and beyond postop.
   - Sit tall with the legs together. Lean back and place the palms on the mat with the arms straight and wider than the hips. Point the fingers away. Bend the knees to a mountain shape, hugging the legs together. Lift the heels and slightly touch the mat with the toes.
   - Lift the chest away from the forearms. Maintain a neutral spine with the chest lifted and the gaze straight forward, the shoulder blades lengthened toward the hips, and the collarbones open.
   - Inhale to prepare. Exhale and rotate the knees as one unit to the right, rolling toward the outside of the little toe. Rotate back to center then rotate to the left. Rotate back to the center and then rotate to the right. Exhale, drawing the abdominals in and up, and lift the legs to the ceiling on the diagonal from the right rotation.
   - Bend the knees back into the right rotation and then rotate left, right, left, and exhale and extend the legs toward the ceiling on the diagonal.
   - Keep the torso square and stable. Think of pulling the opposite hip back toward the mat when you extend the legs on a diagonal toward the ceiling.
   - Repeat 5 times.
3. For the hip, perform a modified cancan on the forearms for at least 1 year postop.

Look for . . . Encourage

- The torso lifted and stable throughout the movement
- Heart center lifted
- Knees slightly flexed with a pad between them when extending out on the diagonal as needed
- Neutral spine throughout the movement
- Sit bones on the mat
- Abdominals drawn in and up

Be aware of . . . Prevent

- Hyperextension of the lumbar spine
- Loss of neutral spine
- Sinking between the shoulders
- Loss of core control

Primary Muscles Activated

Abdominals, shoulder complex, rectus femoris, vastus medialis, vastus intermedius, vastus lateralis, sartorius, pectineus, tensor fasciae latae, iliopsoas, adductor magnus, adductor longus, adductor brevis, gracilis, biceps femoris, semitendinosus, semimembranosus, popliteus, gastrocnemius, plantaris, piriformis, gluteus medius, gluteus minimus, gluteus maximus, obturator internus, obturator externus, quadratus femoris, gemellus inferior, gemellus superior, tibialis posterior, soleus

Swimming

Timeline: 3 to 6 months and 6 months and beyond postop

Appropriate for: knee and hip

Location: a floor mat or a raised mat as needed; a raised mat for a bilateral knee or hip replacement as needed for up to 6 months postop

Instructions for Swim Prep

- Lie prone on the mat with the arms extended long overhead and parallel. Keep the arms wider than shoulder-width apart. Turn the palms slightly in toward each other or face the mat with the palms.
- Extend the legs parallel and hip-distance apart. Feel the tops of the toenails on the mat, deepen the pubic bone toward the mat, and slightly engage the gluteus muscles and hamstrings.
- Draw the abdominals in and up; feel as though you could shoot air between the mat and the belly button, lifting the waistline from the mat.
- Glide the shoulders away from ears and toward the hip points.
- Inhale and lift the right arm and left leg *(a)*. Hold for 2 counts, exhale, and lower.
- Inhale and lift the left arm and right leg *(b)*. Hold for 2 counts, exhale, and lower.
- Repeat 2 times on each side.

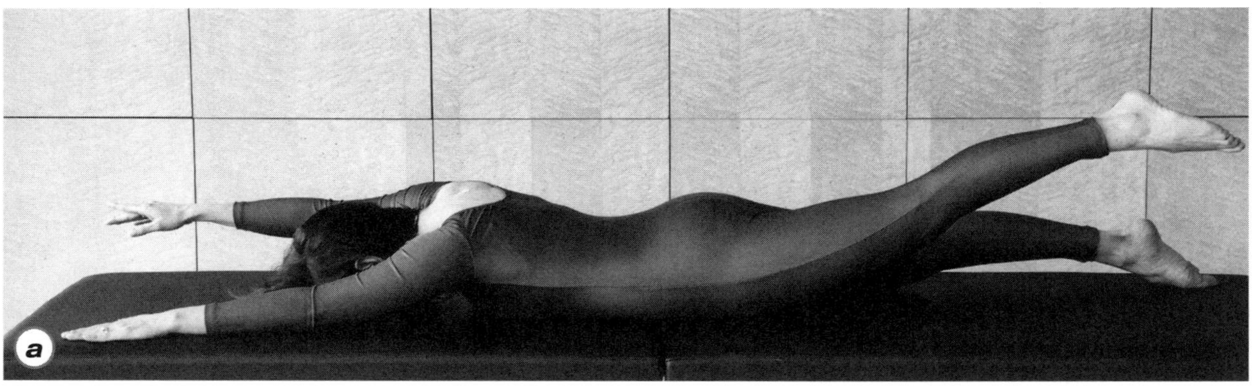

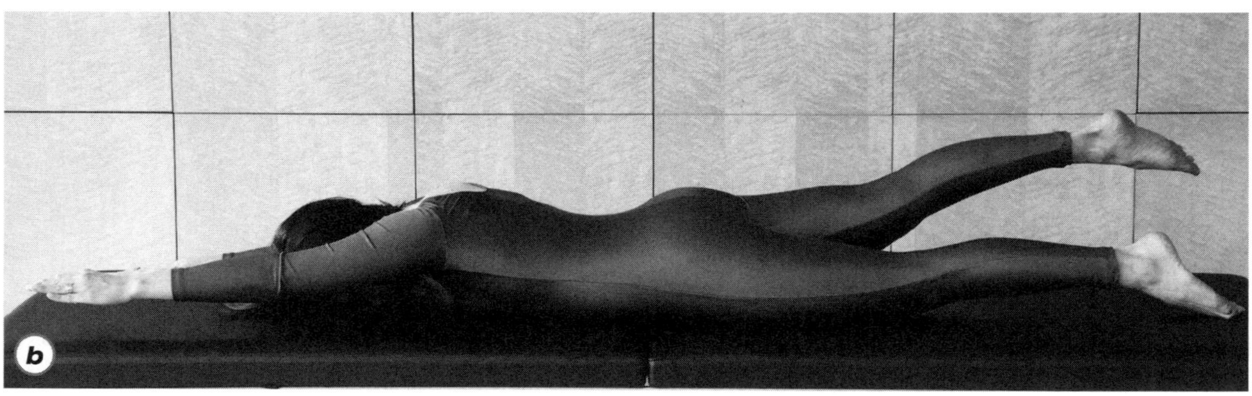

Instructions for Progression Toward Full Swimming

- Inhale, lift the head up in line with the spine, and lift both arms and both legs out of the water.
- Imagine you are looking into a mirror on the mat.
- Exhale, lift the right arm and left leg a little higher, and then switch, lifting the left arm and right leg a little higher. Switch, switch, switch and gradually pick up the pace.
- Inhale and exhale smoothly.
- Keep an even rhythm and pace.
- Repeat 2 to 3 sets of 8 counts.

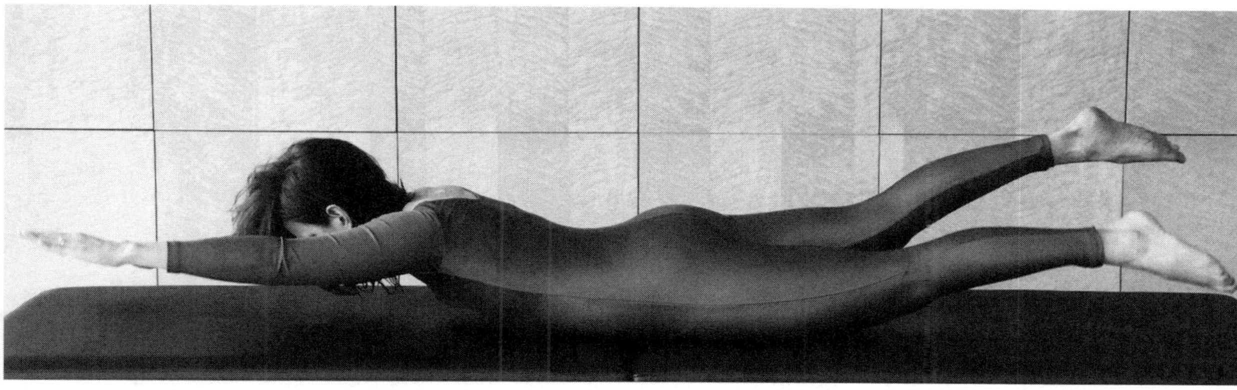

Option

Make a pillow with the hands and place them under the forehead. Only do the leg portion of the exercise. Place a folded towel or mat under the hips and abdominal area for comfort.

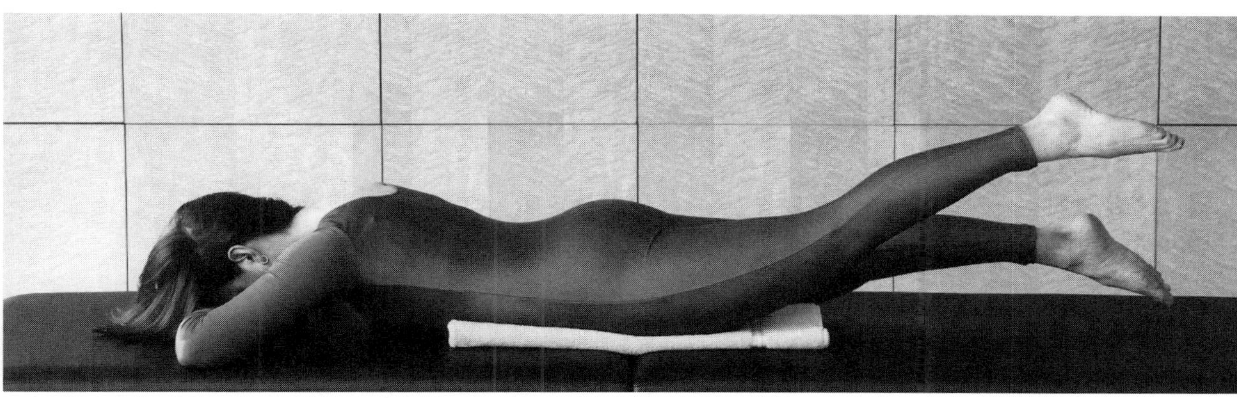

(continued)

Swimming *(continued)*

Look for . . . Encourage

- Head follows the alignment of the spine
- Shoulders glide toward the hip points as the body lengthens up
- Abdominals drawn in and up
- Opposition through movement

Be aware of . . . Prevent

- Hyperextension of the lumbar spine
- Hyperextension of the neck
- Dropping the head
- Loss of core control
- Moving only the lower leg when performing the full movement
- Body rocking side to side with the movement
- Loss of shoulder alignment

Primary Muscles Activated

Abdominals, splenius capitis, splenius cervicis, transversospinalis group, erector spinae group, quadratus lumborum (assists), intertransversarii, interspinalis, latissimus dorsi, gluteus maximus, gluteus medius (posterior portion), adductor magnus (ischiocondylar part), biceps femoris, semitendinosus, semimembranosus, rectus femoris, vastus medialis, vastus intermedius, vastus lateralis, tensor fasciae latae, tibialis posterior, gastrocnemius, plantaris, soleus

Hip Circle (Modified)

Restrictions: not applicable for hip at 3 to 6 months postop; perform corkscrew on page 182

Timeline: 3 to 6 months and 6 months and beyond postop

Appropriate for: knee

Timeline: 6 months and beyond postop

Appropriate for: hip

Location: a floor mat or a raised mat as needed; a raised mat for a bilateral knee or hip replacement as needed for up to 6 months postop

Instructions

- Sit tall with the legs together. Lean back and place the forearms on the mat with the palms down and the fingers pointing toward the hips. The fingertips should rest slightly under the hips.
- Bend the knees into a mountain shape. Place a small, soft ball between the legs at the ankles. Inhale and lift the heels and slightly touch the floor with the toes. Exhale and draw the abdominals in and up. Extend the legs to ceiling.
- Lift the chest away from the forearms. Keep a neutral spine, open collarbones, and shoulders gliding toward the hips. Gaze forward.
- Prepare to make small circles on the ceiling with both legs moving as one unit.
- Visualize a large clock on the ceiling. Inhale to prepare. Exhale and draw the abdominals in and up. Circle the legs as one unit to 3 o'clock, 6 o'clock, 9 o'clock, and then back up to 12 o'clock.
- Pause and then reverse. Inhale to prepare. Exhale to 9 o'clock, 6 o'clock, 3 o'clock, and then back up to 12 o'clock.
- Keep the circle the size of a large clock on the ceiling.
- Keep the hips square and stable.
- **Hip:** Only perform the hip circle 6 months and beyond postop. Maintain the precautions of 115° of hip flexion.
- Repeat 5 times each direction.

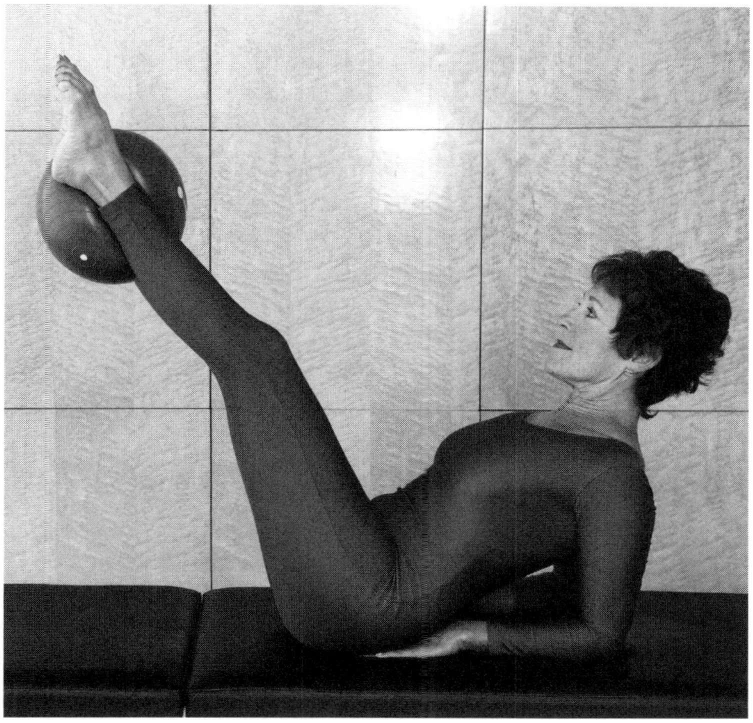

(continued)

Hip Circle (Modified) *(continued)*

Options

1. Place a small pad between the knees and keep a small bend in the knees when you extend the legs.
2. Perform the movement with the legs together with no ball.
3. For 6 months postop and beyond, try the knee-only option.
   - Sit tall with the legs together. Lean back and place the palms on the mat with the arms straight out on an angle slightly greater than hip-distance apart. Point the fingers away from the hips.
   - Perform the hip circle as just described.

Look for . . . Encourage

- Torso lifted and stable throughout the movement
- Circle size that maintains pelvic stability and the abdominals drawn in and up
- Legs circling as one unit, hugging to the midline of the body
- Thinking of pulling the opposite hip back as the legs circle in each direction

Be aware of . . . Prevent

- Sinking between the shoulders
- Hyperextension of the lumbar spine
- Loss of core control and pelvic stability
- Loss of shoulder alignment

Primary Muscles Activated

Abdominals, shoulder complex, rectus femoris, sartorius, pectineus, tensor fasciae latae, iliopsoas, gracilis, adductor magnus, adductor longus, adductor brevis, gracilis, vastus medius, vastus lateralis, vastus intermedius, gluteus maximus, gluteus medius, gluteus minimus, tibialis posterior, soleus, gastrocnemius, plantaris

Leg Pull (Modified)

Restrictions: not applicable for hip at 3 to 6 months postop; perform pre-Pilates supine leg lifts on page 53

Timeline: 3 to 6 months and 6 months and beyond postop

Appropriate for: knee

Timeline: 6 months and beyond postop

Appropriate for: hip

Location: a floor mat or a raised mat as needed; a raised mat for a bilateral knee or hip replacement as needed for up to 6 months postop

Instructions

- Sit tall with the legs together and hugging to the midline of the body. Point the toes. Lean back and place the forearms on the mat with the palms down and the fingers pointing toward the hips. Place a rolled-up towel under the knees as needed.
- Lift the chest away from the forearm. Gaze forward. Maintain a neutral spine, open collarbones, and shoulders gliding down the back toward the hips.
- Draw the abdominals in and up.
- Inhale to prepare. Exhale and lift the right leg off the mat, pointing the toe to the ceiling *(a)*. Inhale and flex the foot, reaching through the heel *(b)*, and lower the leg back down to the mat. Barely touch the mat and point the toe and kick the leg back up.

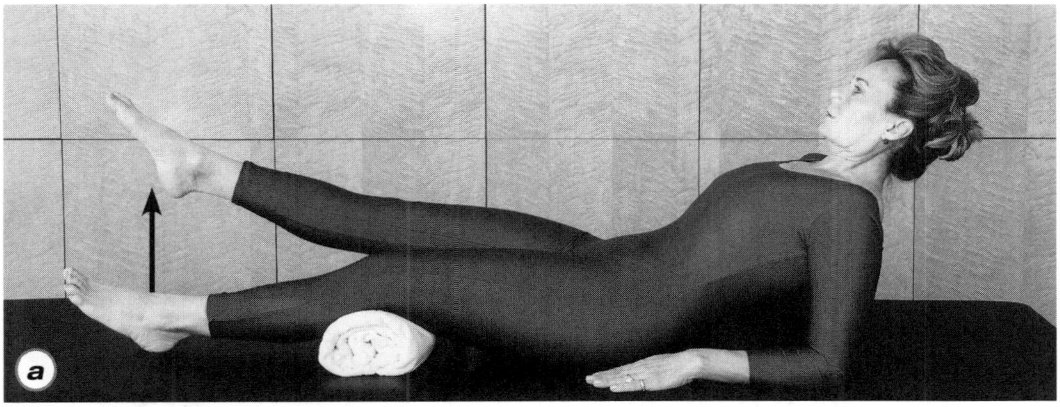

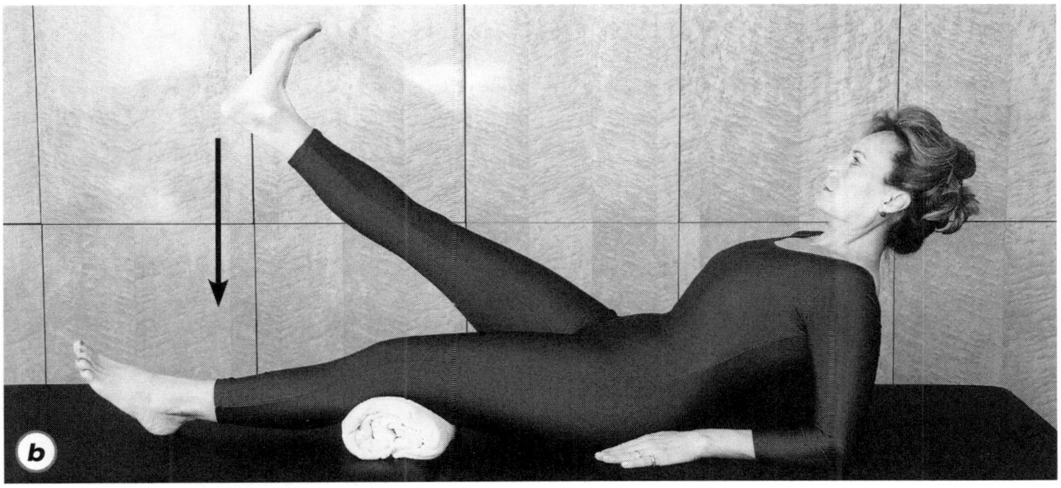

(continued)

Leg Pull (Modified) *(continued)*

- Repeat the kick 3 times. Switch legs and repeat.
- Keep both hips stable on the mat without movement.
- Think of lengthening out of the hip as you kick the leg up toward the ceiling. Shoot an arrow of energy out of the toe toward the ceiling and an arrow of energy though the hip into the mat to create opposition.
- **Knee and hip:** Place a rolled-up towel under the knees. Slightly flex or bend the knees as needed to prevent overuse of the hip flexors.
- Note: While the modified leg pull is not a difficult exercise, for hip and knee replacements, the flexion of the hip when lifting the long lever leg can excessively recruit the hip flexors, which can lead to stress and inflammation. It is best to wait until 6 months after hip arthroplasty to incorporate this exercise into a routine.

Options

1. Place a roller behind the back to rest the forearms on to perform the exercise. Bend the knees as needed.

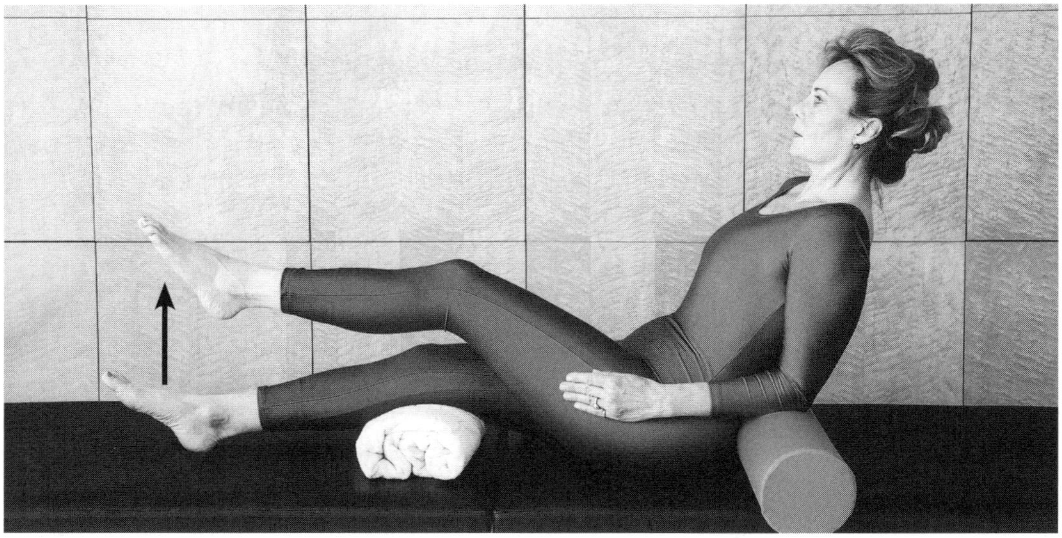

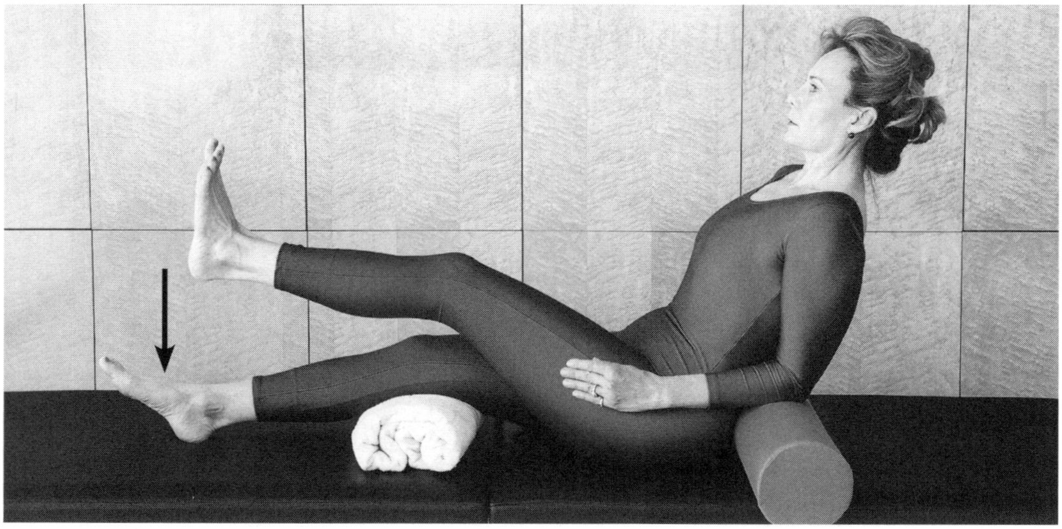

2. Do a leg pull with a lift up and hold portion of the movement.

- Sit tall with the legs together and hugging to the midline of the body. Point the toes. Lean back and place the hands on the mat with the palms down and the fingers pointing toward the hips. Open the arms a little wider than the hips.
- Inhale and lift up; hold the plank position with the chest lifted. Maintain a neutral spine, open collarbones, and shoulders gliding down the back toward the hips. Gaze forward.
- Draw the abdominals in and up. Breathe naturally.
- Hold for 10 counts; exhale and lower back to the mat.
- Repeat 3 times.

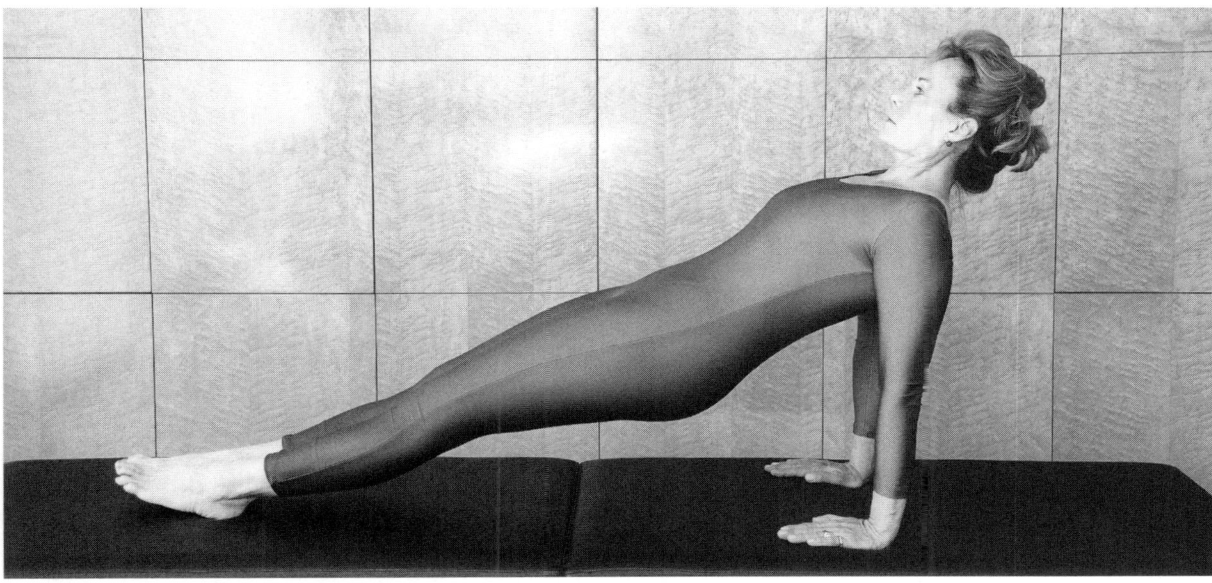

(continued)

Leg Pull (Modified) *(continued)*

Look for . . . Encourage

- Shoulders gliding down the back
- Forward gaze
- Chest lifted
- Thinking of arms planted in cement
- Sit bones glued to the mat and stable pelvis
- Abdominals drawn in and up
- Pelvic stability

Be aware of . . . Prevent

- Feet rolling in, out, or apart
- Hyperextension of the lumbar spine
- Hyperextension of the knees
- Sinking of chest between the shoulders
- Stress and strain of the hip flexors
- Loss of core control
- Loss of pelvic stability with the movement

Primary Muscles Activated

The primary muscles activated depend on the chosen option. The primary muscles include the following: Abdominals, shoulder complex, rectus femoris, sartorius, pectineus, iliopsoas, gracilis, adductor longus, adductor brevis, biceps femoris, semimembranosus, semitendinosus, gluteus maximus, gluteus medius (posterior portion), adductor magnus (ischiocondylar part), vastus medius, vastus lateralis, vastus intermedius, gastrocnemius, soleus, plantaris, tibialis anterior, tibialis posterior

Side Stretch

Timeline: 3 to 6 months and 6 months and beyond postop

Appropriate for: knee and hip

Location: a floor mat or a raised mat as needed; a raised mat for a bilateral knee or hip replacement as needed for up to 6 months postop

Instructions

- Sit tall on a moon box or the mat.
- Lengthen the legs out on the mat with a slight bend in the knees.
- Keep the head and shoulders and hips in alignment.
- Start by sitting tall with the arms extended out to the sides, reaching for each wall. Bring the right arm up next to the ear with the palm facing the head. The left arm stays out in line with the shoulder, pointing to the wall *(a)*.
- Inhale to prepare. Exhale and bring the right arm up and over as the left hand reaches for the mat *(b)*.
- Bend the left arm as needed or allow the left arm to slide along the mat as the right arm reaches up and over toward the left, creating a side stretch on the right side of the body.
- Hold for a count of 5 and then slowly return back to the starting position *(c)*.
  - The right hip flows toward the mat during the entire movement.
  - Keep the right shoulder blade flowing toward the right hip even though you are extending the arm up and over on a diagonal line.
  - Think of arching up and over the rainbow.
- Breathe into the right lung when leading back to the starting position.
- Repeat 3 times and then reverse and stretch the left side.
- **Hip and knee:** Place a moon box, barrel, or folded towel under hips for comfort. Place a rolled-up mat under the knees as needed.

(continued)

Side Stretch *(continued)*

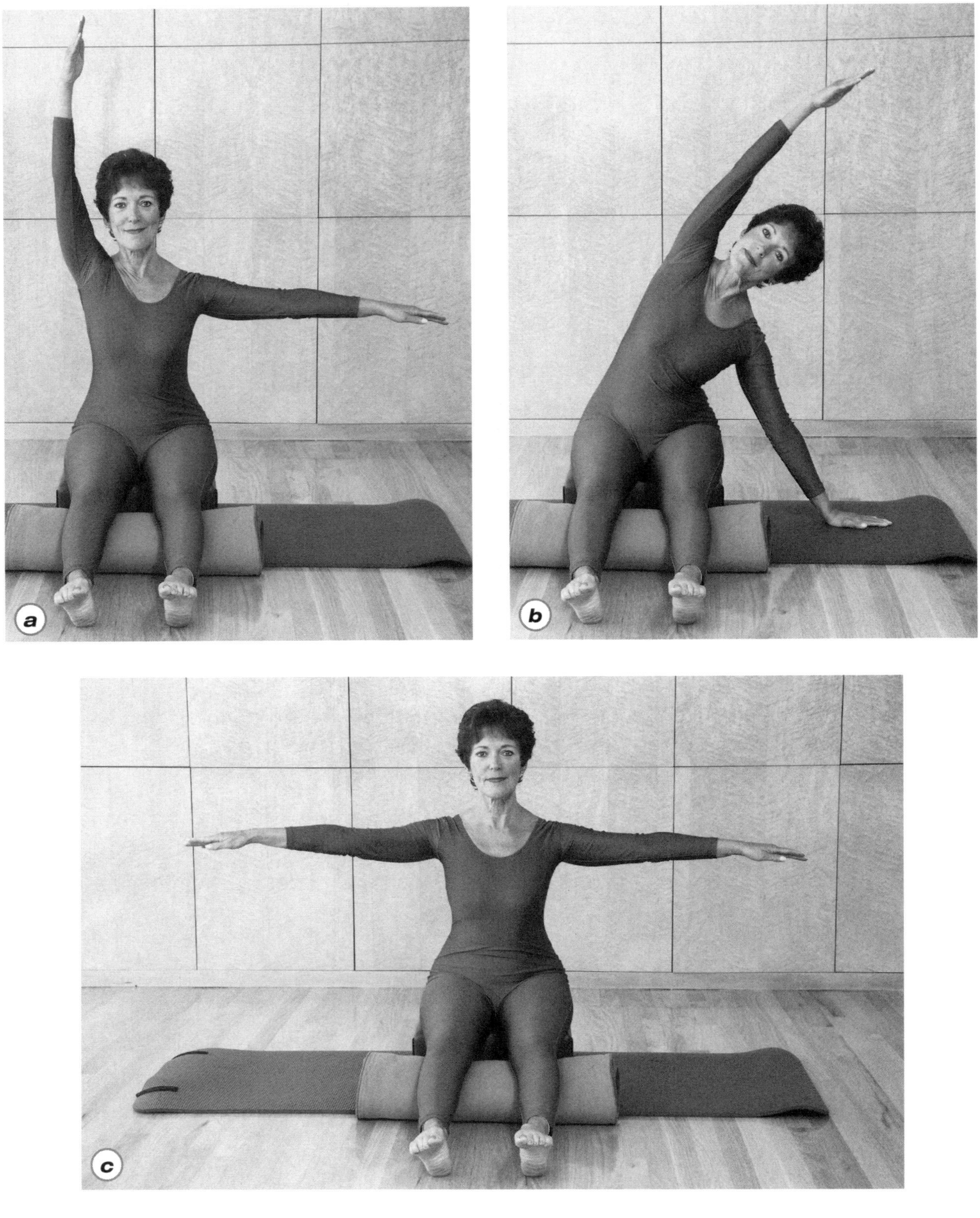

Option

Perform the exercise with the legs crossed.

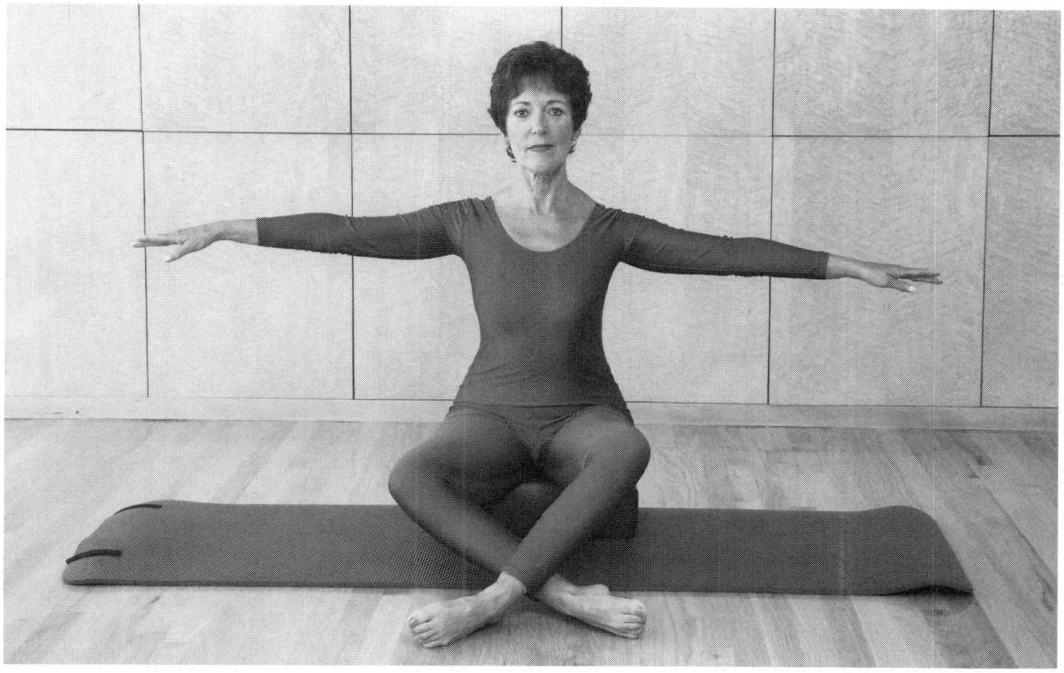

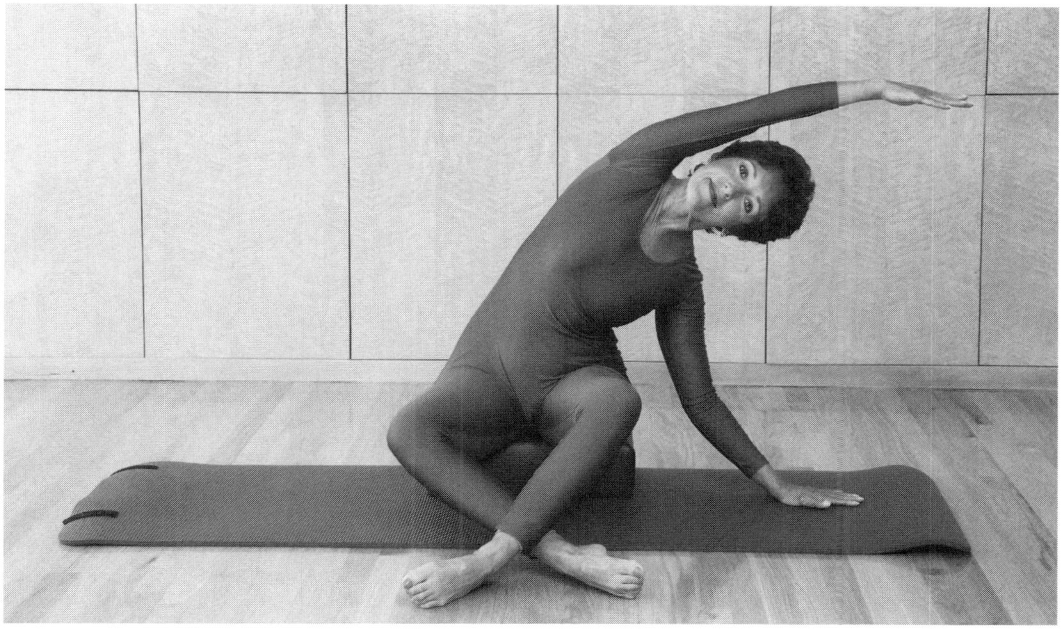

(continued)

Look for . . . Encourage

- Shoulders gliding toward the hip
- Hip deepening into mat during the extension up and over to the opposite side
- Forward gaze
- A long arch in the body
- Visualize a cactus on the mat that you are rounding up and over.

Be aware of . . . Prevent

- Bending the arm that is extending up and over
- Loss of alignment when bending to the side
- Leading back with the arm instead of the lateral spine
- Loss of abdominal engagement with the movement
- Loss of lateral alignment

Primary Muscles Activated

Abdominals, shoulder complex, quadratus lumborum, erector spinae group, intertransversarii, latissimus dorsi

Serratus Push-Up (Modified)

Restrictions: not applicable for knee 3 to 6 months postop

Timeline: 3 to 6 months and 6 months and beyond postop

Appropriate for: hip

Timeline: 6 months and beyond postop

Appropriate for: knee

Location: a floor mat or a raised mat as needed; a raised mat for a bilateral knee or hip replacement as needed for up to 6 months postop

Instructions

- Get down on all fours on the mat. Make sure the knees are under the hips and the palms are directly under the shoulders, fingers pointing forward. The legs are parallel and hip-distance apart.
- Lower down to the right forearm and then to the left forearm. Make fists with the hands and join the forearms into a triangle, with the fists touching each other. Keep the elbows in line with the shoulders.
- Walk forward on the elbows, lowering the hips toward the floor, making a diagonal line from the shoulders to the hips and knees. Stay on the knees with the toes touching the floor. Make sure the elbows are directly under the shoulders *(a)*.
- Draw the abdominals in and up. Engage the gluteus muscles and hamstrings.
- Inhale and lower the chest toward the mat, drawing the shoulder blades together as if you were squeezing an acorn *(b)*. Exhale and lift the chest away from the mat, pressing the shoulder blades apart *(c)*. Feel as though you are sending the shoulder blades up to touch the ceiling.
- **Knee:** Perform this exercise 6 months and beyond postop only. Place a towel or mat under the knees as needed.
- Repeat 5 times, rest, and then repeat another set of 5.
- Finish by moving back into all fours to stretch the lower spine. Draw the abdominals in and up and round the back into flexion. Inhale back to neutral.

(continued)

Serratus Push-Up (Modified) *(continued)*

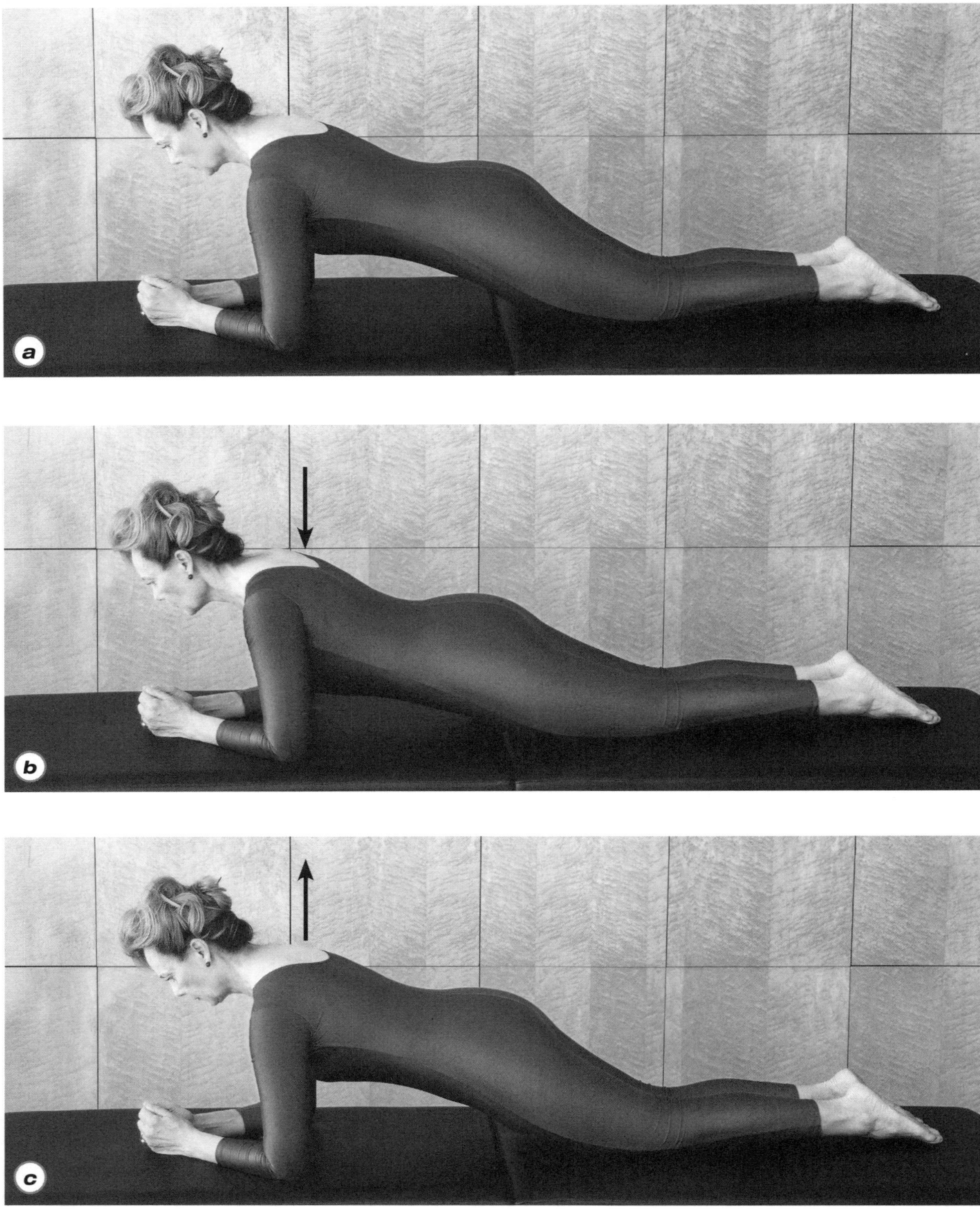

Look for . . . Encourage

- The head following the alignment of the spine
- Shoulders gliding toward the hips
- Feeling as if a sling were under the torso, suspending the torso from the ceiling
- Navel snapped to the spine

Be aware of . . . Prevent

- The head lowering out of alignment like a broken flower bud
- The torso sinking to the mat
- Hyperextension of the lumbar spine
- Loss of core control
- Loss of shoulder alignment

Primary Muscles Activated

Shoulder complex, abdominals, anterior and posterior serratus, erector spinae group, transversospinalis group, splenius capitis, splenius cervicis, quadratus lumborum (assists), intertransversarii, interspinalis, triceps, biceps, deltoid, latissimus dorsi, biceps femoris, semitendinosus, semimembranosus, gluteus maximus, gluteus medius (posterior portion) adductor magnus (ischiocondylar part)

Serratus Push-Up

Restrictions: not applicable for knee and hip 3 to 6 months postop

Timeline: 6 months and beyond postop

Appropriate for: knee and hip

Location: a floor mat or a raised table as needed

Instructions

- Get down on all fours on the mat. Make sure the knees are under the hips and the palms are directly under the shoulders, with the fingers pointing forward. The legs are parallel and hip-distance apart.
- Lower down to the right forearm and then to the left forearm. Make fists with the hands and join the forearms into a triangle, with the fists touching each other. Keep the elbows in line with the shoulders.
- Extend the right foot back in a straight line and place the ball of the foot on the mat with the toes. Bring the left foot back to meet the right *(a)*.
- Hug the legs to the midline of the body. Keep the balls of the feet in line with the heels.
- Draw the abdominals in and up. Engage the gluteus muscles and hamstrings.

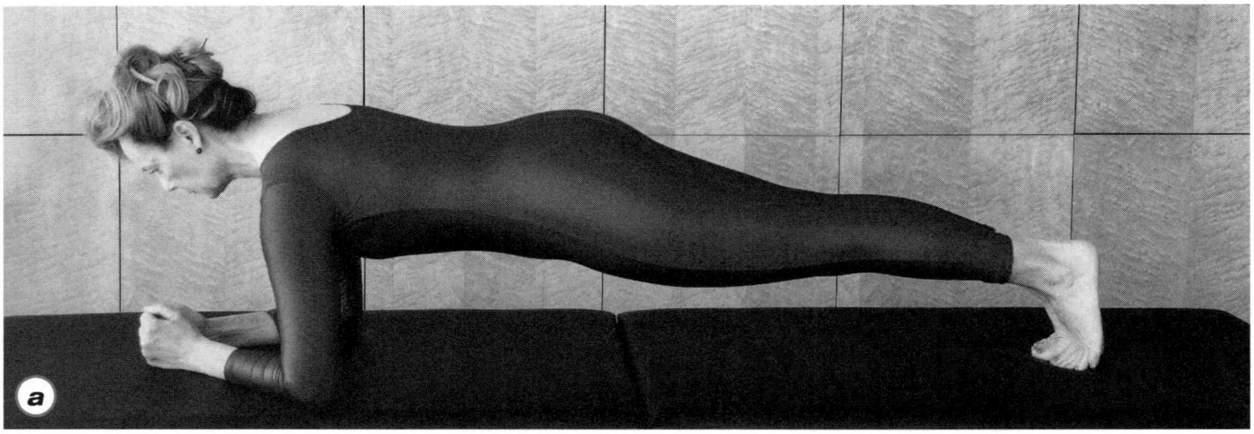
a

- Inhale and lower the chest toward the mat, drawing the shoulder blades together as if you were squeezing an acorn *(b)*. Exhale and lift the chest away from the mat, pressing the shoulder blades apart *(c)*. Feel as if you were sending the shoulder blades up to touch the ceiling.
- Repeat 5 times, rest, and then repeat another set of 5.
- Finish by moving back to all fours to stretch the lower spine. Draw the abdominals in and up and round the back in flexion. Inhale back to neutral.

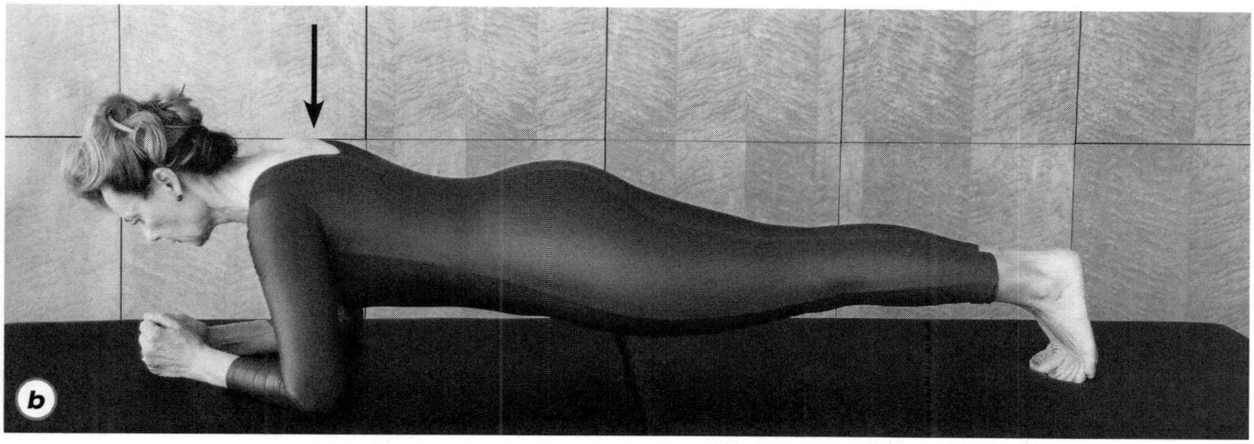
b

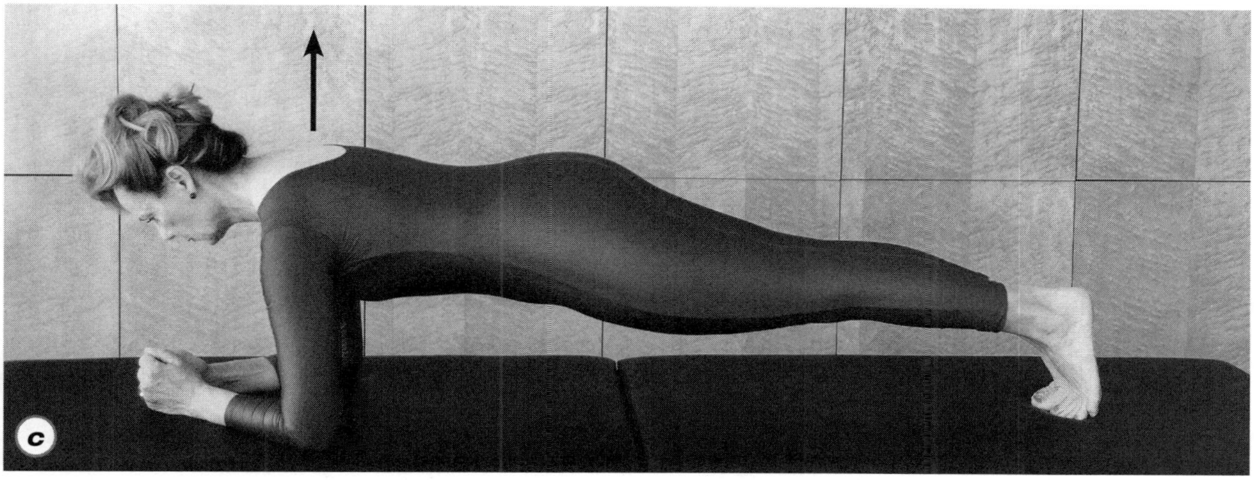
c

(continued)

Options

1. Use a towel or pad under the knees as needed for getting into the full forearm plank position.
2. Continue with the modified serratus push-up as needed.

Look for . . . Encourage

- The head following the alignment of the spine
- Shoulders gliding toward the hips
- Feeling as if a sling were under the torso, suspending the torso from the ceiling
- Navel snapped to the spine

Be aware of . . . Prevent

- The head lowering out of alignment like a broken flower bud
- The torso sinking to the mat
- Loss of core control
- Hyperextension of the lumbar spine
- Loss of shoulder alignment

Primary Muscles Activated

Shoulder complex, abdominals, anterior and posterior serratus, erector spinae group, transversospinalis group, splenius capitis, splenius cervicis, quadratus lumborum (assists), intertransversarii, interspinalis, triceps, biceps, deltoid, latissimus dorsi, biceps femoris, semitendinosus, semimembranosus, gluteus maximus, gluteus medius (posterior portion) adductor magnus (ischiocondylar part), vastus medius, vastus intermedius, vastus lateralis, tensor fasciae latae, tibialis anterior

Push-Up (Modified)

Restriction: not applicable for knee 3 to 6 months postop

Timeline: 3 to 6 months and 6 months and beyond postop

Appropriate for: hip

Timeline: 6 months and beyond postop

Appropriate for: knee

Location: a floor mat or a raised mat as needed; a raised mat for a bilateral knee or hip replacement as needed for up to 6 months postop

Instructions

- Get down on all fours on the mat. Make sure the knees are under the hips and the hands are under the shoulders, with the fingers pointing forward. The legs are parallel and hip-distance apart.
- Staying on the knees, walk the hands out to create a diagonal line from the shoulders to the hips. Stay on the knees with the toes slightly touching the floor. Keep the hands directly under the shoulders. Hug the elbows toward the rib cage of the body *(a)*.
- Draw the abdominals in and up (drawing the waistline toward the spine). Engage the gluteus muscles and hamstrings.

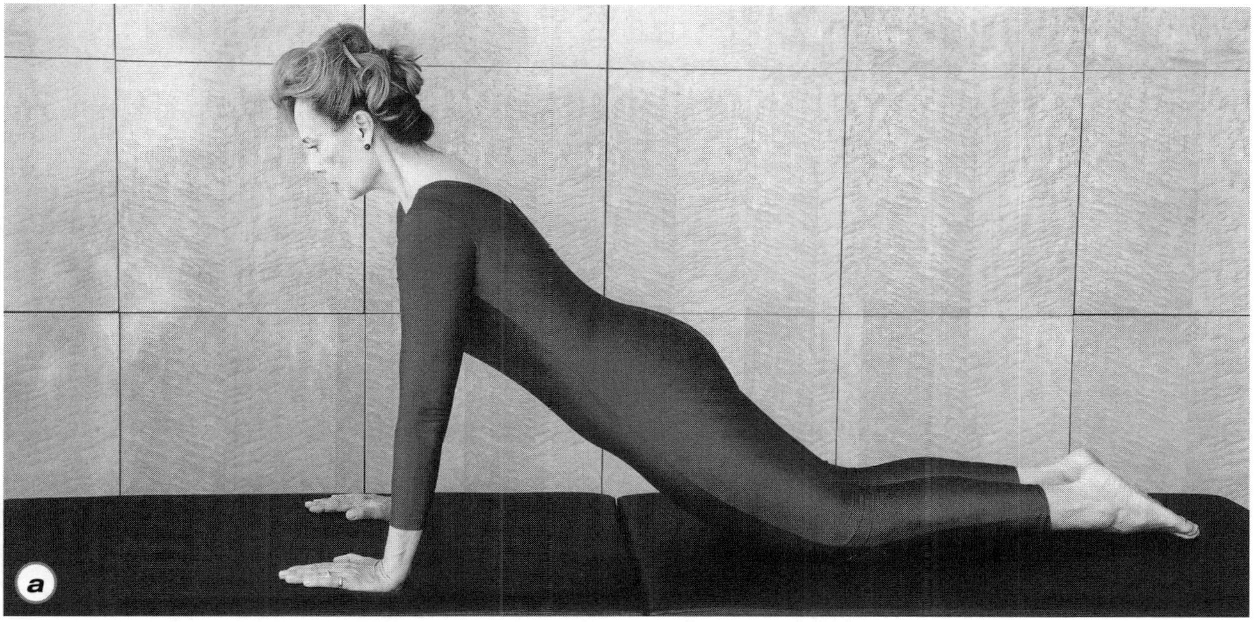

(continued)

Push-Up (Modified) *(continued)*

- Inhale and bend the elbows, lowering the torso toward the mat *(b)*. The elbows stay close to the rib cage. Only lower down to where you can maintain the stability of the torso in the diagonal line. Exhale and press back up to a straight arm. Feel as if you were pressing the hands away from the shoulders.

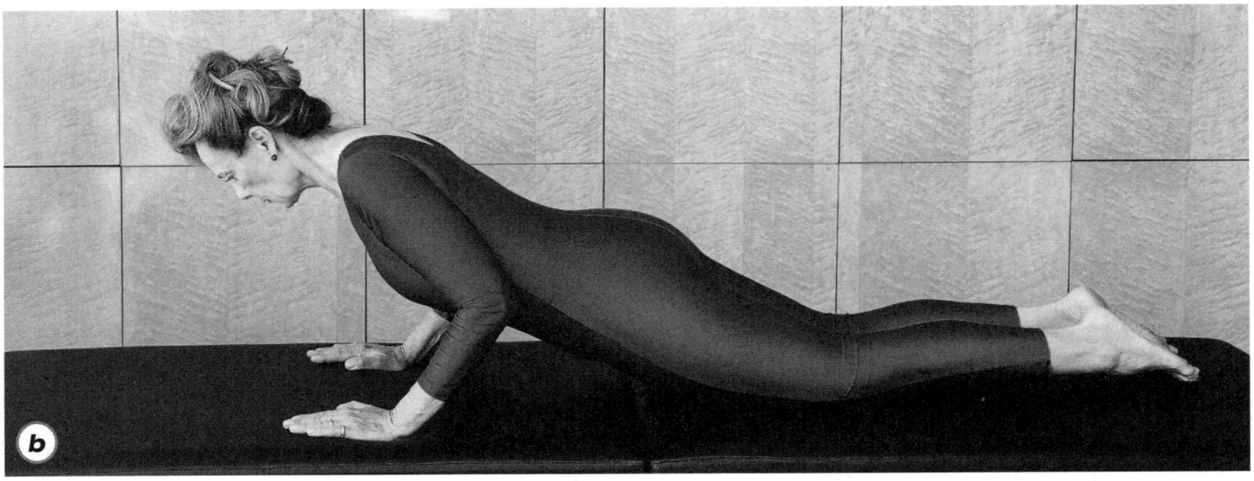
b

- Perform the movement by flexing the elbows toward the feet. Keep the gaze slightly ahead on the mat.
- **Knee:** Perform this exercise 6 months and beyond postop only. Place a towel or mat under the knees as needed.
- Repeat 5 times, rest, and then repeat another set of 5.
- Finish by moving back into all fours to stretch the lower spine. Draw the abdominals in and up and round the back in flexion. Inhale back to neutral.

Look for . . . Encourage

- The head following the alignment of the spine
- Shoulders gliding toward the hips
- Feeling as if a sling were under the torso, suspending the torso from the ceiling
- Navel snapped to the spine, abdominals drawn in and up
- Torso stability

Be aware of . . . Prevent

- The head lowering out of alignment like a broken flower bud
- The torso sinking to the mat
- Loss of core control
- Hyperextension of the lumbar spine
- Leading back up with the hips
- Loss of shoulder alignment

Primary Muscles Activated

Shoulder complex, triceps, biceps, deltoid abdominals, erector spinae group, transversospinalis group, splenius capitis, splenius cervicis, quadratus lumborum (assists), intertransversarii, interspinalis, latissimus dorsi, biceps femoris, semitendinosus, semimembranosus, gluteus maximus, gluteus medius (posterior portion) adductor magnus (ischiocondylar part)

Push-Up

Restrictions: not applicable for knee and hip 3 months postop

Timeline: 6 months and beyond postop

Appropriate for: knee and hip

Location: a floor mat or a raised table as needed

Instructions

- Get down on all fours on the mat. Make sure the knees are under the hips and the hands are under the shoulders, with the fingers pointing forward.
- Extend the right foot back in a straight line and place the ball of the foot with the toes on the mat (keep the heel in line with the toes). Bring the left foot back to meet the right. The legs are parallel and hugging to the midline or slightly apart. Keep the palms directly under the shoulders. Keep the elbows hugging to the sides of the rib cage *(a)*.
- Create one long line from the shoulders to the feet.
- Draw the abdominals in and up, pulling the waistline up toward the spine. Engage the gluteus muscles and hamstrings.

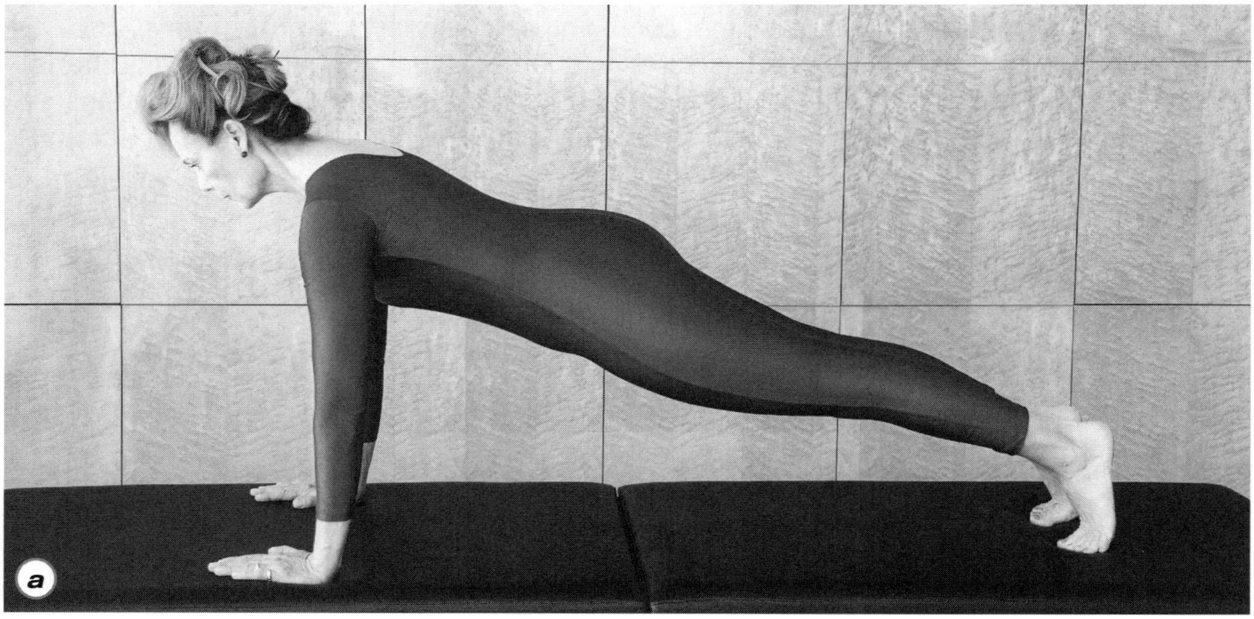

a

- Inhale and bend the elbows, lowering the torso toward the mat *(b)*. The elbows stay close to the rib cage. Only lower down to where you can maintain the stability of the torso in the slight diagonal line. Exhale and press back up to a straight arm. Feel as if you were pressing the hands away from the shoulders, lifting the torso toward the ceiling.

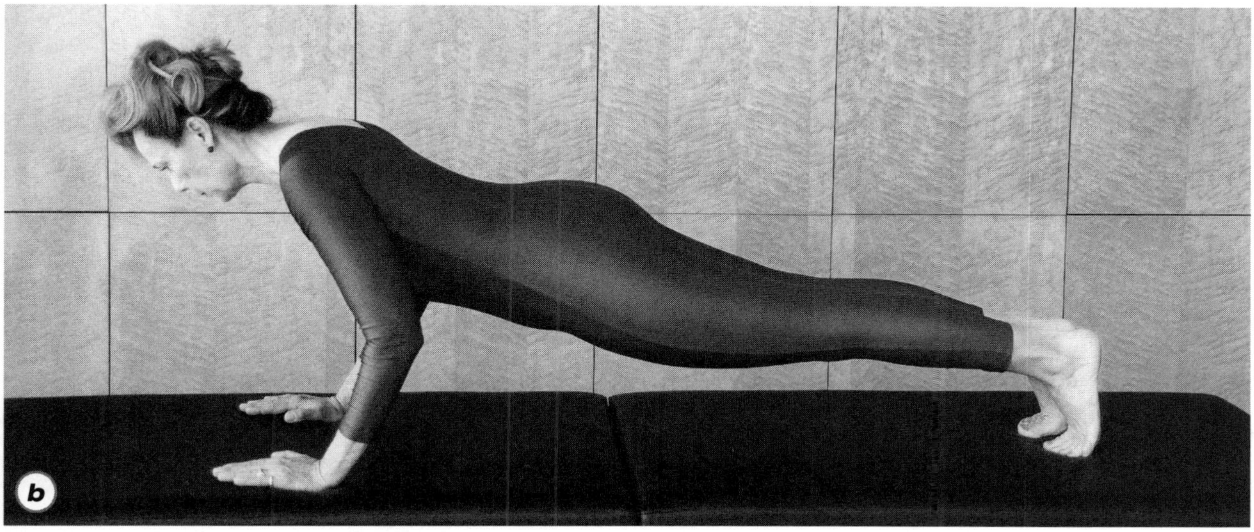

- Repeat 5 times, rest, and then repeat another set of 5.
- Finish by moving back into all fours to stretch the lower spine. Draw the abdominals in and up and round the back into flexion. Inhale back to neutral.

(continued)

Options

1. Place the hands slightly in front of the shoulders and farther out to the sides. When you bend the elbows, let them flow out instead of into the sides of the body.
2. Use a towel or pad under the knees as needed to get into position.
3. Continue with the modified push-up as needed.

Look for . . . Encourage

- The head following the alignment of the spine
- Shoulders gliding toward the hips
- Feeling as if a sling were under the torso, suspending the torso from the ceiling
- Navel snapped to the spine, abdominals drawn in and up
- The elbows close to the rib cage when bending
- Torso stability

Be aware of . . . Prevent

- The head lowering out of alignment like a broken flower bud
- The torso sinking to the mat
- Loss of core control
- Hyperextension of the lumbar spine
- Leading back up with the hips
- Loss of shoulder alignment

Primary Muscles Activated

Shoulder complex, abdominals, triceps, biceps, deltoid, erector spinae group, transversospinalis group, splenius capitis, splenius cervicis, quadratus lumborum (assists), intertransversarii, interspinalis, latissimus dorsi, biceps femoris, semitendinosus, semimembranosus, gluteus maximus, gluteus medius (posterior portion) adductor magnus (ischiocondylar part), vastus medius, vastus intermedius, vastus lateralis, tensor fasciae latae, tibialis anterior

chapter 6

Pilates Mat Side Kick Series

The side kick series (SKS) exercises and variations are extremely important for a client with a hip or knee syndrome or arthroplasty. During these exercises, the core of the body is the stabilizing unit while the legs are worked with precision and control. Because this series is so important to the ROM, flexibility, and strength of the muscles surrounding the joints of the hip, knee, and pelvis, each exercise variation for each postop milestone is described in detail with pictures. Clients can advance to the next stage based on their postop timeline and their ability to maintain core control and stability, maintain disassociation, and tolerate the ROM required to execute the exercise correctly.

In the early stages of introducing the Pilates exercises, select only 3 to 5 of the side kick variations and use minimal repeats. Remember, the ligaments surrounding the joint of a client with a knee or hip replacement have been moved, possibly cut, and possibly debrided. So the work needs to be slow and steady in order to rebuild the strength and stability of the joint. Introducing Pilates preoperatively is a wonderful way to build muscle memory and create a smoother postoperative recovery.

The setup and execution of the SKS exercises for a client with a knee or hip syndrome depend on the client's available ROM and ability to move without pain. These clients should start slowly with minimal repeats and utilize shorter lever lengths (bringing the leg or legs closer to the joint). Use towels, pads, soft balls, and yoga blocks to assist with positioning the client for movement and to support adjacent joints. The exercises that follow always point back to the setup, depending on whether it is from the long-lever (pages 265 to 269) or short-lever options (pages 303 to 307). The possible body positions for each lever length and timeline offer several choices for each setup. Select the setup based on the individual needs of the client—the best setup allows the client to move without pain and access the best ROM. The following lists of SKS exercises outline which exercises correspond to each lever option.

Long-Lever Side Kick Series

1. Body position: setup for long-lever series for 6 weeks to 3 months postop
   - Up and down
   - Front and back
   - Little circle
   - Internal and external rotation
   - Inner-thigh lift
   - Inner-thigh circle
2. Body position: setup for long-lever series for 3 to 6 months and beyond postop
   - Up and down
   - Front and back
   - Little circle
   - D-circle
   - Internal and external rotation
   - Bicycle
   - Scissors
   - Parallel leg lift
   - Lift, lift, lower, lower
   - 90° long-leg lift
   - 90° long-leg circle
   - Inner-thigh lift
   - Inner-thigh circle

Short-Lever Side Kick Series

1. Body position: setup for short-lever series for 6 weeks to 3 months postop
   - 90° bent-knee lift and lower
   - 90° bent-knee circle
   - 90° bent-knee touch
2. Body position: setup for short-lever series for 3 to 6 months and beyond postop
   - 90° bent-knee lift and lower
   - 90° bent-knee circle
   - 90° bent-knee touch
   - 90° bent-knee rotation

The first section of this chapter presents the setup for the long-lever SKS at each postoperative milestone. Starting on page 303, the setup for the short-lever SKS at each postoperative milestone is presented. Following the setups for both the long-lever and short-lever SKS are descriptions and pictures of each exercise and variation utilizing the postop setup described.

Each exercise presented in this chapter shows the setup and action of the movement with several options. The instructions also include what to look for and encourage and what to be aware of and prevent. The primary muscles of the movement are listed, with emphasis on the muscles that are activated or stabilized from the pelvis, hip, and knee.

> All exercises should be performed under the guidance of a qualified Pilates instructor and with referral from the operative physician. The client's needs, restrictions, and ROM recommendations should be specified by the physician and followed accordingly. These guidelines may vary from the protocols that follow, and the protocols should be modified based on the individual's needs and the surgeon's preferences.

Long-Lever Body Position Setup

Timeline: 6 weeks to 3 months postop

Appropriate for: knee and hip

Location: a raised mat, hip height

Instructions

- Lie on one side with the hips and shoulders stacked evenly on the back edge of the mat. Hinge from the hip and bring both legs to the front corner of the mat. Bend the bottom leg into a right angle, keeping the knee in line with the hip and the ankle in line with the knee. For support, place the top hand, with the fingers wide, 6 inches (15 centimeters) in front of the body between the sternum and the navel. Press into the heel of the hand.
- Rest the head on the bottom arm, a pad, or a small ball. Keep the head and arm in line with the shoulders and hips.
- Draw the abdominals in and up, feeling light in the waist as if you could shoot air between the waist and the mat.
- Breathe with an even flow of inhaling and exhaling.
- **Knee and hip:**
  - Keep the working leg parallel, with the knee and toe pointing to the other side of the room.
  - Keep the knee slightly flexed or bent to shorten the lever length.
  - Do not let the leg cross the midline of the body. Use a yoga block, pillow, or barrel to place the working leg in order to maintain this position. Rest between repeats as needed as shown here.

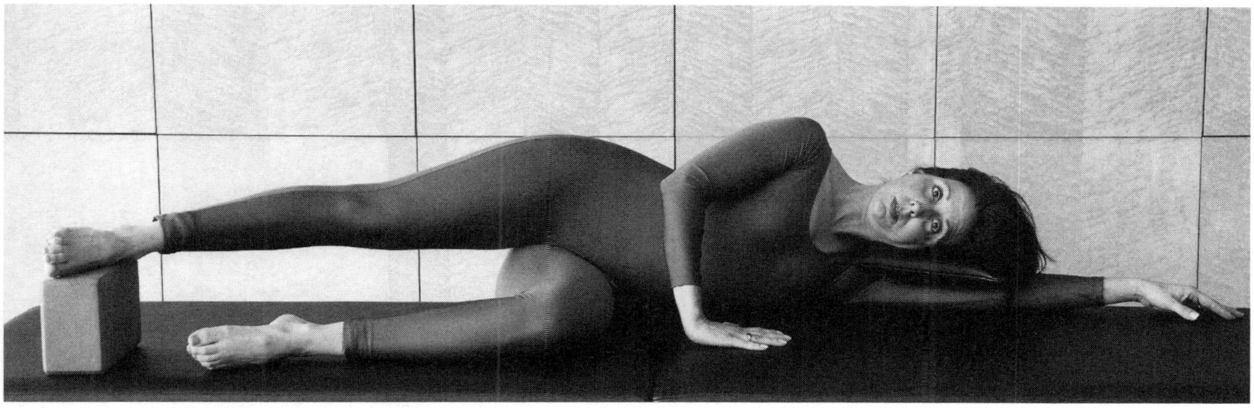

(continued)

Setup Options

1. Place a towel under the hip or knee as needed to decrease pressure on the joint.

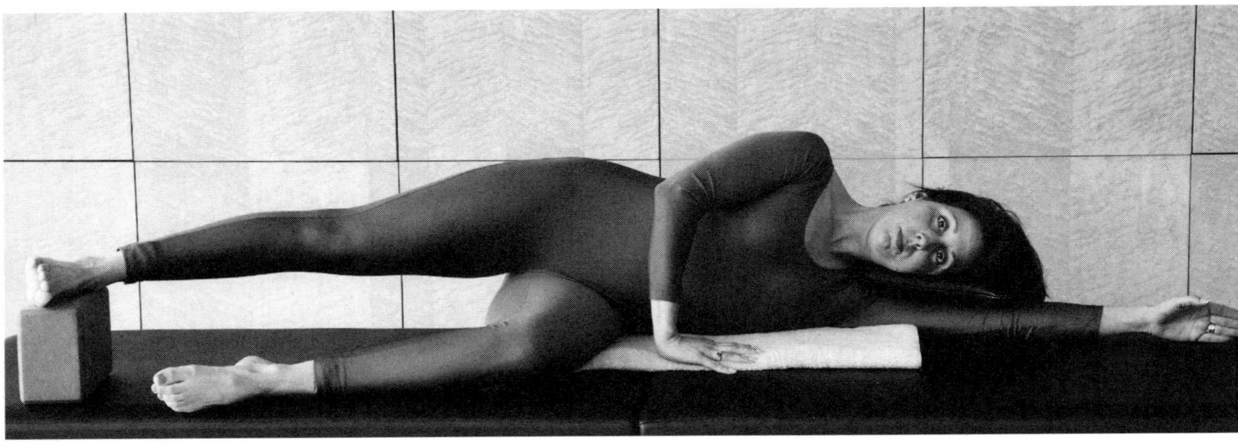

2. Bend the bottom arm and prop the head on the hand. Keep the arm in line with the spine.

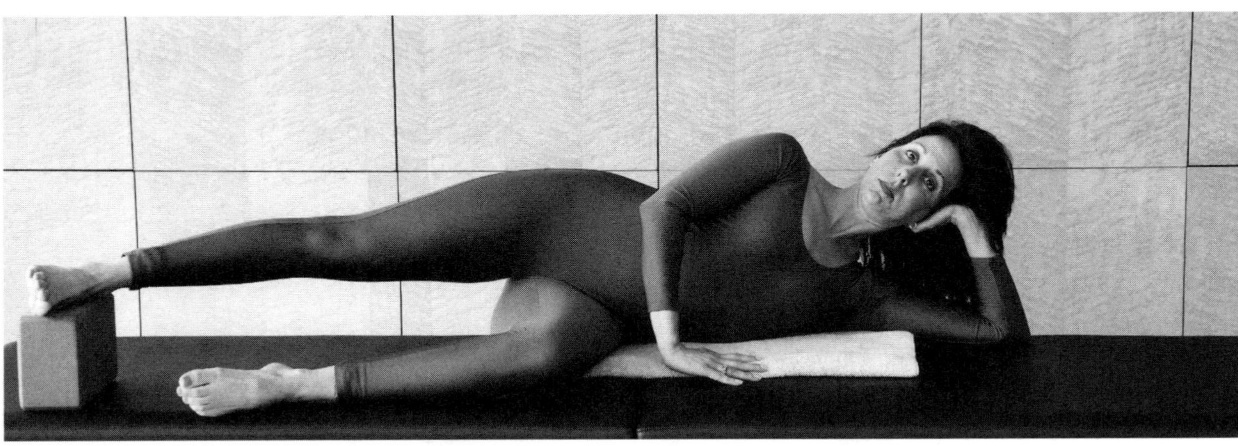

3. Place the top hand on a small, soft ball or Pilates ring to challenge the torso stability.

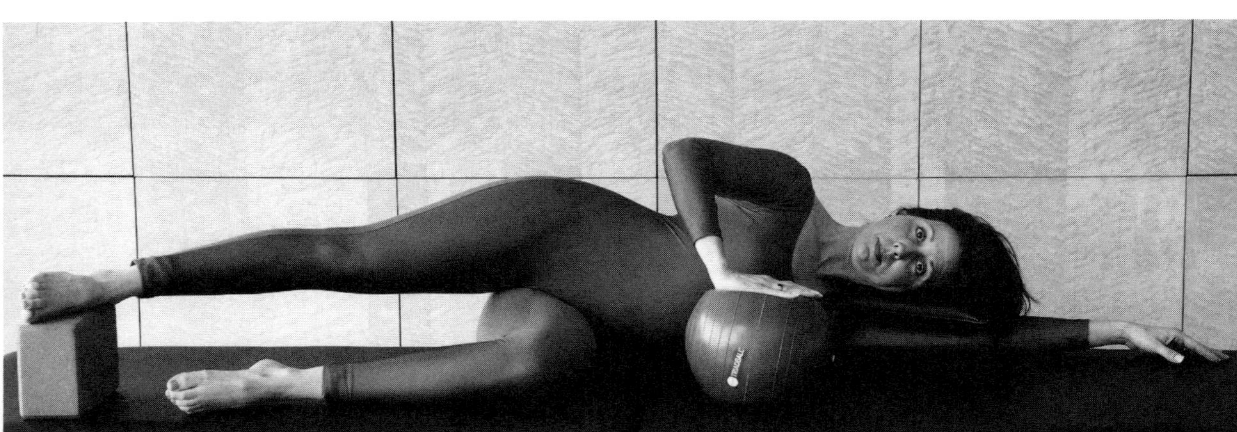

LONG-LEVER BODY POSITION SETUP

Timeline: 3 to 6 months and 6 months and beyond postop

Appropriate for: knee and hip

Location: a floor mat or a raised mat as needed; a raised mat for a bilateral knee or hip replacement if needed

Instructions

- Lie on one side with the hips and shoulders stacked evenly on the back edge of the mat. Hinge from the hip and bring both legs to the front corner of the mat. For support, place the top hand 6 inches (15 centimeters) in front of the body between the sternum and the navel. Press into the heel of the hand. Prop the head up on the bottom hand and arm. Keep the arm in line with the spine.
- Stabilize the bottom leg by lengthening out of the hip and imprinting the lateral edge of the foot onto the mat.
- Draw the abdominals in and up, feeling light in the waist as if you could shoot air between the waist and the mat.
- Breathe with an even flow of inhaling and exhaling.
- **Knee and hip:**
  - Keep the working leg parallel, with the knee and the toe pointing to the other side of the room.
  - Keep the knee slightly flexed or bent to shorten the lever length as needed.

(continued)

Long-Lever Body Position Setup *(continued)*

Setup Options

1. Continue to use a towel under the joint as needed.

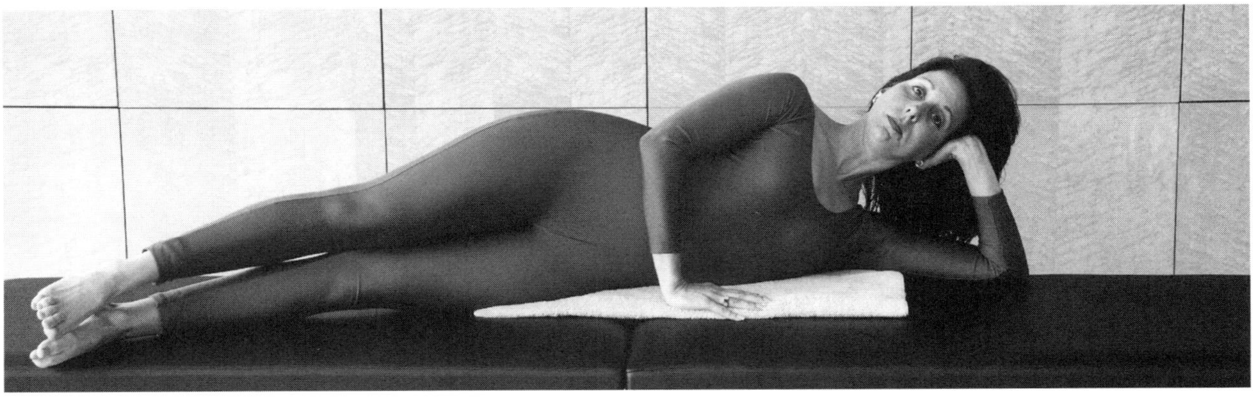

2. Lie down on the biceps as needed.

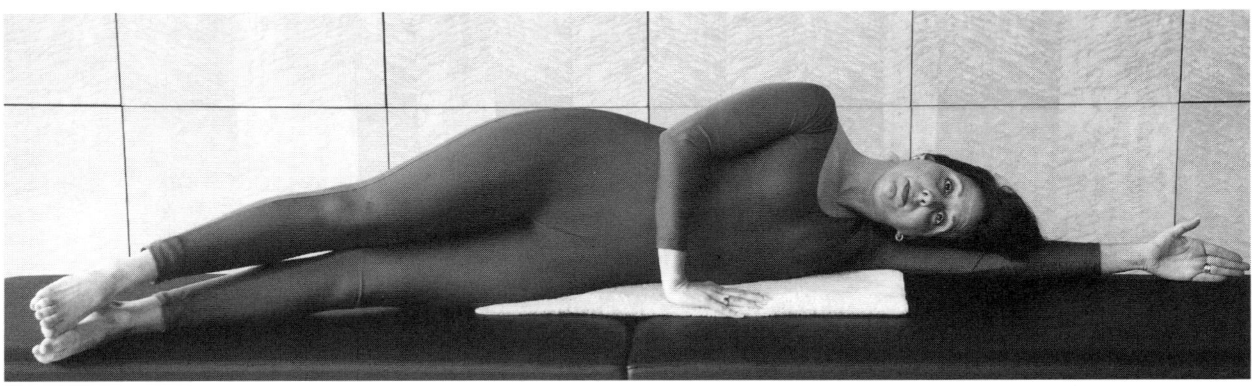

3. For an advanced challenge, bend the top arm and place the hand behind the head. Stay long through the torso with the elbow in line with the spine.

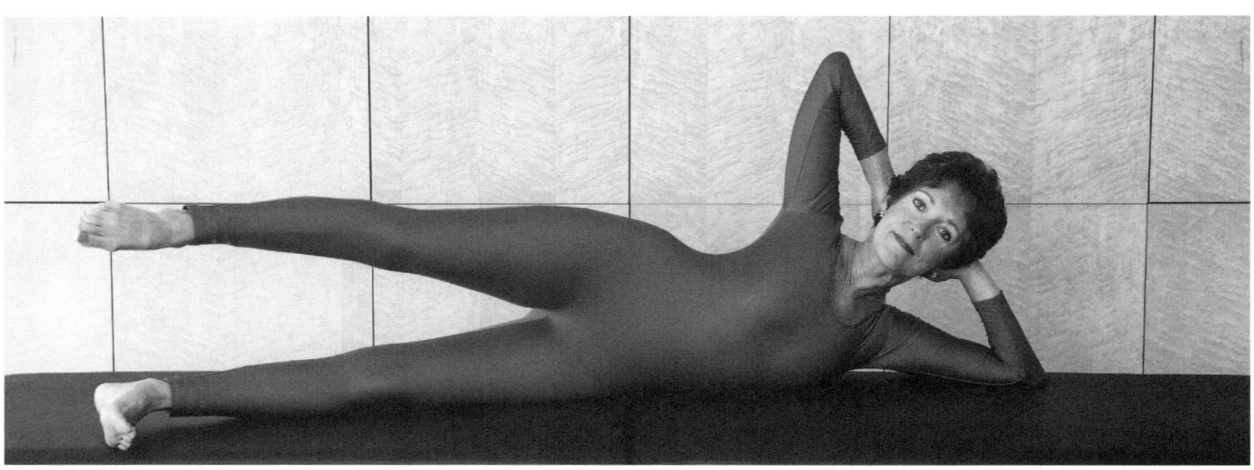

4. Place the top hand on a small, soft ball or Pilates ring to challenge the stability of the torso.

Look for . . . Encourage

- The torso remains very stable while the legs work with precision and control
- Lengthening out of the hip with movement
- Creating opposition through movement
- Maintaining a neutral spine
- Lifting the waistband by drawing the abdominals in and up
- The shoulders and hips are stacked and in line with the back edge of the mat
- The shoulders gliding toward the hips away from the ears
- The ROM of the leg is based on the individual's ability to stabilize the core and work within a comfortable ROM
- Disassociation of the head of the femur from the acetabulum (stable pelvis with a flowing movement of the working leg)
- For 3 to 6 months and beyond, the base leg lengthens out of the hip and the lateral edge of the foot is imprinted into the mat to keep the bottom leg engaged
- For 3 to 6 months and beyond, the knee is bent to shorten the lever as needed
- Keep the arm the head is resting on in line with the stacked hips and shoulders

Be aware of . . . Prevent

- Arching (hyperextension) of the lumbar spine
- Hyperextension of the knee
- Torso instability, movement of the torso with the leg through each movement
- Loss of core control
- Loss of the hip–hip and shoulder–shoulder alignment on the back edge of the mat

Note

The pointers on what to encourage and prevent that are listed here apply to all of the following long-lever series movements described in this chapter.

Up and Down

Timeline: 6 weeks to 3 months postop

Appropriate for: knee and hip

Location: a raised mat, hip height

Instructions

- Select the most appropriate setup option (see pp. 265-266).
- Draw the abdominals in and up.
- Start the movement by resting the top leg on a yoga block *(a)*.
- Lift the top leg up to hip height and point the toes *(b)*. Work toward lifting the leg to 45°, flex the foot, and slowly lower to the starting position *(c)*. Float the leg up and resist the leg as you lower it.

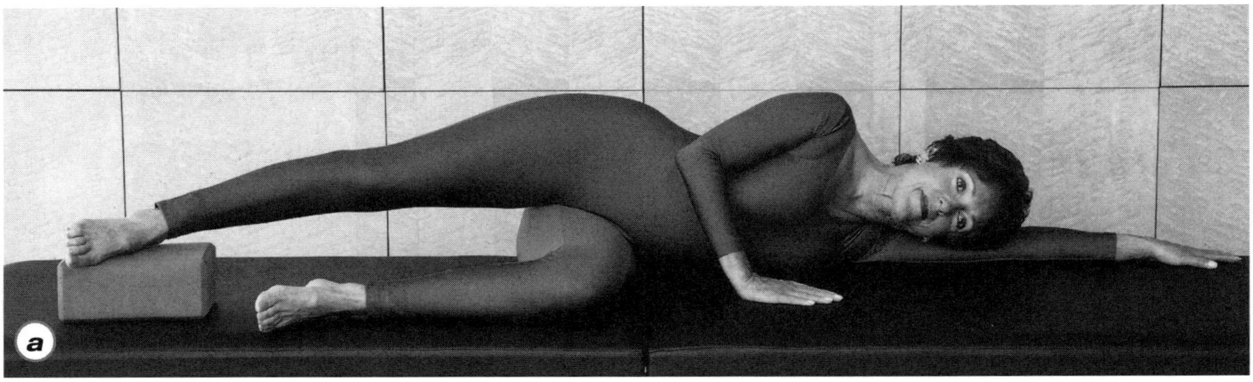

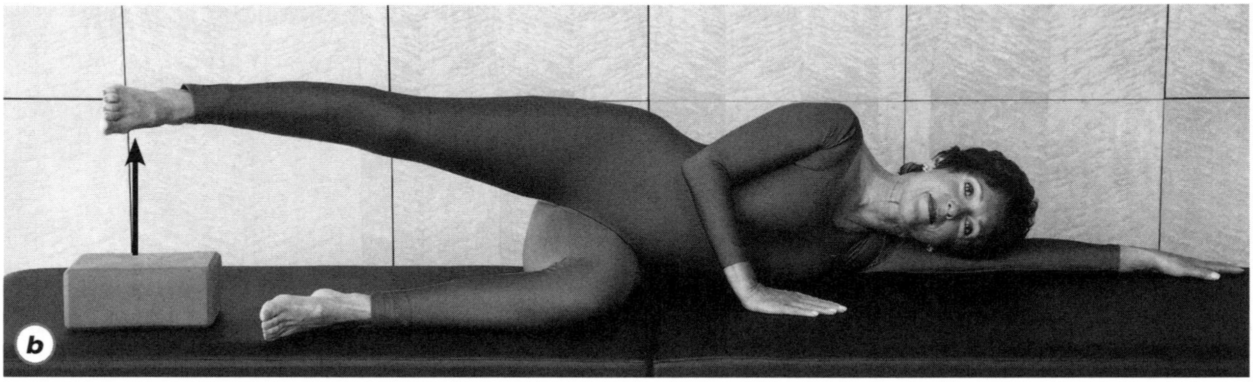

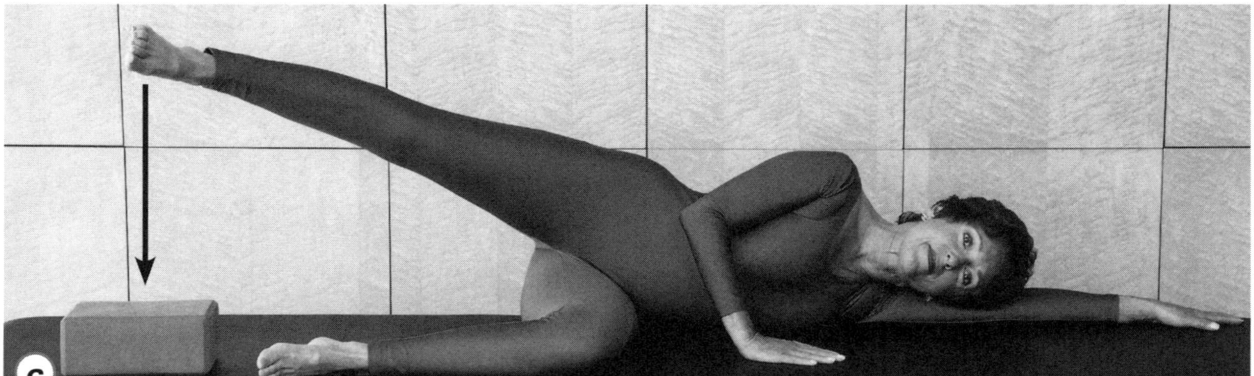

- Breathe with an even flow of inhaling and exhaling.
- Repeat 5 times and then reverse the action. Flex up and point down 5 times.
- When performing the movement, maintain a stable torso. Imagine reaching for the opposite wall with the foot.
- **Knee and hip:** Keep the leg parallel, with the knee and toe on the same plane. The knee remains soft. Do not turn the foot out externally. Do not let the hip cross the midline of the body.

Option

Use a towel and a small, soft ball for extra support and to challenge the stability of the core.

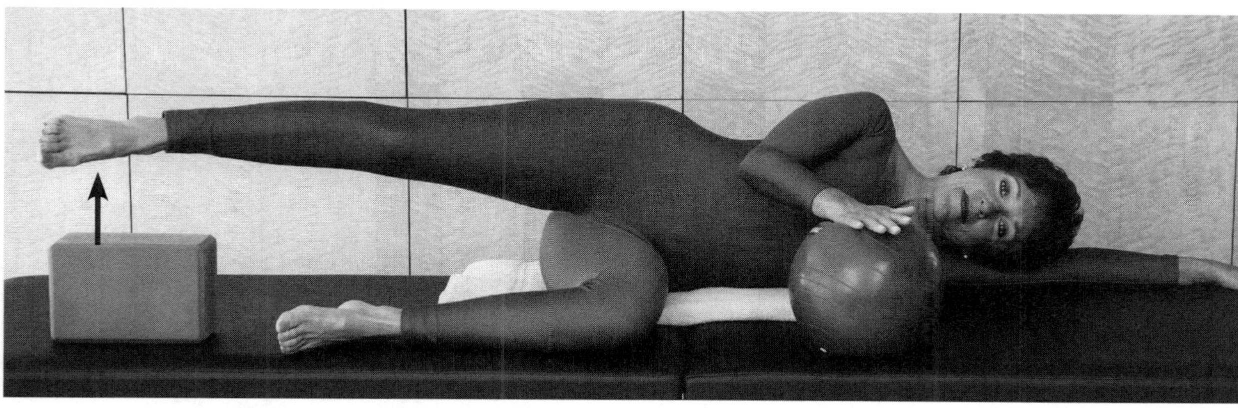

(continued)

UP AND DOWN

Timeline: 3 to 6 months and 6 months and beyond postop

Appropriate for: knee and hip

Location: a raised mat for a bilateral hip or knee replacement if needed for up to 6 months postop, then a floor mat or raised table as needed

Instructions

- Select the most appropriate setup option (see pp. 265-269).
- Lift the top leg to hip height and point the toes *(a)*. Keep the leg parallel and lift it up as tolerated *(b).* Flex the foot and lower slowly to the starting position. Float the leg up and resist the leg when lowering it.
- Breathe with an even flow of inhaling and exhaling.
- Repeat 8 times, pointing up and flexing down. Then reverse 8 times, flexing up and pointing down.
- When performing the movement, keep the torso stable. Imagine reaching for the opposite wall with the foot.
- **Knee and hip:** Keep the leg parallel, with the knee and toe on the same plane. Do not turn the foot out externally. The knee remains soft.

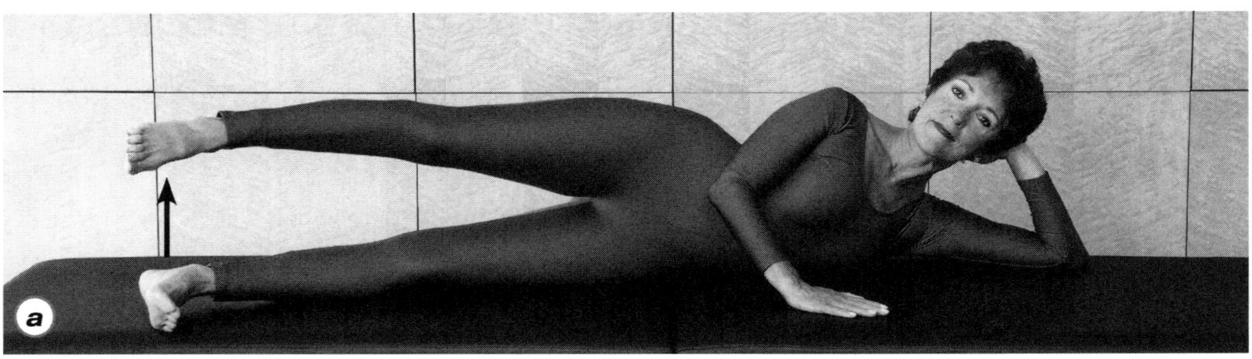

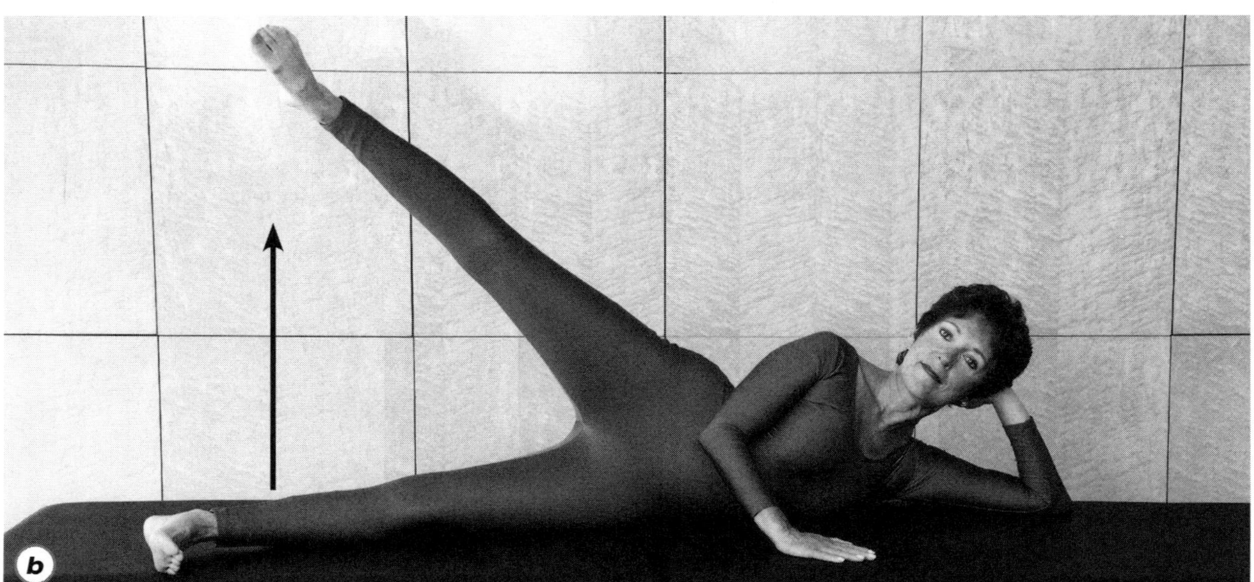

Options

1. Place both hands behind the head.

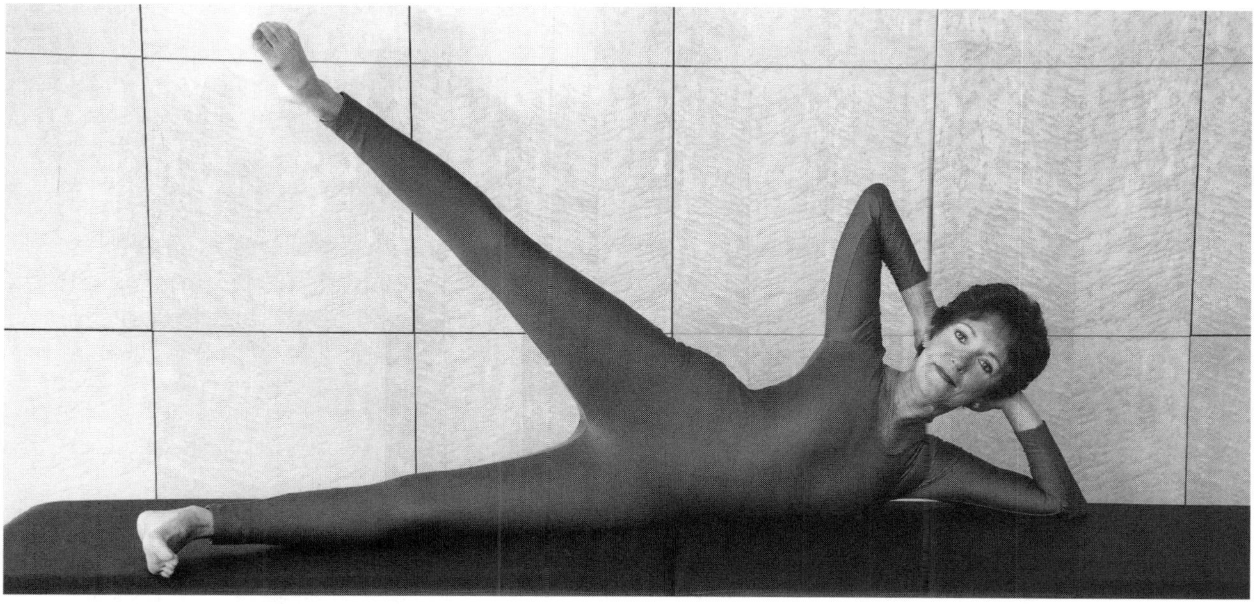

2. Place the hand on a Pilates ring with a slight external rotation of the leg.

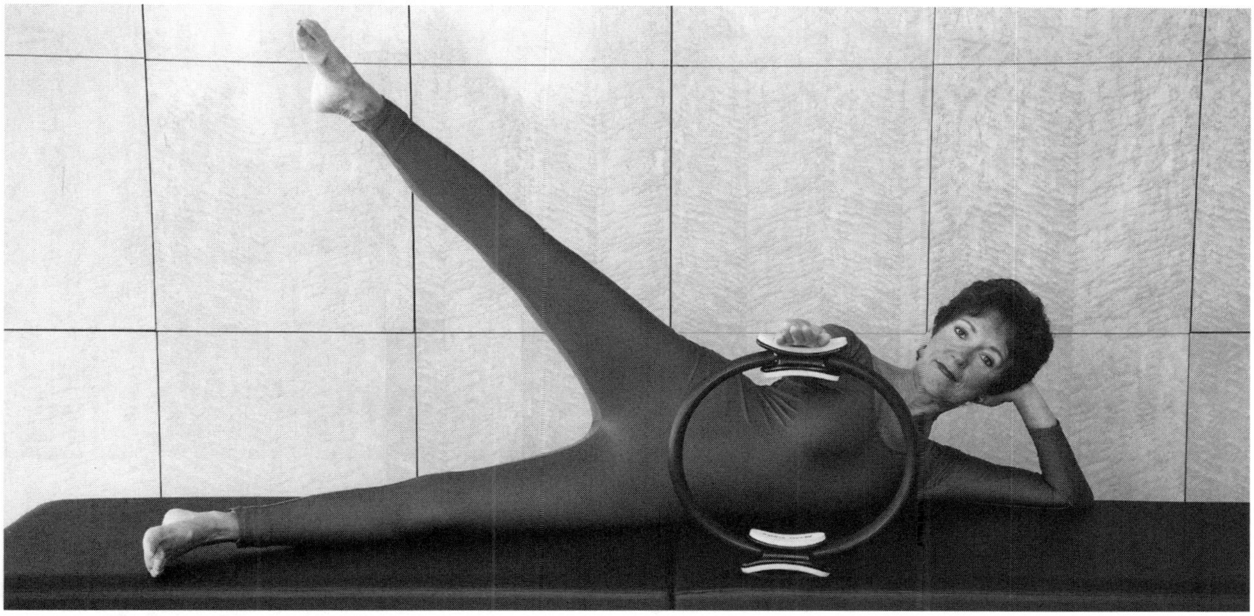

Primary Muscles Activated

Abdominals, gluteus maximus, gluteus medius, gluteus minimus, rectus femoris, sartorius, tensor fasciae latae, pectineus, adductor magnus, adductor longus, adductor brevis, gracilis, gastrocnemius, biceps femoris, semimembranosus, semitendinosus, vastus medius, vastus lateralis, vastus intermedius, ankle flexors, ankle extensors, popliteus, plantaris, soleus, tibialis posterior, tibialis anterior

Front and Back

Timeline: 6 weeks to 3 months postop
Appropriate for: knee and hip
Location: a raised mat, hip height

Instructions

- Select the most appropriate setup option (see pp. 265-266).
- Lift the top leg to hip height and bend the knee to 45° to 90° of flexion with the foot relaxed to shorten the lever length *(a)*. Keep the leg in a flexed position throughout the movement. Inhale and move the working leg to the front up to 90° of hip flexion *(b)*. Exhale and extend the leg, in the same flexed position, back in line with the body at hip height *(c)*. Bring the flexed leg back to start position *(d)*.
- Breathe with an even flow of inhaling and exhaling.
- Repeat 6 to 8 times.
- When performing the movement, keep the torso stable. Reduce the ROM if the upper body is moving with the movement of the leg.
- **Knee and hip:** Keep the leg parallel. Do not let the hip cross the midline of the body. Place a towel, pillow, or pad between the legs to keep the thigh at hip height as needed.
- Keep a yoga block or barrel available to rest the leg on between sets.

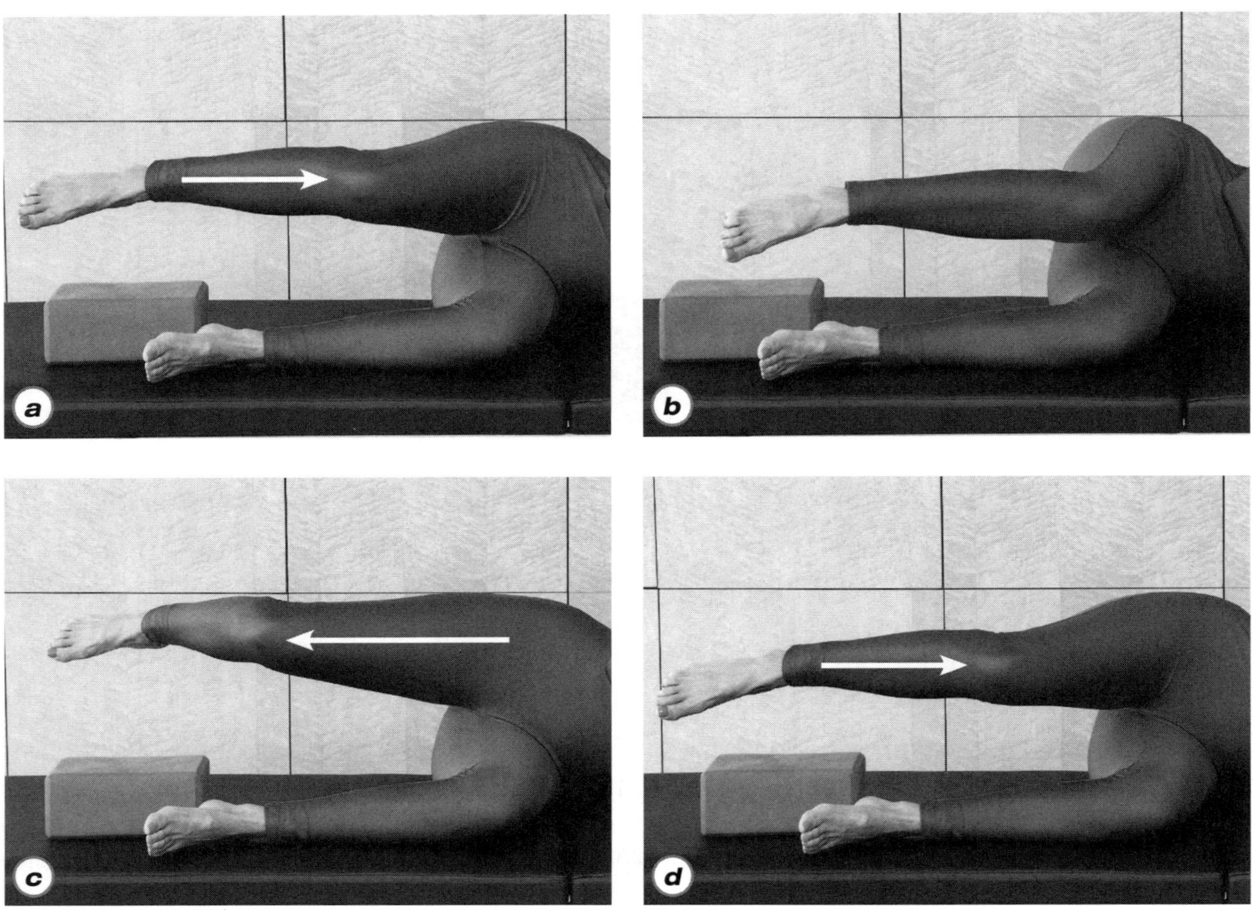

Option

Provided that you can keep the leg up at hip height, lengthen the working leg to a long lever, lengthening out of the hip to perform the movement. Inhale and hinge from the hip, bringing the leg up to 90° of flexion. Exhale and extend the leg back in line with the body.

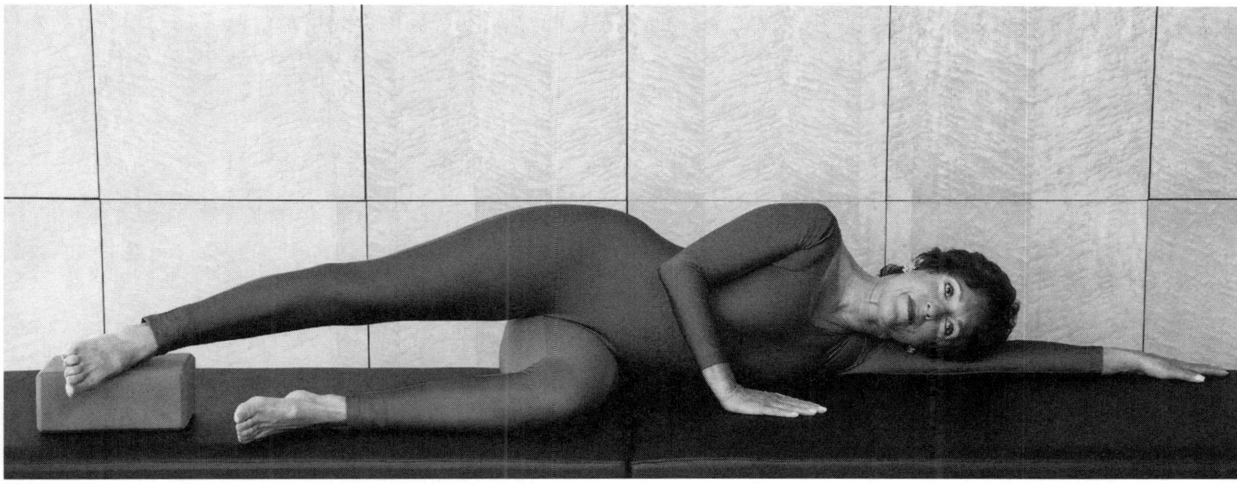

(continued)

FRONT AND BACK

Timeline: 3 to 6 months and 6 months and beyond postop

Appropriate for: knee and hip

Location: a floor mat or a raised mat as needed; a raised mat for a bilateral knee or hip replacement as needed

Instructions

- Select the most appropriate setup option (see pp. 267-268).
- Lift the top leg up to hip height and flex the foot. Inhale and hinge from the hip, bringing the working leg toward the navel only. Place a small, soft ball under the hand and towel under the hip joint if necessary.
- Exhale, point the toe, and bring the leg behind the stationary leg at hip height into extension with no turn out of the foot externally. Lengthen long out of the hip. Keep the leg at hip height from the front to the back.
- Flex the foot forward and double pulse the leg (kick, kick) and then point the foot and lengthen to the back as tolerated without moving the torso of the body.
- Breathe with an even flow of inhaling and exhaling.
- Repeat 8 to 10 times.
- Keep the frame of the leg on the same height throughout the entire movement.
- Make sure the torso stays very still and stable. Reduce the ROM if the torso moves with the movement of the leg.
- **Knee and hip:** Keep the leg parallel, with the knee and foot pointing to the other side of the room. Keep the knee slightly flexed. Bend the working leg as needed to shorten the lever length.

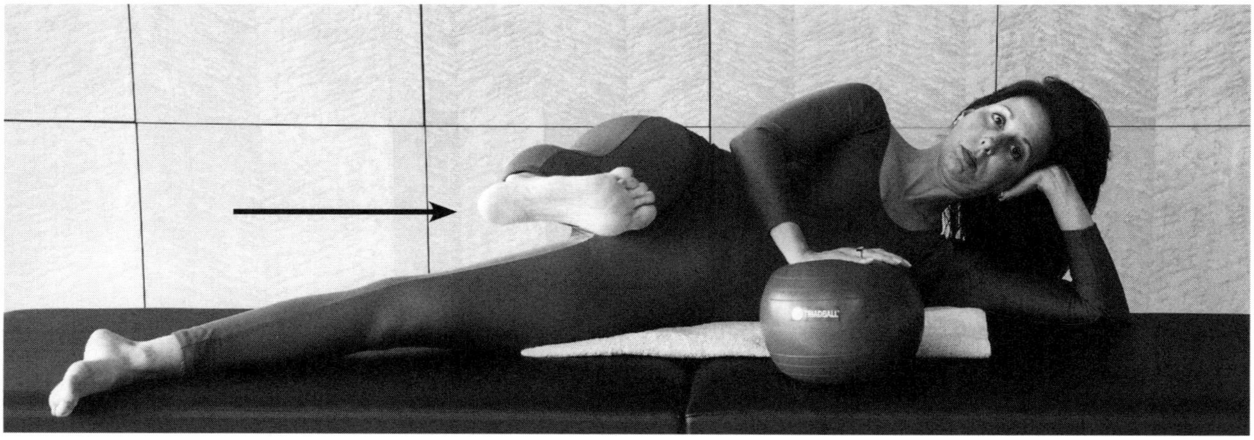

Options

1. Perform the front and back movements with the bottom leg lengthened out on the mat. Rest the head on the arm and place a towel under the hip joint as needed.

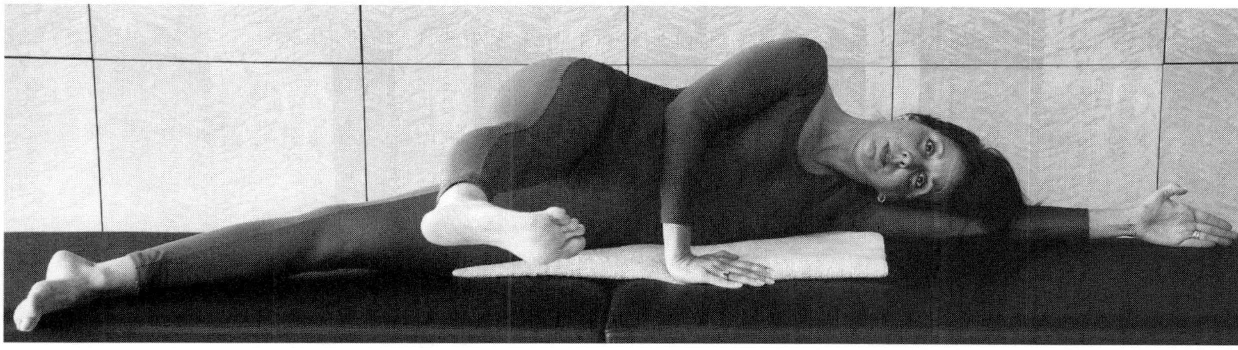

2. Bend the bottom leg while performing the front and back movements. Rest the head on the arm as a pillow and provide a soft ball for the hand to press into. Use a towel under the hip joint as needed.

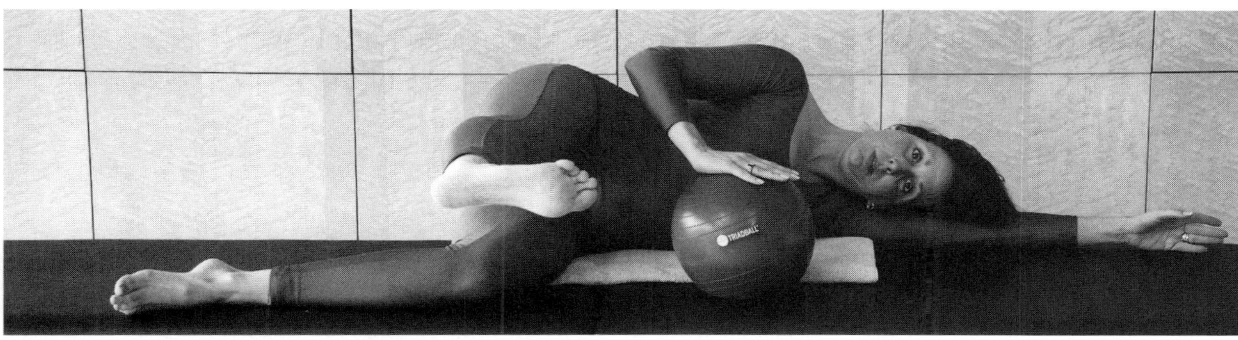

3. Use a Pilates ring while performing the front and back movements by pressing the hand with the fingers long into the ring, keeping the shoulders away from the ears.

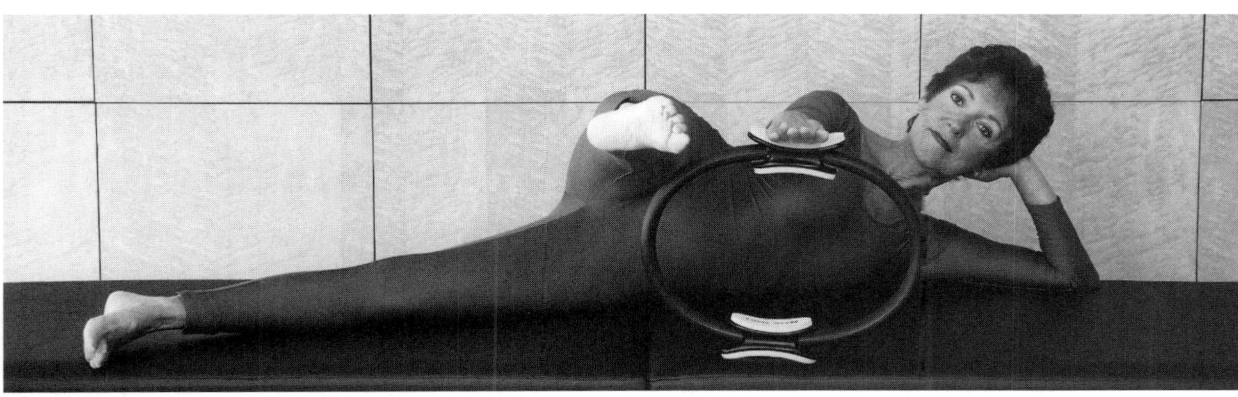

Primary Muscles Activated

Abdominals, rectus femoris, sartorius, pectineus, iliopsoas, gluteus maximus, gluteus medius, biceps femoris, semitendinosus, semimembranosus, tensor fasciae latae, adductor magnus, adductor longus, adductor brevis, gracilis, popliteus, gastrocnemius, plantaris, vastus intermedius, vastus medialis, vastus lateralis, piriformis, soleus, tibialis anterior, tibialis posterior

Little Circle

Timeline: 6 weeks to 3 months postop
Appropriate for: knee and hip
Location: a raised mat, hip height

Instructions

- Select the most appropriate setup option (see pp. 265-266).
- Draw the abdominals in and up.
- Lift the top leg to hip height, and point the toes. Begin to draw a small circle with the toes. Accentuate the motion at the top of the circle.
- Circle from the hip.
- Breathe with an even flow of inhaling and exhaling.
- Repeat 5 circles in each direction.
- When performing the movement, make sure the upper body stays stable. Imagine reaching for the opposite wall with the foot to create length.
- **Knee and hip:** Keep the leg parallel, with the knee and toe pointing to the other side of the room. Keep the knee slightly bent and soft. Do not let the hip cross the midline of the body.

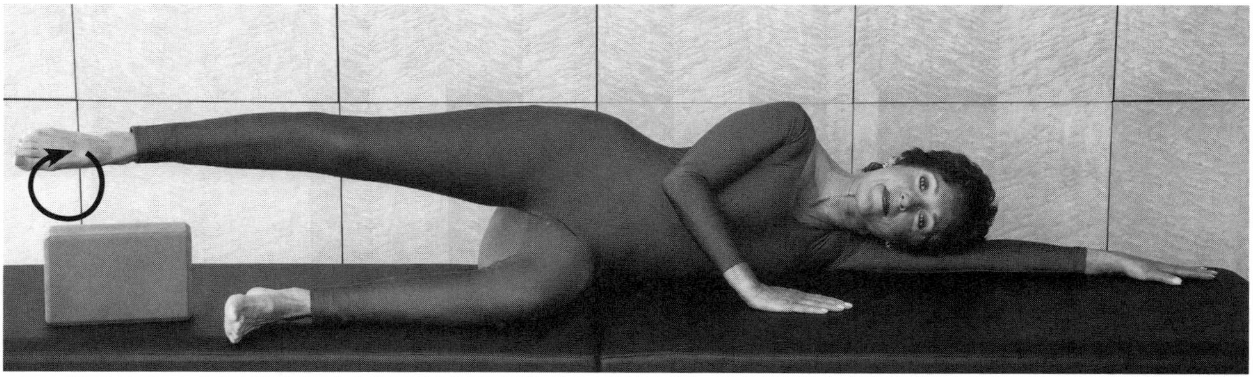

Option

Place the hand on a small, soft ball to challenge the core stability and use a towel for comfort.

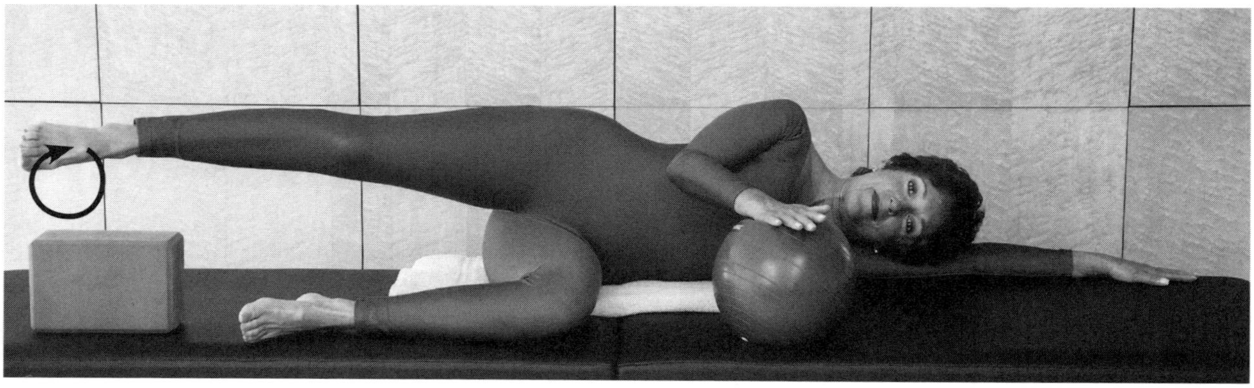

LITTLE CIRCLE

Timeline: 3 to 6 months and 6 months and beyond postop

Appropriate for: knee and hip

Location: a floor mat or a raised mat as needed; a raised mat for a bilateral knee or hip replacement as needed

Instructions

- Select the most appropriate setup option (see pp. 267-268).
- Draw the abdominals in and up.
- Lift the top leg to hip height and point the toes. Draw a small circle with the toes. Accentuate the motion at the top of the circle. You can place one hand on the mat *(a)* or both hands behind the head *(b)*.

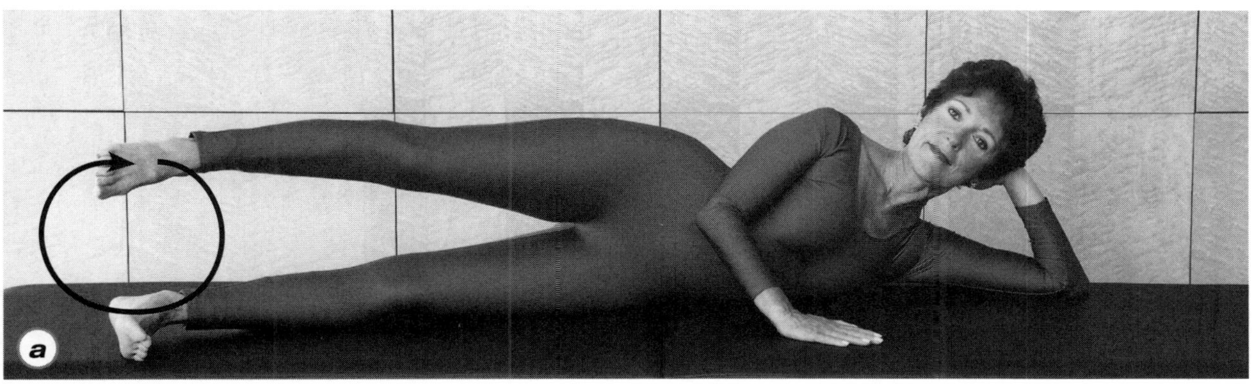

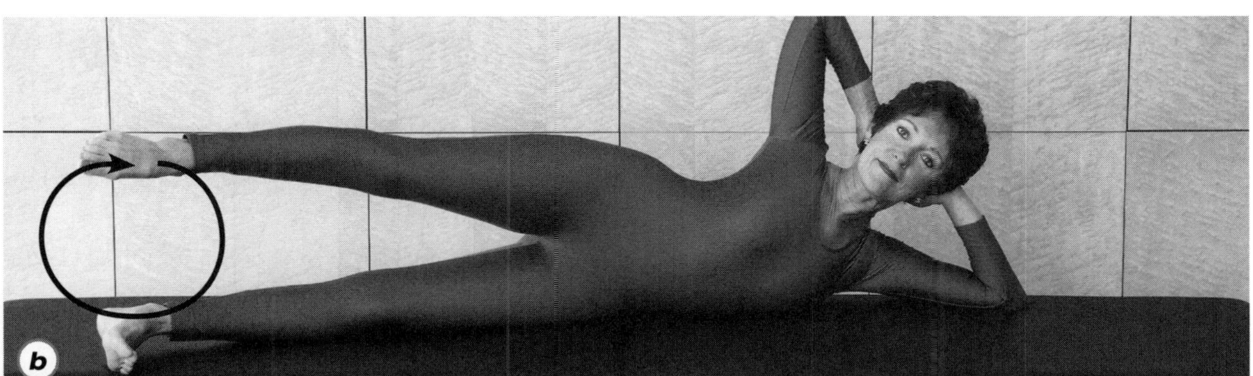

(continued)

Little Circle *(continued)*

- Circle from the hip.
- Reverse in the opposite direction.
- Breathe with an even flow of inhaling and exhaling.
- Perform 8 to 10 circles in each direction.
- When performing the movement, make sure the upper body stays stable. Imagine reaching for the opposite wall with the foot to create length.
- **Knee and hip:** Keep the leg parallel, with the knee and toe pointing to the other side of the room. The knee remains soft.

Primary Muscles Activated

Abdominals, rectus femoris, iliopsoas, sartorius, pectineus, gracilis, biceps femoris, semitendinosus, semimembranosus, gluteus medius, tensor fasciae latae, gluteus minimus, gluteus maximus, adductor magnus, adductor longus, adductor brevis, vastus intermedius, vastus medialis, vastus lateralis, tibialis posterior, gastrocnemius, soleus, plantaris

D-Circle

Restrictions: not applicable for knee or hip at 6 weeks postop; perform the D-circle no earlier than 3 months postop

Timeline: 3 to 6 months and 6 months and beyond postop

Appropriate for: knee and hip

Location: a floor mat or a raised mat as needed; a raised mat for a bilateral knee or hip replacement as needed

Instructions

- Select the most appropriate setup option (see pp. 267-268). This movement can be performed with a Pilates ring, as is shown here *(a)*.
- Lift the top leg beyond hip height, and then lift the leg as high as tolerated. Point the toes *(b)*. Make the first half of a large circle *(c)*, return back to the start *(d)*, and repeat. The movement looks like a large letter *D*.
- Breathe with an even flow of inhaling and exhaling.
- Repeat 5 times in each direction.
- When performing the movement, keep the torso stable. Imagine reaching for the opposite wall with the foot to create length.
- **Knee and hip:** Keep the leg parallel, with the knee and toe on the same plane. Keep the knee slightly flexed.

(continued)

D-Circle *(continued)*

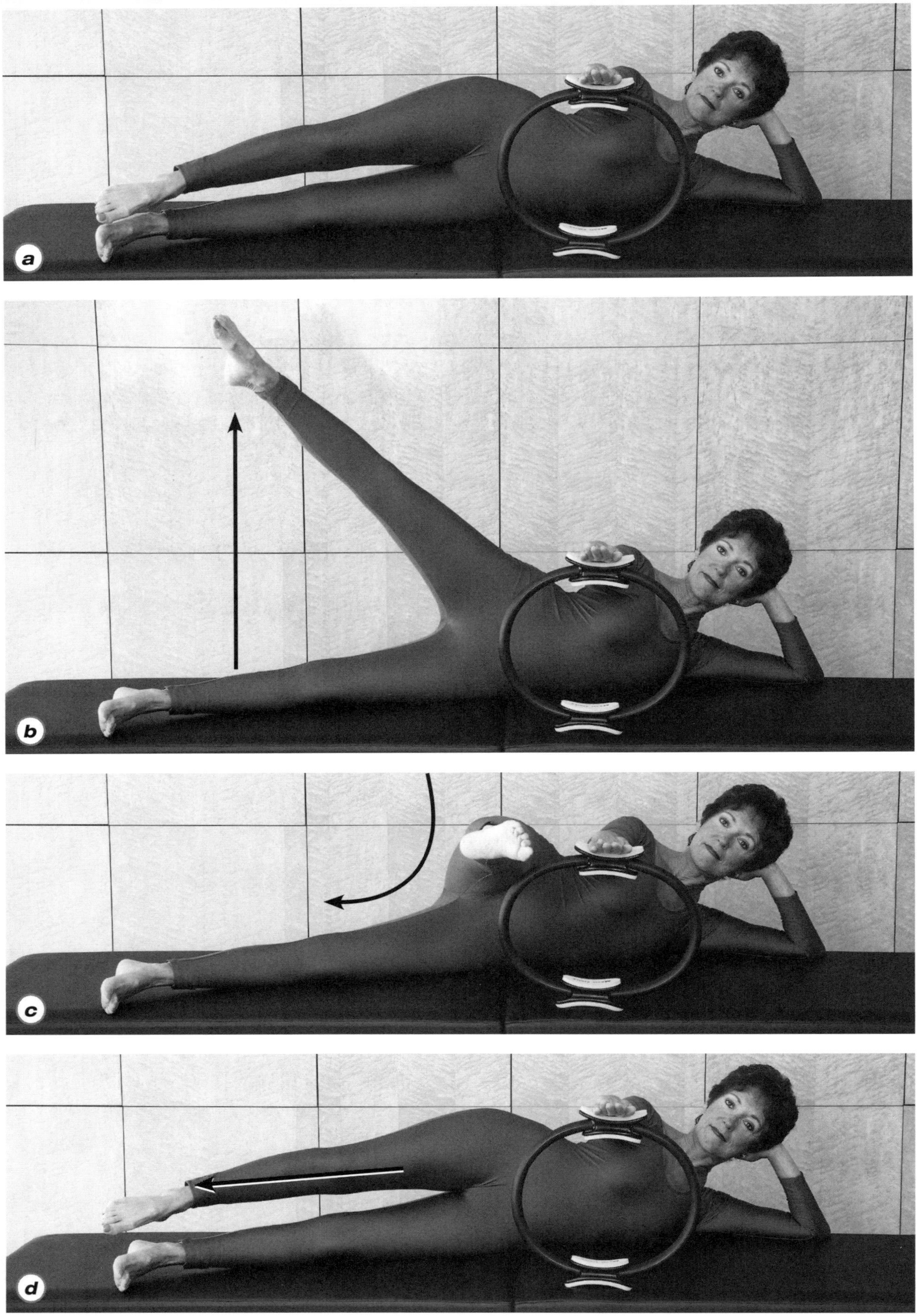

Primary Muscles Activated

Abdominals, rectus femoris, iliopsoas, sartorius, pectineus, gracilis, biceps femoris, semitendinosus, semimembranosus, gluteus medius, tensor fasciae latae, gluteus minimus, gluteus maximus, adductor magnus, adductor longus, adductor brevis, vastus intermedius, vastus medialis, vastus lateralis, tibialis posterior, gastrocnemius, soleus, plantaris

Internal and External Rotation

Timeline: 6 weeks to 3 months postop
Appropriate for: knee and hip
Location: a raised mat, hip height

Instructions

- Select the most appropriate setup option (see pp. 265-266).
- Draw the abdominals in and up.
- Lift the top leg to hip height and flex the foot *(a)*. Rotate the foot, ankle, knee, and hip up and point the toes toward the ceiling *(b)*. Rotate the hip, knee, ankle, and foot back to parallel. The energy of the movement flows through to the heel and beyond.

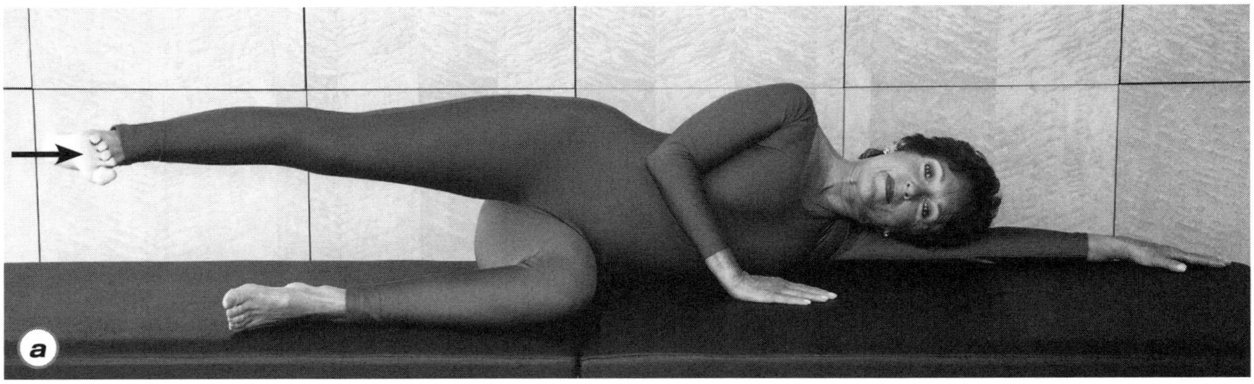

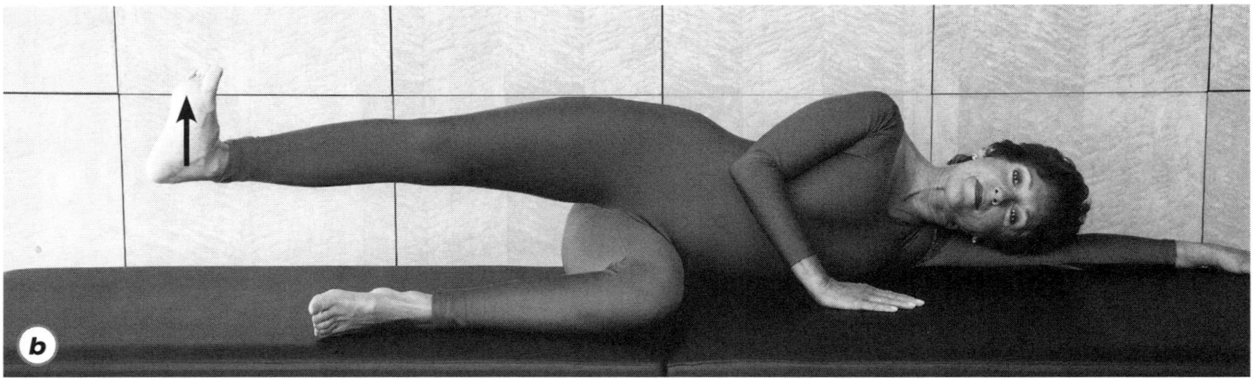

- Breathe with an even flow of inhaling and exhaling.
- Repeat 5 times.
- When performing the movement, make sure the upper body stays stable and the abdominals remain engaged.
- **Knee and hip:** Keep the leg parallel, with the knee and toe on the same plane to start the exercise. The knee is slightly flexed. Do not let the hip cross the midline of the body. Use a yoga block, barrel, or study pillows to rest the leg between sets as needed.
- **Hip:** Limit external rotation to 20°.

INTERNAL AND EXTERNAL ROTATION

Timeline: 3 to 6 months and 6 months and beyond postop

Appropriate for: knee and hip

Location: a floor mat or a raised mat as needed; a raised mat for a bilateral knee or hip replacement as needed

Instructions

- Select the most appropriate setup option (see pp. 267-268).
- Draw the abdominals in and up.
- Lift the top leg to hip height and flex the foot *(a)*. Rotate the foot, ankle, knee, and hip up and point the toes toward ceiling *(b)*. Rotate the hip, knee, ankle, and foot to parallel *(c)* and then down, pointing the toes toward the floor *(d)*. The energy of the movement flows through to the heel and beyond.
- Breathe with an even flow of inhaling and exhaling.
- Repeat 8 times.
- When performing the movement, make sure the upper body stays steady and the abdominals remain engaged.
- **Knee:** Keep the leg parallel, with the knee and toe pointing to the other side of the room to start the exercise. The knee remains slightly flexed.
- **Hip:** Slightly bend the knee with the movement. Limit external and internal rotation to 20° for up to 6 months, then 30° for 6 months and beyond.

(continued)

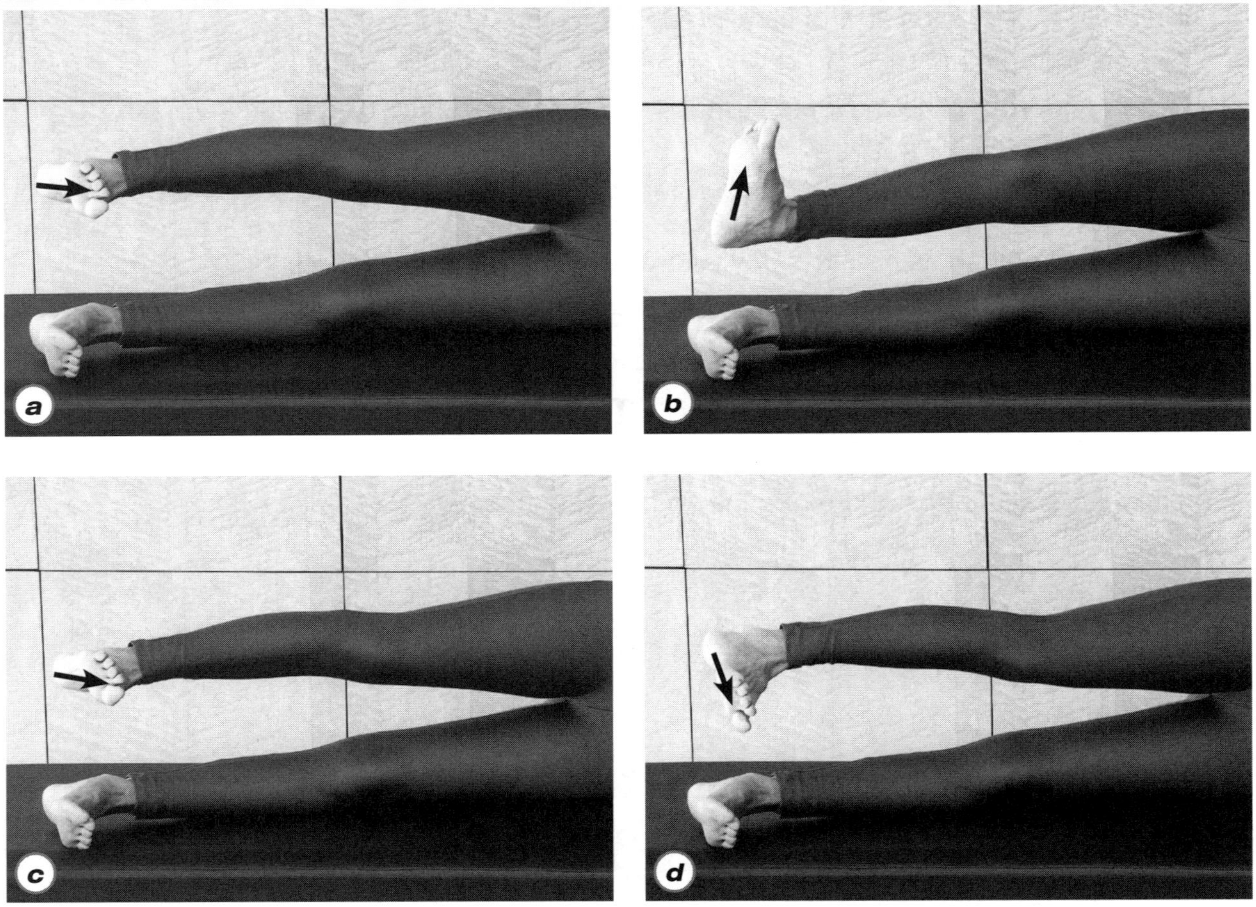

Option

The internal and external rotation can be performed with the head resting on the biceps or propped up on the forearm with the top hand on the mat or behind the head. Keep lengthening out of the hip and the feeling of keeping the waistline lifted from the mat throughout the movement.

Primary Muscles Activated

Abdominals, rectus femoris, iliopsoas, gluteus medius, tensor fasciae latae, gluteus minimus, gluteus maximus, sartorius, adductor magnus, adductor longus, adductor brevis, piriformis, gemellus superior, gemellus inferior, obturator internus, obturator externus, quadratus femoris, pectineus, gracilis, vastus medialis, vastus intermedius, vastus lateralis, tibialis anterior, hamstrings are stretched (biceps femoris, semitendinosus, semimembranosus)

Bicycle

Restrictions: not applicable for the knee or hip at 6 weeks to 3 months postop

Timeline: 3 to 6 months and 6 months and beyond postop

Appropriate for: knee and hip

Location: a floor mat or a raised mat as needed; a raised mat for a bilateral knee or hip replacement as needed

Instructions

- Select the most appropriate setup option (see pp. 267-268).
- Draw the abdominals in and up.
- Lift the top leg to hip height. Bring the leg to the front of the body to the waist only, and hold the leg at this point *(a)*. Bend the knee as tolerated toward the chest *(b)*, and keep this leg position as you start to extend from the hip. Bring the leg to the back wall, leading the foot to the buttocks *(c-d)*. Straighten the leg toward the back wall *(e)*, bring the straight leg all the way back around to the front *(a)*, and begin again. (The photos used here show approximately 110° of hip flexion.)
- The flow is as follows: knee to chest, knee to knee, heel to buttocks, leg to back wall, and leg all the way back around to the front.
- Repeat in the opposite direction; start with the leg extended back to the wall. The flow is as follows: heel to buttocks, knee to knee, knee to chest, leg all the way back.
- Breathe with an even flow of inhaling and exhaling.
- Repeat 4 times in each direction.
- When performing the movement, make sure the upper body remains stable. Reduce the ROM if there is movement in the torso. Try to imagine reaching for the opposite wall with the foot for length.
- **Knee:** Bend the knee as tolerated and watch for hyperextension of the knee when the leg is extended.
- **Hip:** Do not let the leg drop across the midline within the movement. The working leg comes up only toward the waist to start the movement. Bend the knee to the chest, keeping 110° of hip flexion for up to 6 months postop and then 115° of hip flexion for 6 months postop and beyond. Extend the leg to slightly behind the midline of the body, with no external rotation of the leg.
- There should be *no* external rotation of the knee and hip when the leg extends back.

Option

Place the stabilizing hand on a ball or behind the head to increase the challenge of performing the movement with a stable torso.

(continued)

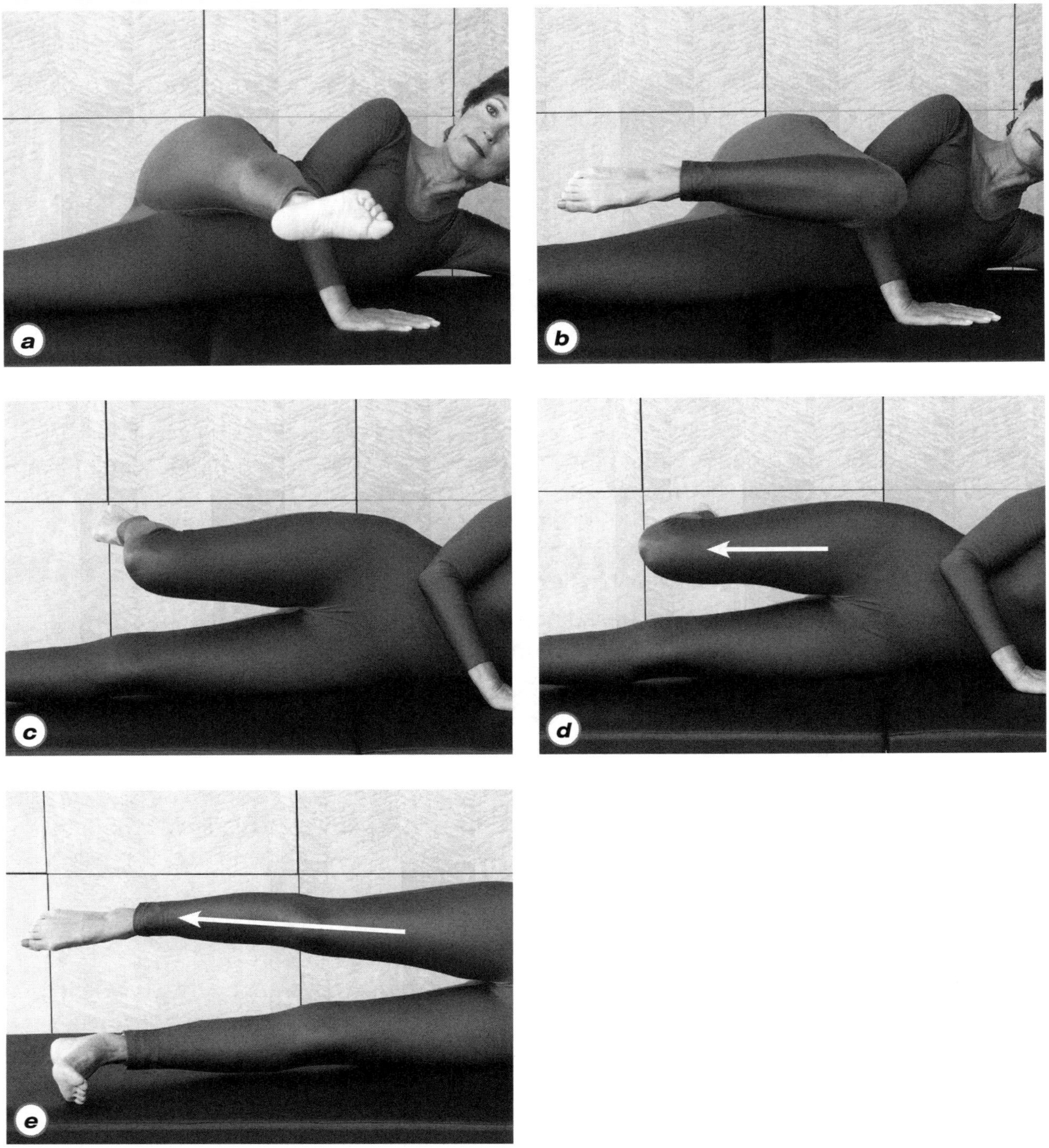

Primary Muscles Activated

Abdominals, rectus femoris, vastus medialis, vastus lateralis, vastus intermedius, sartorius, pectineus, iliopsoas, gluteus maximus, gluteus medius, gluteus minimus, biceps femoris, semitendinosus, semimembranosus, gracilis, popliteus, gastrocnemius, plantaris, tensor fasciae latae, adductor magnus, adductor longus, adductor brevis, gracilis, piriformis, ankle extensors, tibialis posterior, soleus

Scissors

Restrictions: not applicable for knee or hip at 6 weeks to 3 months postop

Timeline: 3 to 6 months and 6 months and beyond postop

Appropriate for: knee and hip

Location: a floor mat or a raised mat as needed; a raised mat for bilateral knee or hip replacement as needed

Instructions

- Select the most appropriate setup option (see pp. 267-268).
- Bring both legs back toward the midline of the body at least 25° forward of the hips.
- Draw the abdominals in and up.
- Lift the top leg to hip height and point the toes. Bring the top leg back and the bottom leg forward in the opposite direction, hinging from the hip. Keep the movement slow and controlled, so that the legs are cutting through the air like a pair of scissors and switch *(a-b)*.

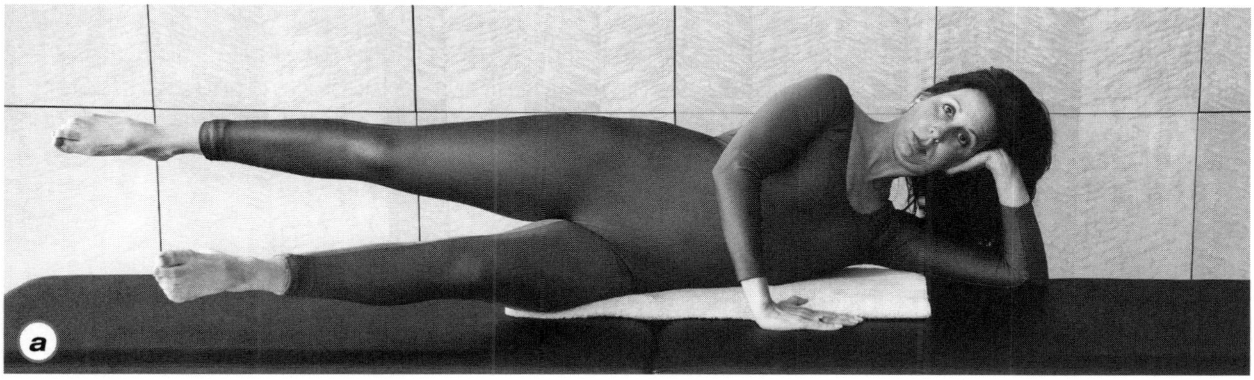
a

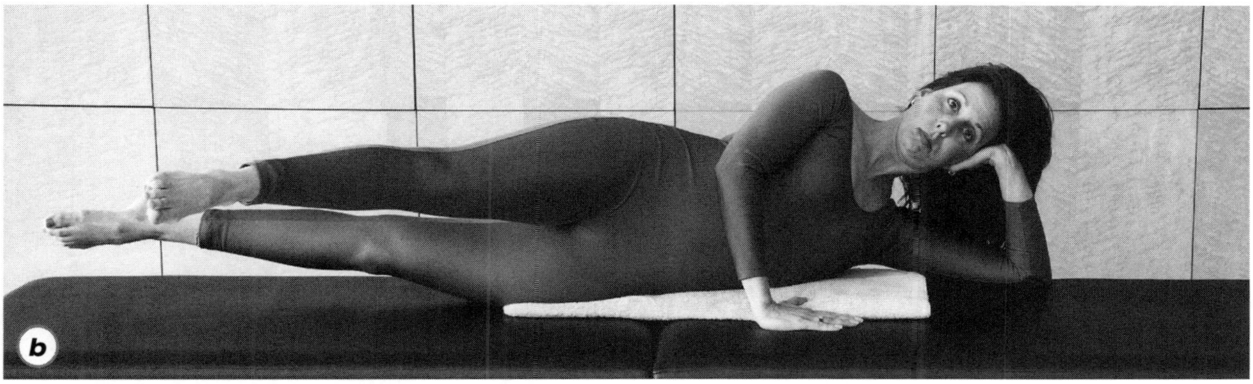
b

(continued)

Scissors *(continued)*

- Breathe with an even flow of inhaling and exhaling.
- Repeat 8 times in each direction.
- Keep the torso steady and the abdominals engaged. Imagine reaching for the opposite walls with the foot and lengthen out of the hip. Think of opposition, with an arrow of energy shooting through the crown of the head and another arrow of energy shooting through each foot.
- **Knee:** Keep the knees soft. Imagine 5° to 10° of flexion with the extension of the legs.
- **Hip:** Keep the movement small, slow, and controlled as tolerated. Place a pad or a towel under the hip on the mat. Keep the legs parallel and hip height. Keep a slight extension of the leg beyond the midline of the body, with soft knees and no external rotation of the leg.

Option

The scissors can be performed with the head resting on the biceps or propped up on the forearm with the top hand on the mat or behind the head. Keep lengthening out of the hip and feel as if you were lifting the waistline from the mat throughout the movement.

Primary Muscles Activated

Abdominals, rectus femoris, sartorius, pectineus, iliopsoas, gluteus maximus, gluteus medius, biceps femoris, semitendinosus, semimembranosus, adductor magnus, adductor longus, adductor brevis, gracilis, vastus medialis, vastus lateralis, vastus intermedius, tensor fasciae latae, tibialis posterior, gastrocnemius, plantaris, soleus

Parallel Leg Lift

Restrictions: not applicable for knee or hip at 6 weeks postop

Timeline: 3 to 6 months and 6 months and beyond postop

Appropriate for: knee and hip

Location: a floor mat or a raised mat as needed; a raised mat for a bilateral knee or hip replacement as needed

Instructions

- Select the most appropriate setup option (see pp. 267-268).
- Bring both legs back toward the midline of the body, keeping them at least 25° forward of the hips.
- Draw the abdominals in and up.
- Lift the top leg up to hip height and point the toes. Bring the bottom leg up to meet the top leg. Hug both legs to the midline of the body. Lift and lower both legs together without letting the legs touch the mat between repetitions *(a-b)*. Lift slowly and resist to lower.

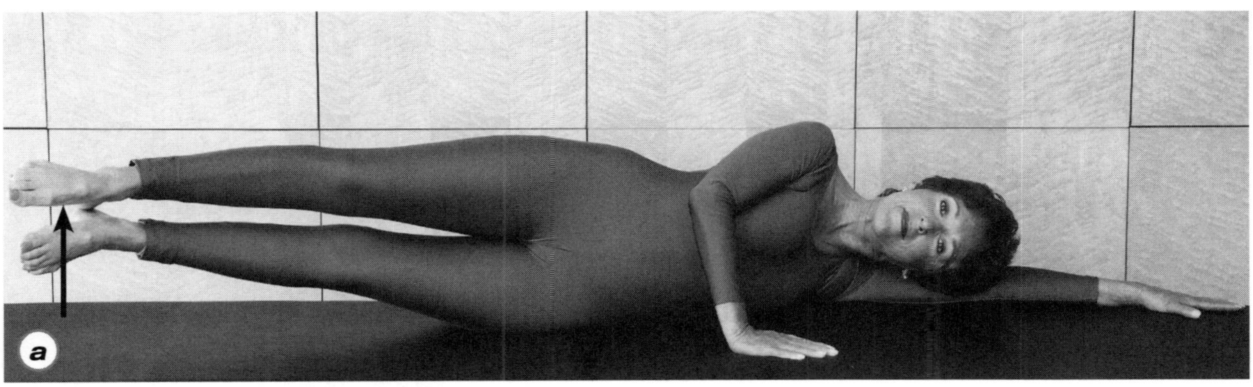

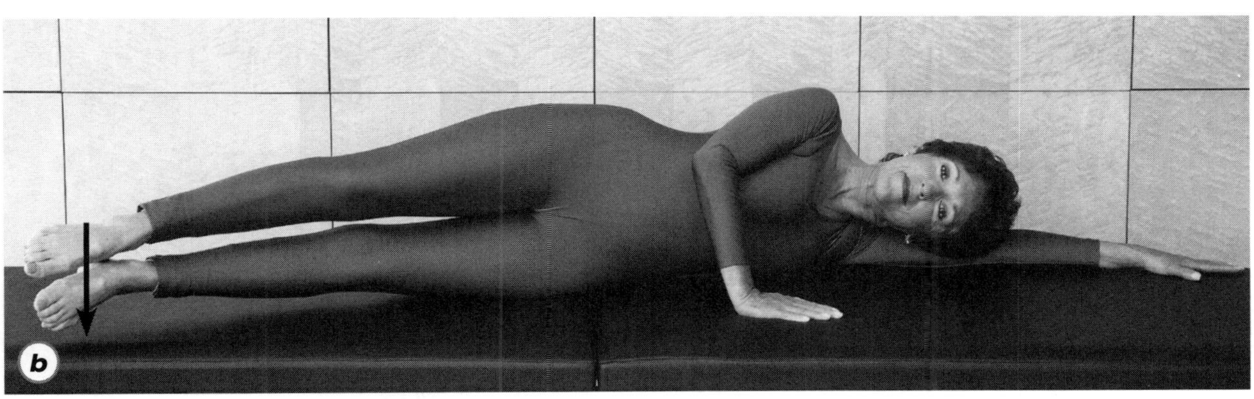

(continued)

Parallel Leg Lift *(continued)*

- Breathe with an even flow of inhaling and exhaling.
- Repeat 8 times.
- Keep the torso steady and the abdominals engaged. Imagine reaching for the opposite wall with the feet to create length.
- **Knee:** Keep the knees slightly flexed.
- **Hip:** Place a pad or a towel under the hip on the mat as needed. Keep the legs parallel.

Option

The parallel leg lifts can be performed with the head resting on the biceps or propped up on the forearm with the top hand on the mat or behind the head. Keep lengthening out of the hip and feel as if you were lifting the waistline from the mat throughout the movement.

Primary Muscles Activated

Abdominals, rectus femoris, iliopsoas, vastus medialis, vastus lateralis, vastus intermedius, gluteus maximus, gluteus medius, gluteus minimus, tensor fasciae latae, pectineus, sartorius, adductor magnus, adductor longus, adductor brevis, gracilis, pectineus, gastrocnemius, soleus, ankle extensors, plantaris, tibialis posterior

Lift, Lift, Lower, Lower

Restrictions: not applicable for knee or hip at 6 weeks postop

Timeline: 3 to 6 months and 6 months and beyond postop

Appropriate for: knee and hip

Location: a floor mat or a raised mat as needed; a raised mat for a bilateral knee or hip replacement as needed

Instructions

- Select the most appropriate setup option (see pp. 267-268).
- Bring both legs back toward the midline of the body, keeping them at least 25° forward of the hips *(a)*.
- Draw the abdominals in and up.
- Lift the top leg to hip height and point the toes *(b)*. Bring the bottom leg up to meet the top leg *(c)*. Hug both legs to the midline of the body.
- Lower the bottom leg *(d)* and then the top leg *(e)*. Lift the top leg and then the bottom leg to meet the top.
- The flow is lift, lift, lower, lower. The legs stay lifted a few inches (centimeters) from the mat throughout the movement.
- Breathe with an even flow of inhaling and exhaling.
- Repeat 8 times.
- Keep the torso steady and the abdominals engaged. Imagine reaching for the opposite wall with the feet for length.
- **Knee:** Keep the knee slightly flexed.
- **Hip:** Place a pad or a towel under the hip on the mat, and keep the legs parallel.

(continued)

Lift, Lift, Lower, Lower *(continued)*

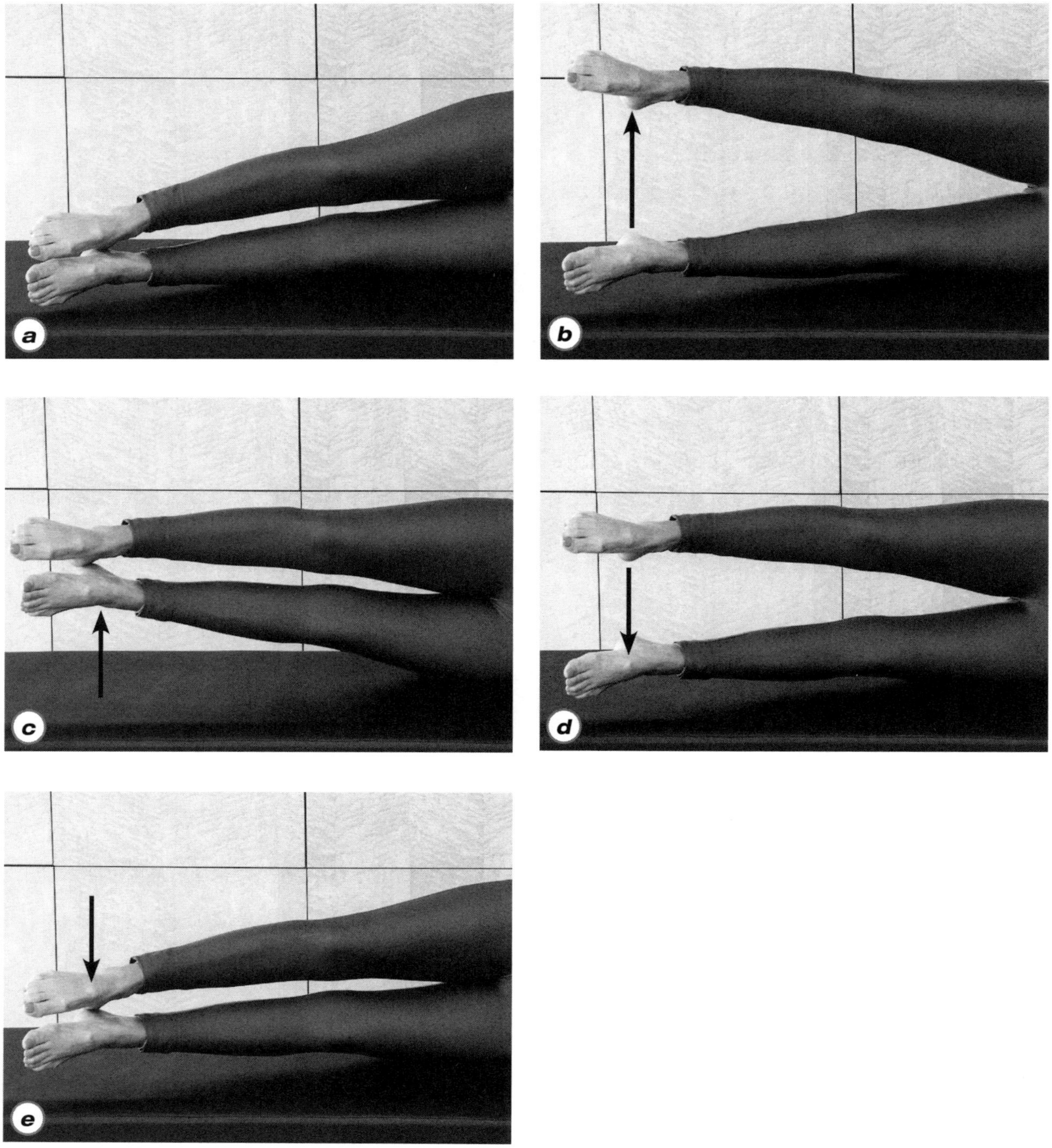

Options

1. Lift the top leg to hip height, point the toes, and bring the bottom leg up to meet the top leg. Hug both legs to the midline of the body. Lift and lower the bottom leg only while keeping the top leg steady. Meet and greet. Repeat 8 times.
2. Lift the top leg to hip height, point the toes, and bring the bottom leg up to meet the top leg. Hug both legs to the midline of the body. Lift and lower the top leg only while keeping the lower leg steady. Repeat 8 times. This is a challenging option.
3. The lift, lift, lower, lower and its variations can be performed with the head resting on the biceps or propped up on the forearm with the top hand on the mat or behind the head. Keep lengthening out of the hip and feel as if you were lifting the waistline from the mat throughout the movement.

Primary Muscles Activated

Abdominals, rectus femoris, iliopsoas, vastus medialis, vastus lateralis, vastus intermedius, gluteus maximus, gluteus medius, gluteus minimus, tensor fasciae latae, pectineus, sartorius, adductor magnus, adductor longus, adductor brevis, gracilis, pectineus, gastrocnemius, soleus, ankle extensors, plantaris, tibialis posterior

90° Long-Leg Lift and 90° Long-Leg Circle

Restrictions: not applicable for knee or hip at 6 weeks to 3 months postop or at 3 to 6 months postop

Timeline: 6 months and beyond postop
Appropriate for: knee and hip

Location: a floor mat or a raised mat as needed

Instructions for 90° Long-Leg Lift

- Select the most appropriate setup option (see pp. 267-268).
- Bend the bottom leg into a right angle, extend the top leg out in line with the body *(a)*. Bring the top leg forward and in line with the bottom thigh of the bent leg; keep it parallel to the floor. The hip, knee, and ankle are on the same line extended from the hip and the foot is flexed *(b)*. Draw the hip back as you extend the foot in opposition. Think of an arrow of energy pointing to the wall behind the hip and another arrow of energy pointing through the toe toward the wall.
- Draw the abdominals in and up.
- Lift and lower the leg 6 to 8 inches (15-20 centimeters). Keep the movement small and controlled *(c-d)*.

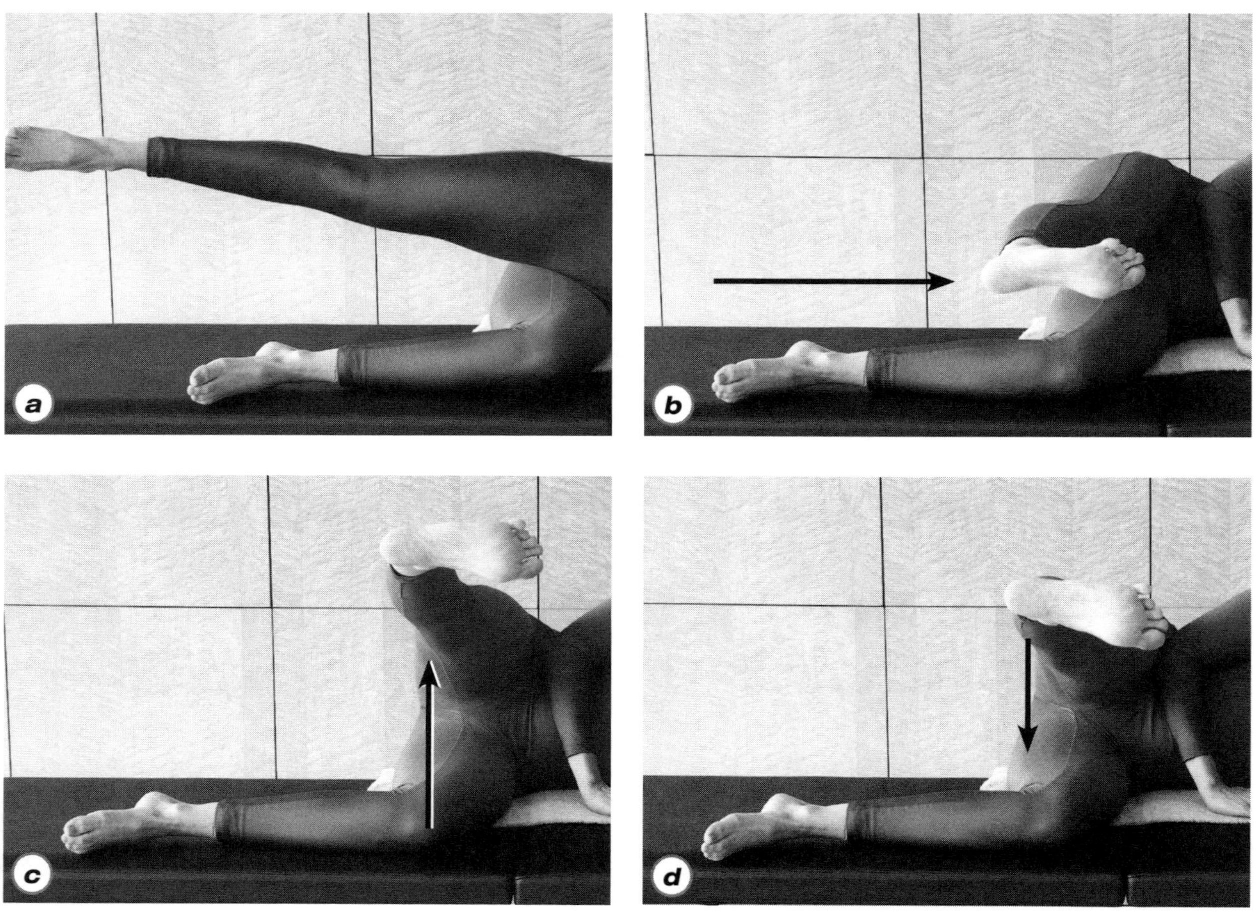

- Breathe with an even flow of inhaling and exhaling.
- Repeat 8 times.
- Bend the knee of the working leg as needed to take the stress off the abductors.

Instructions for 90° Long-Leg Circle

- Select the most appropriate setup option (see pp. 267-268).
- While the bottom leg stays bent at a right angle, extend the top leg out in line with the body.
- Circle the leg in both directions. Make the circles small and concise and accentuate the top of the movement.
- Breathe with an even flow of inhaling and exhaling.
- Repeat 8 times in both directions.
- Bend the knee of the working leg as needed to take the stress off the abductors.

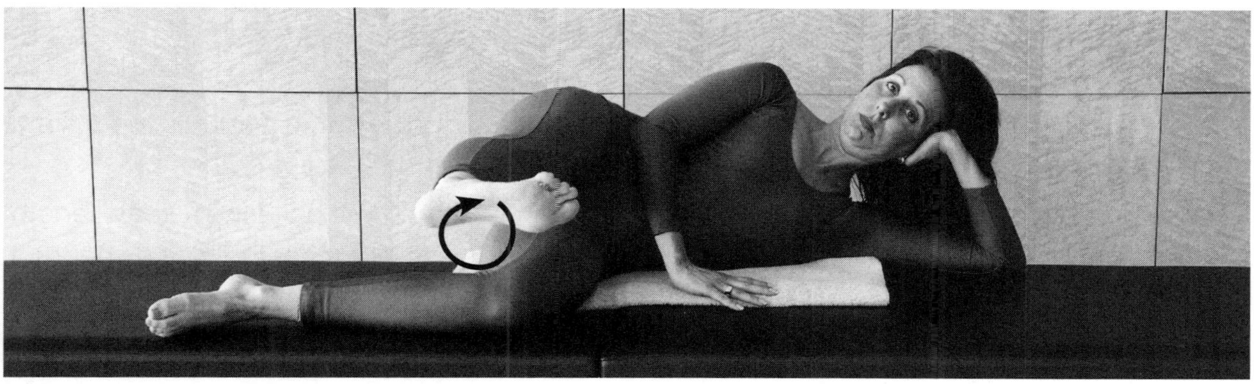

Option

Lift and lower the leg and then bring the leg forward toward the face 3 to 4 inches (8-10 centimeters) and then return it to the starting position. The flow is lift, lower, front, back. Repeat 6 to 8 times.

Primary Muscles Activated

Abdominals, rectus femoris, iliopsoas, sartorius, pectineus, gracilis, gluteus maximus, tensor fasciae latae, gluteus minimus, gluteus medius, adductor magnus, adductor longus, adductor brevis, biceps femoris, semitendinosus, semimembranosus, popliteus, gastrocnemius, plantaris, vastus medialis, vastus intermedius, vastus lateralis, piriformis, tibialis anterior

Inner-Thigh Lift and Inner-Thigh Circle

Timeline: 6 weeks to 3 months postop

Appropriate for: knee and hip

Location: a raised mat, hip height

Instructions for Inner-Thigh Lift

- Lie on one side with the hips and shoulders stacked up evenly on the back edge of the mat. Hinge from the hips and bring both legs to the front corner. For support, place the top hand, with the fingers wide, 6 inches (15 centimeters) in front of the body between the sternum and the navel.
- Rest the head on the bottom arm, a pad, or a small, soft ball.
- Bend the top leg into a right angle with a maximum of 90° of flexion from the chest. Place the knee on a yoga block; a small, soft ball; or sturdy pillows to keep the bent leg the width of the hip. The leg needs to be supported with no pressure on the knee or hip. The bottom leg is extended out to the front corner of the mat.
- Draw the abdominals in and up.
- Lift and lower the bottom leg toward the midline of the body with the foot relaxed *(a-b)*.
- Repeat 6 times.
- Keep the torso steady. Imagine reaching for the opposite wall with the leg to create length.
- **Knee and hip:** Keep the knee slightly flexed and place a towel under the hips as needed.

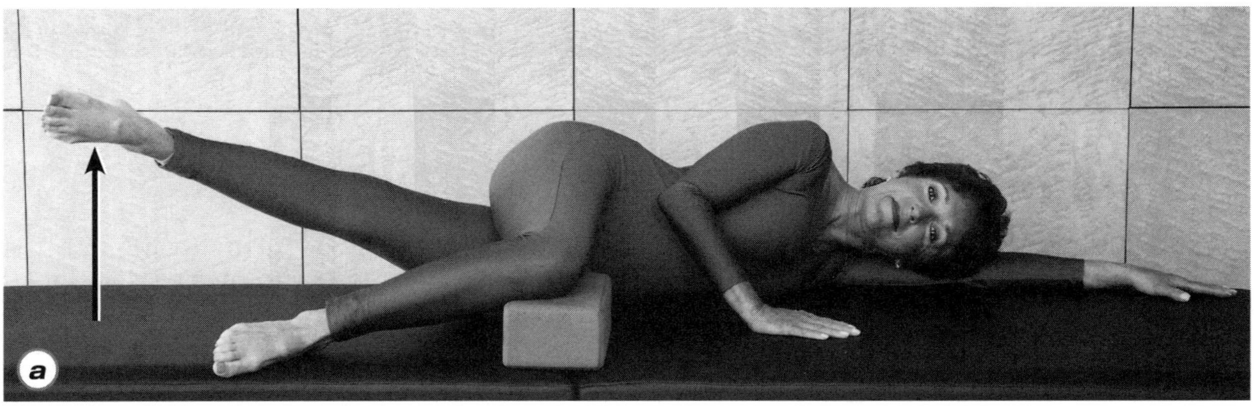

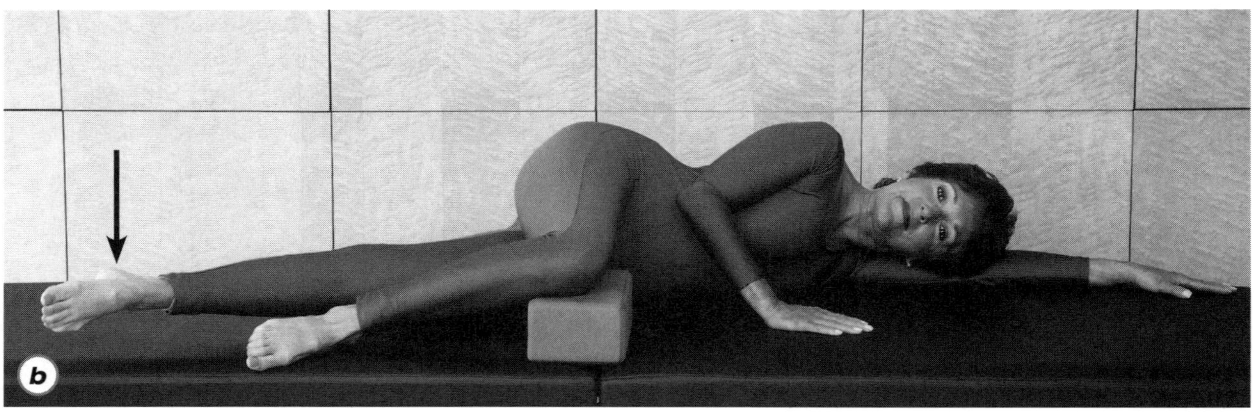

Instructions for Inner-Thigh Circle

- Position the body as described for the inner-thigh lift.
- Lift the bottom leg to hip height and make small circles in both directions. Keep the foot relaxed.
- Repeat 6 times in each direction.
- Keep the torso stable. Imagine reaching for the opposite wall with the foot for length.

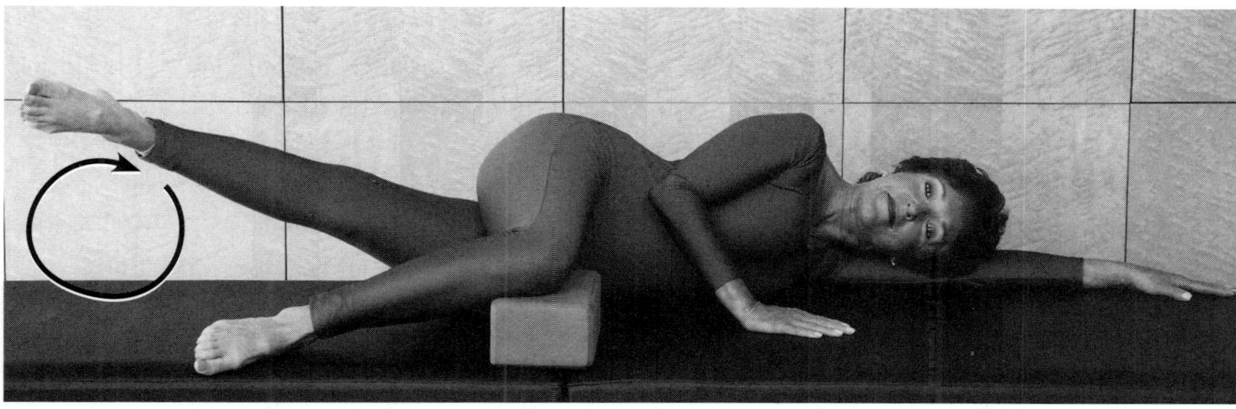

(continued)

INNER-THIGH LIFT AND INNER-THIGH CIRCLE

Timeline: 3 to 6 months and 6 months and beyond postop

Appropriate for: knee and hip

Location: a floor mat or a raised mat as needed; a raised mat for a bilateral knee or hip replacement as needed

Instructions for Inner-Thigh Lift

- Lie on one side with the hips and shoulders stacked up evenly on the back edge of the mat. Hinge from the hips and bring both legs to the front corner of the mat. For support, place the top hand, with the fingers wide, 6 inches (15 centimeters) in front of the body between the sternum and the navel.
- Bend the bottom elbow and prop the head on the hand. Draw the waistline up from the mat.
- Bend the top leg into a right angle with a maximum of 90° of flexion from the chest. Rest the knee on a yoga block; small, soft ball; or sturdy pillows to keep the bent leg the width of the hip. The leg needs to be supported with no pressure on the knee or hip. The bottom leg is extended out to the front corner of the mat.
  - Photo *(a)* shows the use of one small, soft ball.
  - Photo *(b)* shows the use of two small, soft balls.
- Draw the abdominals in and up.
- Lift and lower the bottom leg toward the midline of the body. Keep the foot relaxed *(c)*.
- Repeat 10 times.
- Keep the torso stable. Imagine reaching for the opposite wall with the leg to create length.

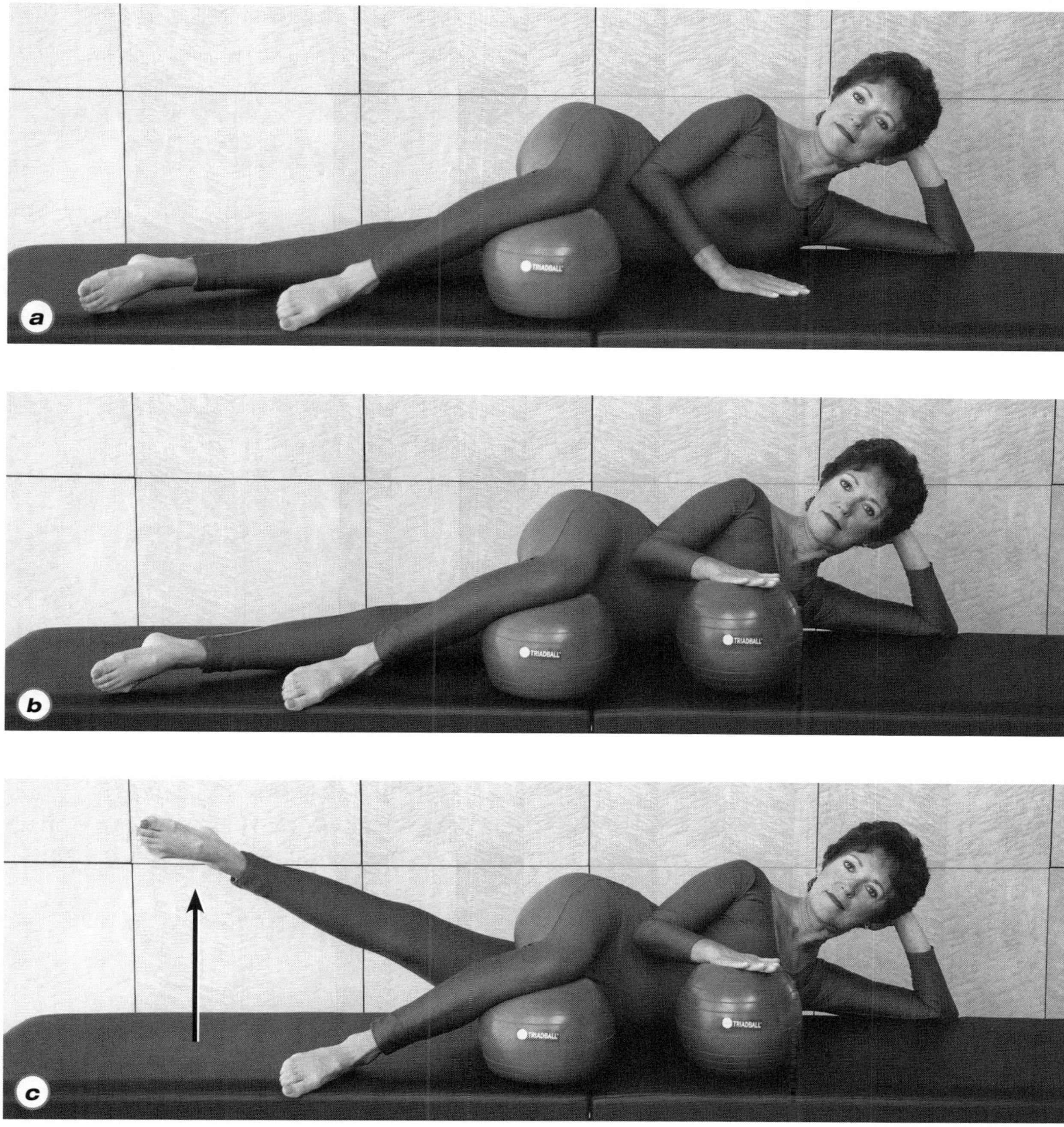

(continued)

Instructions for Inner-Thigh Circle

- Position the body as described for the inner-thigh lift (see p. 298).
- Lift the bottom leg to hip height and make small circles in both directions. Keep the foot relaxed.
- Repeat 6 times in each direction.
- Keep the torso stable. Imagine reaching for the opposite wall with the foot for length.

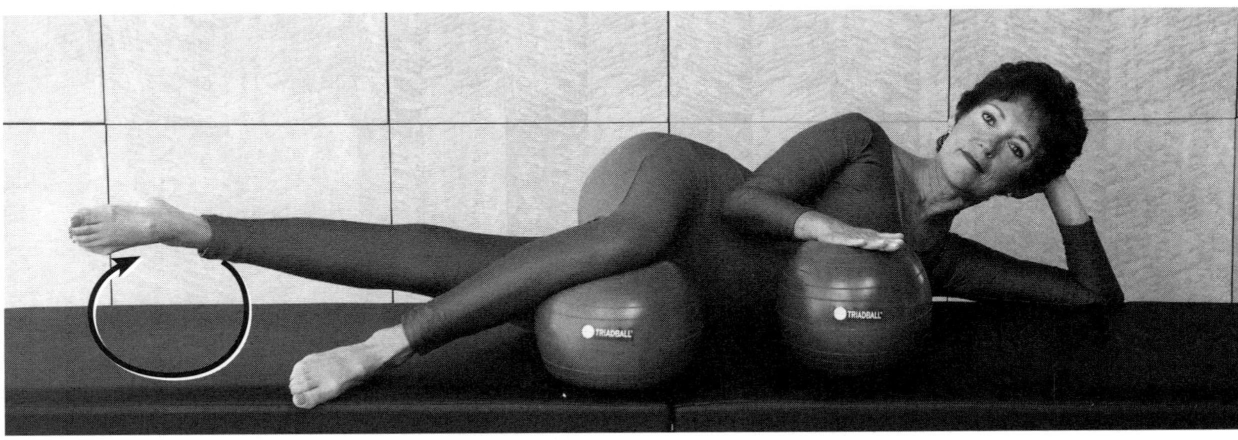

Options

1. For the thigh lifts, pulse the bottom leg up for a count of 6 and repeat 1 time.
2. For the thigh lifts, lift the bottom leg, bring it up 4 to 5 inches (10-13 centimeters), bring it forward toward the waist, return it back, lift it up higher, and then lower it to the starting position. The flow is front, back, up, and down. Repeat 8 times.

Primary Muscles Activated

Abdominals, rectus femoris, iliopsoas, sartorius, pectineus, gracilis, tensor fasciae latae, adductor magnus, adductor longus, adductor brevis, biceps femoris, semitendinosus, semimembranosus, popliteus, gastrocnemius, plantaris, vastus medialis, vastus intermedius, vastus lateralis

Short-Lever Body Position Setup

Timeline: 6 weeks to 3 months postop
Appropriate for: knee and hip
Location: a raised mat, hip height

Instructions

- Lie on one side with the hips and shoulders stacked evenly on the back edge of the mat. Bring both legs to the front corner of the mat. Then bend both legs into a tabletop position, keeping the knees in line with the hip and the shins in line with the front edge of the mat. For support, place the top hand, with the fingers wide, 6 inches (15 centimeters) in front of the body between the sternum and the navel. Press into the heel of the hand.
- Rest the head on the bottom arm, a pad, or a ball.
- Place a small pad or towel between the knees as needed for comfort.
- Draw the abdominals in and up, lifting the waistband from the mat.
- **Knees:** Bend the knees as tolerated into a side-lying tabletop position.
- Breathe with an even flow of inhaling and exhaling.

Setup Options

1. Place a thick pad between the knees to keep space between the legs and to keep the knee as close to hip level as possible.

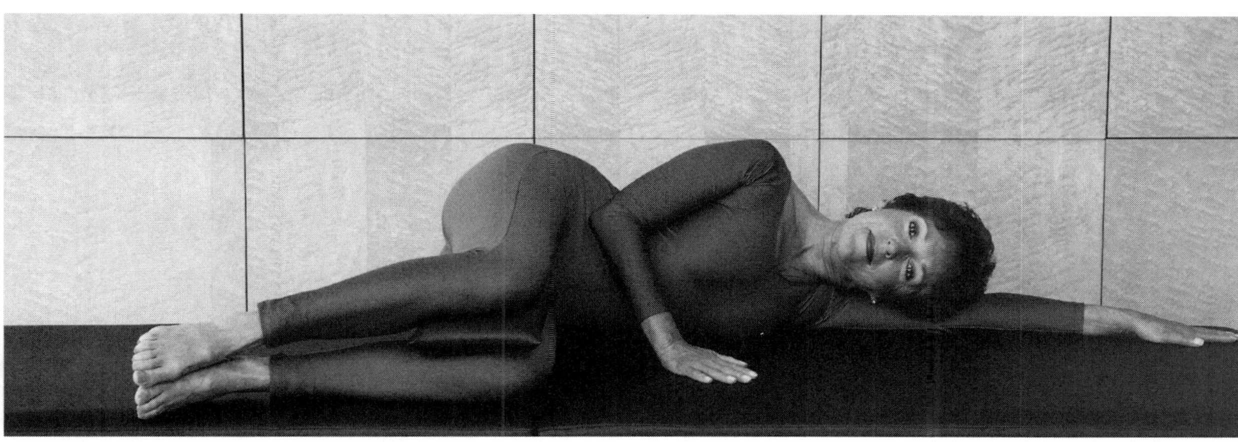

(continued)

Short-Lever Body Position Setup *(continued)*

2. Rest the head on the ball as a pillow and place a pad between the knees.

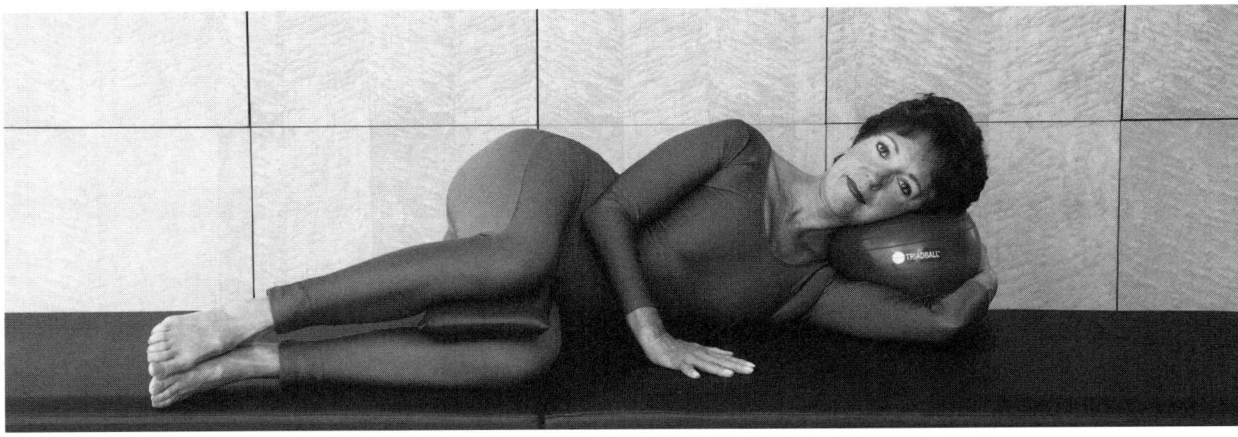

3. Use two soft balls and a pad between the knees.

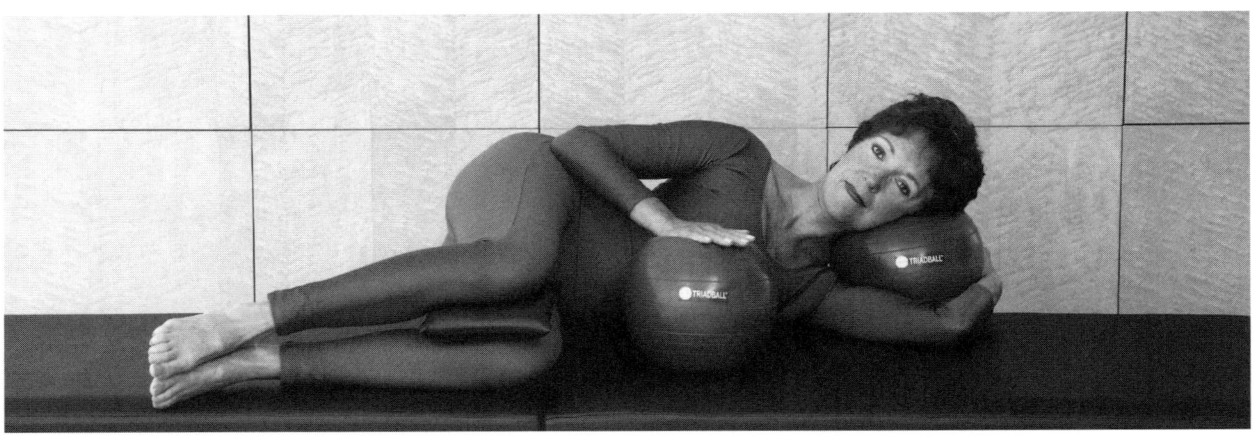

SHORT-LEVER BODY POSITION SETUP

Timeline: 3 to 6 months and 6 months and beyond postop

Appropriate for: knee and hip

Location: a floor mat or a raised mat as needed; a raised mat for a bilateral knee or hip replacement as needed

Instructions

- Lie on one side with the hips and shoulders stacked evenly on the back edge of the mat. Bring both legs to the front corner of the mat. Bend the knees and bring the legs to a tabletop position, with the knees in line with the hips and the shins in line with the front edge of the mat. For support, place the top hand 6 inches (15 centimeters) in front of the body between the sternum and the navel. Press into the heel of the hand.
- Prop the head up on the bottom hand and arm.
- Draw the abdominals in and up.
- Breathe with an even flow of inhaling and exhaling.

Setup Options

1. Prop the head on the hand and arm.

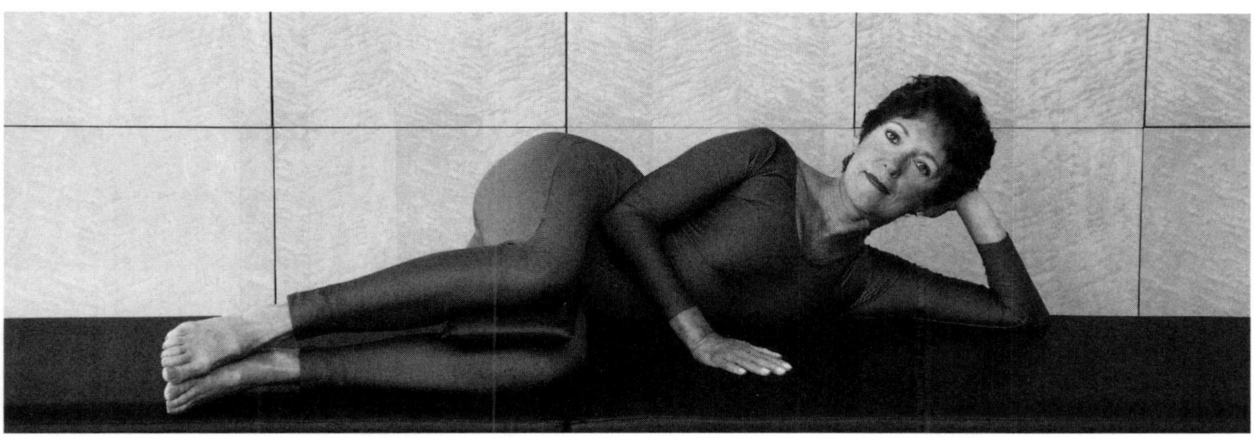

(continued)

Short-Lever Body Position Setup *(continued)*

2. Prop the head on the hand and arm, and then bend the top arm and place the hand behind the head.

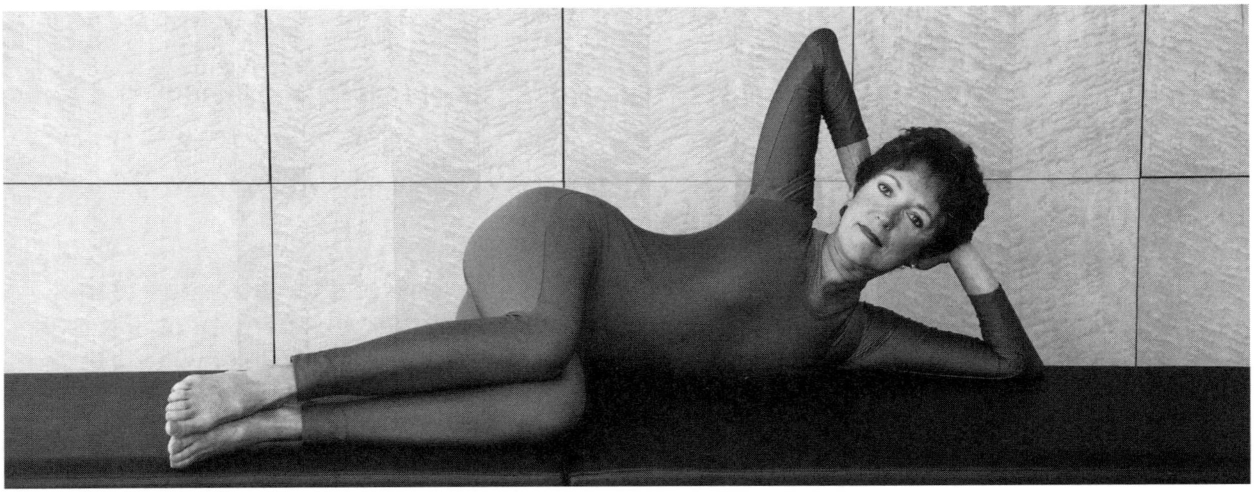

3. Place the top hand on a ball or Pilates ring while performing the movement.

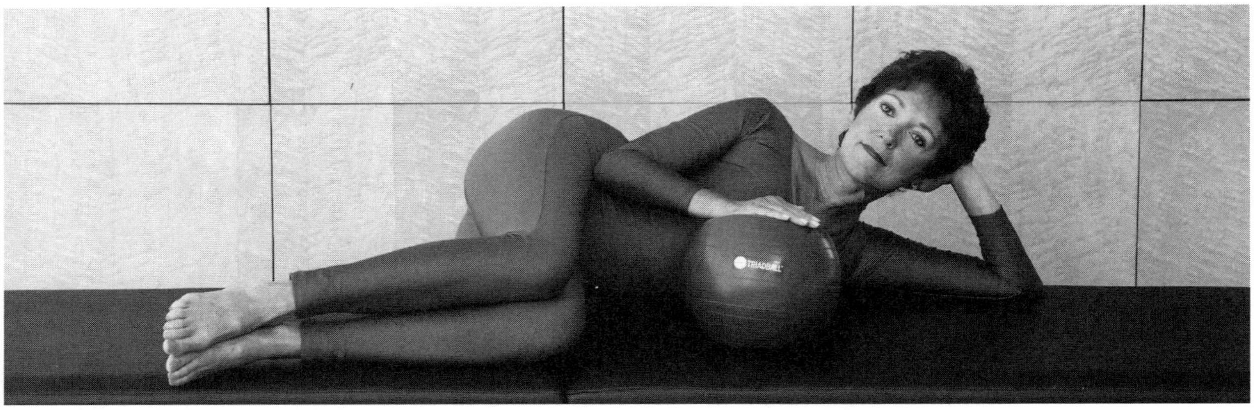

Look for . . . Encourage

- Hips and shoulders stacked on the back edge of the mat and in line with the spine (hip over hip, shoulder over shoulder)
- The bottom arm that the head is resting on should be in line with the stacked shoulders and hips
- The heel in line with the knee
- Creation of opposition by thinking of drawing the hip away from the knee with movement
- Abdominals drawn in and up
- Shoulders gliding toward the hips
- Disassociation of the head of the femur from the acetabulum (stable pelvis with a flowing movement of the working leg)

Be aware of . . . Prevent

- Dropping the heel lower than the knee
- Top hip falling forward and away from the midline of the body
- Loss of core control with movement
- Loss of neutral spine with movement

Note

The pointers on what to encourage and prevent that are listed here apply to all of the following short-lever series movements described in this chapter.

90° Bent-Knee Lift and Lower and 90° Bent-Knee Circle

Timeline: 6 weeks to 3 months postop

Appropriate for: knee and hip

Location: a raised mat, hip height

Instructions for 90° Bent-Knee Lift and Lower

- Select the most appropriate setup option (see pp. 303-304).
- Draw the abdominals in and up.
- With the legs in side-lying tabletop position *(a)*, lift the top leg parallel 4 to 6 inches (10-15 centimeters) from the lower leg *(b)*. Then return to the starting position. Keep the knee and ankle at the same height as you lift and lower.
- Lift the leg only to the point that the pelvis stays steady.
- Breathe with an even flow of inhaling and exhaling.
- Lift and lower slowly and keep the movement controlled.
- Repeat 6 times.
- **Knee:** Bend the knees as tolerated into the side-lying tabletop position. Keep a thick pad between the knees.
- **Hip:** Keep the hip in line with the knee and place a pad, towel, or pillow between the knees to rest on between repeats.

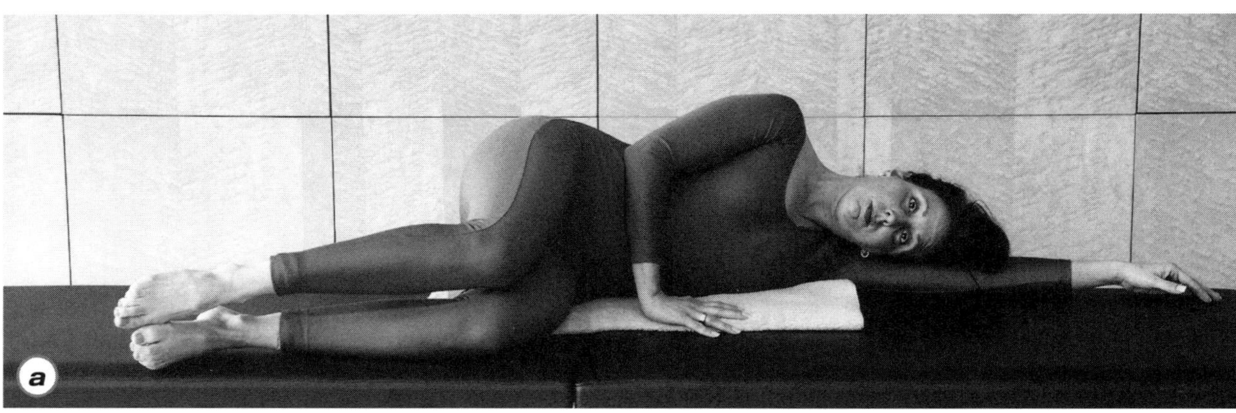

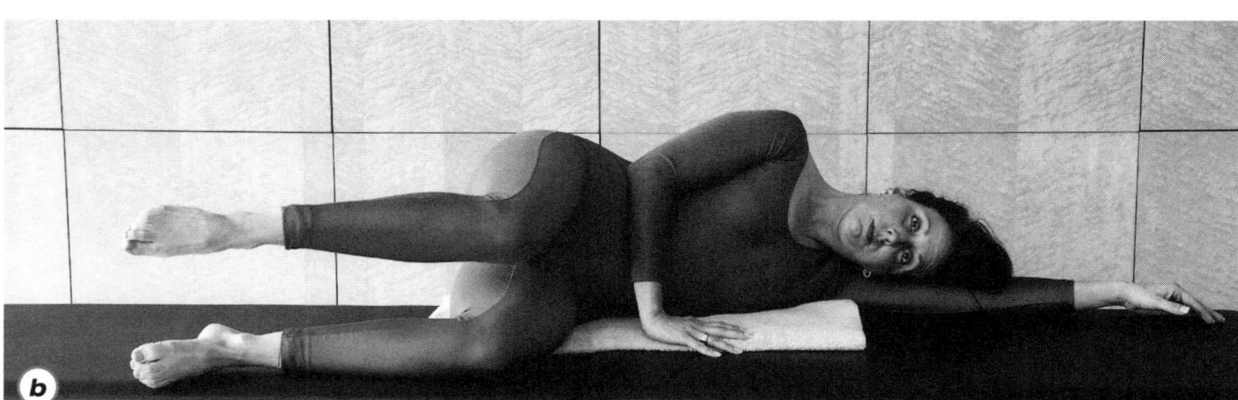

Instructions for 90° Bent-Knee Circle

- With the legs in side-lying tabletop position, lift the top leg parallel to the lower leg and only slightly higher than hip height.
- Begin to make small circles.
- Breathe with an even flow of inhaling and exhaling.
- Circle from the hip, keeping the movement slow and controlled.
- Repeat 6 times and then reverse the direction.
- **Knee:** Bend the knees as tolerated into the side-lying tabletop position.
- **Hip:** Keep the hip in line with the knee and place a pad, towel, or pillow between the knees to rest on between repeats.

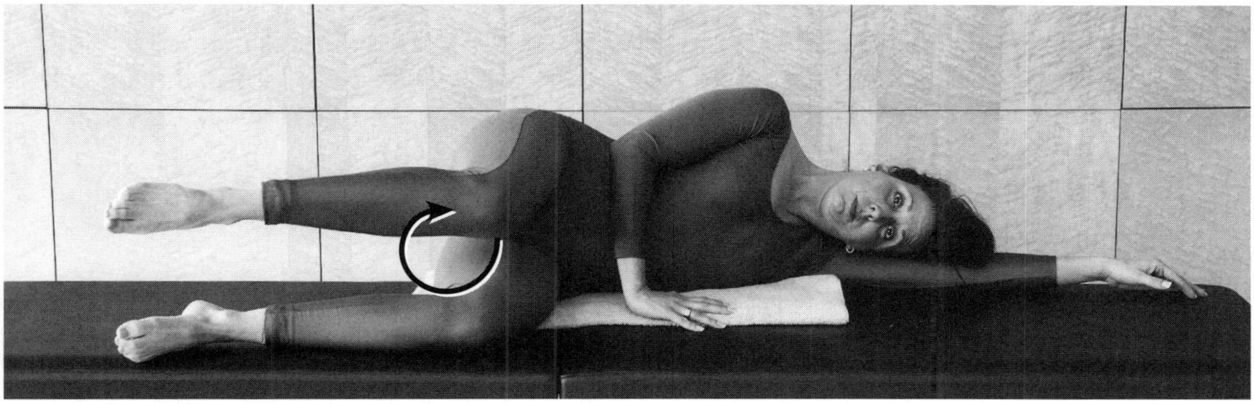

(continued)

SIDE KICK SERIES

90° BENT-KNEE LIFT AND LOWER AND 90° BENT-KNEE CIRCLE

Timeline: 3 to 6 months and 6 months and beyond postop

Appropriate for: knee and hip

Location: a floor mat or a raised mat as needed; a raised mat for a bilateral knee or hip replacement as needed

Instructions for 90° Bent-Knee Lift and Lower

- Select the most appropriate setup option (see pp. 305-306).
- Draw the abdominals in and up.
- With the legs in side-lying tabletop position *(a)*, lift the top leg parallel about 8 inches (20 centimeters) from the bottom leg and then lower the top leg *(b)*. Keep the leg active throughout all of the repeats. Keep the knee and ankle at the same height as you lift and lower.
- Lift the leg only to the point that the pelvis stays steady and stacked.
- Keep the movement slow and controlled.
- Breathe with an even flow of inhaling and exhaling.
- Repeat 10 times.
- **Knee:** Bend the knees as tolerated into the side-lying tabletop position.
- **Hip:** Keep the hip in line with the knee.

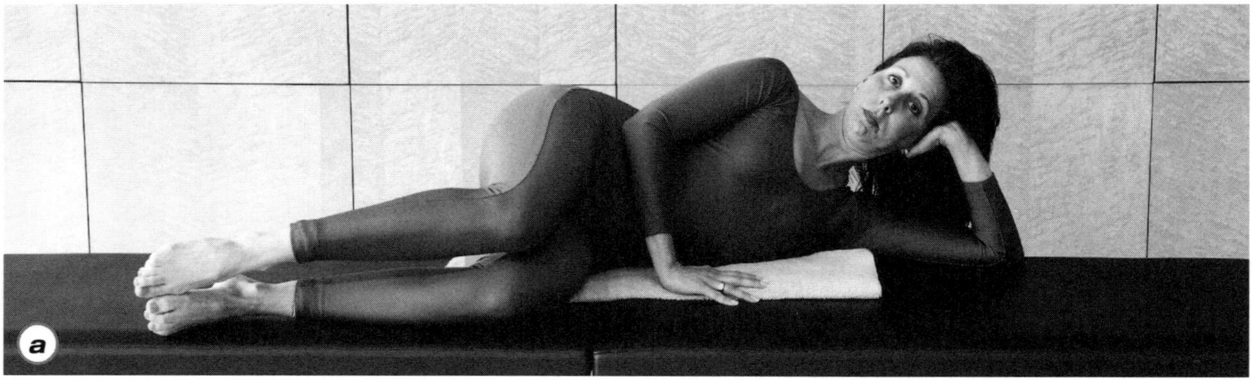

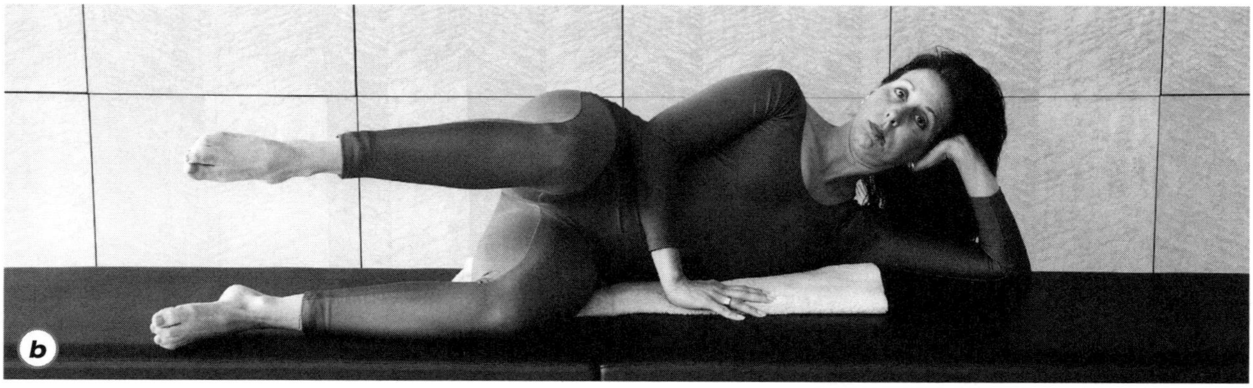

Instructions for 90° Bent-Knee Circle

- Select the most appropriate setup option (see pp. 305-306).
- Draw the abdominals in and up.
- With the legs in a side-lying tabletop position, lift the top leg parallel to the lower leg and only slightly higher than hip height.
- Begin to make small circles the size of a dinner plate.
- Circle from the hip.
- Repeat 6 times and then reverse the direction.

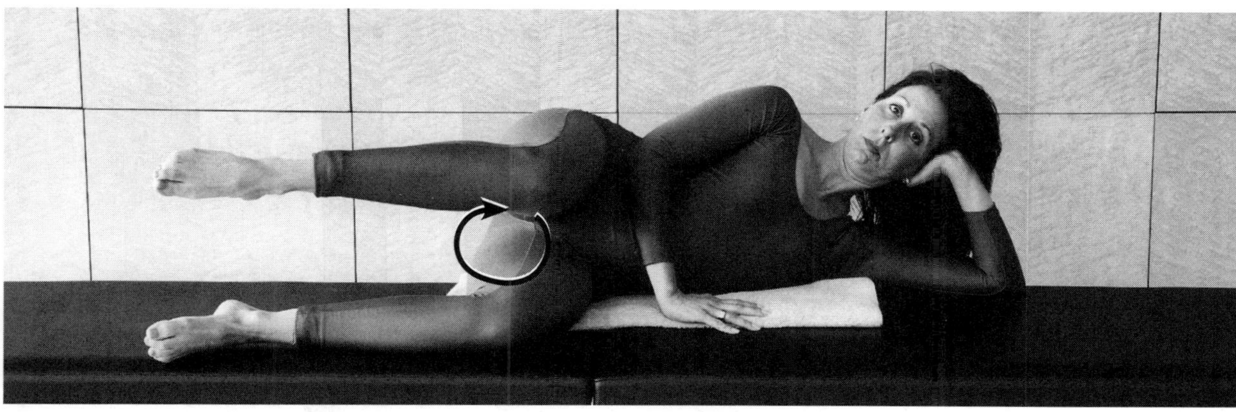

Option

With the legs in side-lying tabletop position, lift the top leg parallel to the lower leg and only slightly higher than hip height. Bring the knee toward the nose and then return it to the starting position. Lift the leg higher and then lower it to the starting position. The flow is up, front, back, up higher, down to start. Repeat 6 to 10 times.

Primary Muscles Activated

Abdominals, rectus femoris, iliopsoas, sartorius, pectineus, gracilis, biceps femoris, semitendinosus, semimembranosus, gluteus medius, tensor fasciae latae, popliteus, gastrocnemius, plantaris, gluteus minimus, gluteus maximus, gluteus medius, adductor magnus, adductor longus, adductor brevis, piriformis

90° Bent-Knee Touch

Timeline: 6 weeks to 3 months postop

Appropriate for: knee and hip

Location: a raised mat, hip height

Instructions

- Select the most appropriate setup option (see pp. 303-304).
- With the legs in side-lying tabletop position, press the medial edge of the bottom foot to the medial edge of the top foot *(a)*. Slide the feet back a few inches (centimeters) toward the buttocks.
- Draw the abdominals in and up.
- Lift the top knee away from the bottom knee a few inches as tolerated *(b)*, and then lower slowly to the starting position.

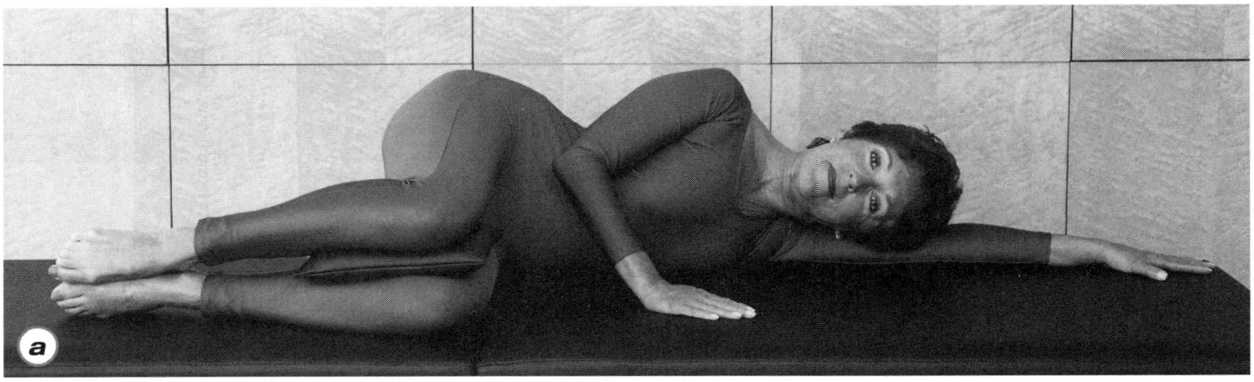

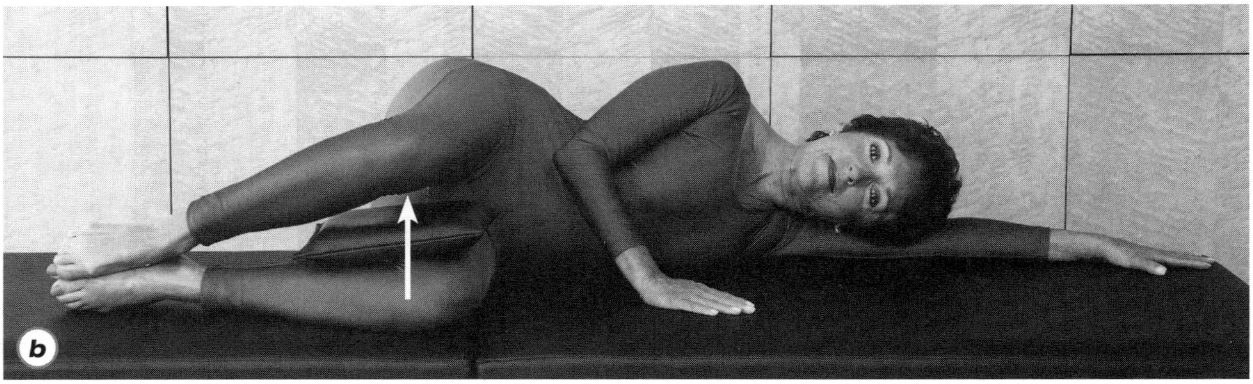

- Open and close the knees, keeping the sides of the feet glued together during the movement.
- Keep the torso steady. Do not let the top hip flow back out of alignment when lifting the knee.
- Breathe with an even flow of inhaling and exhaling.
- Repeat 6 times. Keep the movement slow and controlled.
- **Knee:** Bend the knees as tolerated into the side-lying tabletop position.
- **Hip:** Use a towel under the hips as needed. For 6 weeks to 2 months postop, keep the ROM small. Start with no more than 20° of external rotation and then work up to a maximum of 30° by 3 months.

(continued)

90° BENT-KNEE TOUCH

Timeline: 3 to 6 months and 6 months and beyond postop

Appropriate for: knee and hip

Location: a floor mat or a raised mat as needed; a raised mat for a bilateral knee or hip replacement as needed

Instructions

- Select the most appropriate setup option (see pp. 305-306).
- With the legs in side-lying tabletop position, press the medial edge of the bottom foot to the medial edge of the top foot *(a)*. Slide the feet back a few inches toward the buttocks.
- Draw the abdominals in and up.
- Lift the top knee away from the bottom knee, up to 8 to 10 inches (20-25 centimeters) as tolerated *(b)*, and then lower slowly to the starting position.

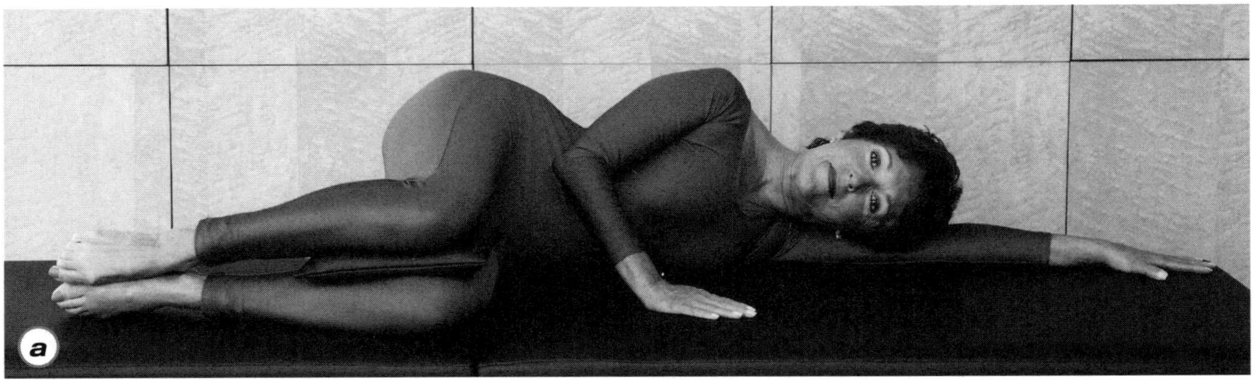

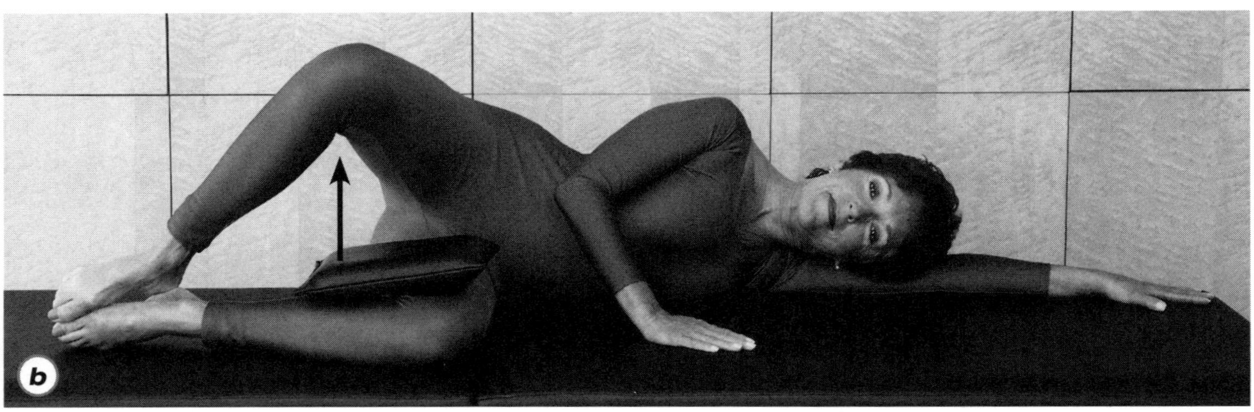

- Breathe with an even flow of inhaling and exhaling.
- Repeat 10 times, keeping the movement slow and controlled.
- Open and close the knees, keeping the sides of the feet glued together during the movement.
- **Hip:** Maintain a maximum of 30° of external rotation.
- Keep the torso steady. Do not let the top hip flow back out of alignment when lifting the knee.

Primary Muscles Activated

Abdominals, rectus femoris, iliopsoas, sartorius, pectineus, gracilis, biceps femoris, semitendinosus, semimembranosus, gluteus medius, tensor fasciae latae, popliteus, gastrocnemius, plantaris, gluteus minimus, gluteus maximus, adductor magnus, adductor longus, adductor brevis, piriformis, gemellus superior, gemellus inferior, obturator internus, obturator externus, quadratus femoris

90° Bent-Knee Rotation

Restrictions: not applicable for the knee or hip at 6 weeks to 3 months postop or 3 months to 6 months postop

Timeline: 6 months and beyond postop

Appropriate for: knee and hip

Location: a floor mat or a raised mat as needed

Instructions

- With the legs in side-lying tabletop position, press the medial edge of the bottom foot to the medial edge of the top foot. Slide the feet back a few inches toward the buttocks.
- Lift the top knee away from the bottom knee *(a)*, and then simultaneously switch and lower the knee while lifting the top foot away from the bottom foot *(b)*.
- Switch, rotating the knee up and the foot down *(c)*.
- Breathe with an even flow of inhaling and exhaling.
- Keep the movement slow and controlled without losing form.
- Repeat 6 times.
- The flow is foot to foot and then knee to knee.
- **Hip:** Limit external and internal rotation to up to 30°.

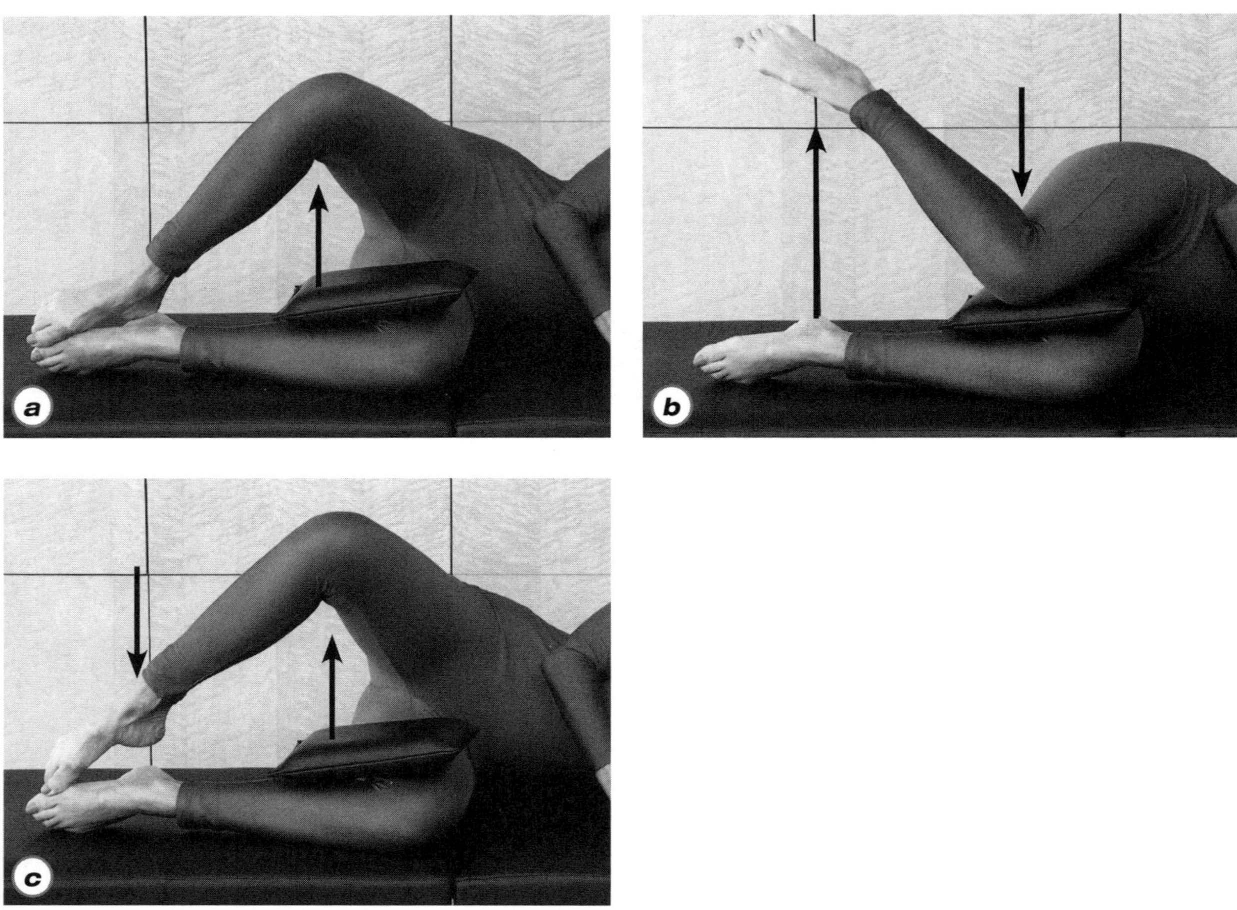

Option

Use a ball under the top hand to challenge core stability.

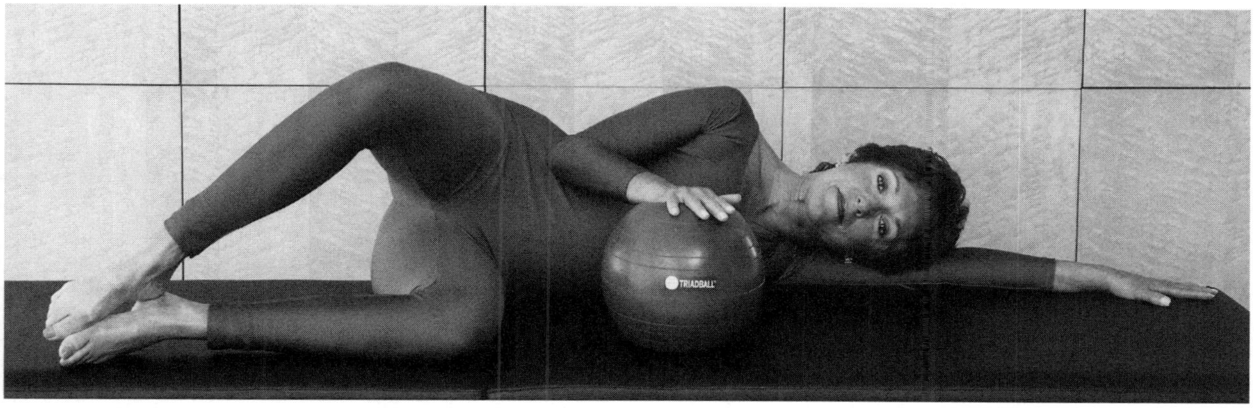

Primary Muscles Activated

Abdominals, rectus femoris, iliopsoas, sartorius, pectineus, gracilis, biceps femoris, semitendinosus, semimembranosus, gluteus medius, tensor fasciae latae, popliteus, gastrocnemius, plantaris, gluteus minimus, gluteus maximus, adductor longus, adductor brevis, adductor magnus, piriformis, gemellus superior, gemellus inferior, obturator internus, obturator externus, quadratus femoris

chapter 7

Pilates Mat Program Sequences

This chapter provides case scenarios and sample Pilates mat program sequences. The sample Pilates sequence for knee syndromes showcases pes bursitis (see chapter 2, p. 20, for a description of this syndrome), while the sample Pilates sequence for hip syndromes showcases trochanteric bursitis (see chapter 1, p. 6, for a description of this syndrome). In addition, there are two complete sample Pilates mat program sequences showcasing joint replacement: one addressing TKA and one addressing THA. Both of the arthroplasty sequences follow a case scenario of osteoarthritis and progress from a preoperative sequence to a sequence for 6 months postop and beyond.

Each sample Pilates sequence begins with a case scenario that details the client's age, gender, and syndrome or operation. The total number of exercises prescribed and the approximate time required to complete the sequence are also listed. Then the exercises comprising the Pilates sequence are listed, along with a thumbnail-sized photo of each exercise and the page number where you can find a complete description of each exercise.

⚠ All exercises should be performed under the guidance of a qualified Pilates instructor and with referral from the operative physician. The client's needs, restrictions, and ROM recommendations should be specified by the physician and followed accordingly. These guidelines may vary from the protocols that follow, and the protocols should be modified based on the individual's needs and the surgeon's preferences.

Pes Bursitis of the Knee

Case scenario: A 50-year-old female with pes bursitis of the right knee has a history of running 4 times per week. It has been 2 months since she has engaged in a strength training or cardiorespiratory exercise routine. She has never taken a Pilates mat class or had private Pilates instruction.

Exercises: 25

Approximate time: 50 minutes

Pre-Pilates Exercises

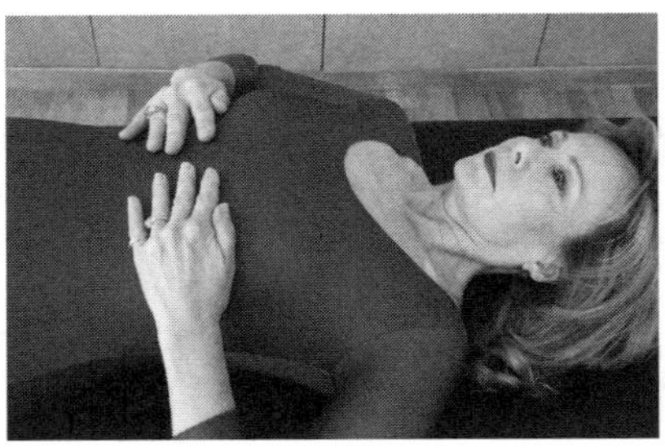

Breathing
Page 39

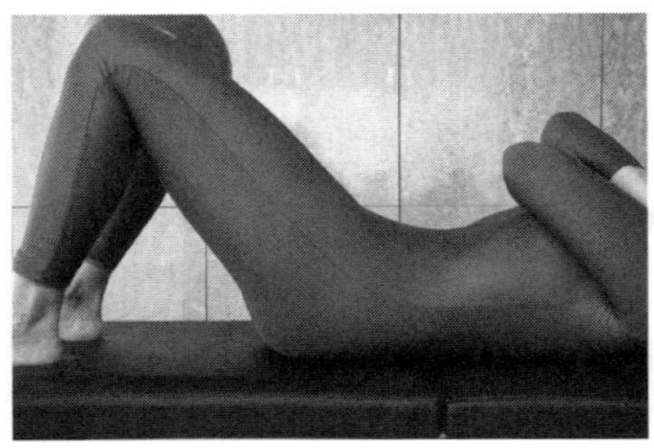

Pelvic curl
Page 45

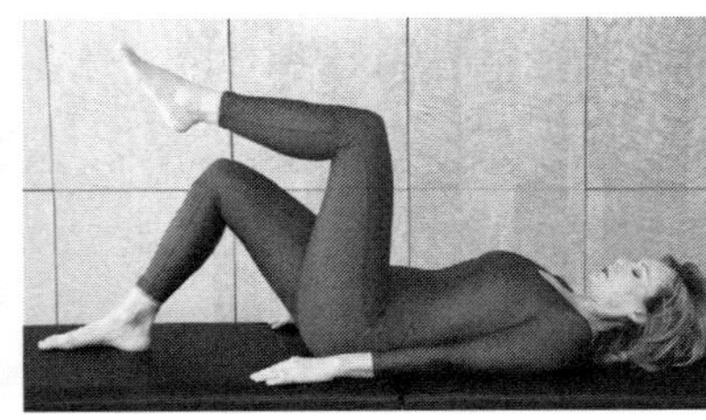

Toe tap
Page 46

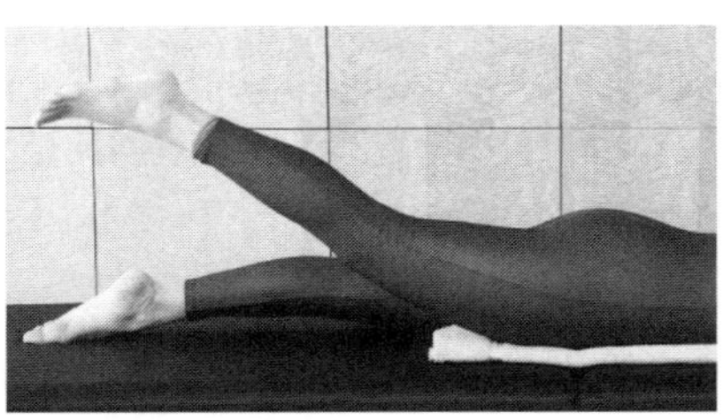

Prone leg lift, version one
Page 56

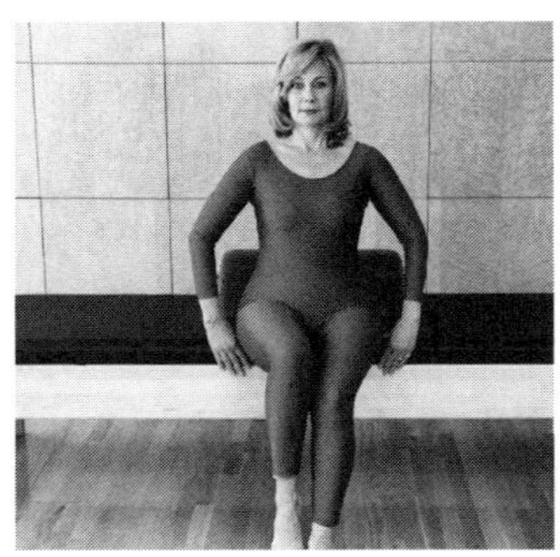

Sitting bent-knee lift, version one
Page 59

Pilates Exercises

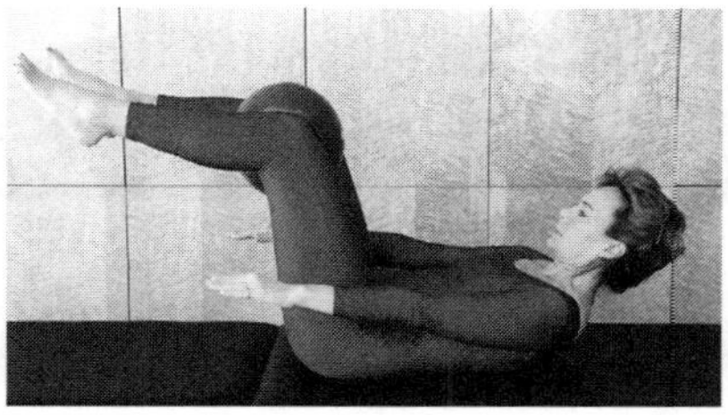

Hundred
Page 135

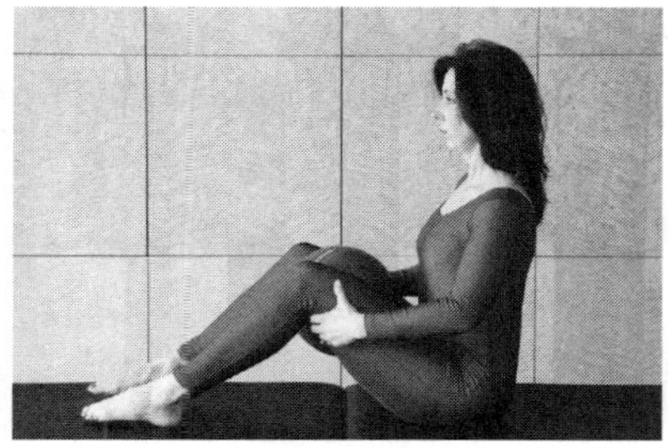

Half roll-down
Page 140

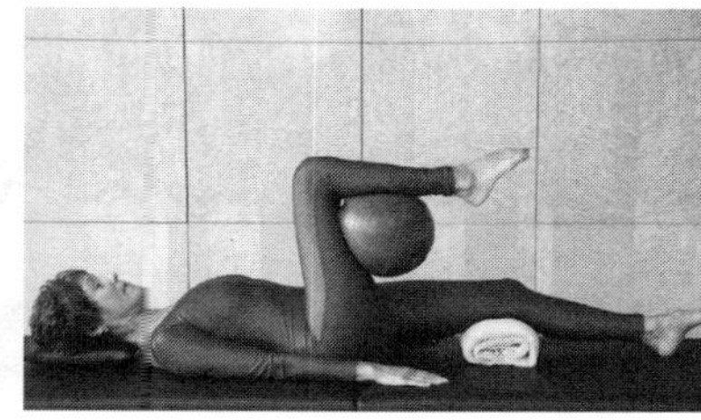

Single-leg circle
Page 81

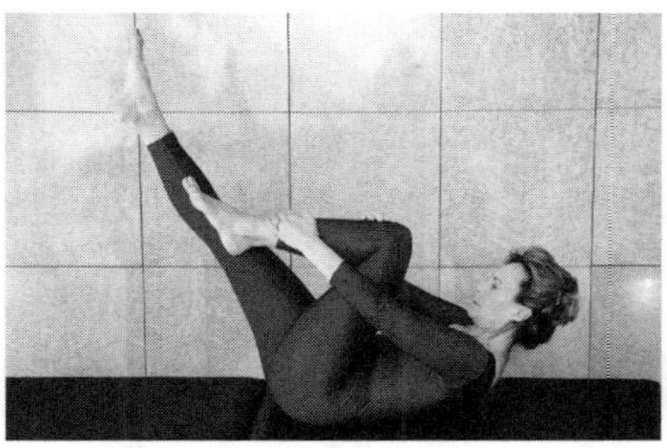

Single-leg stretch
Page 160

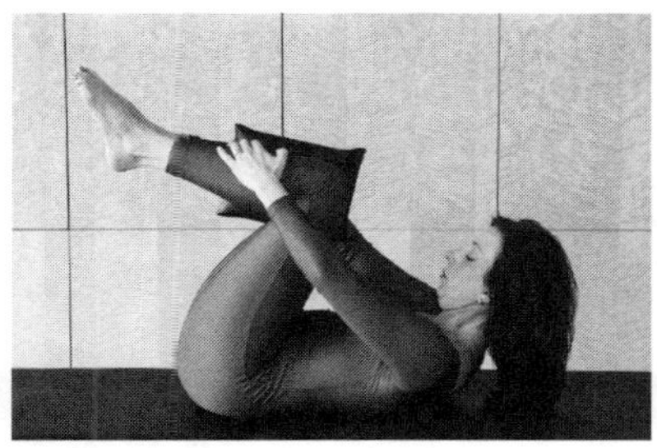

Double-leg stretch
Page 163

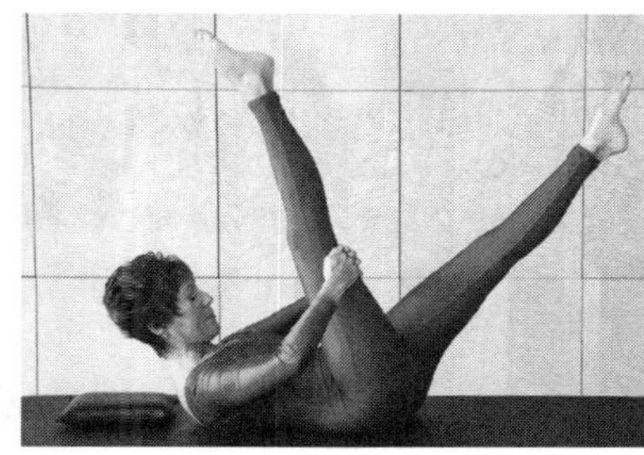

Scissors
Page 90

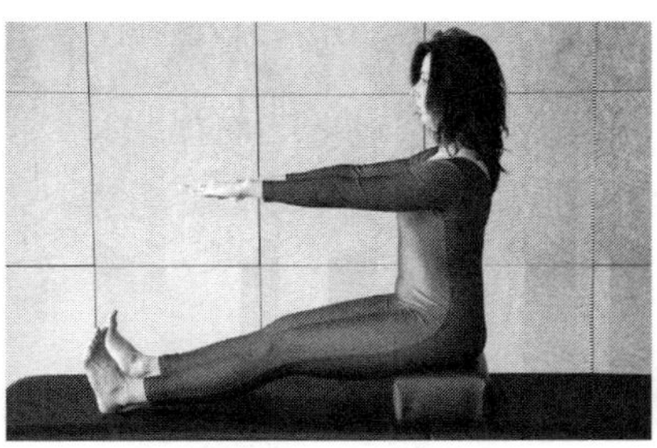

Spine stretch forward
Page 104

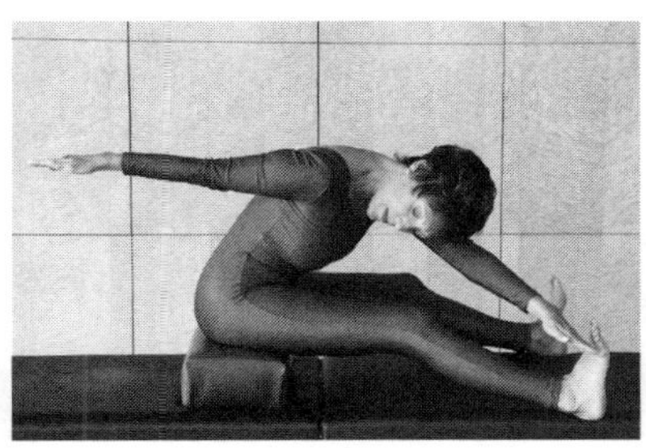

Saw
Page 107

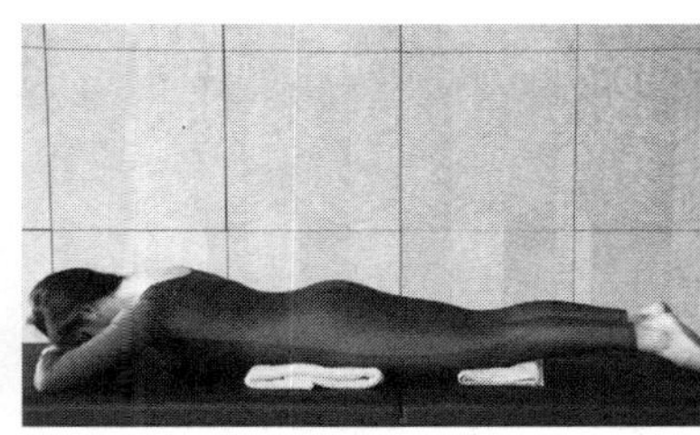

Swan prep
Page 111

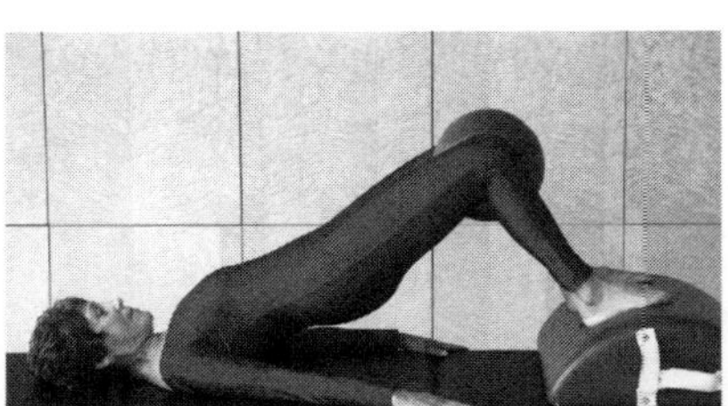

Shoulder bridge (modified)
Page 117

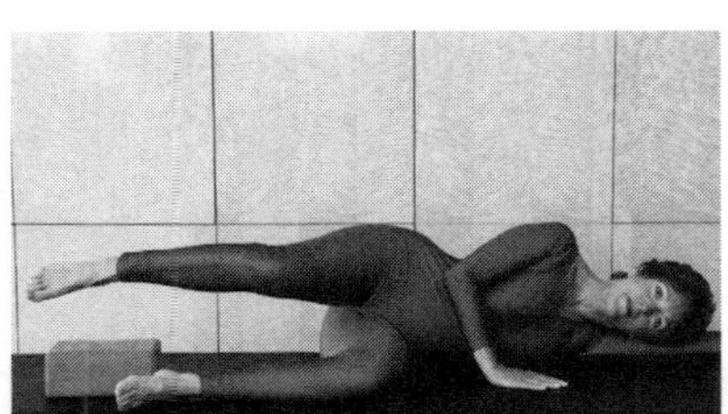

SKS, front and back
Page 274

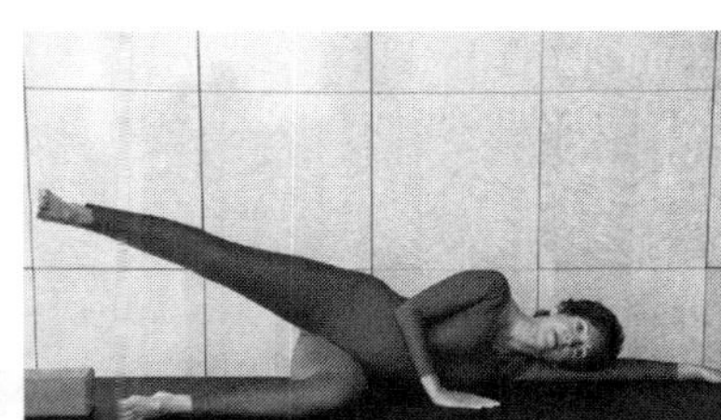

SKS, up and down
Page 270

(continued)

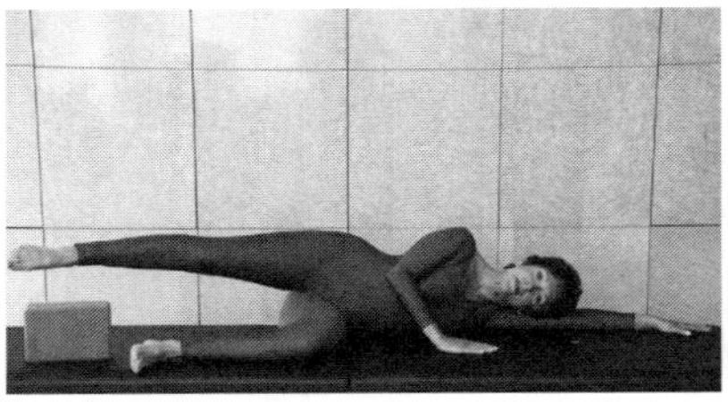

SKS, little circle
Page 278

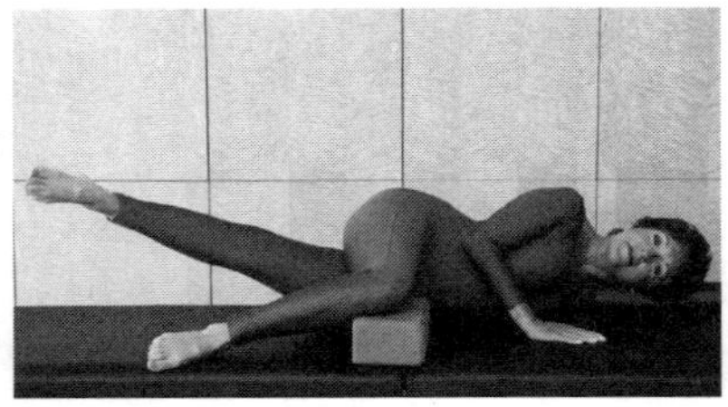

SKS, inner-thigh lift
and inner-thigh circle
Page 298

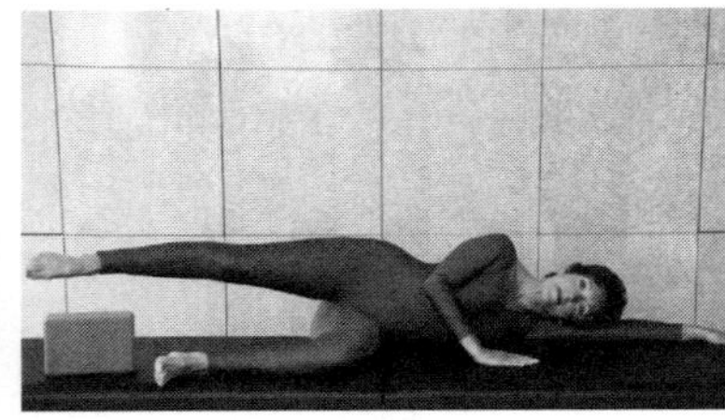

SKS, internal
and external rotation
Page 284

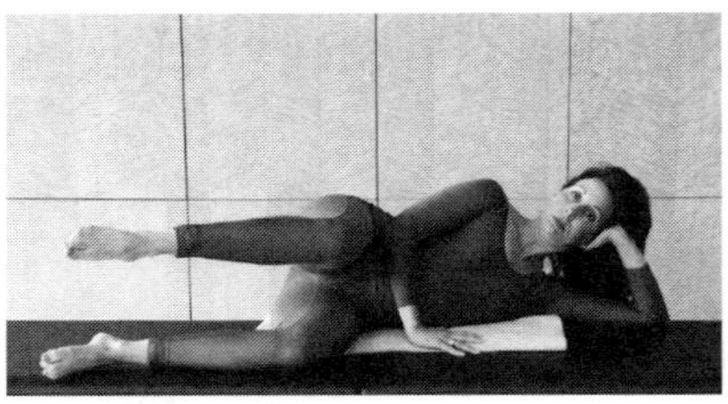

SKS, 90° bent-knee lift
Page 310

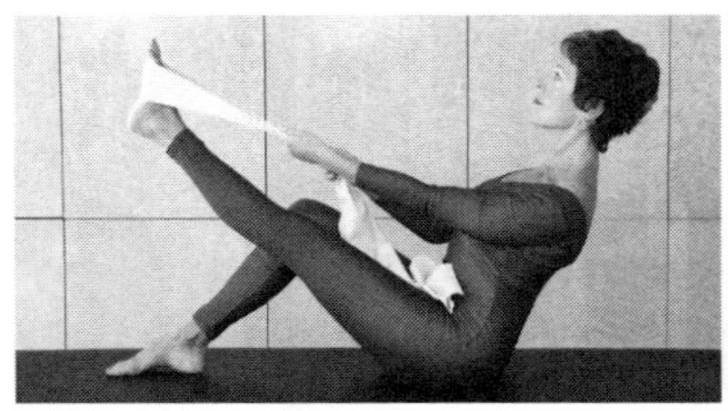

Teaser prep 2
Page 127

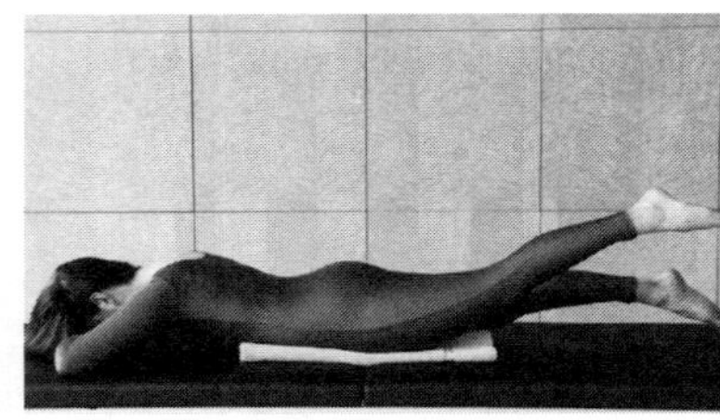

Swim prep
Page 239

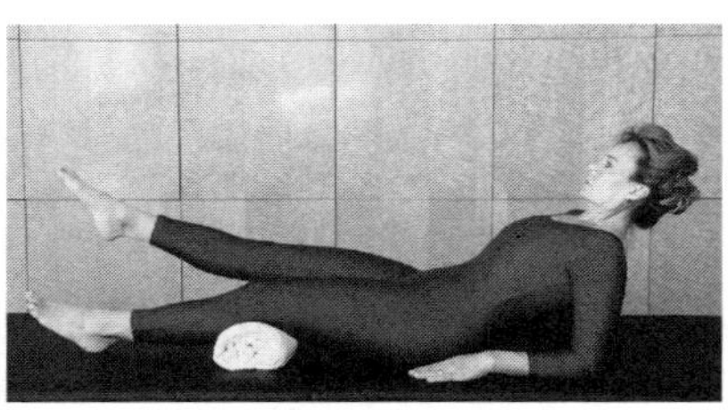

Leg pull (modified)
Page 243

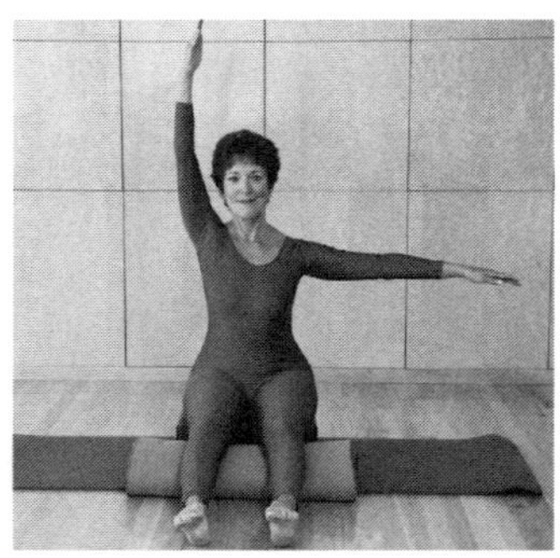

Side stretch
Page 247

Total Knee Replacement (Arthroplasty): Preoperative Program Sequence

Case scenario: A 60-year-old male with osteoarthritis of the right knee walks with pain and uses a cane for assistance. He is scheduled for a TKA in 8 weeks. He is starting a preoperative specified Pilates routine in preparation for the TKA. He has a history of exercising on a routine basis. His exercise program consists of using the recumbent bike for cardiorespiratory training and performing upper-body strength training 3 times per week. He has no history of practicing Pilates.

Exercises: 25

Approximate time: 50 minutes

Pre-Pilates Exercises

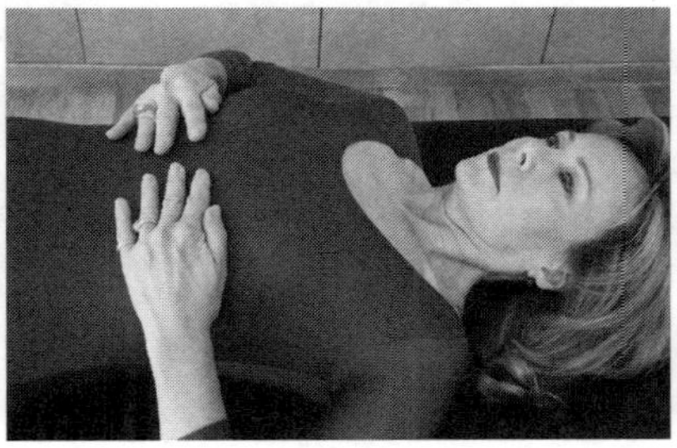

Breathing
Page 39

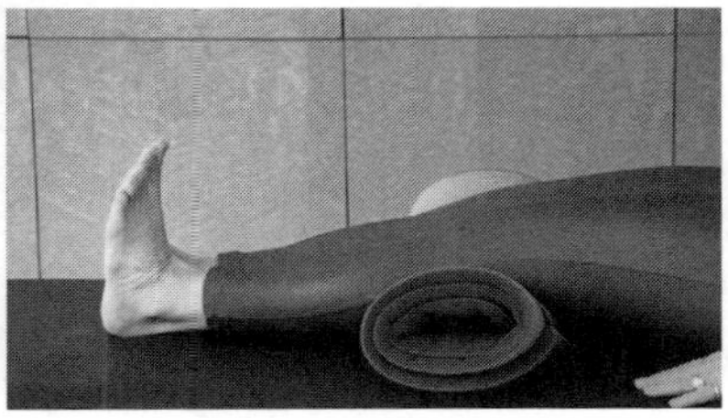

Ankle pump
Page 40

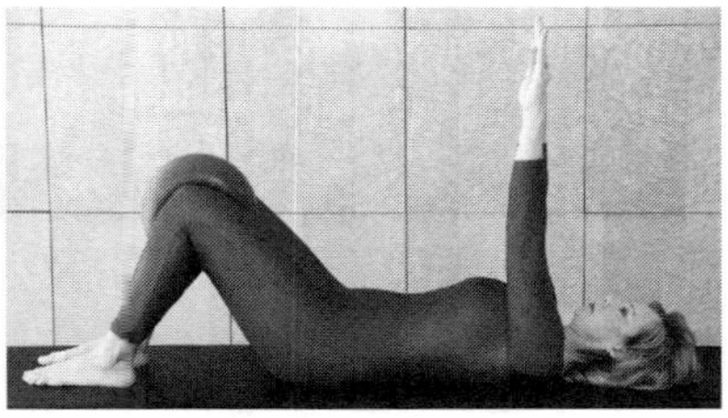

Abdominal prep
Page 48

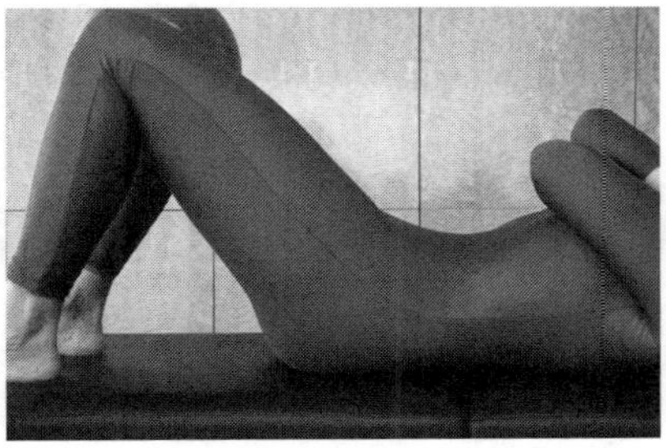

Pelvic curl
Page 45

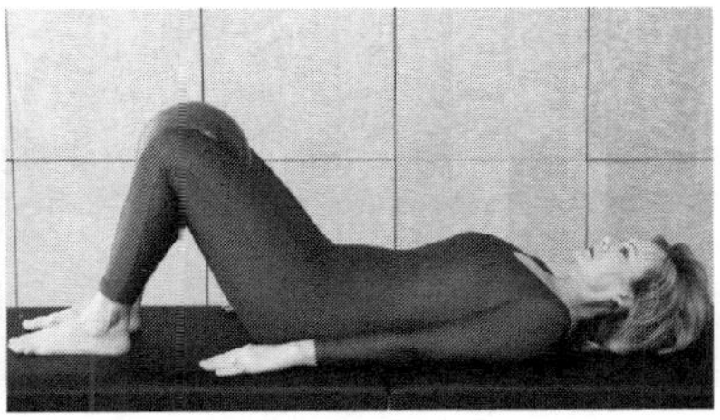

Adductor squeeze
Page 52

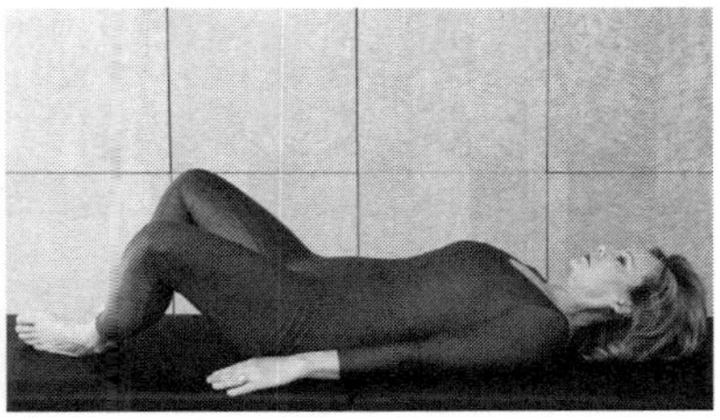

Knee fold, version two
Page 50

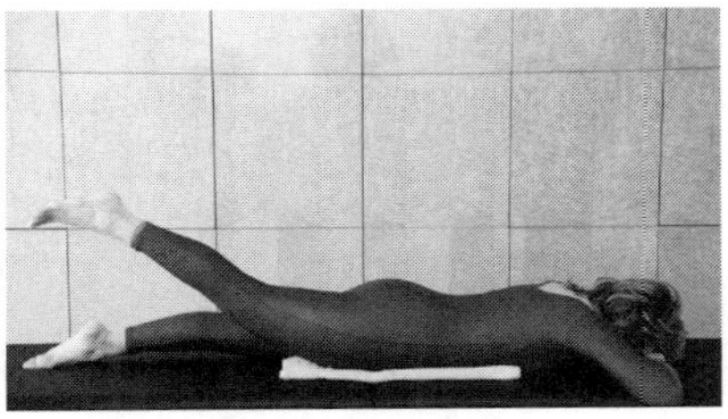

Prone leg lift, version one
Page 56

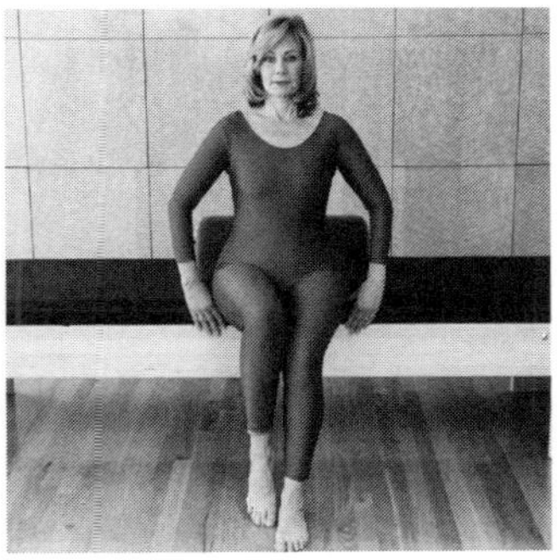

Sitting bent-knee lift,
version one
Page 59

(continued)

Pilates Exercises

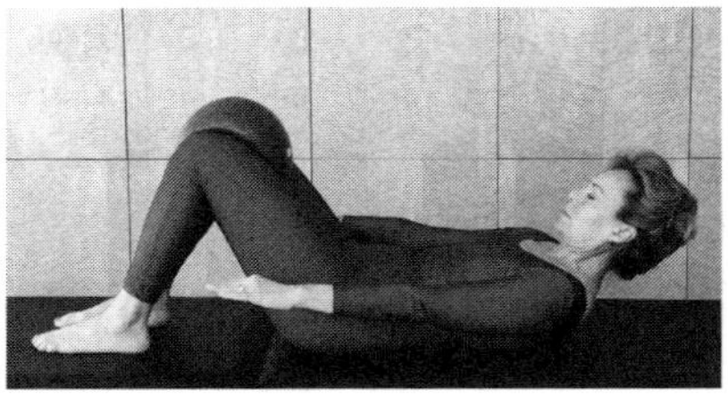

Hundred
Page 69

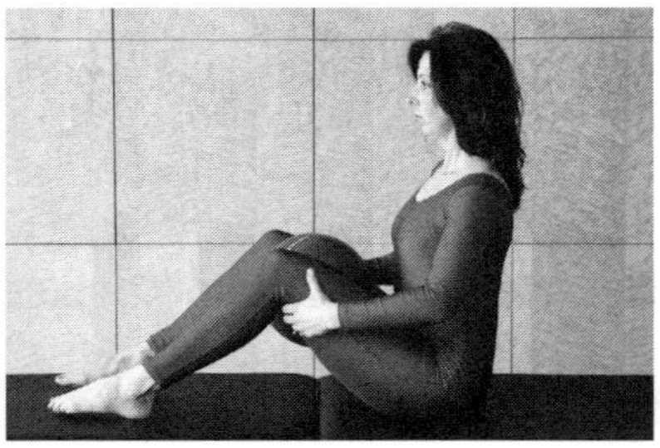

Half roll-down
Page 70

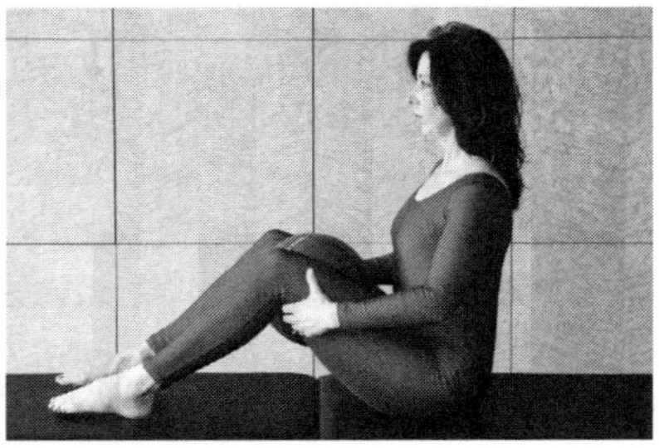

Half roll-up
Page 75

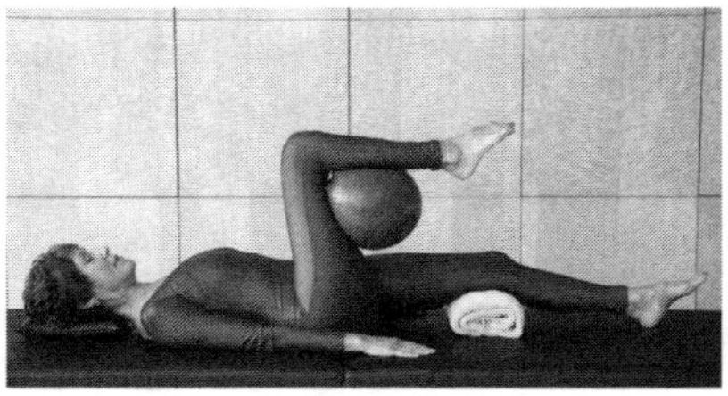

Single-leg circle
Page 81

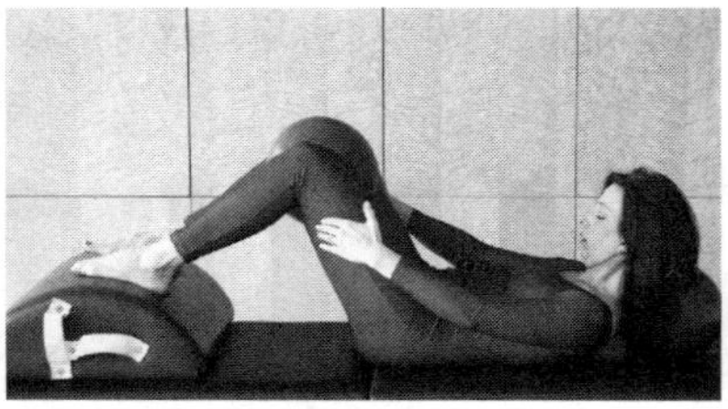

Double-leg stretch
Page 87

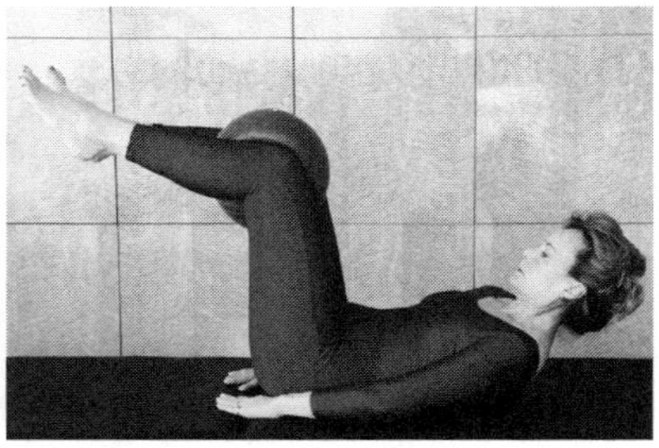

Lower lift
Page 95

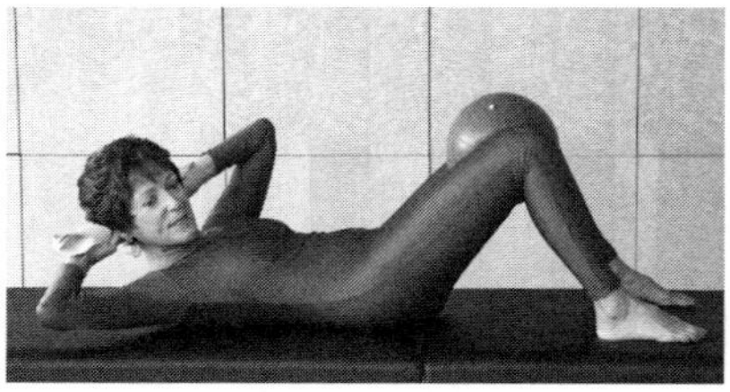

Crisscross
Page 100

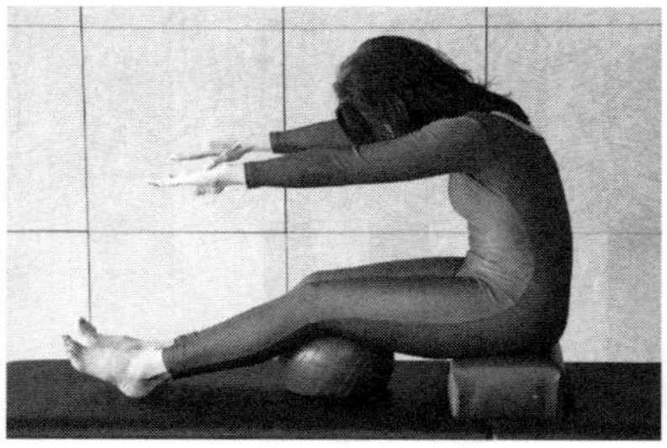

Spine stretch forward
Page 105

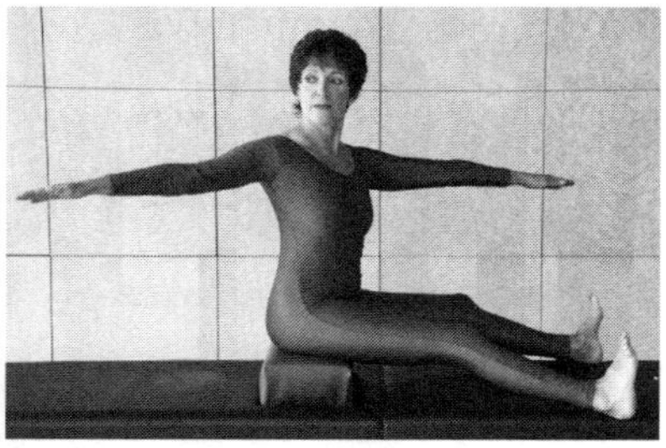

Saw
Page 107

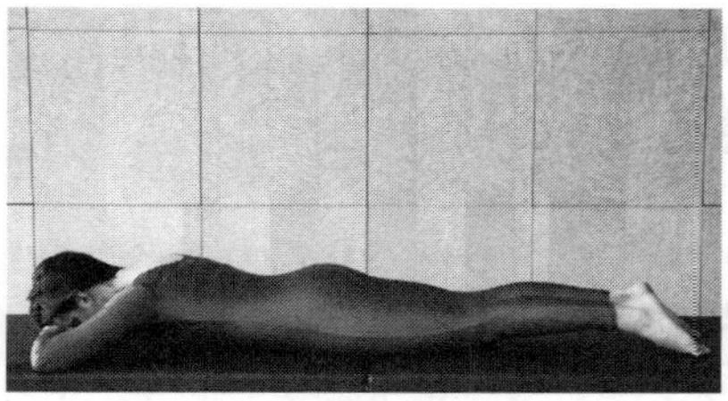

Swan prep
Page 110

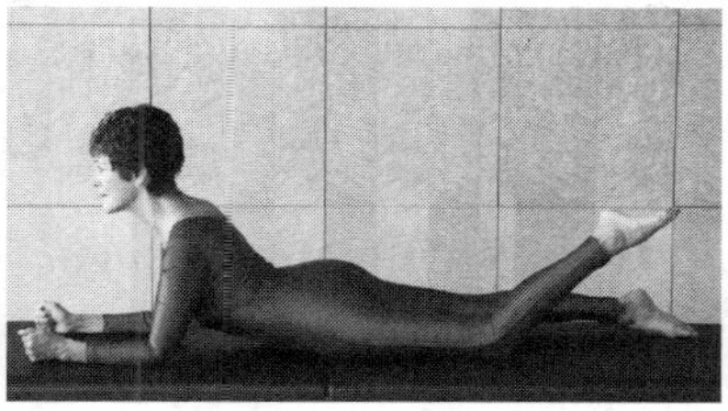

Single-leg kick
Page 113

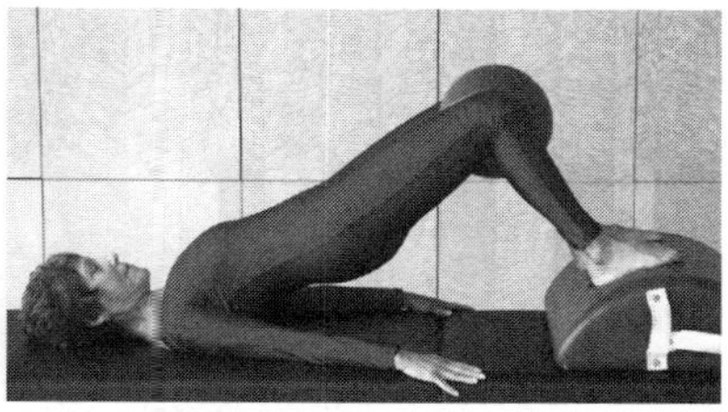

Shoulder bridge (modified)
Page 117

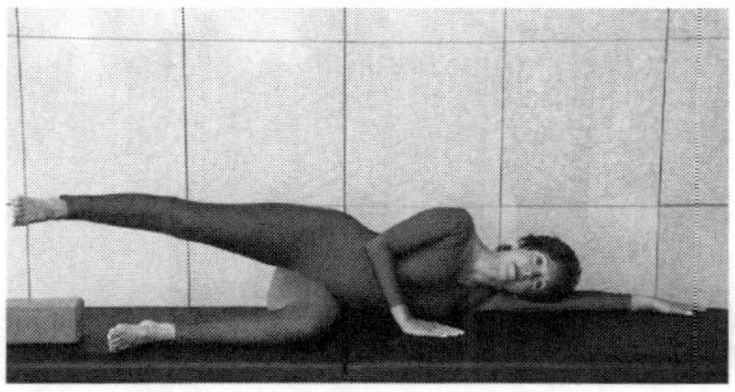

SKS, up and down
Page 270

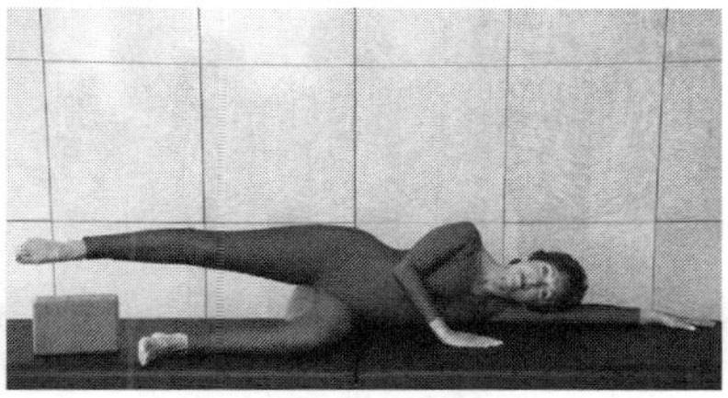

SKS, little circle
Page 278

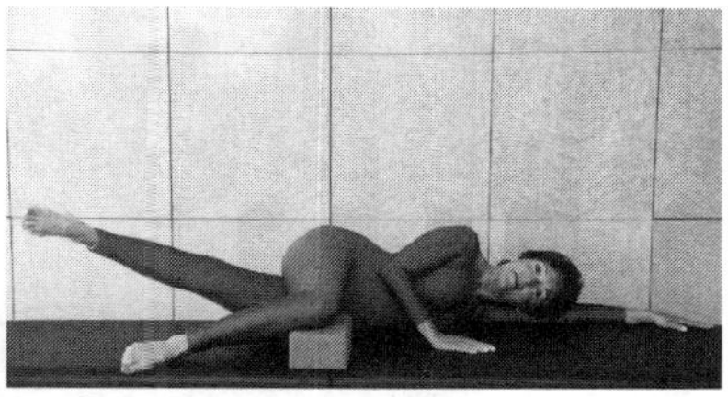

SKS, inner-thigh lift
Page 298

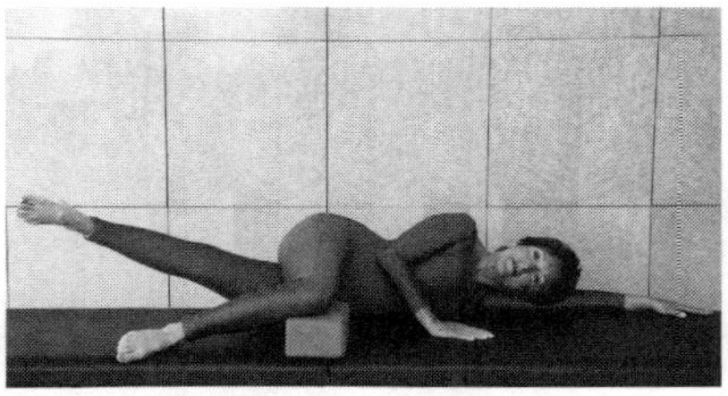

SKS, inner-thigh circle
Page 299

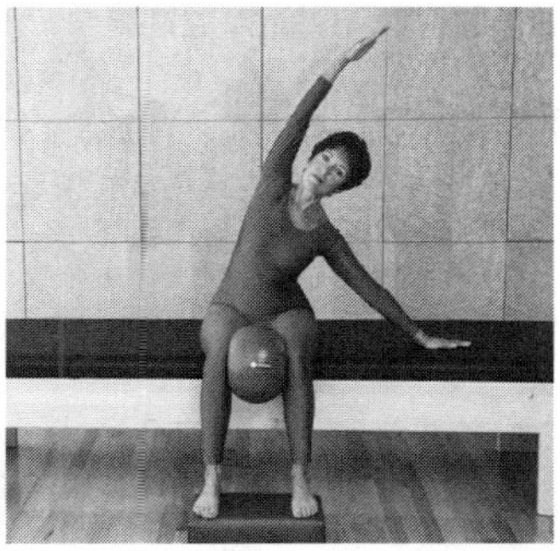

Side stretch
Page 129

Total Knee Replacement (Arthroplasty): Program Sequence for 6 Weeks Postop

Case scenario continued: A 60-year-old male with osteoarthritis of the right knee walked with pain and used a cane for assistance previous to TKA. He finished an 8-week preoperative Pilates routine in preparation for the TKA. He was exercising 3 times a week before surgery. He is now ready to continue Pilates at 6 weeks postoperative.

Exercises: 26

Approximate time: 50 minutes

Pre-Pilates Exercises

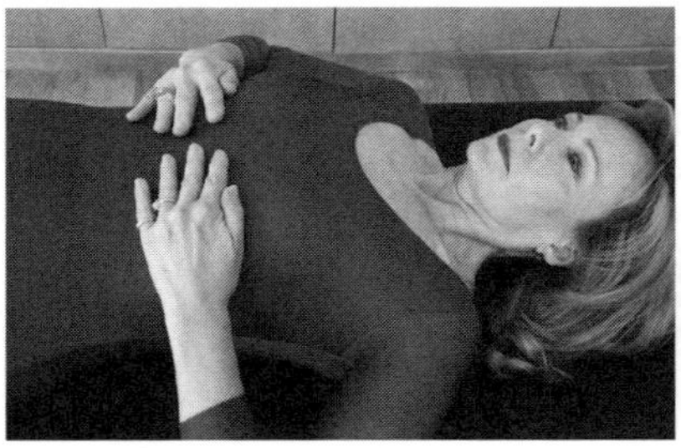

Breathing
Page 39

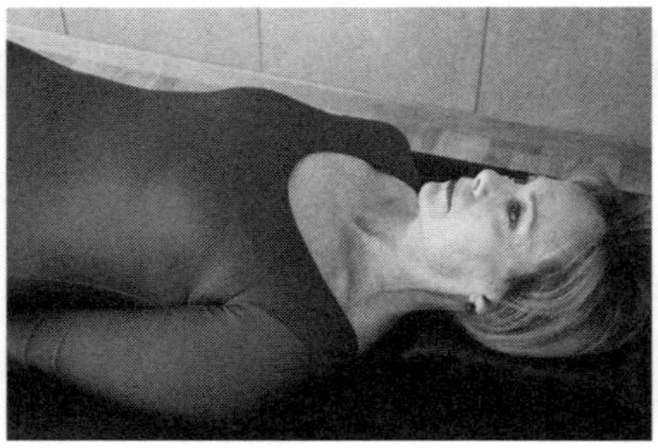

Shoulder roll
Page 44

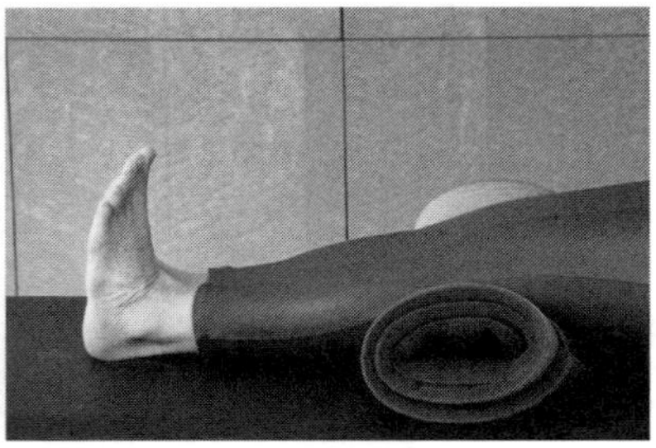

Ankle pump
Page 40

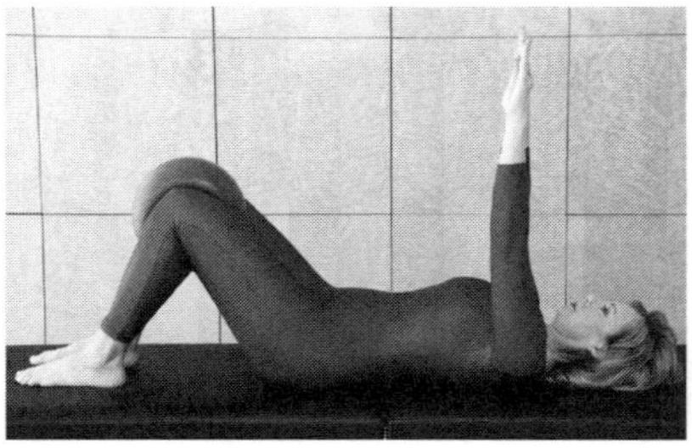

Abdominal prep
Page 48

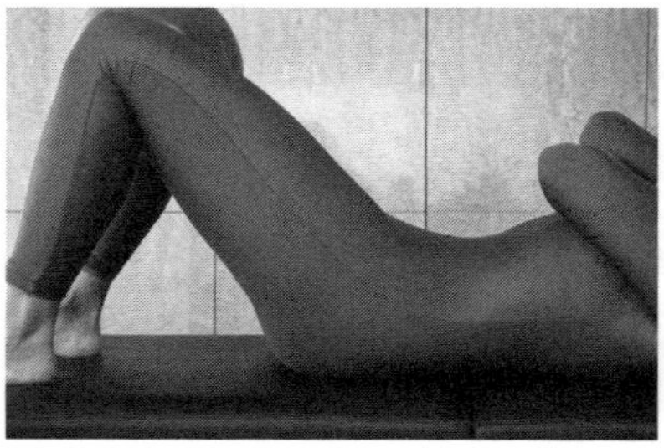

Pelvic curl
Page 45

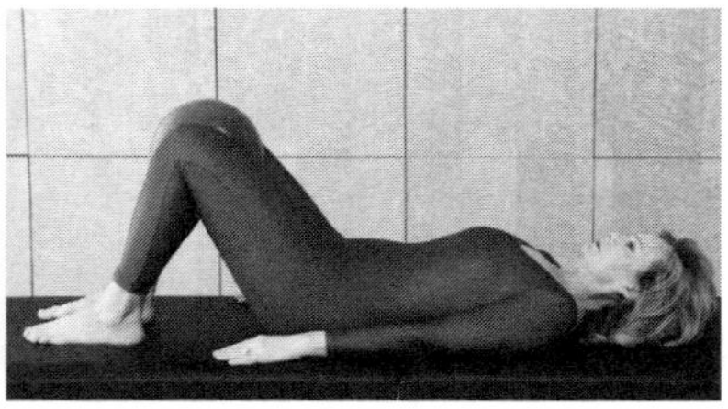

Adductor squeeze
Page 52

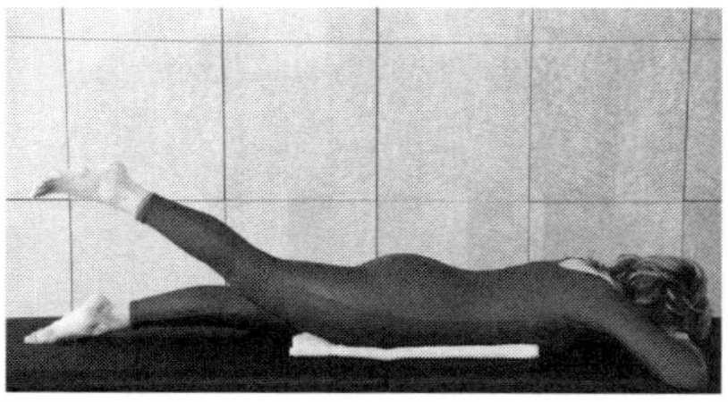

Prone leg lift, version one
Page 56

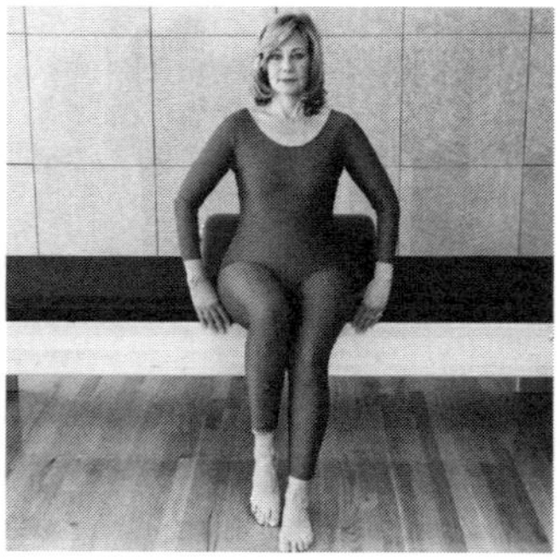

Sitting bent-knee lift, version one
Page 59

Pilates Exercises

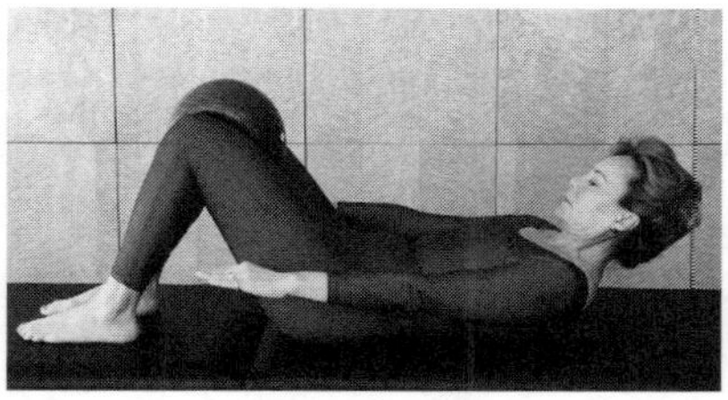

Hundred
Page 69

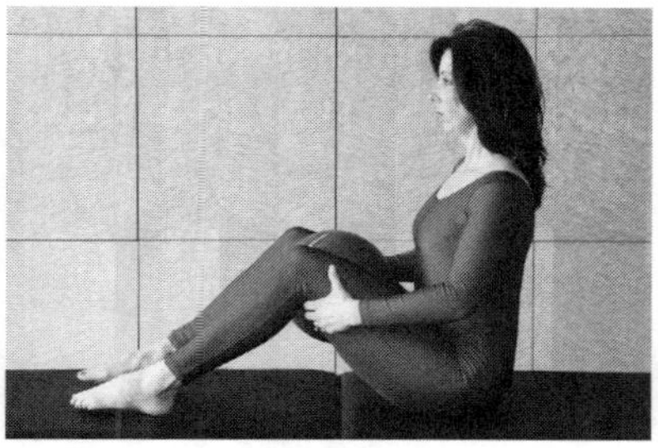

Half roll-down
Page 70

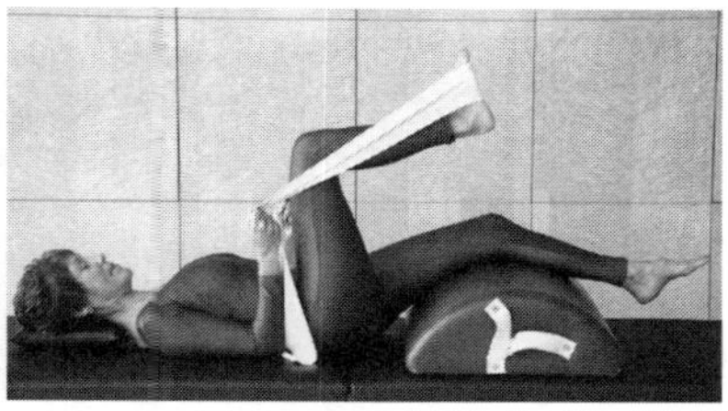

Single-leg circle
Page 80

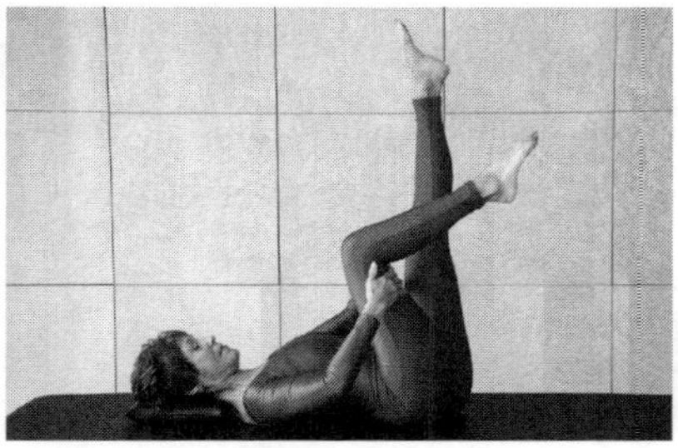

Single-leg stretch
Page 83

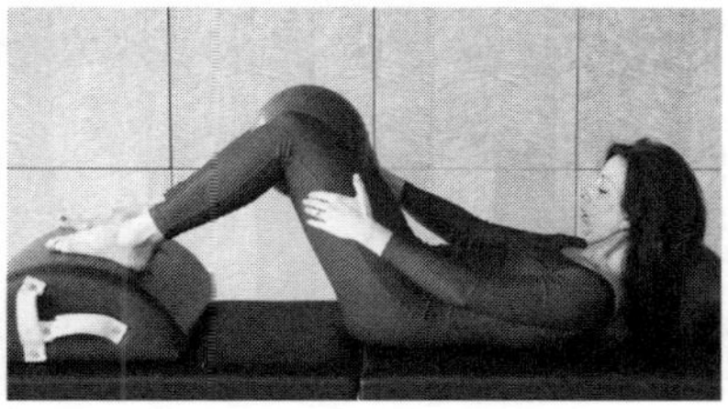

Double-leg stretch
Page 87

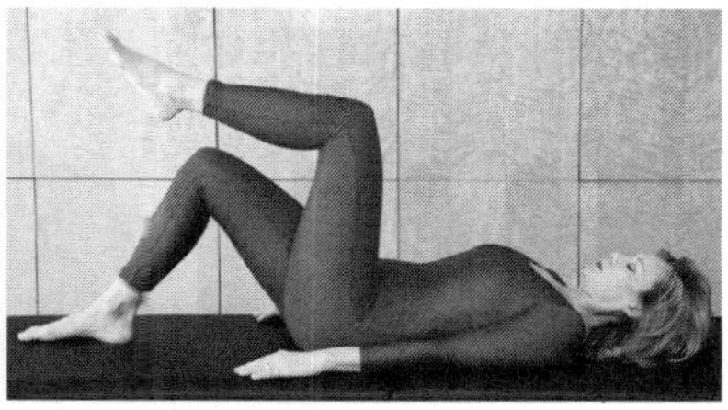

Toe tap, version one
Page 46

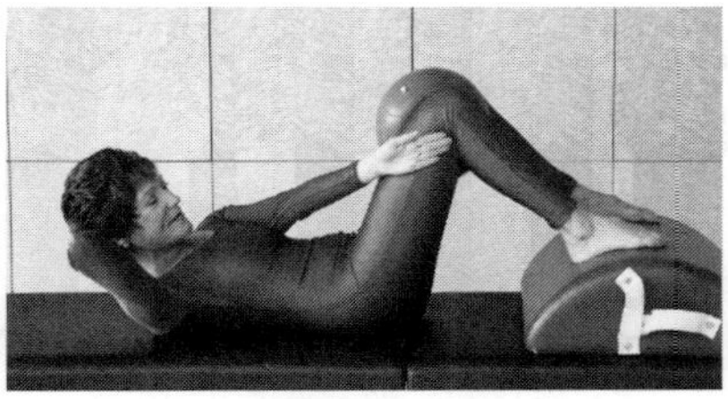

Crisscross
Page 98

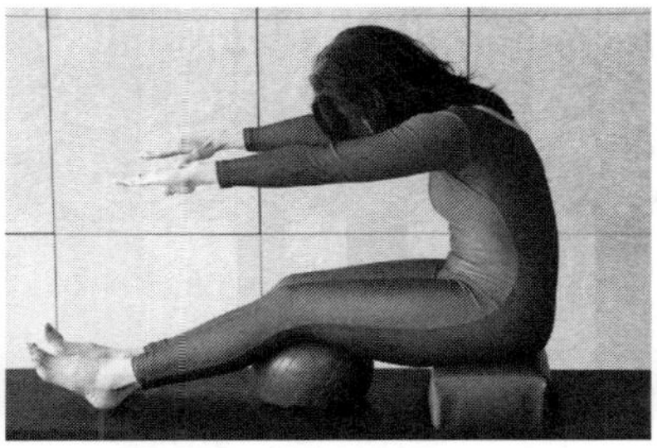

Spine stretch forward
Page 105

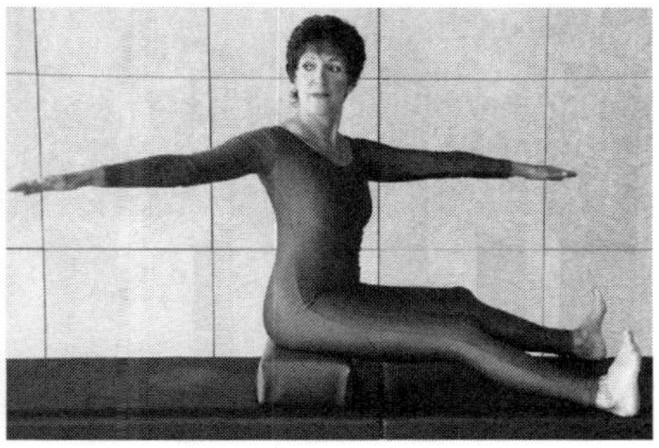

Saw
Page 107

(continued)

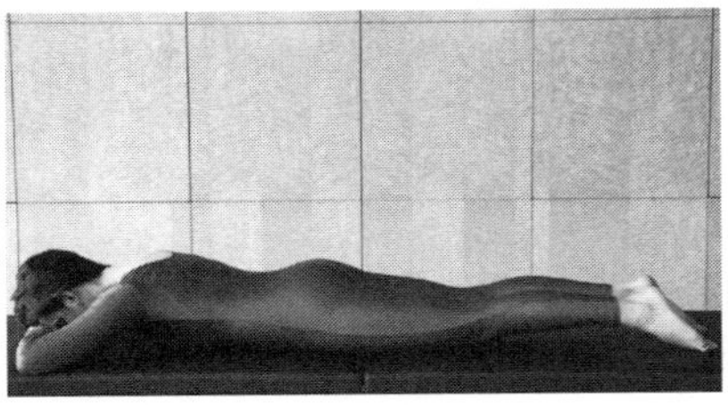

Swan prep
Page 110

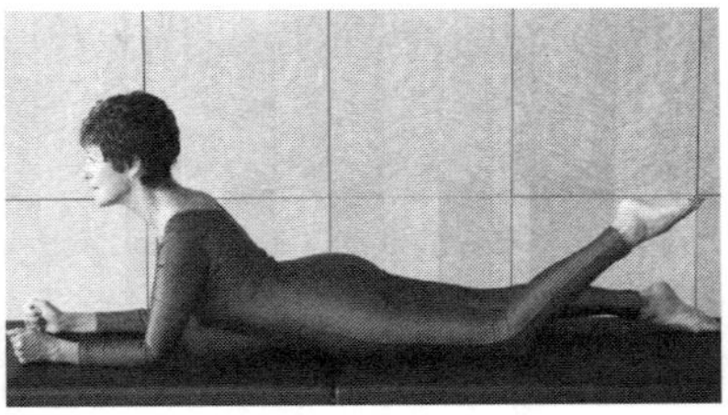

Single-leg kick
Page 113

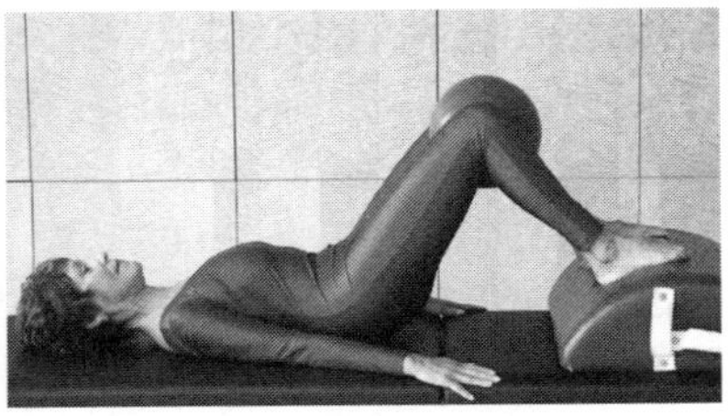

Shoulder bridge (modified)
Page 117

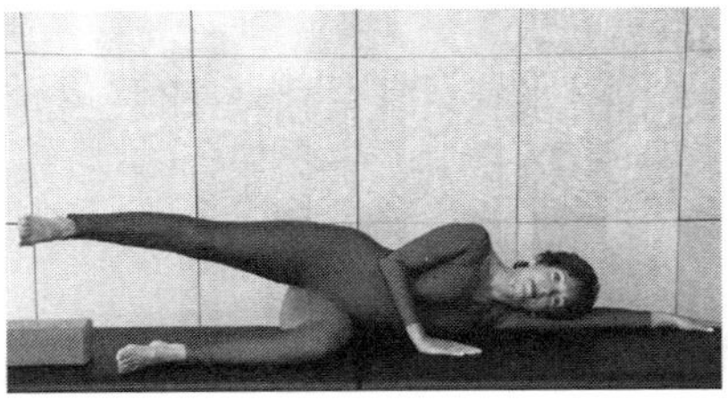

SKS, up and down
Page 270

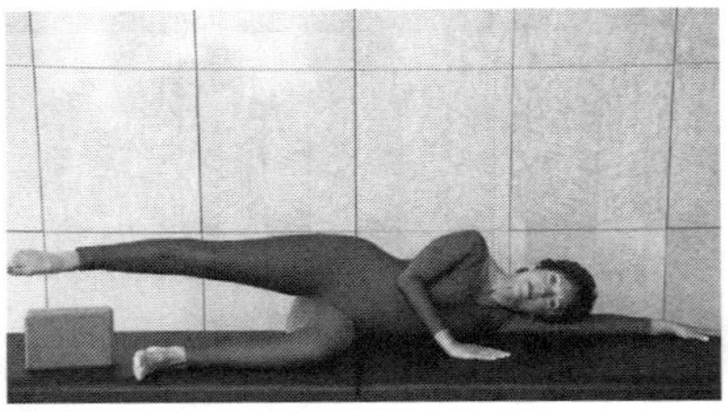

SKS, little circle
Page 278

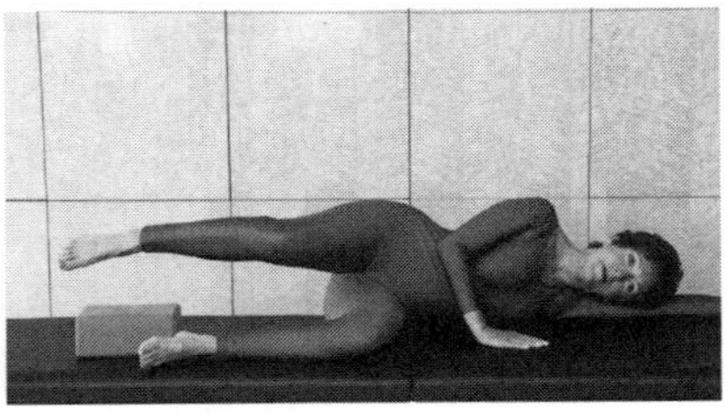

SKS, front and back
Page 274

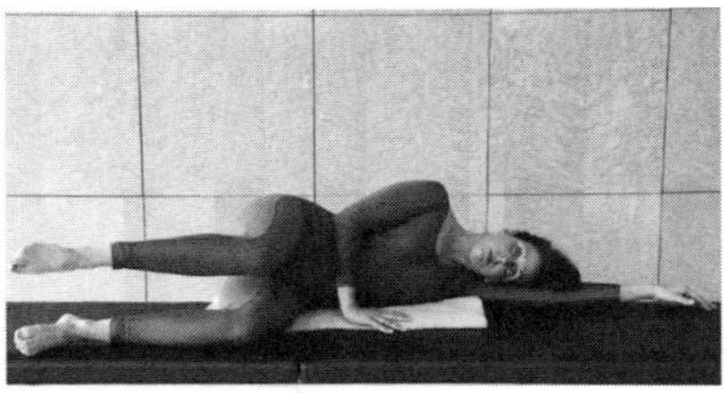

SKS, 90° bent-knee lift and lower
Page 308

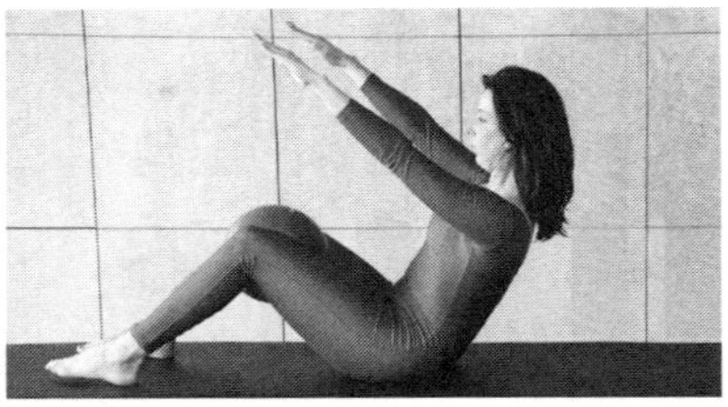

Teaser prep 1
Page 121

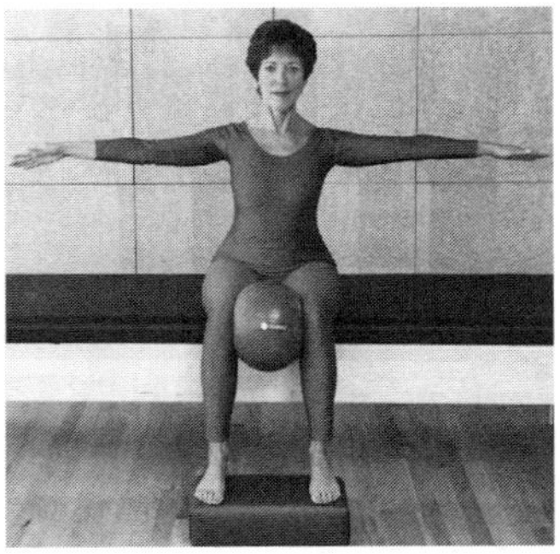

Side stretch
Page 129

Total Knee Replacement (Arthroplasty): Program Sequence for 3 Months Postop

Case scenario continued: A 60-year-old male with osteoarthritis of the right knee walked with pain and used a cane for assistance previous to TKA. He finished an 8-week, 3-times-a-week, preoperative Pilates routine in preparation for the TKA. He has been performing Pilates exercises since 6 weeks postop and is now ready to lessen restrictions and start a program for 3 to 6 months postop.

Exercises: 31

Approximate time: 50 minutes

Pre-Pilates Exercises

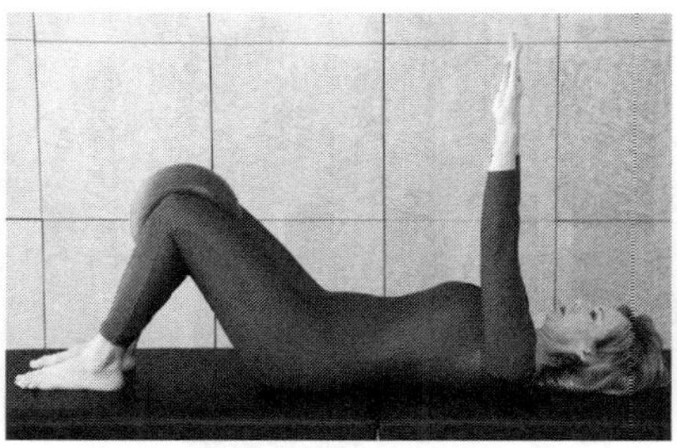

Abdominal prep
Page 48

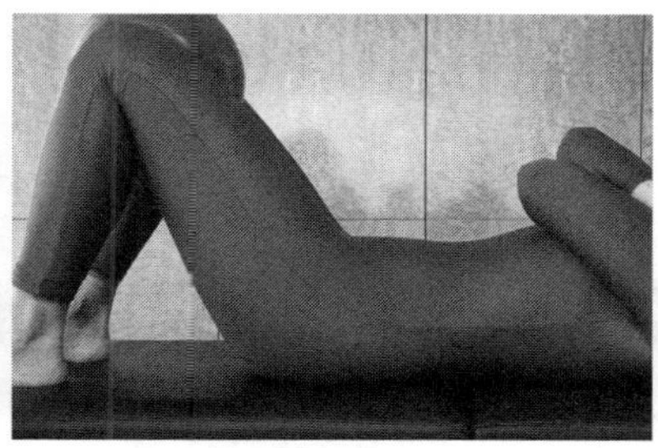

Pelvic curl
Page 45

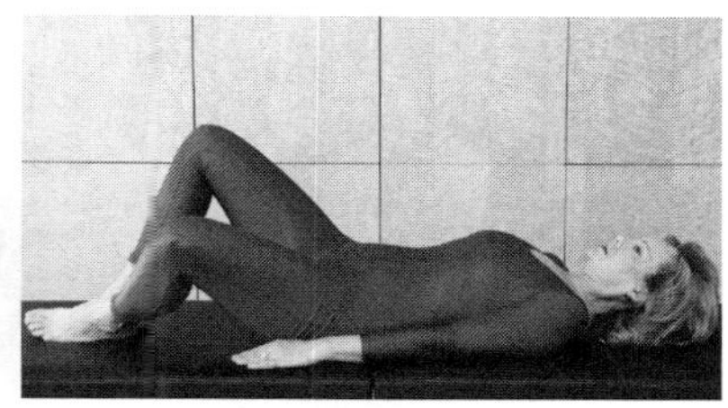

Knee fold
Page 50

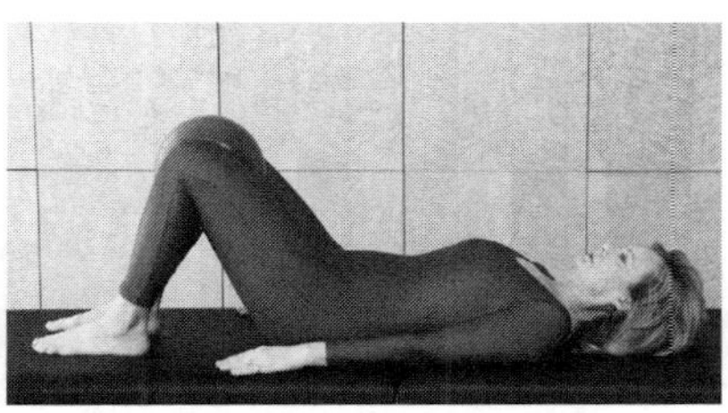

Adductor squeeze
Page 52

(continued)

Pilates Exercises

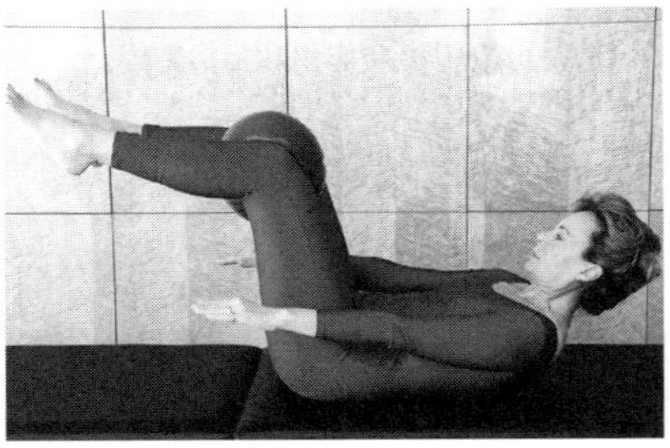

Hundred
Page 135

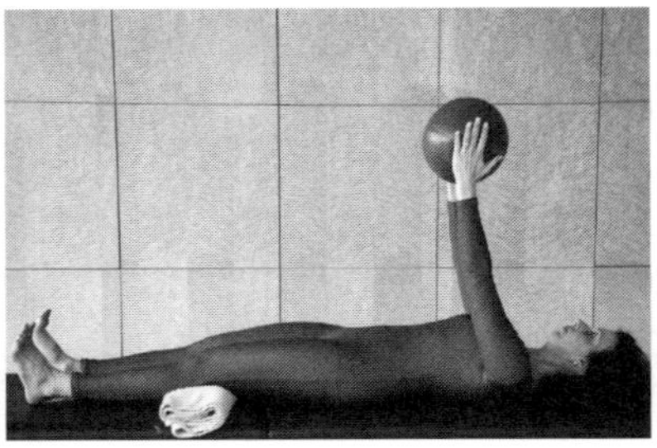

Roll-up
Page 145

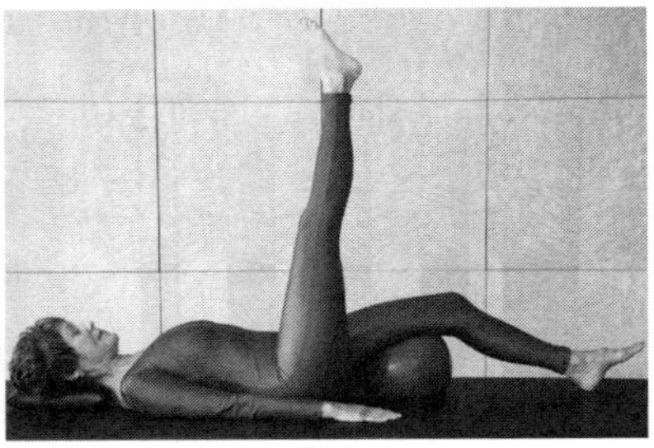

Single-leg circle
Page 152

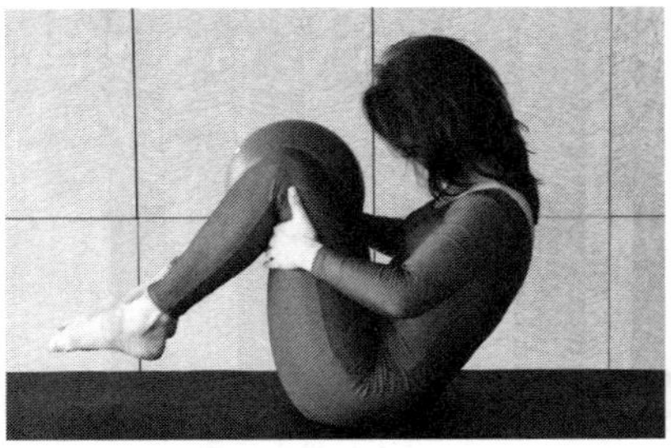

Rolling like a ball
Page 156

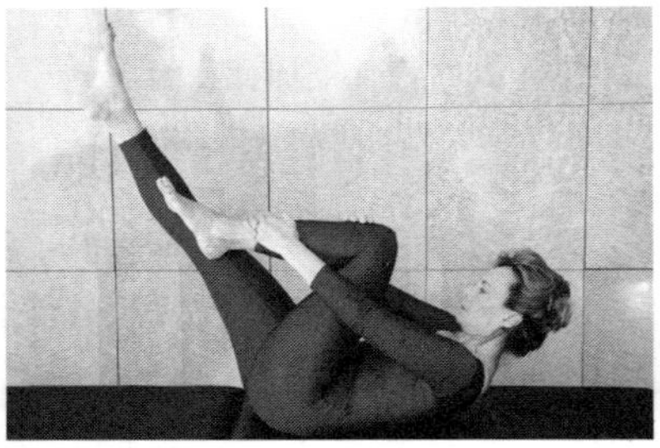

Single-leg stretch
Page 160

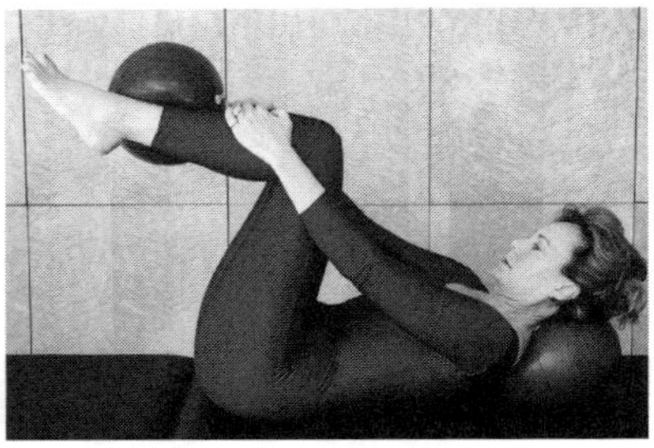

Double-leg stretch
Page 165

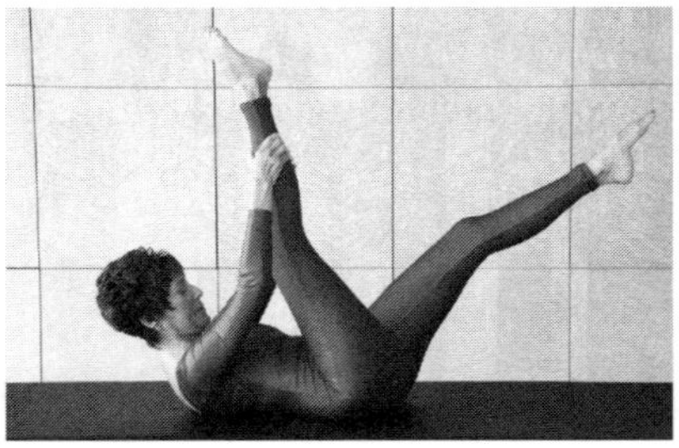

Scissors
Page 168

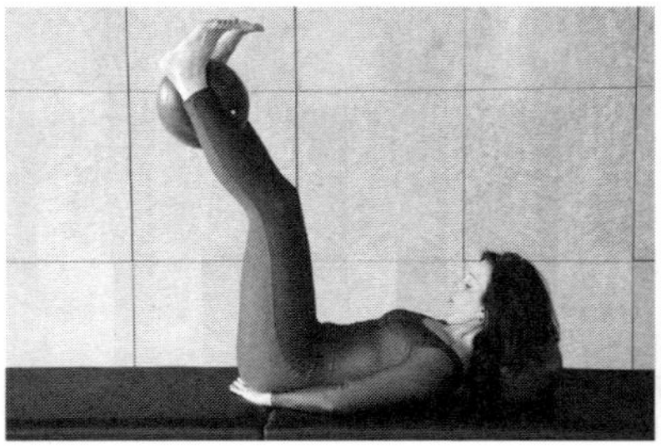

Lower lift
Page 172

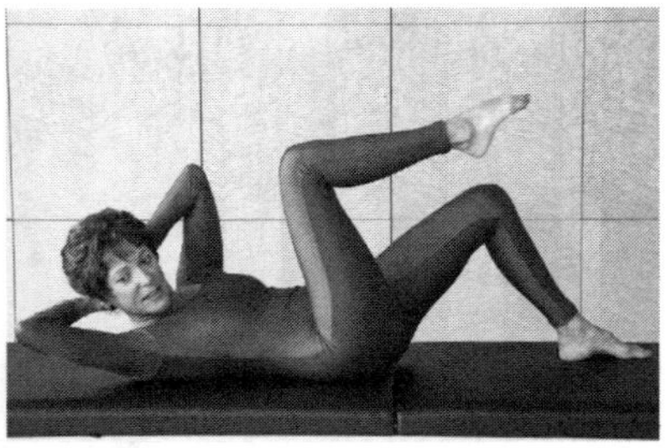

Crisscross, 6 weeks
to 3 months postop version
Page 102

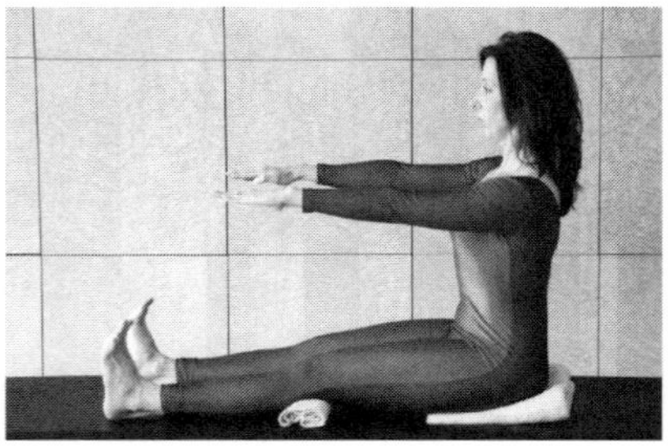

Spine stretch forward
Page 177

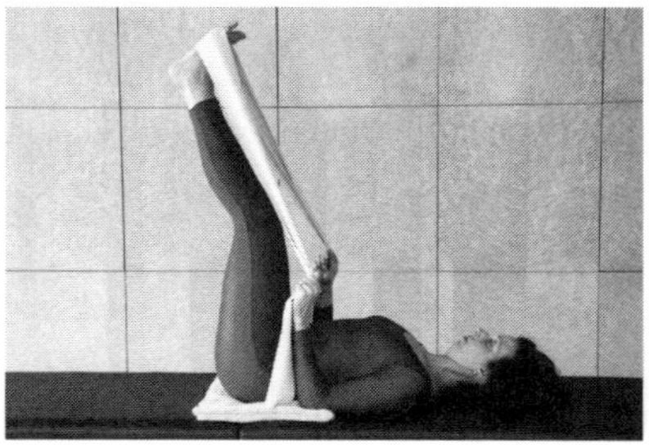

Corkscrew
Page 183

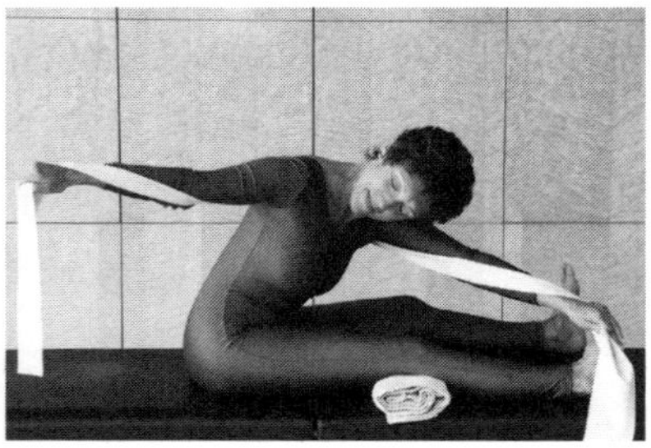

Saw
Page 189

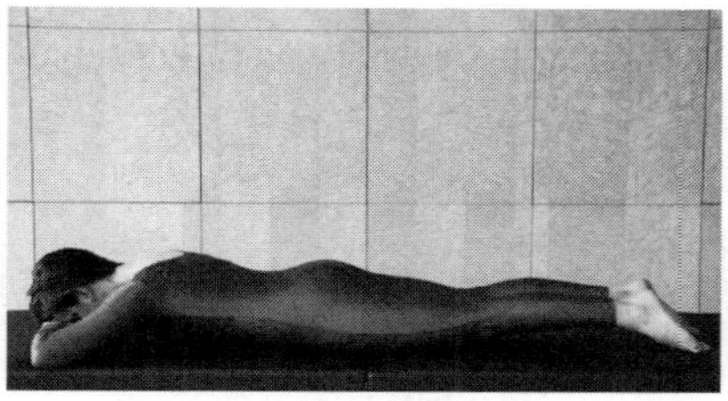

Swan prep
Page 191

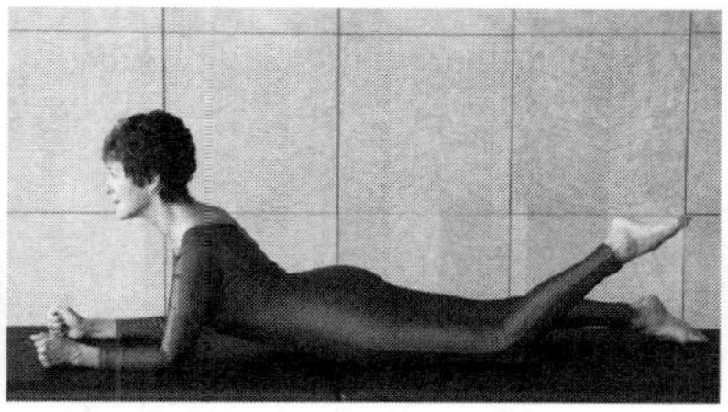

Single-leg kick, 6 weeks to 3 months postop version
Page 113

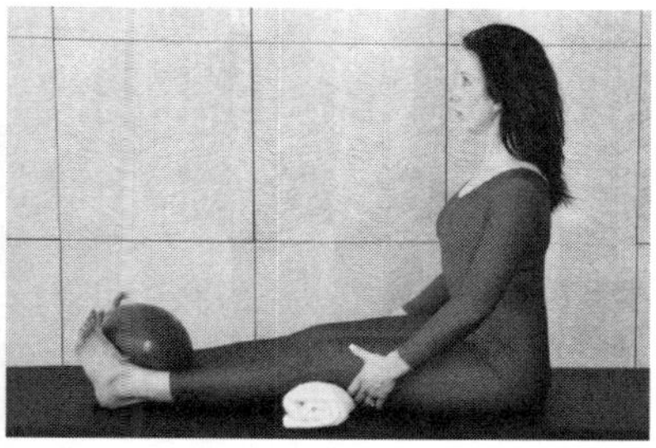

Neck pull (modified)
Page 204

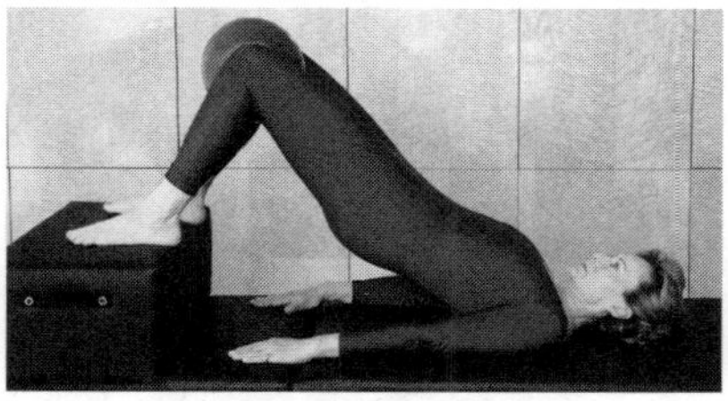

Shoulder bridge (modified)
Page 119

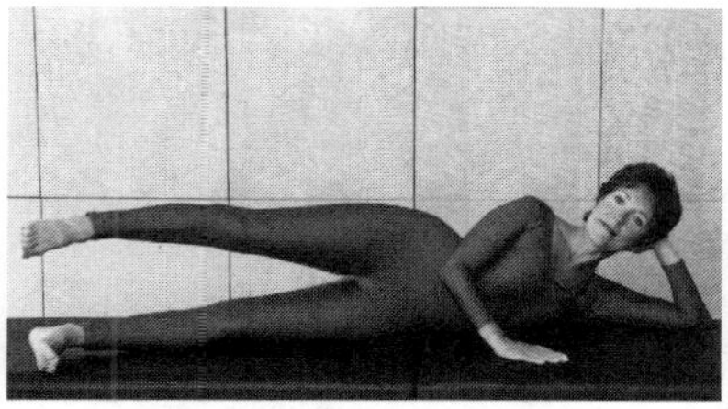

SKS, up and down
Page 272

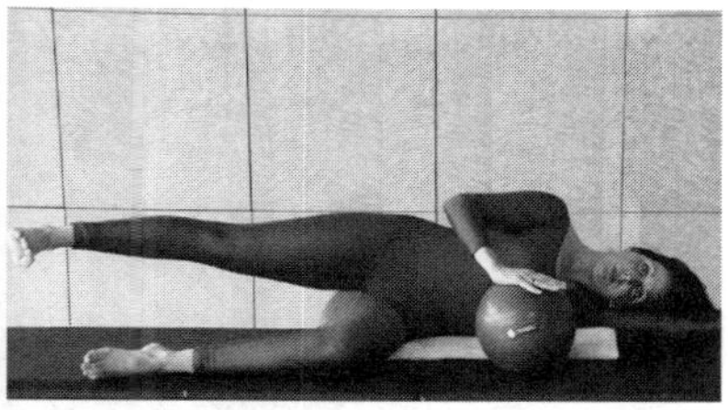

SKS, front and back
Page 277

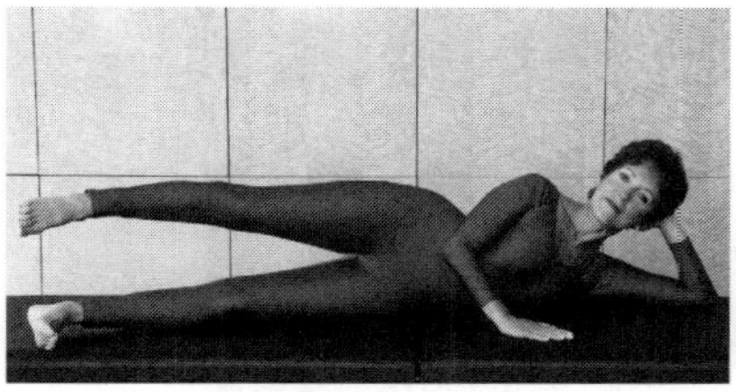

SKS, little circle
Page 279

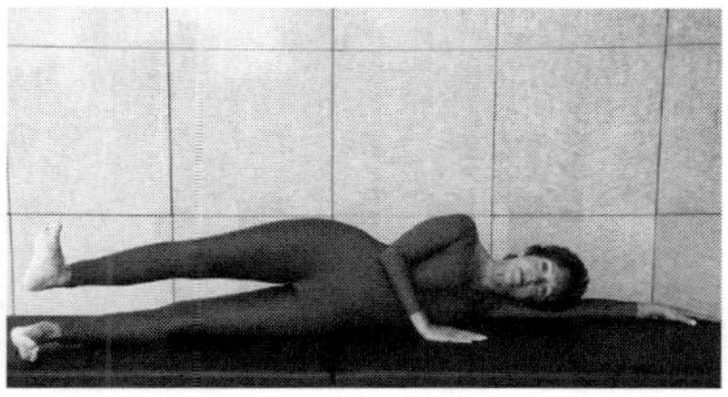

SKS, internal and external rotation, 6 weeks to 3 months postop version
Page 284

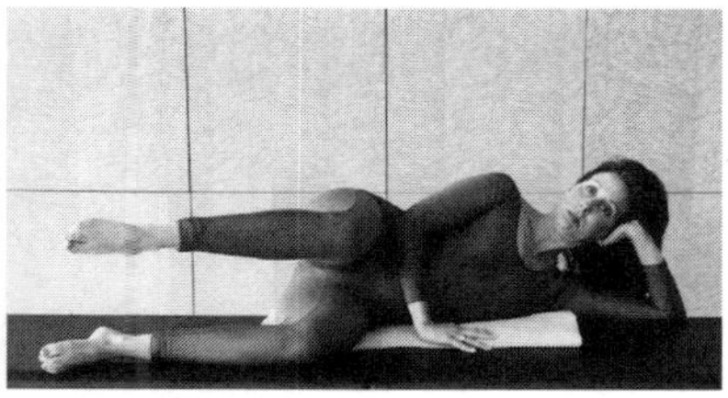

SKS, 90° bent-knee lift and lower
Page 310

(continued)

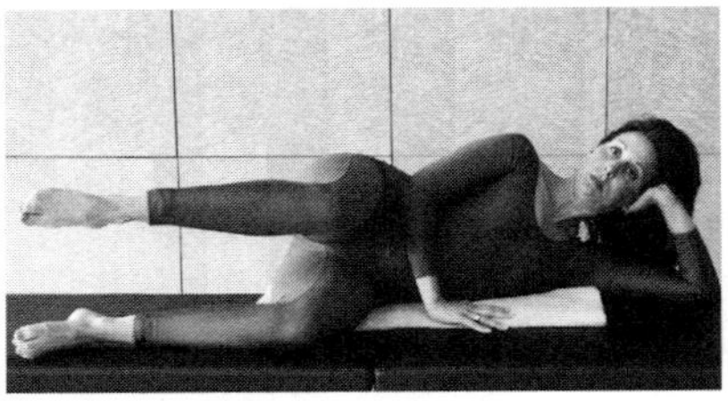

SKS, 90° bent-knee circle
Page 311

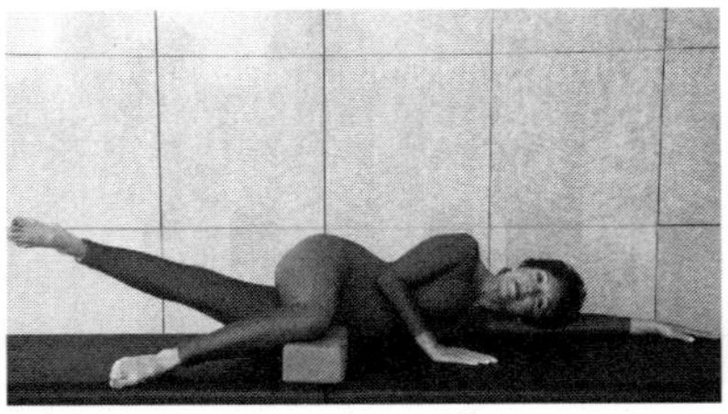

SKS, inner-thigh lift
Page 298

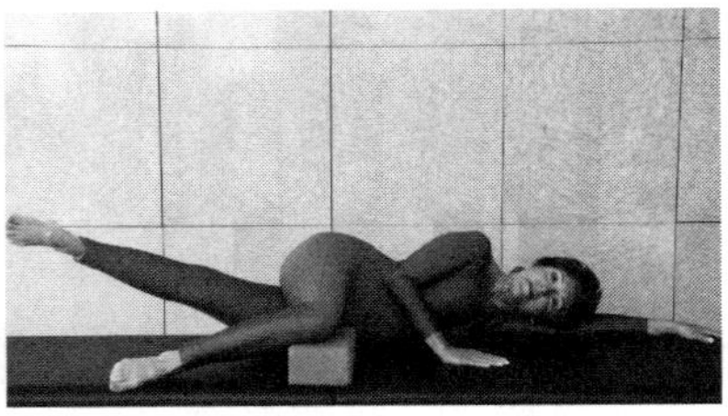

SKS, inner-thigh circle
Page 299

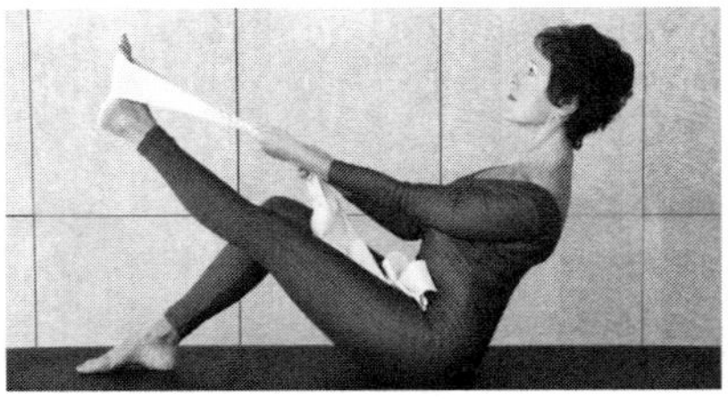

Teaser prep 2
Page 221

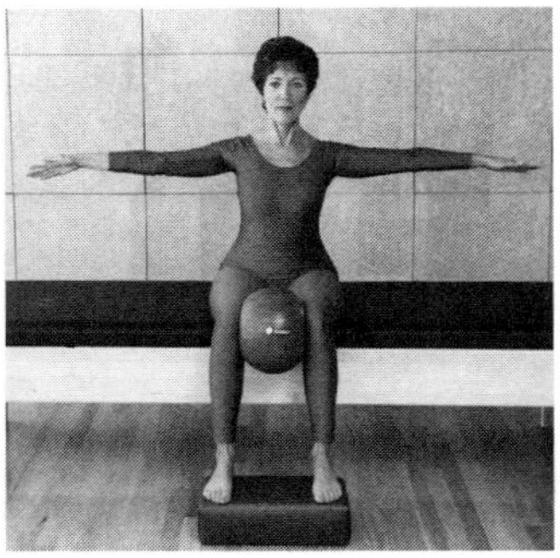

Side stretch
Page 129

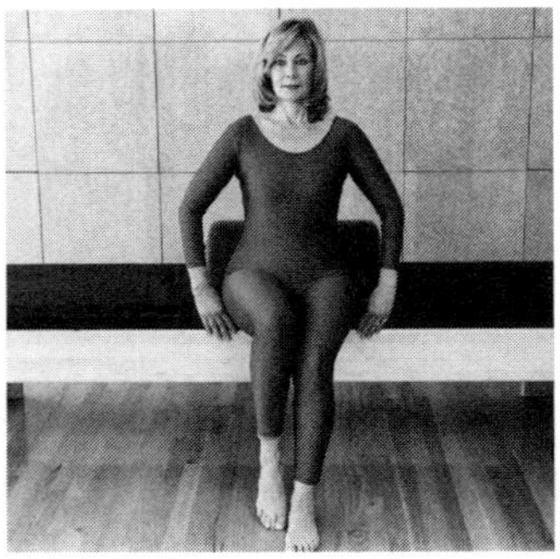

Sitting bent-knee lift,
version one
Page 59

Total Knee Replacement (Arthroplasty): Program Sequence for 6 Months Postop

Case scenario continued: A 60-year-old male with osteoarthritis of the right knee walked with pain and used a cane for assistance previous to TKA. He finished an 8-week pre-operative Pilates routine in preparation for the TKA. He has been performing Pilates mat exercises since 6 weeks postop and is now ready to work toward the ideal movements and begin a program for 6 months postop and beyond.

Exercises: 34

Approximate time: 50 minutes

Pre-Pilates Exercises

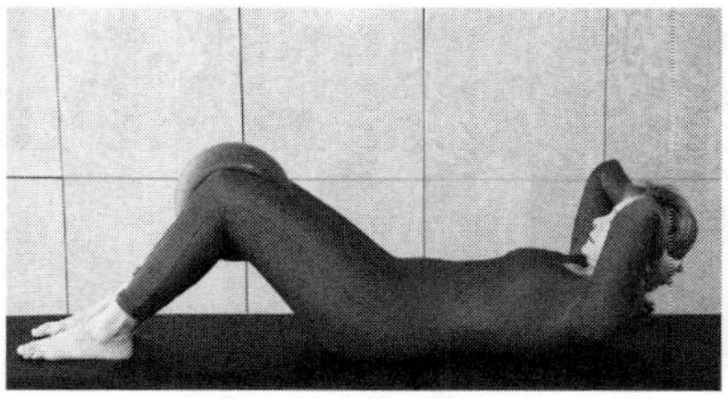

Abdominal prep
Page 48

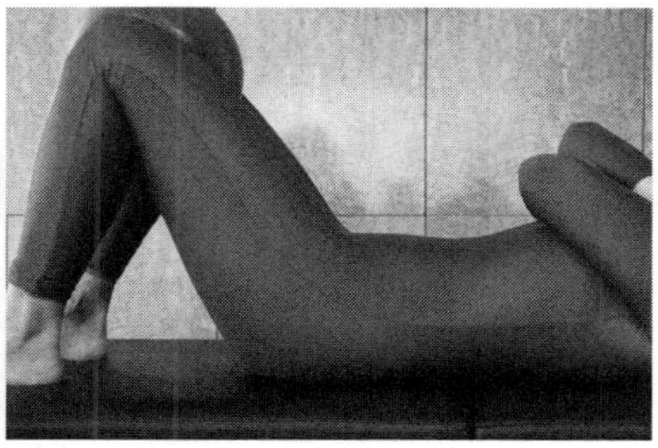

Pelvic curl
Page 45

Pilates Exercises

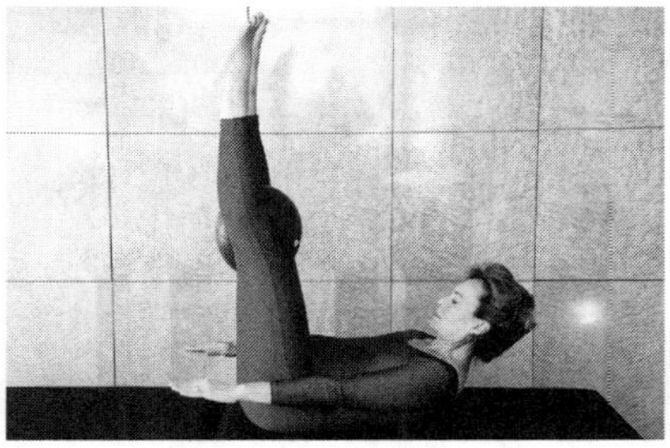

Hundred
Page 137

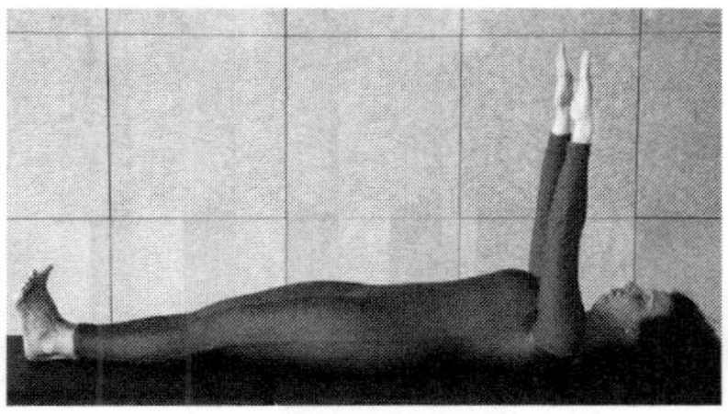

Roll-up
Page 147

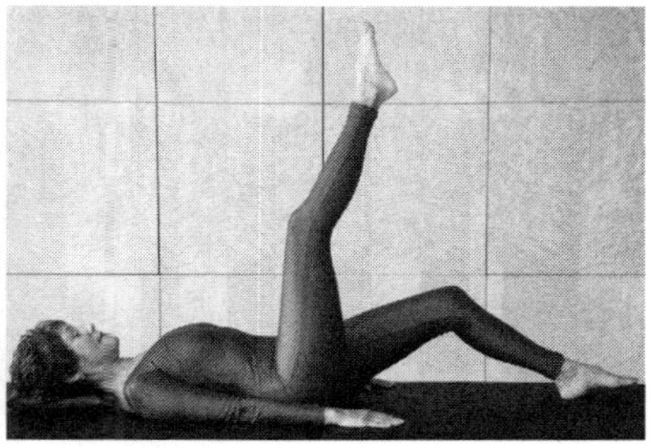

Single-leg circle, 3 to 6 months postop version
Page 150

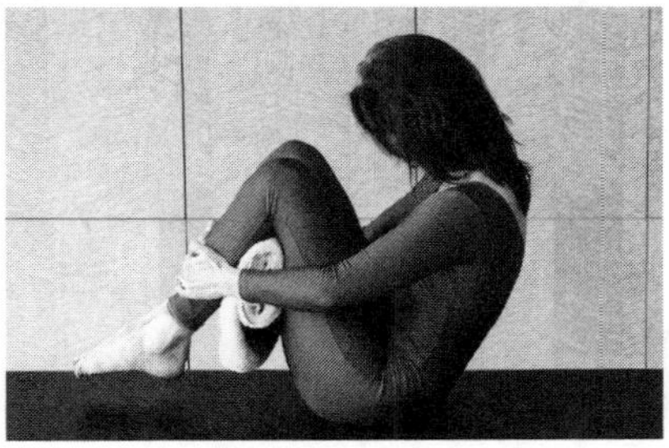

Rolling like a ball
Page 158

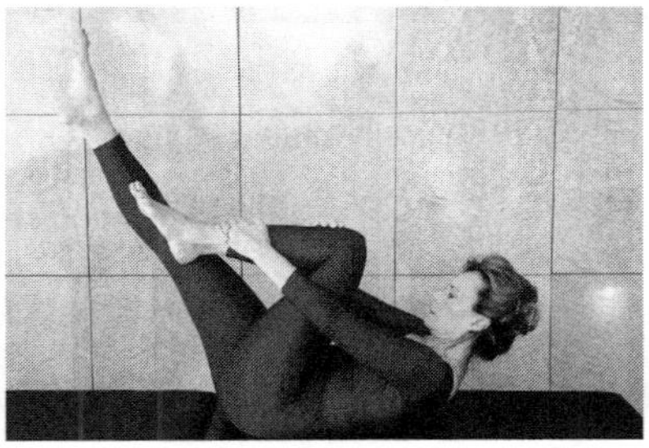

Single-leg stretch
Page 160

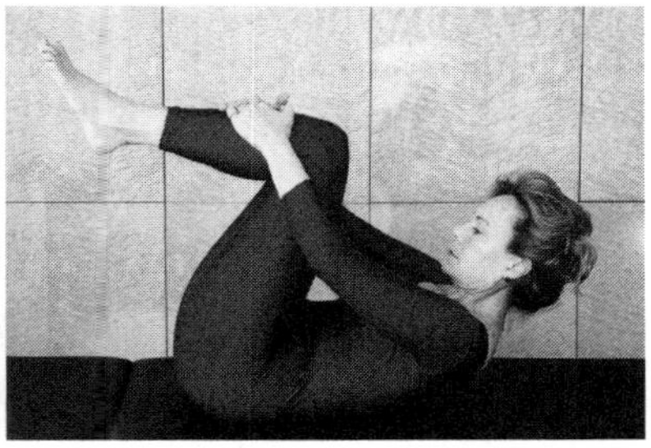

Double-leg stretch
Page 166

(continued)

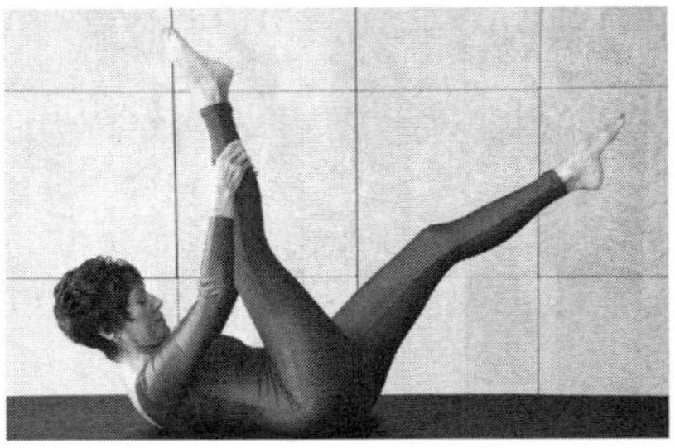

Scissors
Page 168

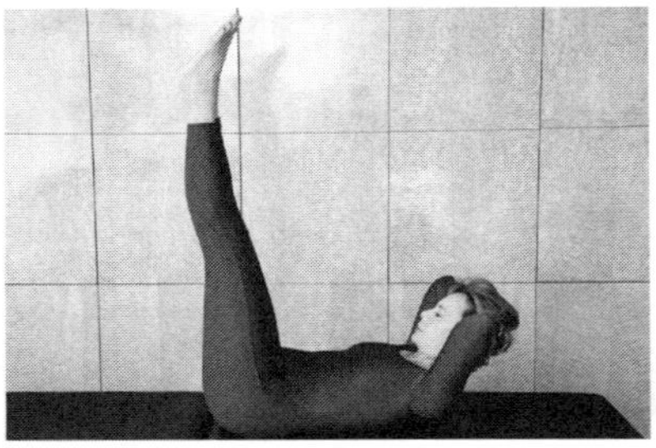

Lower lift
Page 171

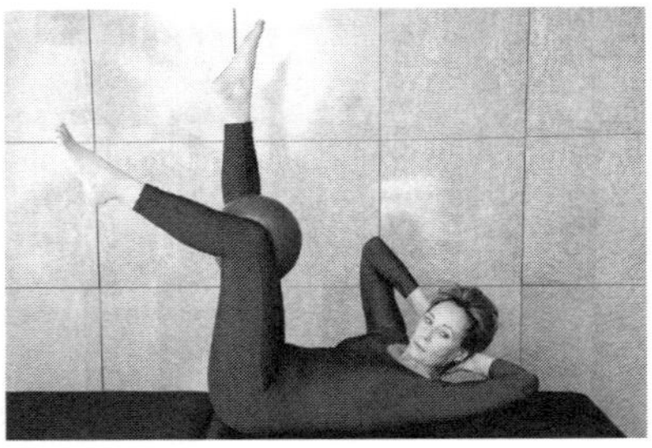

Crisscross
Page 175

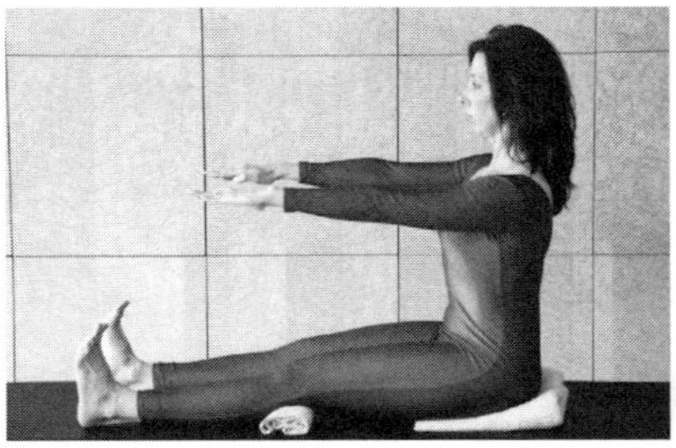

Spine stretch forward,
3 to 6 months postop version
Page 177

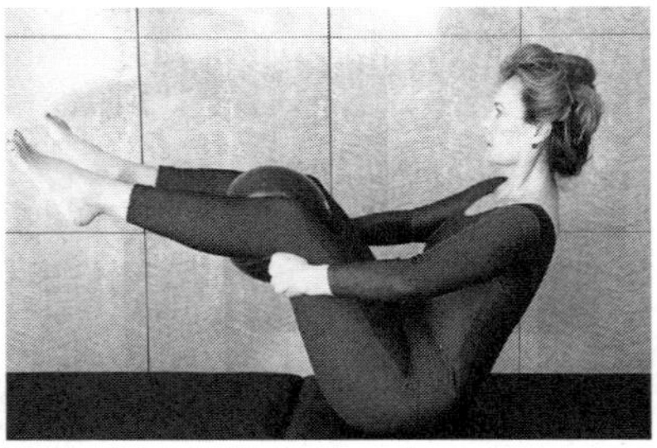

Open-leg rocker
Page 179

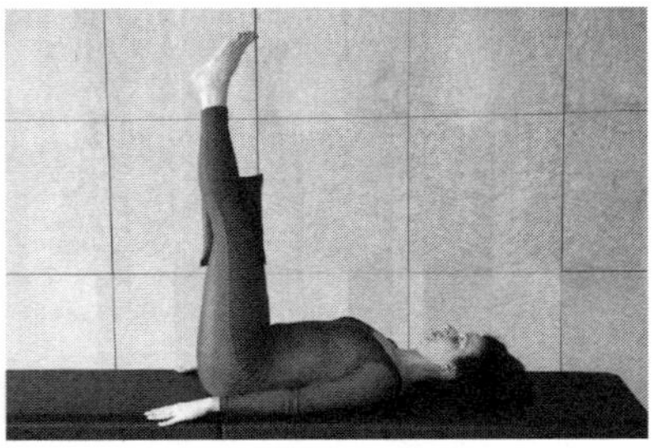

Corkscrew
Page 183

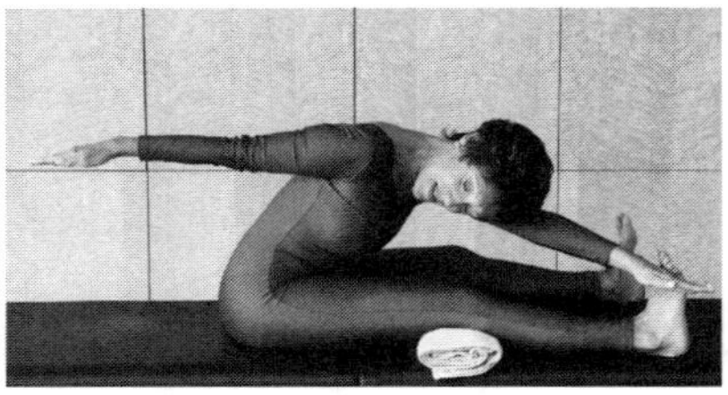

Saw
Page 189

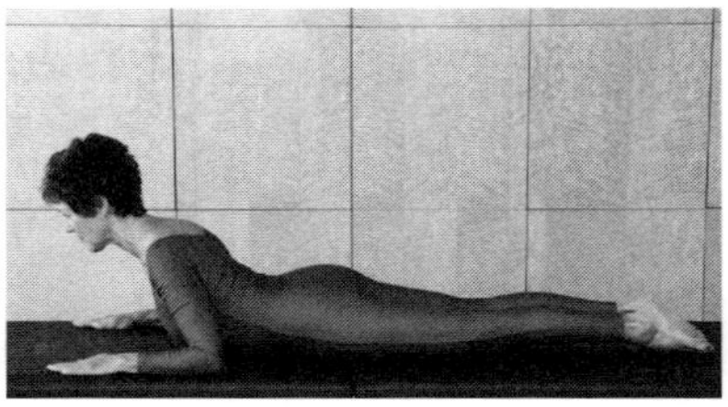

Swan
Page 195

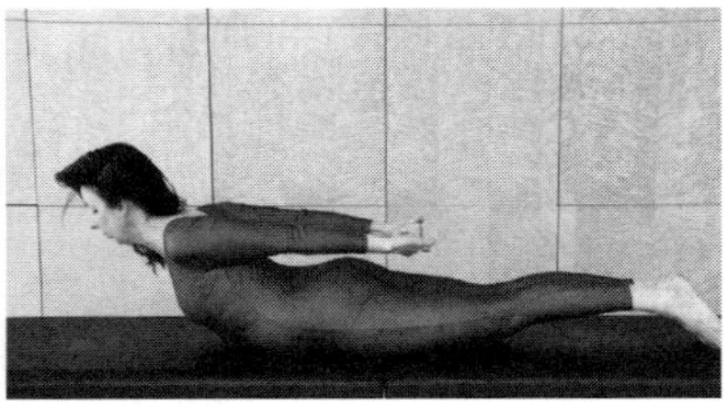

Double-leg kick
Page 198

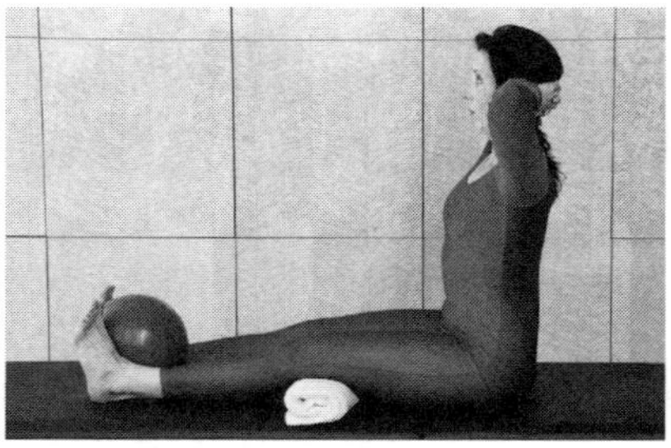

Neck pull
Page 207

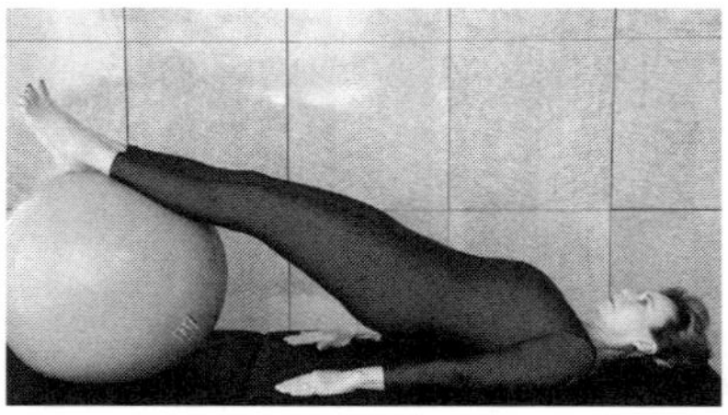

Shoulder bridge
Page 214

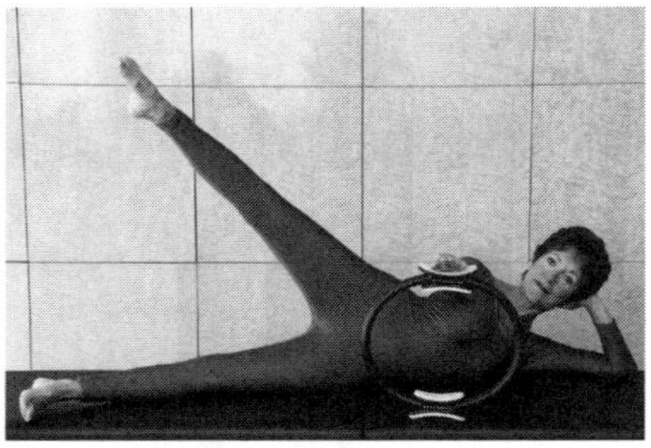

SKS, up and down
Page 273

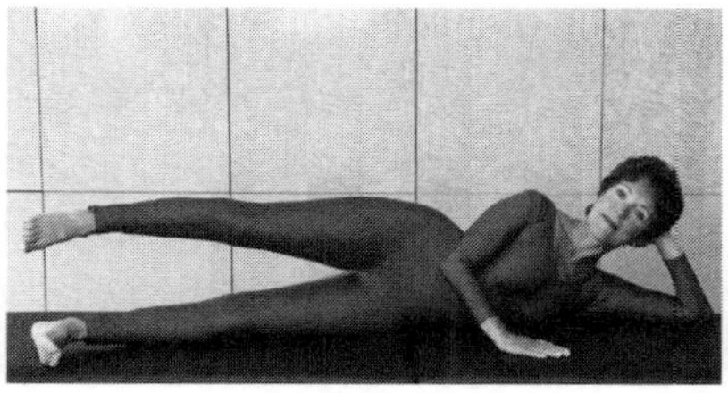

SKS, little circle
Page 279

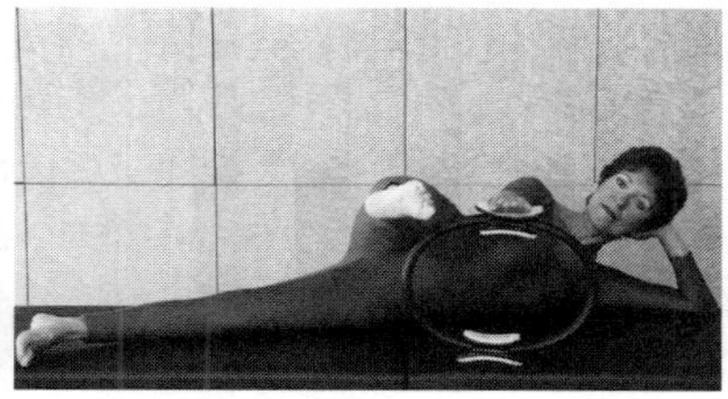

SKS, D-circle
Page 281

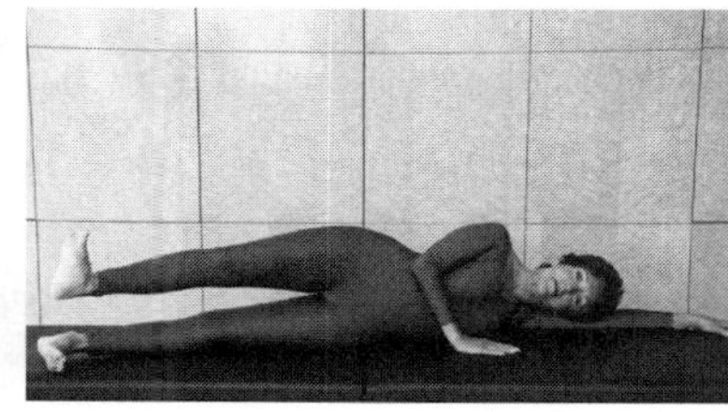

SKS, internal and external rotation, slightly flexed knee
Page 285

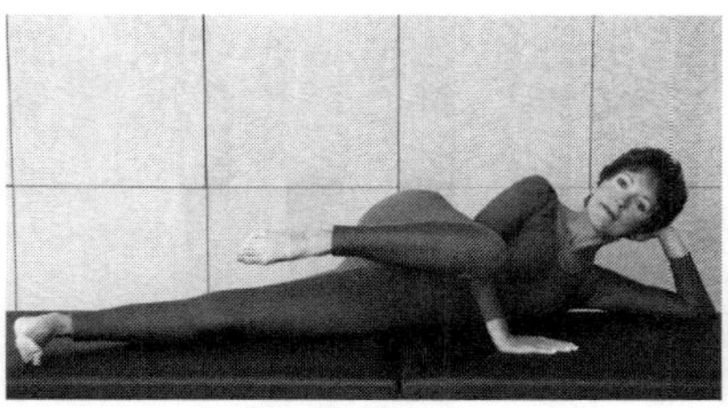

SKS, bicycle
Page 287

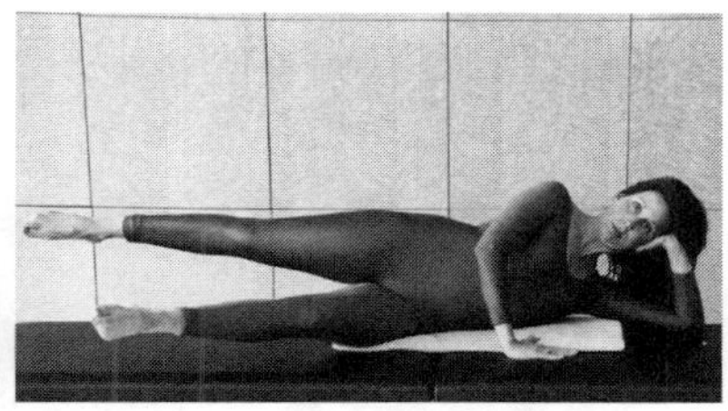

SKS, scissors
Page 289

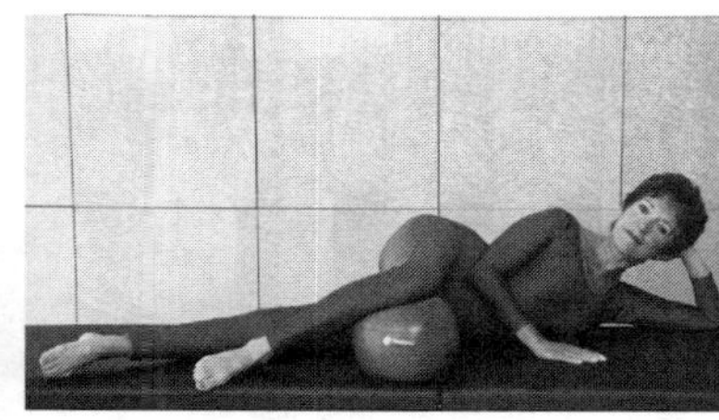

SKS, inner-thigh lift
Page 300

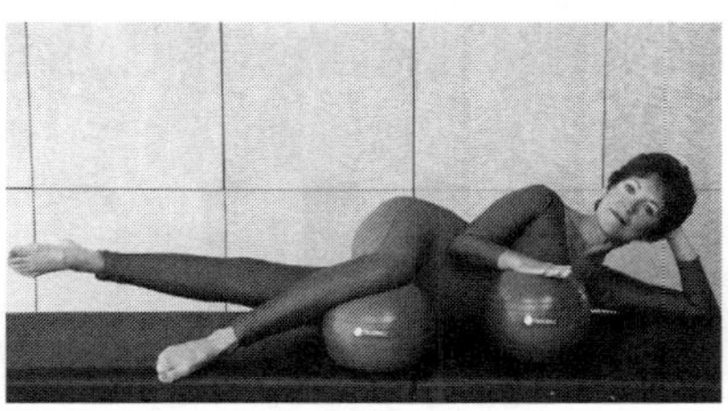

SKS, inner-thigh circle
Page 302

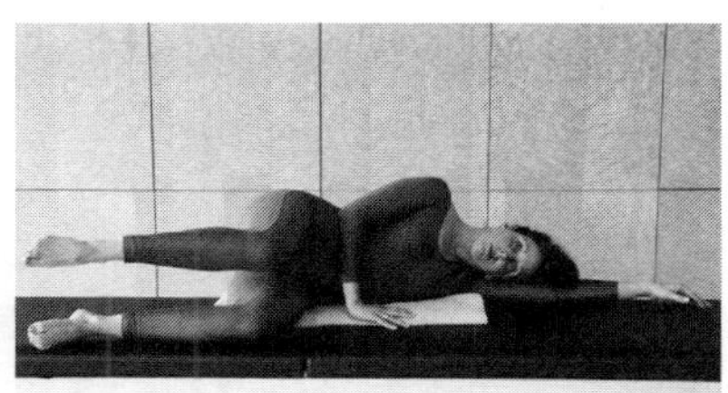

SKS, 90° bent-knee lift and lower
Page 310

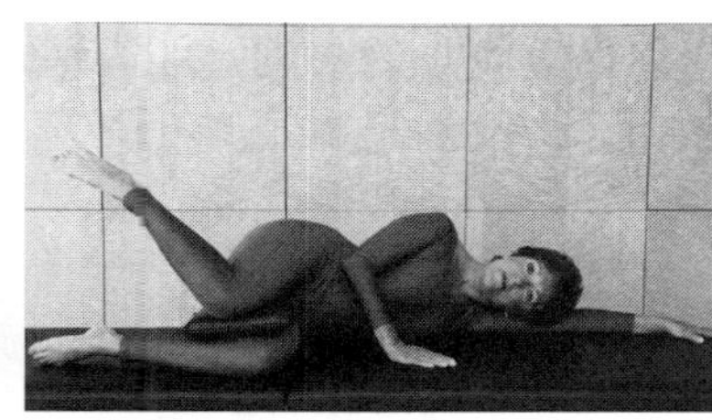

SKS, 90° bent-knee rotation
Page 316

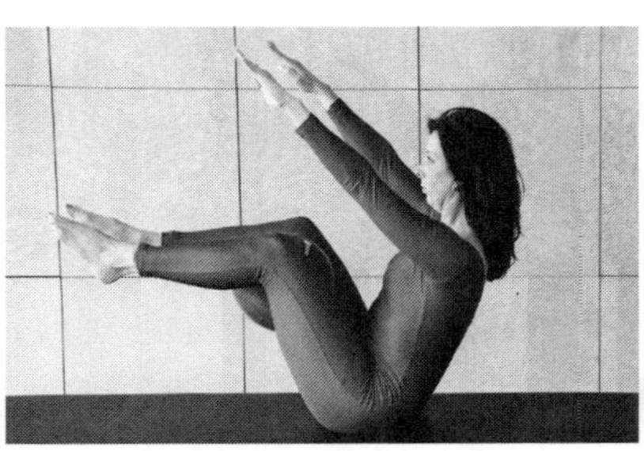

Teaser 1
Page 223

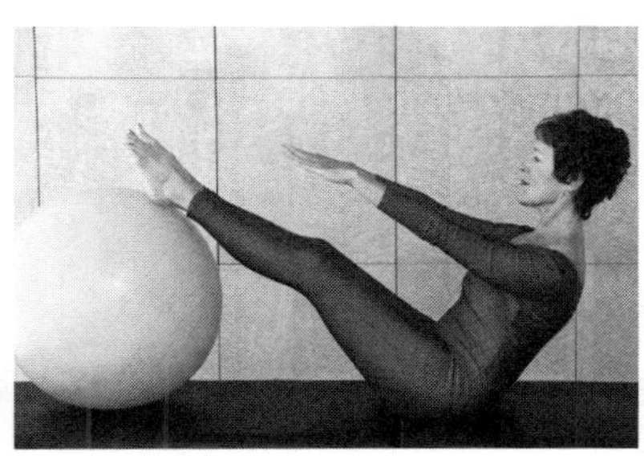

Teaser 2
Page 228

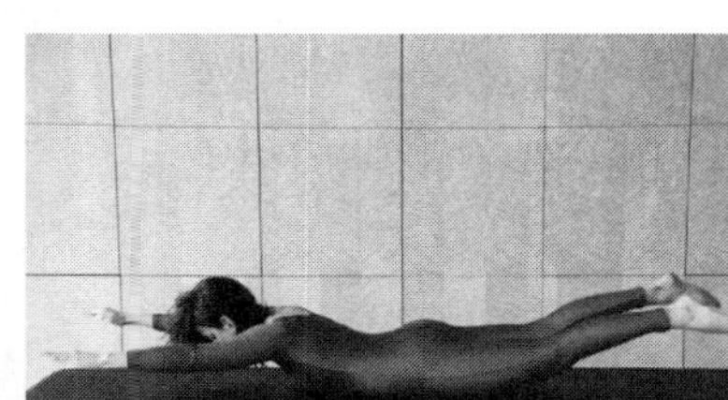

Swimming
Page 239

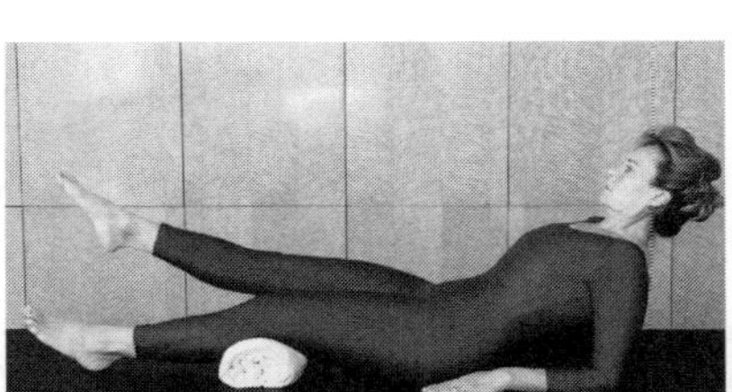

Leg pull (modified)
Page 243

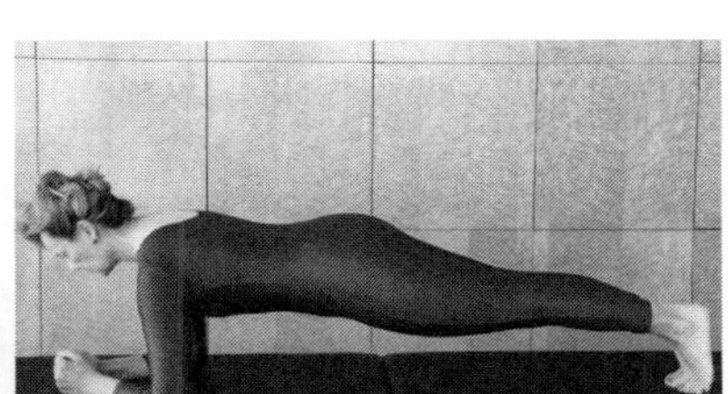

Serratus push-up (modified)
Page 251

Trochanteric Bursitis of the Hip

Case scenario: A 58-year-old female with trochanteric bursitis of the left hip has a history of exercising 3 times per week doing cardiorespiratory and strength training. She took a Pilates mat class on a weekly basis for about 1 year, but it has been at least 6 months since she attended a class at her local gym. She has decided to begin a Pilates program of exercise.

Exercises: 30

Approximate time: 50 minutes

Pre-Pilates Exercises

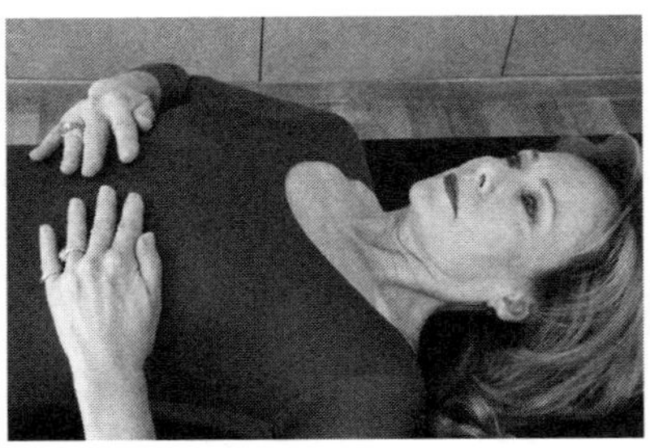

Breathing
Page 39

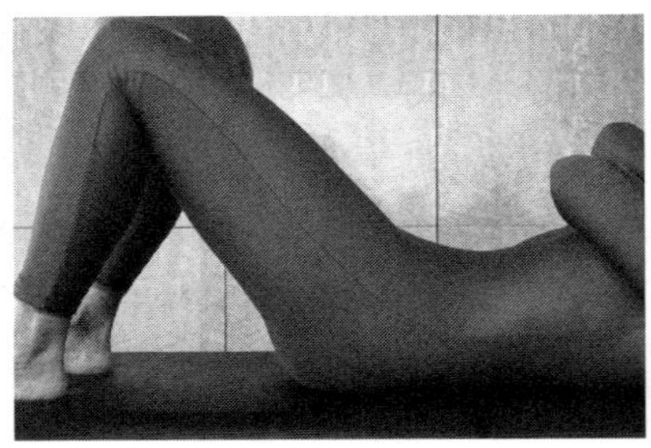

Pelvic curl
Page 45

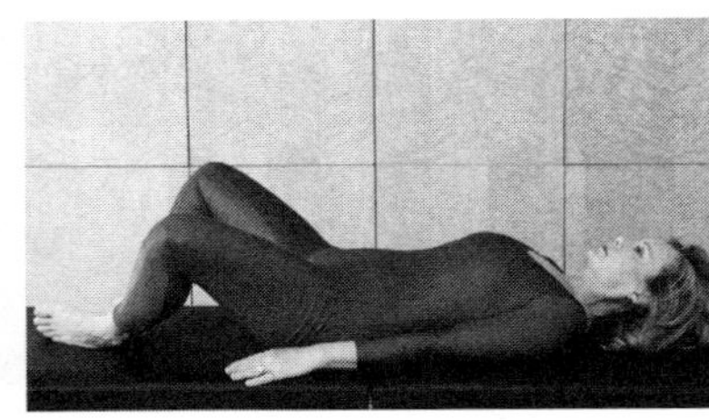

Knee fold
Page 50

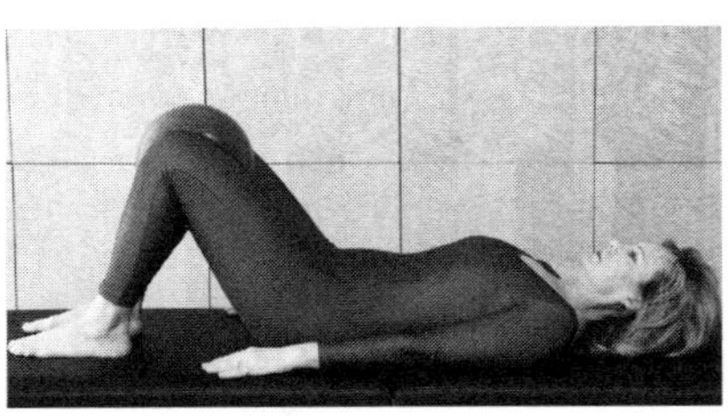

Adductor squeeze
Page 52

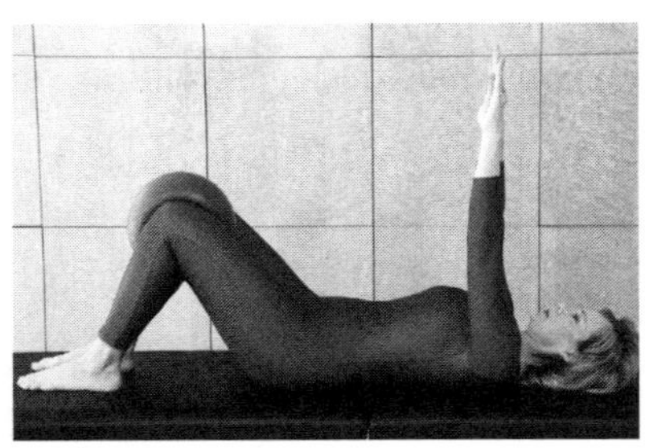

Abdominal prep
Page 48

Pilates Exercises

Note that for the SKS exercises, you will want to use a towel or padding under the hip.

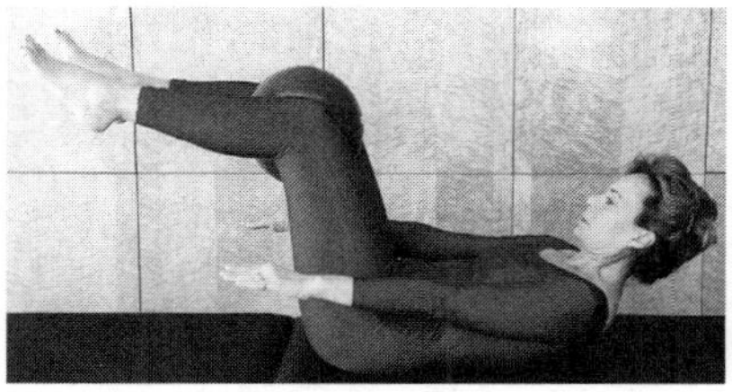
Hundred
Page 135

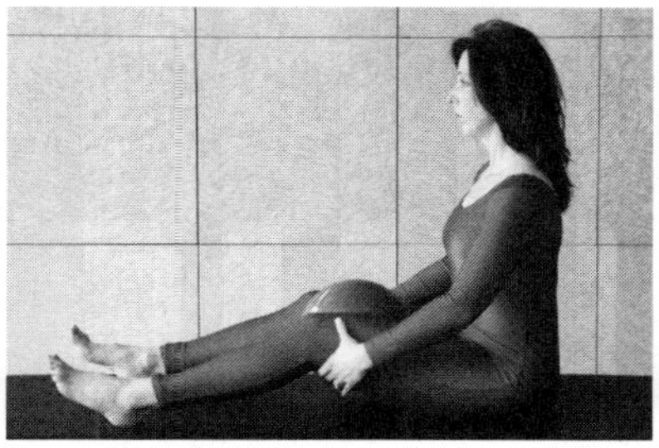
Half roll-up
Page 77

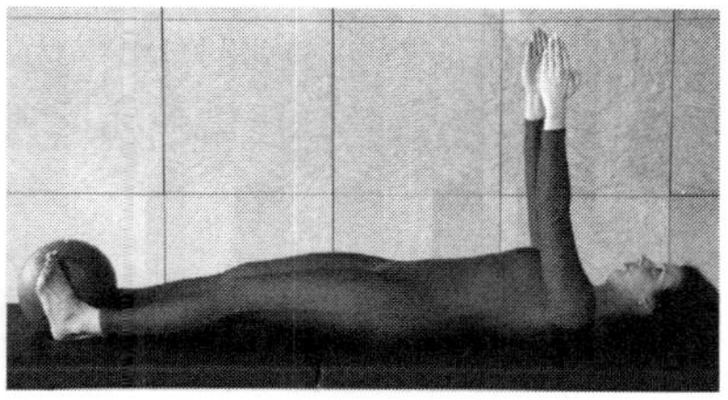
Roll-up
Page 143

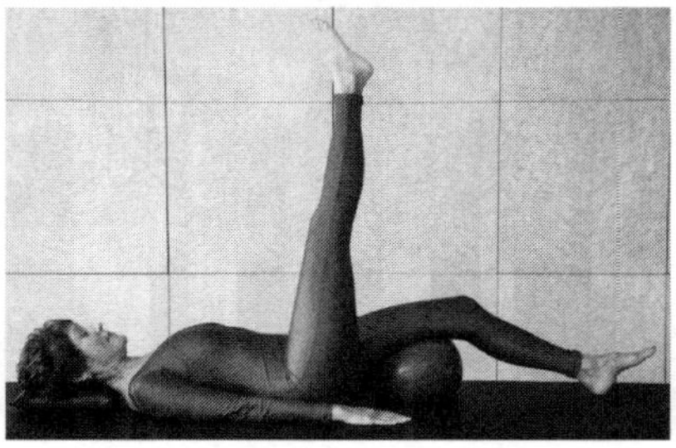
Single-leg circle
Page 152

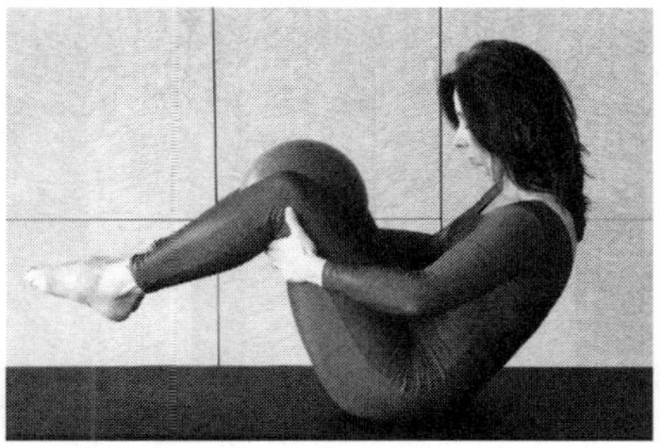
Rolling like a ball
Page 159

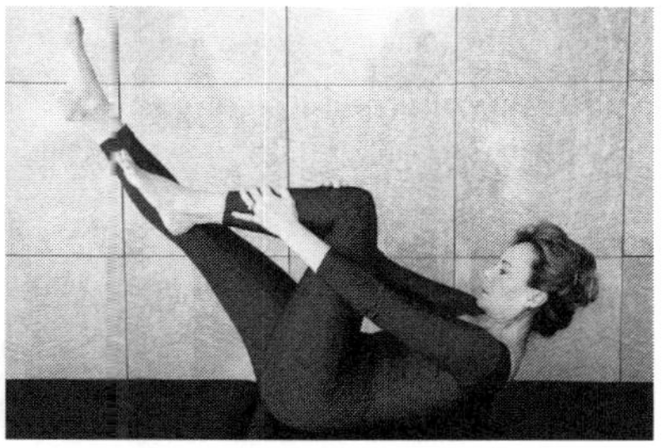
Single-leg stretch
Page 160

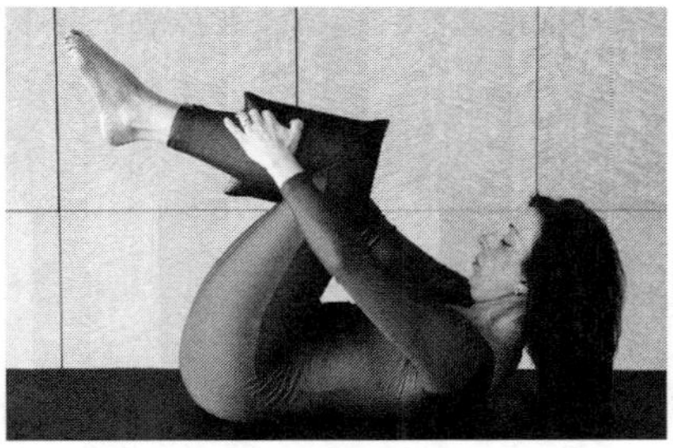
Double-leg stretch
Page 163

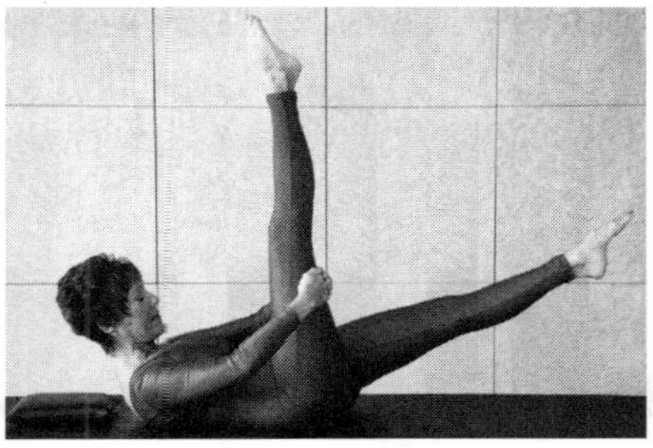
Scissors
Page 90

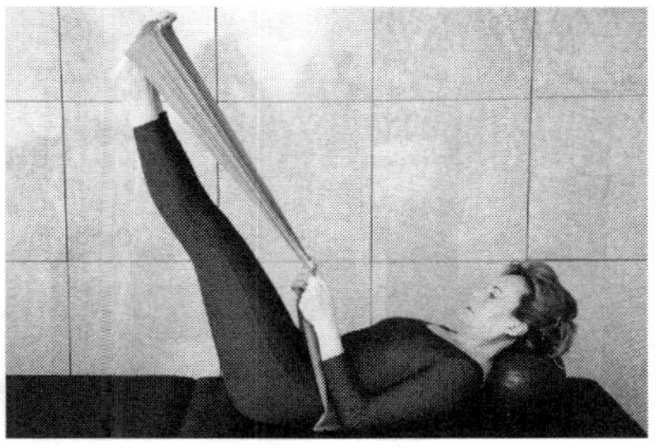
Lower lift
Page 172

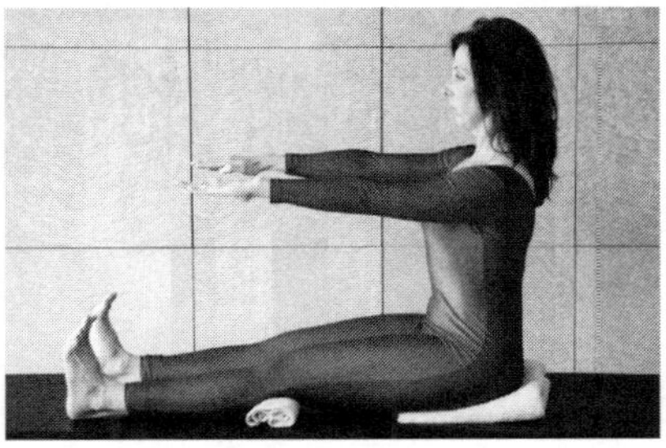
Spine stretch forward
Page 177

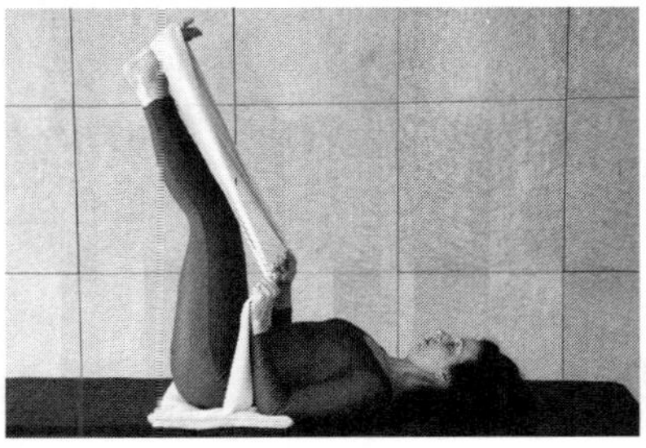
Corkscrew
Page 183

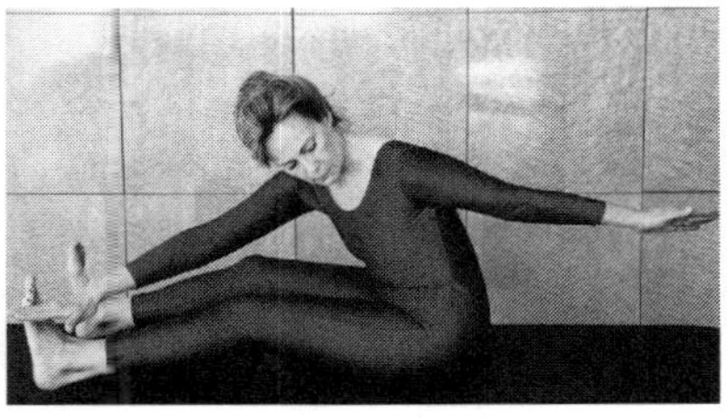
Saw
Page 187

(continued)

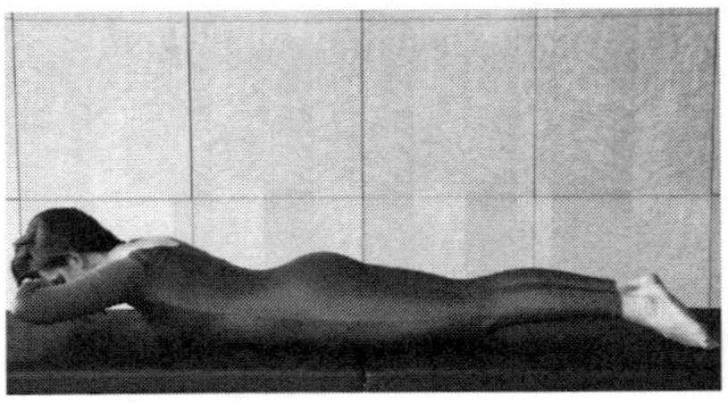

Swan prep
Page 191

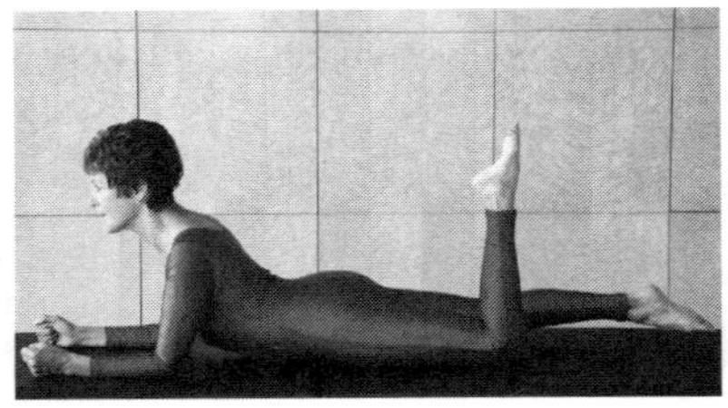

Single-leg kick
Page 196

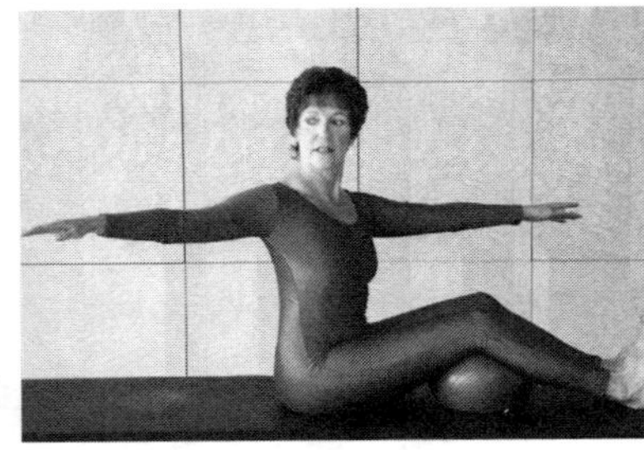

Spine twist
Page 202

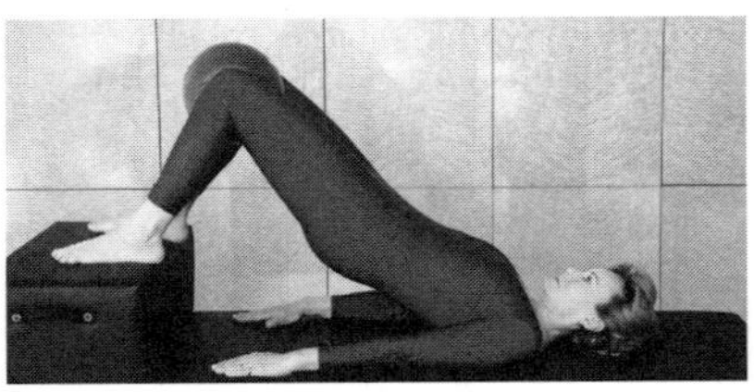

Shoulder bridge (modified)
Page 119

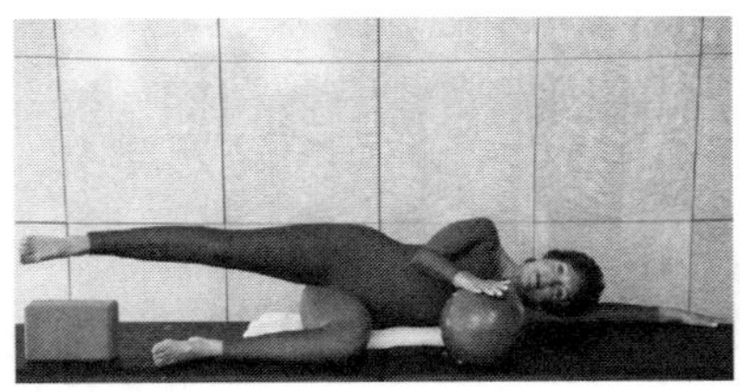

SKS, up and down
Page 270

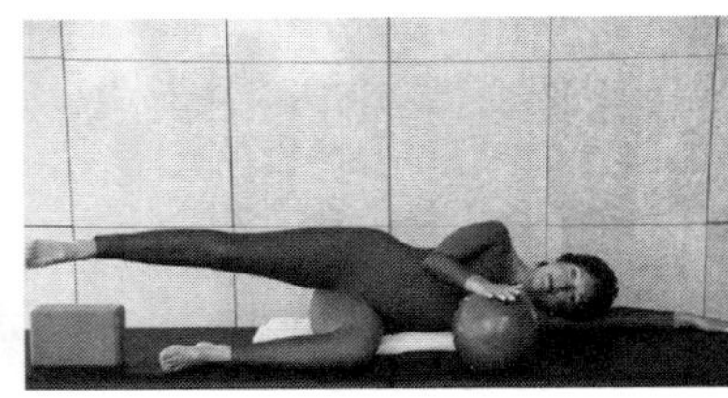

SKS, little circle
Page 278

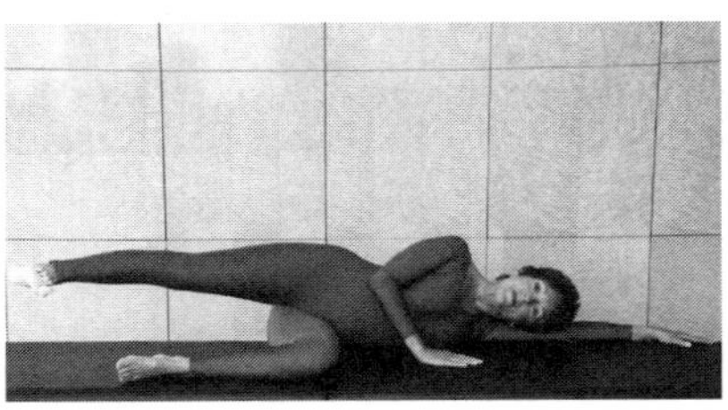

SKS, internal and external rotation, towel under hips
Page 284

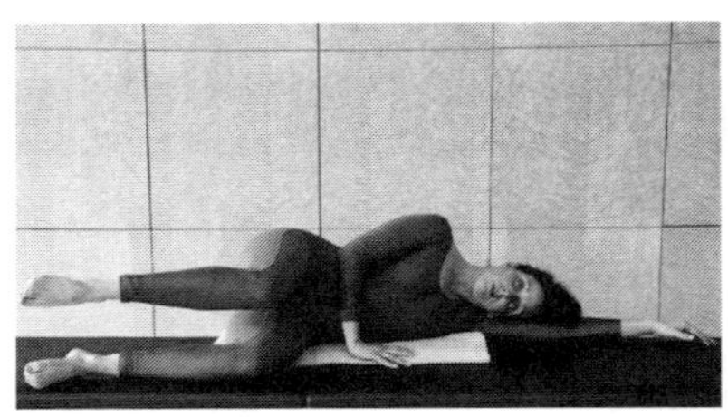

SKS, 90° bent-knee lift and lower
Page 308

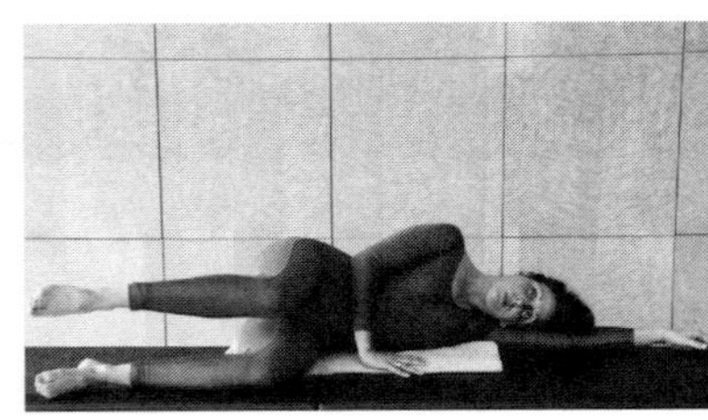

SKS, 90° bent-knee circle
Page 309

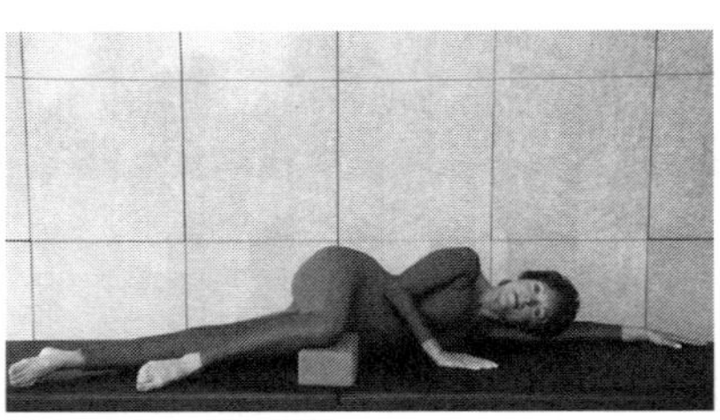

SKS, inner-thigh lift, towel under hips
Page 298

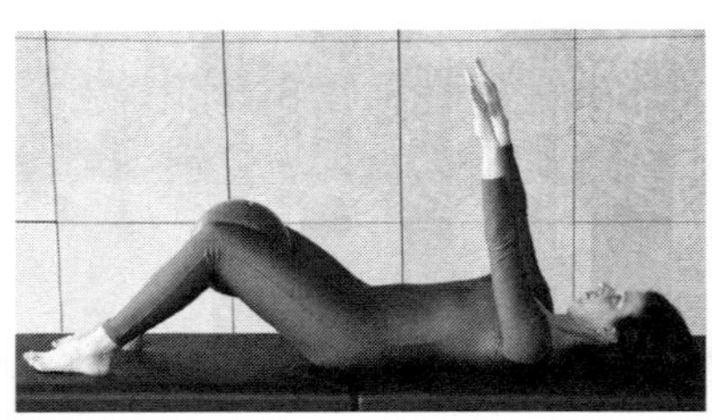

Teaser prep 1
Page 217

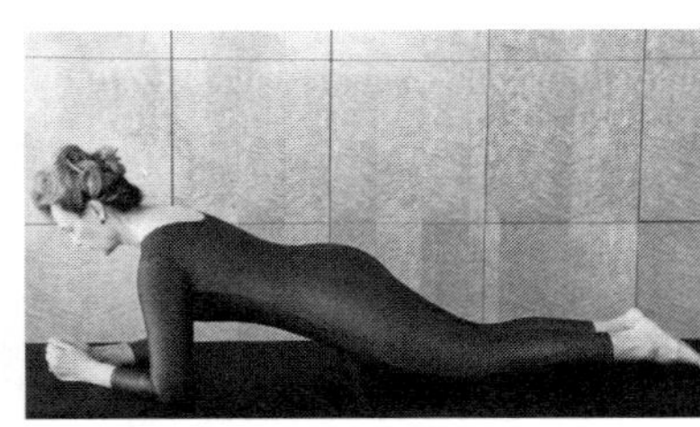

Serratus push-up (modified)
Page 251

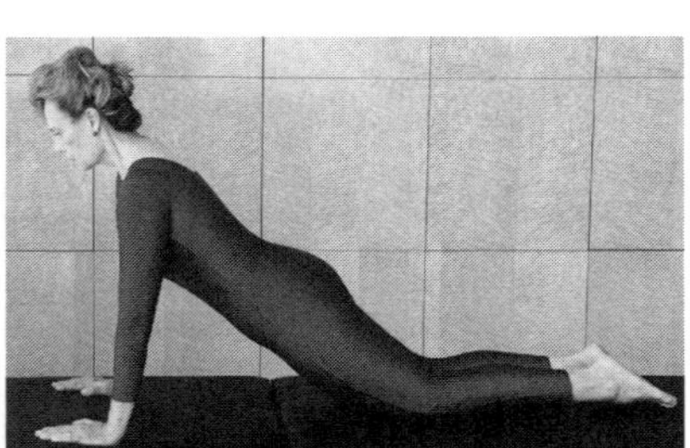

Push-up (modified)
Page 257

Total Hip Replacement (Arthroplasty): Preoperative Program Sequence

Case scenario: A 50-year-old female with osteoarthritis of the hip walks with pain and uses a cane for assistance. She is scheduled for THA in 8 weeks. She is starting a preoperative Pilates routine in preparation for the THA. Her exercise history consists of strength training 2 times per week and using the recumbent bike as tolerated. She attended a Pilates class once a week about 6 months ago.

Exercises: 28

Approximate time: 50 minutes

Pre-Pilates Exercises

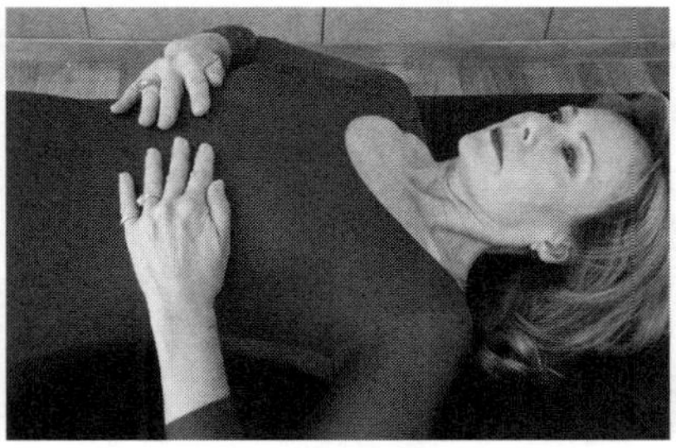

Breathing
Page 39

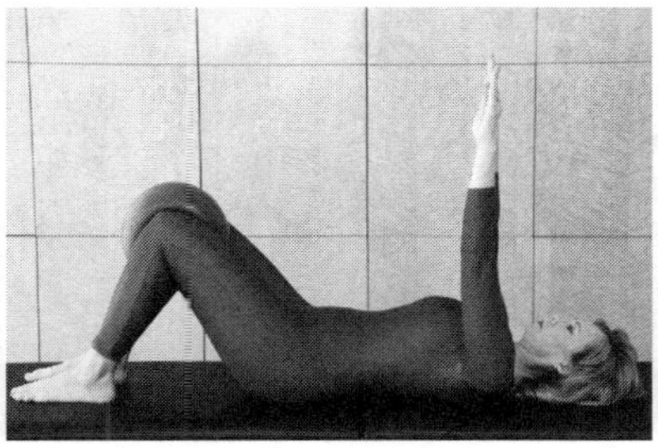

Abdominal prep
Page 48

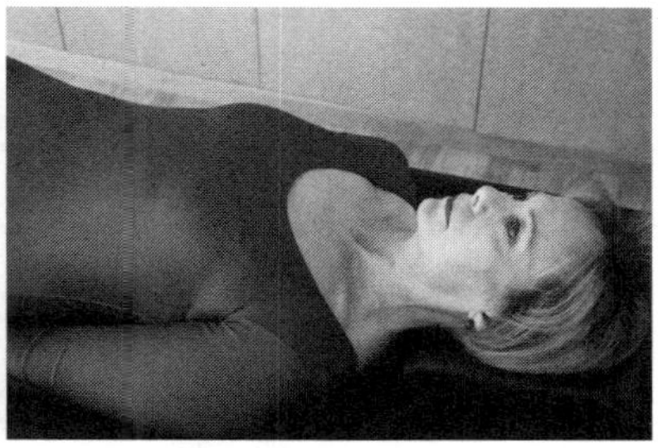

Shoulder roll
Page 44

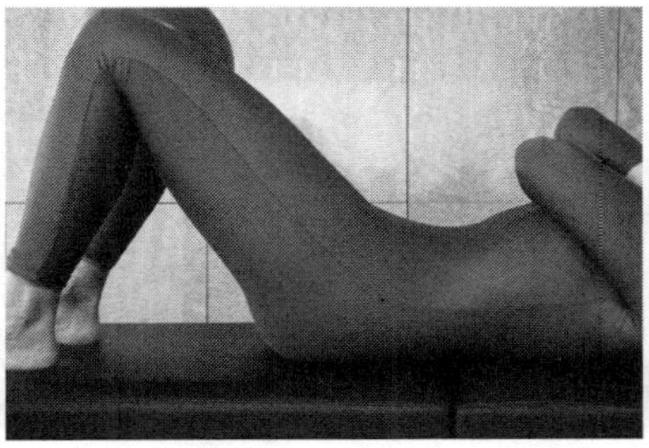

Pelvic curl
Page 45

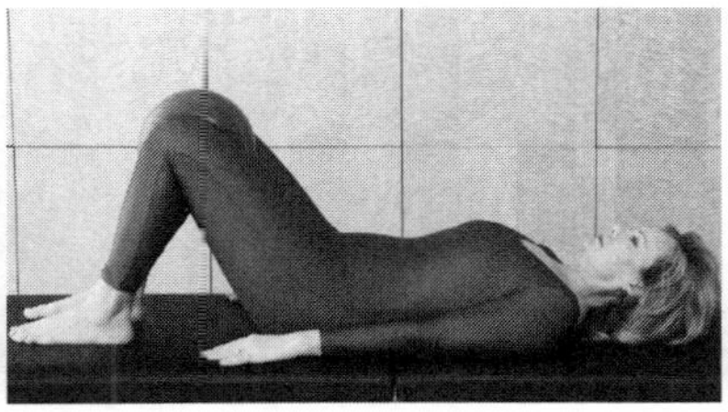

Adductor squeeze
Page 52

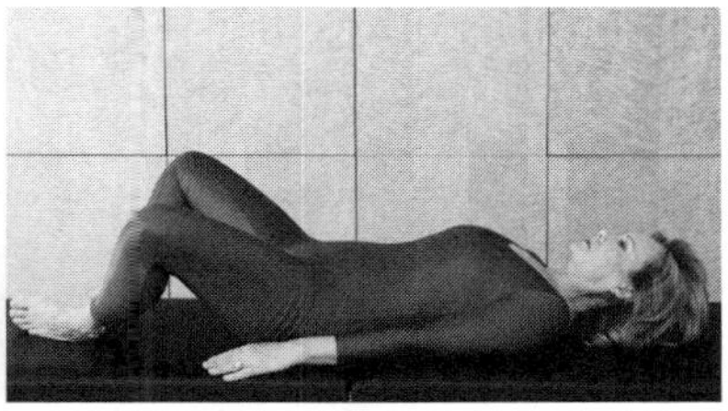

Knee fold
Page 50

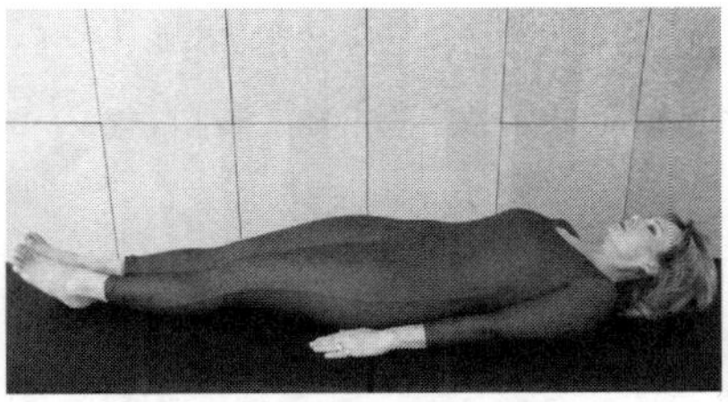

Abduction and adduction
Page 43

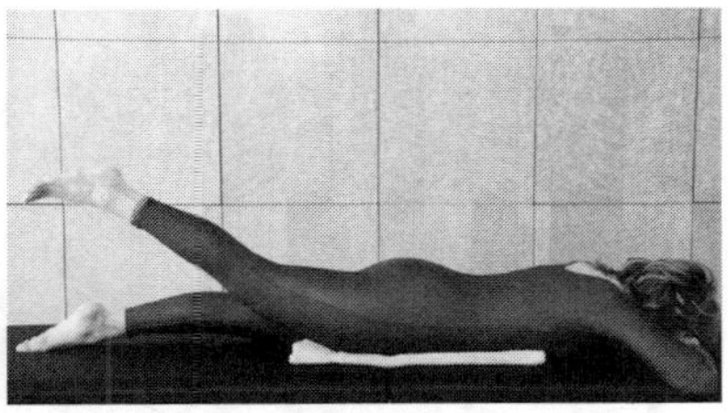

Prone leg lift, version one
Page 56

(continued)

Pilates Exercises

Note that for the SKS exercises, you will want to use a towel or padding under the hip.

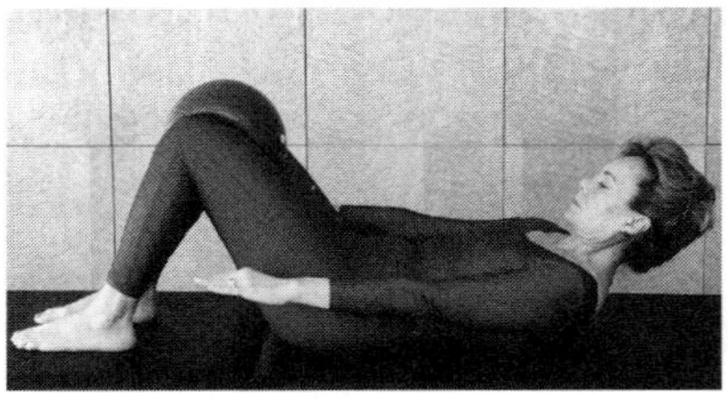
Hundred
Page 69

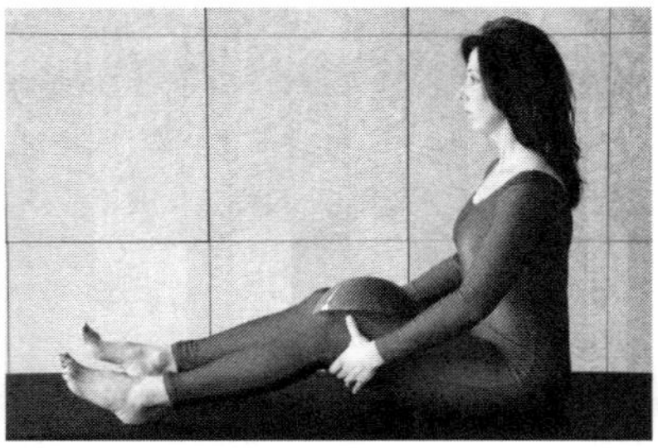
Half roll-down
Page 72

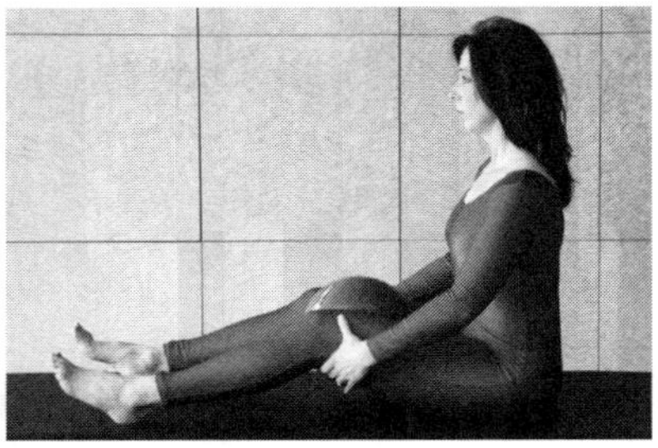
Half roll-up
Page 77

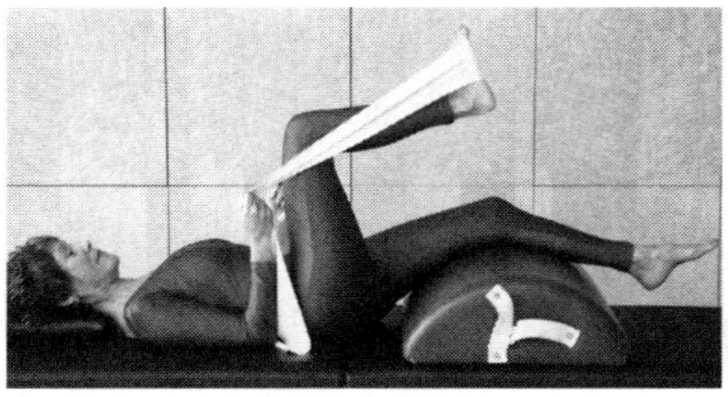
Single-leg circle
Page 80

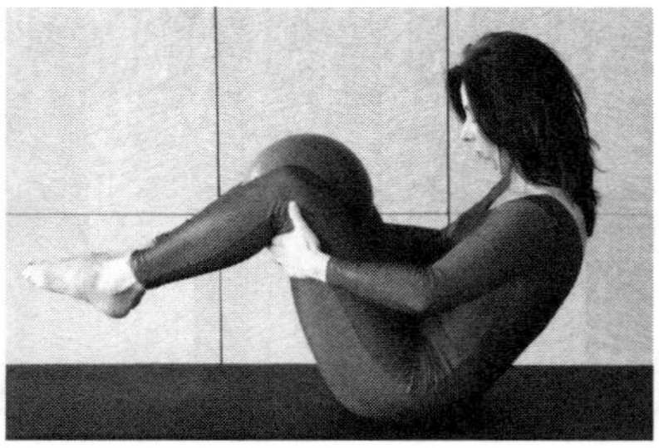
Rolling like a ball
Page 159

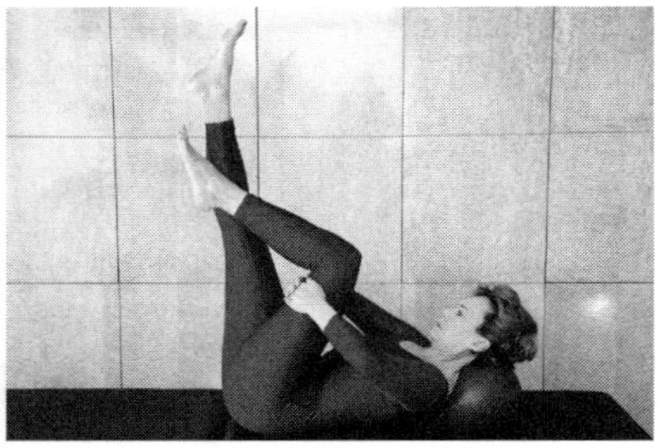
Single-leg stretch
Page 84

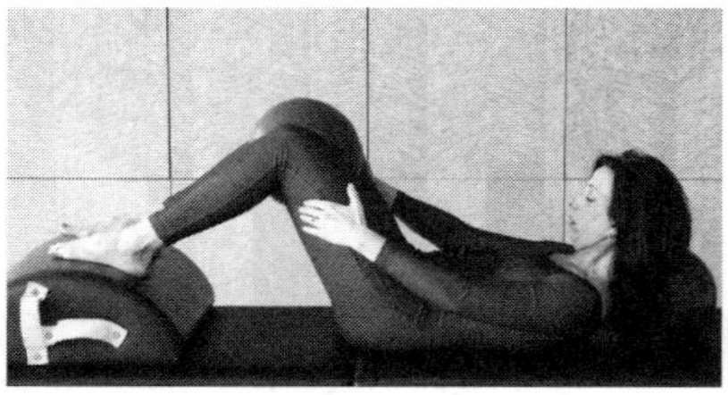
Double-leg stretch
Page 87

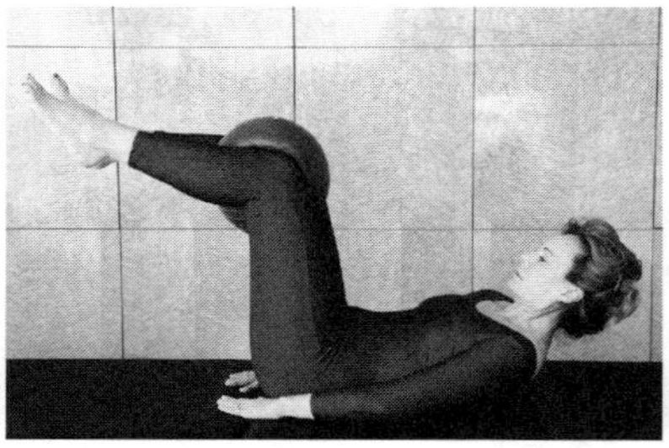
Lower lift
Page 95

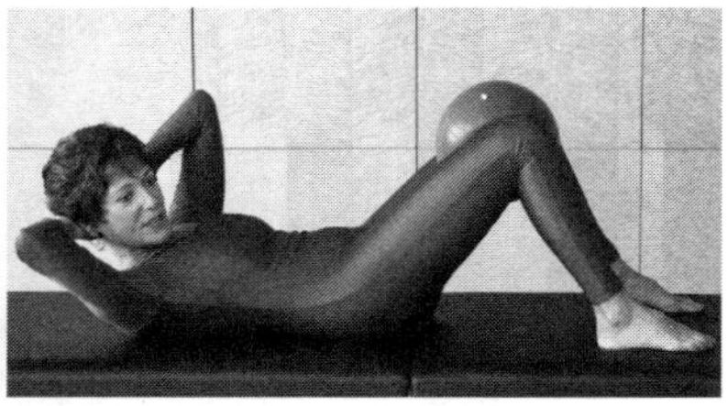
Crisscross
Page 99

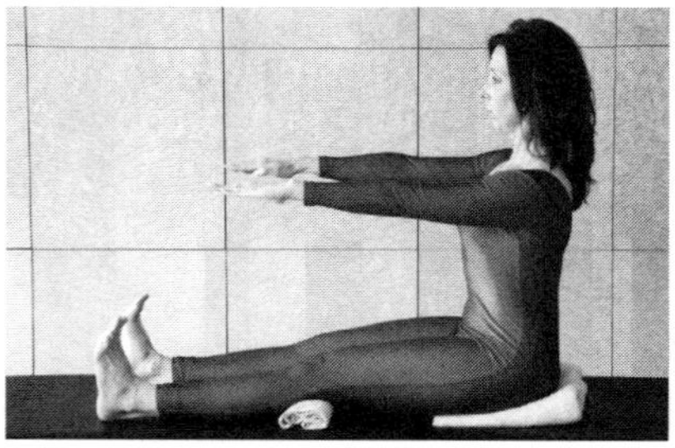
Spine stretch forward
Page 177

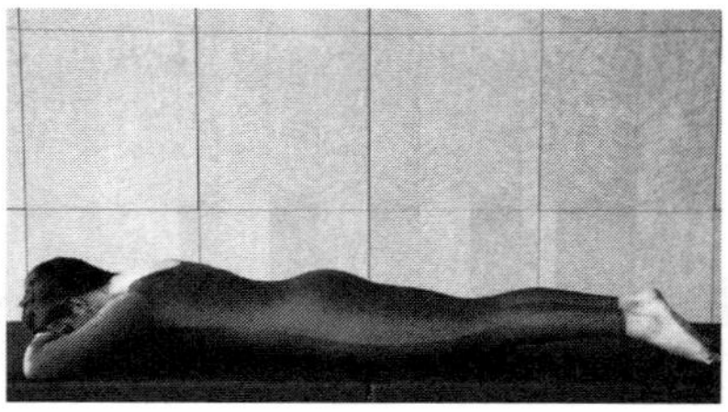
Swan prep
Page 191

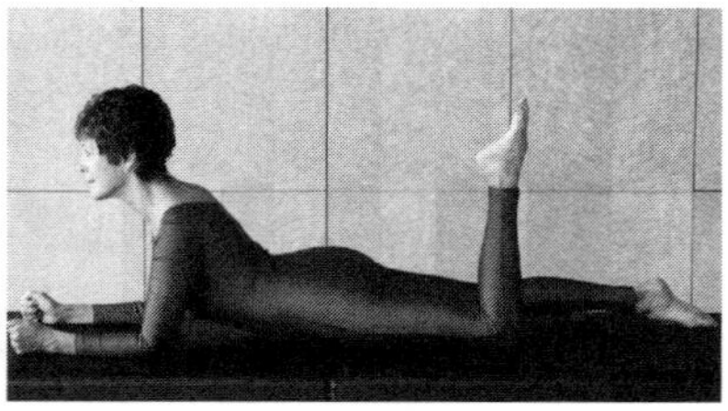
Single-leg kick
Page 196

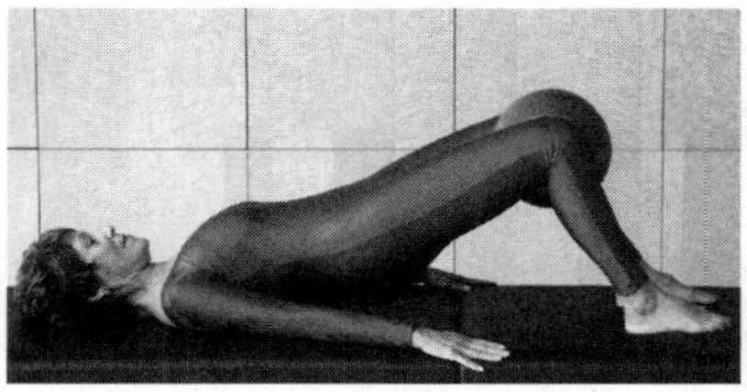
Shoulder bridge (modified)
Page 117

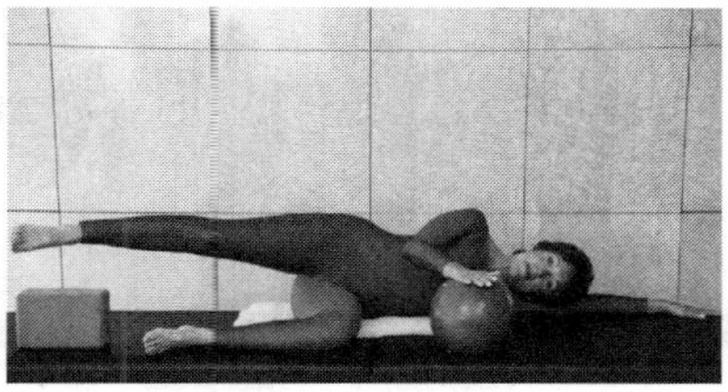
SKS, up and down
Page 271

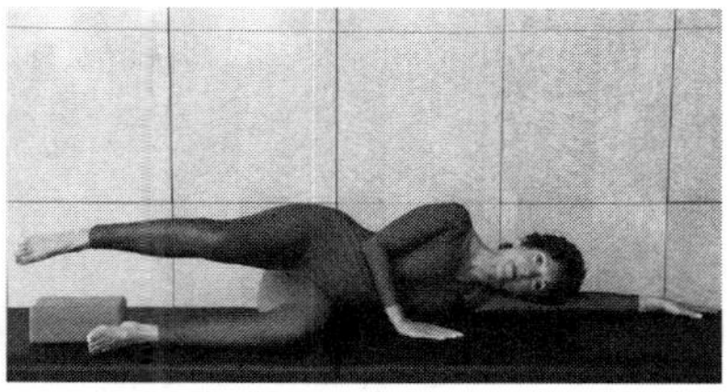
SKS, front and back
Page 274

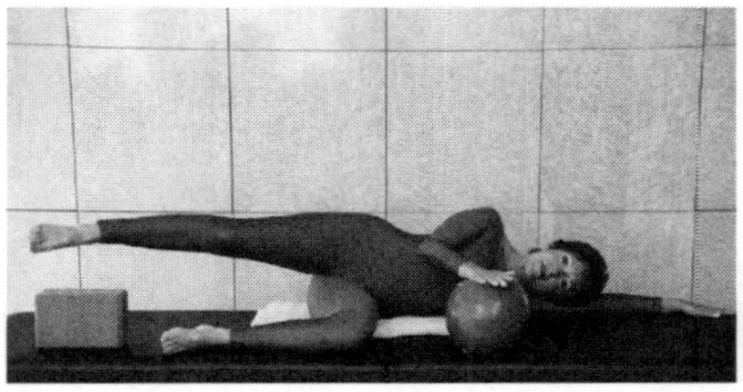
SKS, little circle
Page 278

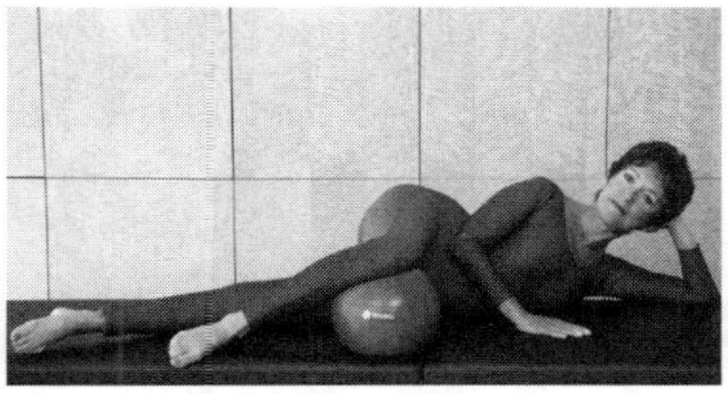
SKS, inner-thigh lift
Page 300

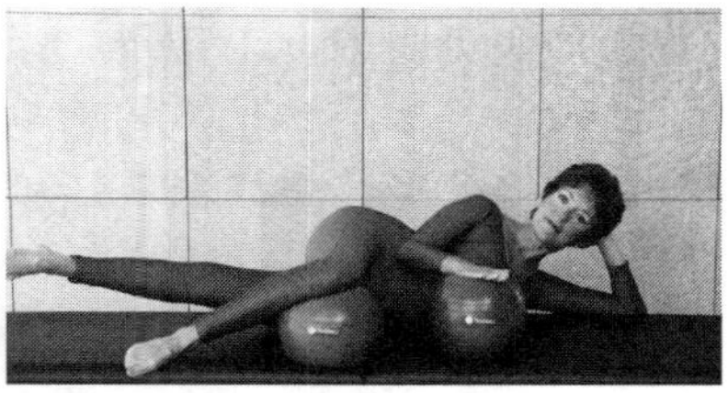
SKS, inner-thigh circle
Page 302

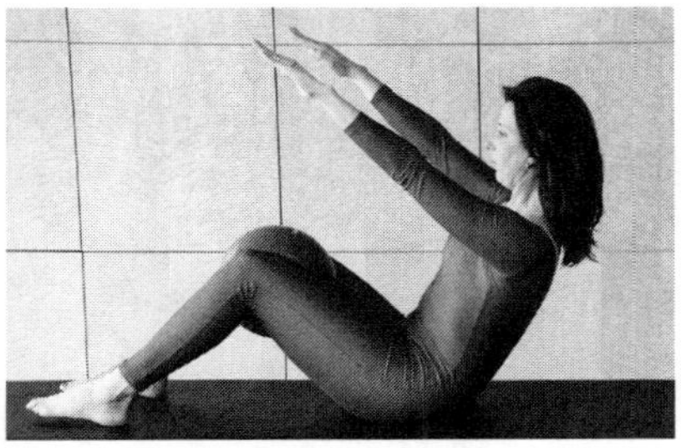
Teaser prep 1
Page 121

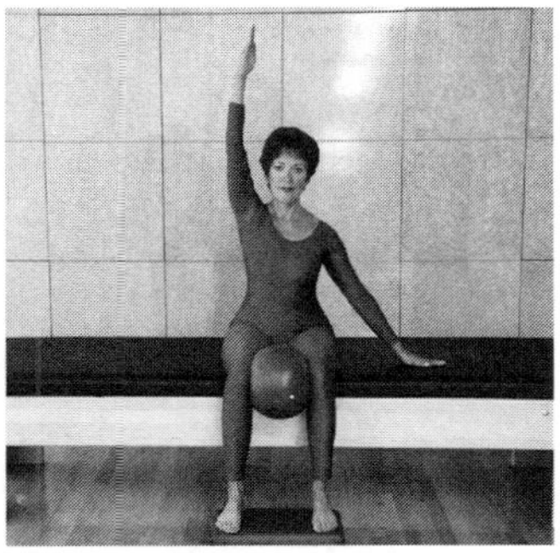
Side stretch
Page 129

Total Hip Replacement (Arthroplasty): Program Sequence for 6 Weeks Postop

Case scenario continued: A 50-year-old female with osteoarthritis of the hip underwent a scheduled THA and is now ready for a specified Pilates mat program for 6 weeks to 3 months postoperative. She completed a preoperative Pilates routine that she followed 3 times a week before surgery.

Exercises: 29

Approximate time: 50 minutes

Pre-Pilates Exercises

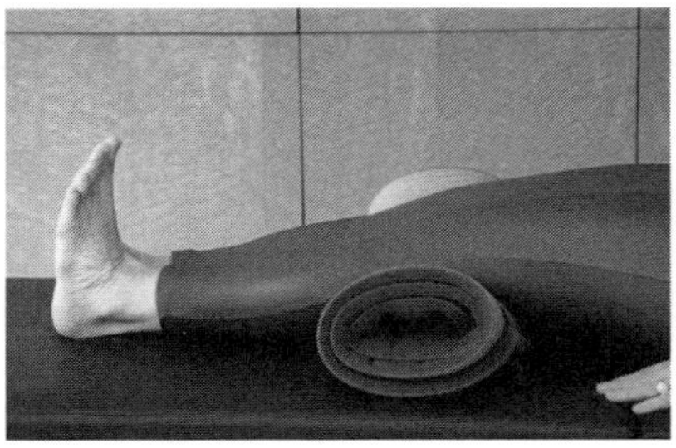

Ankle pump
Page 40

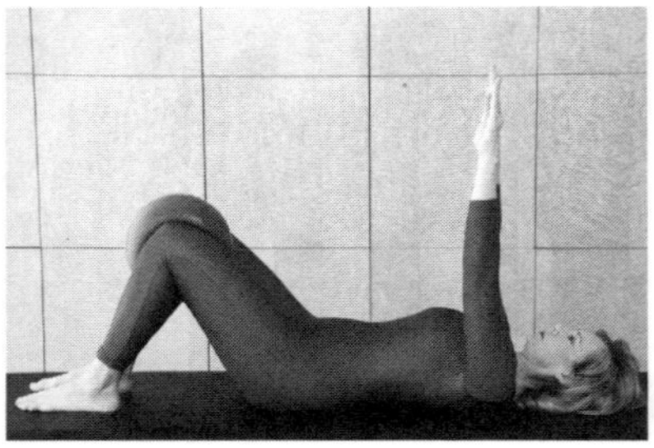

Abdominal prep
Page 48

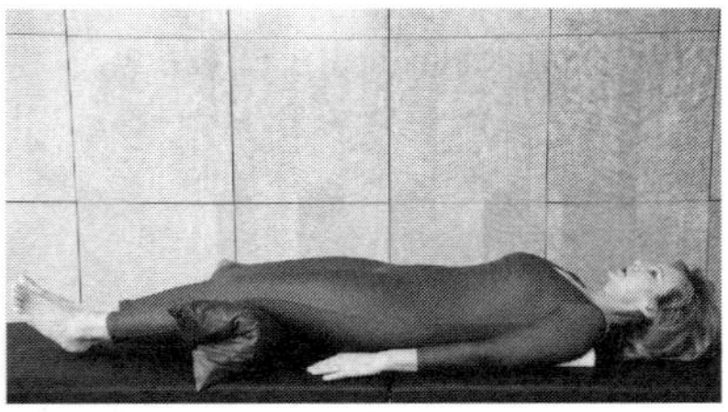

Quadriceps set
Page 41

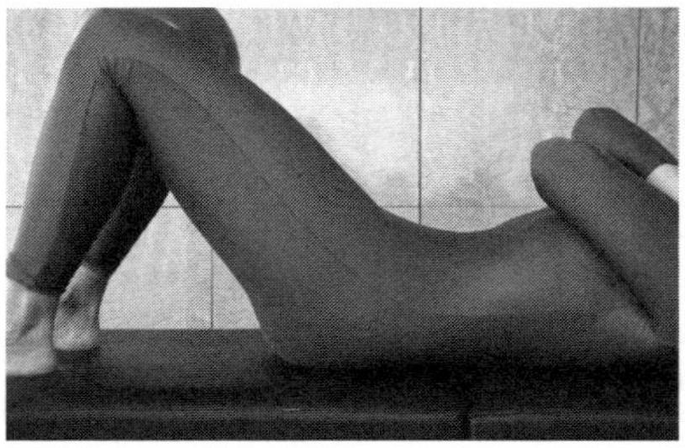

Pelvic curl
Page 45

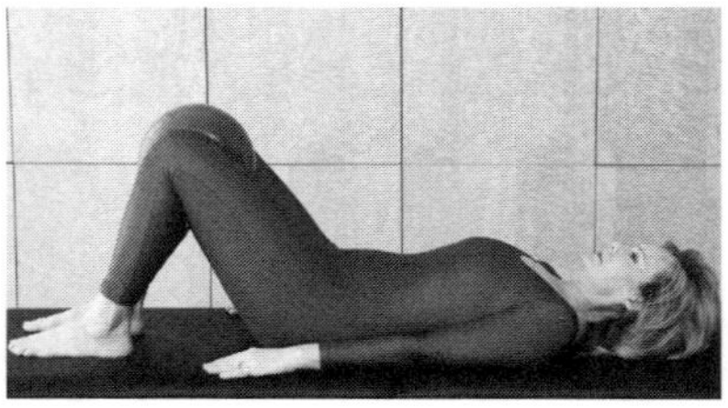

Adductor squeeze
Page 52

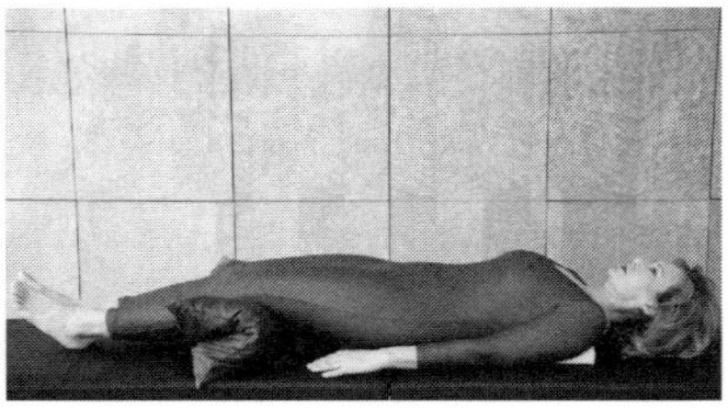

Gluteal set
Page 42

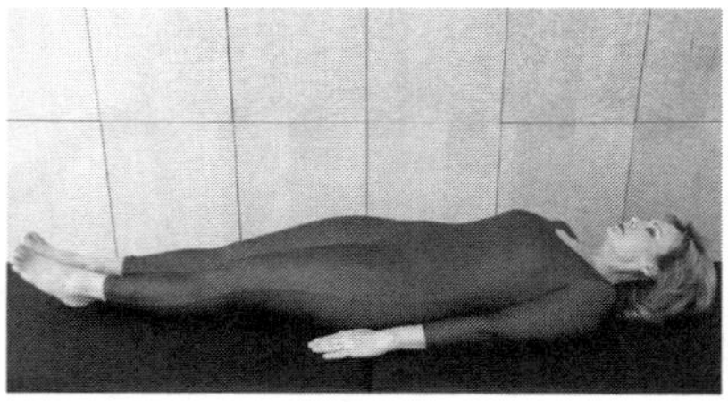

Abduction and adduction
Page 43

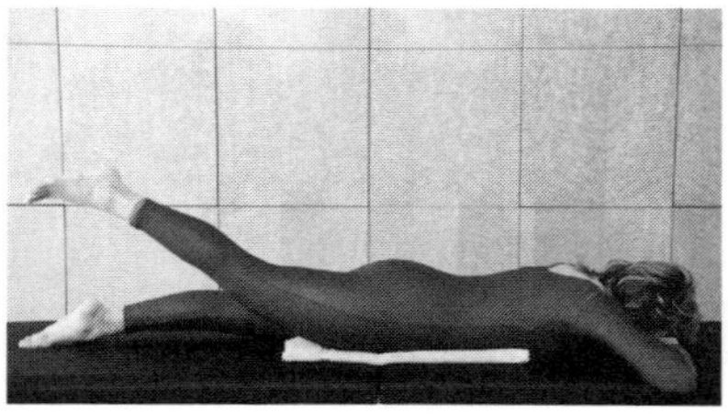

Prone leg lift, version one
Page 56

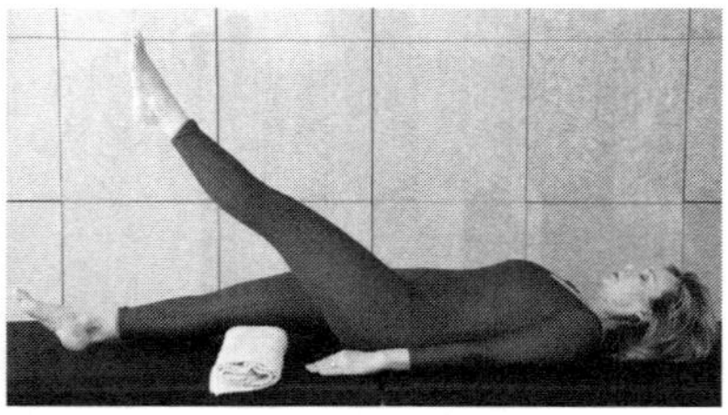

Supine leg lift, version one
Page 53

Pilates Exercises

Note that for the SKS exercises, you will want to use a towel or padding under the hip.

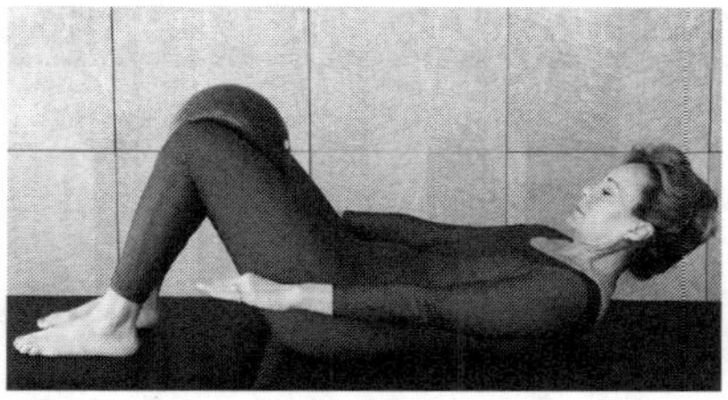

Hundred
Page 69

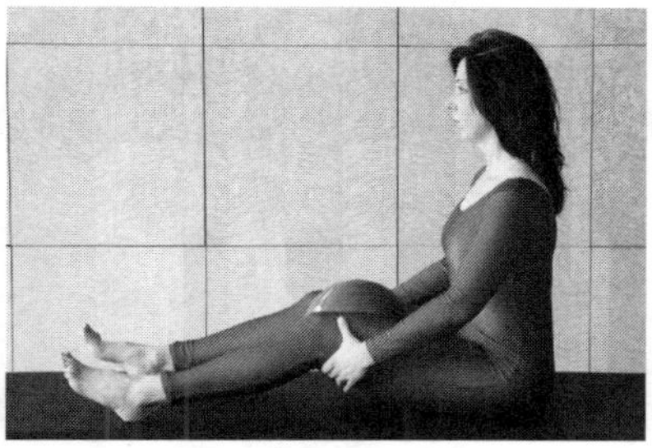

Half roll-down
Page 72

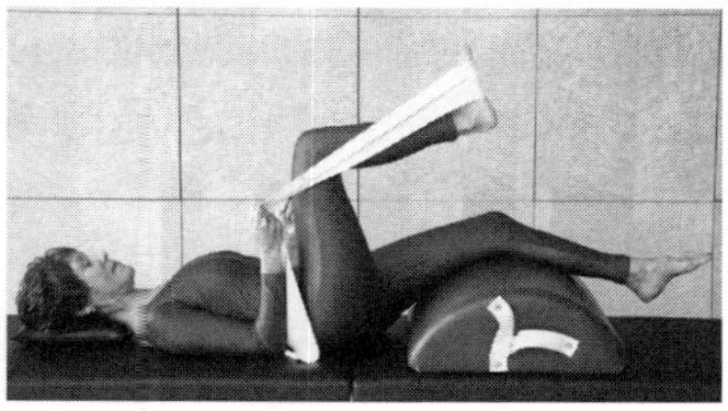

Single-leg circle
Page 80

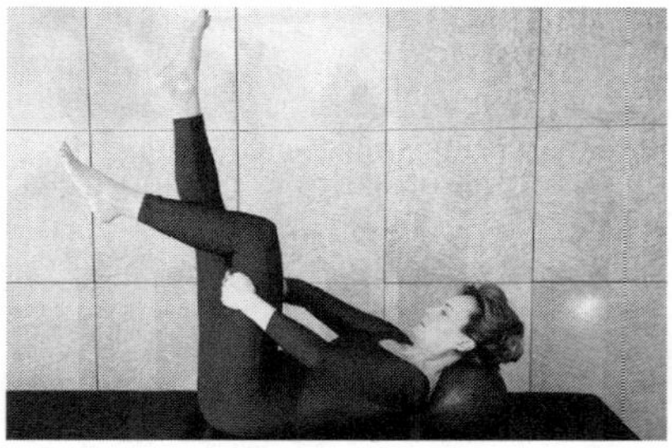

Single-leg stretch
Page 84

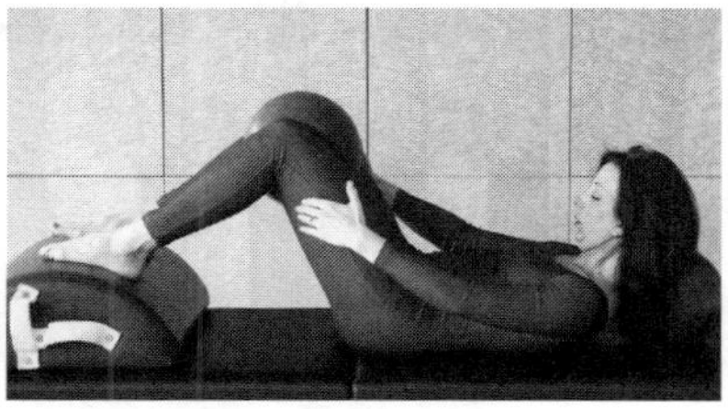

Double-leg stretch
Page 87

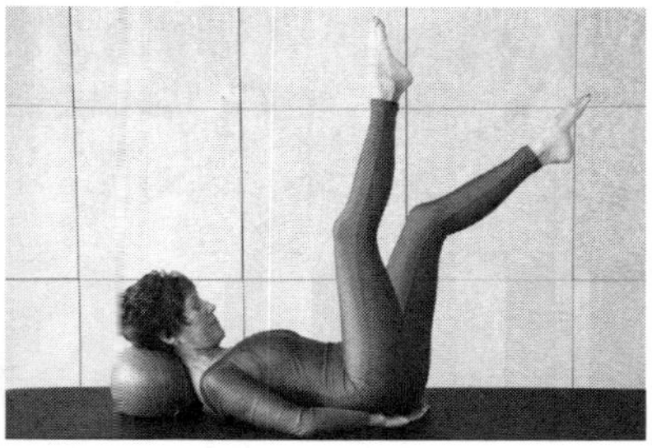

Scissors
Page 92

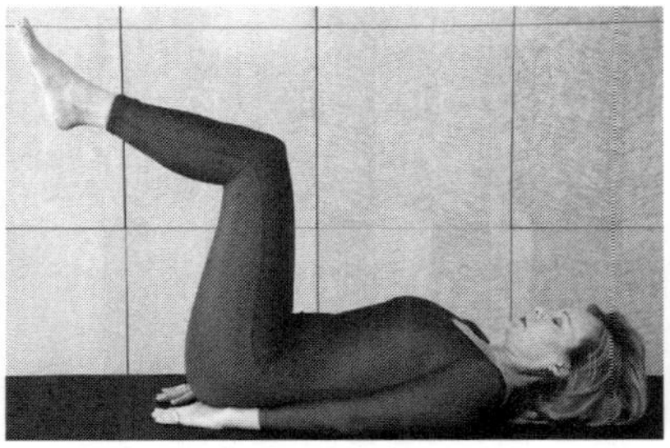

Toe tap
Page 47

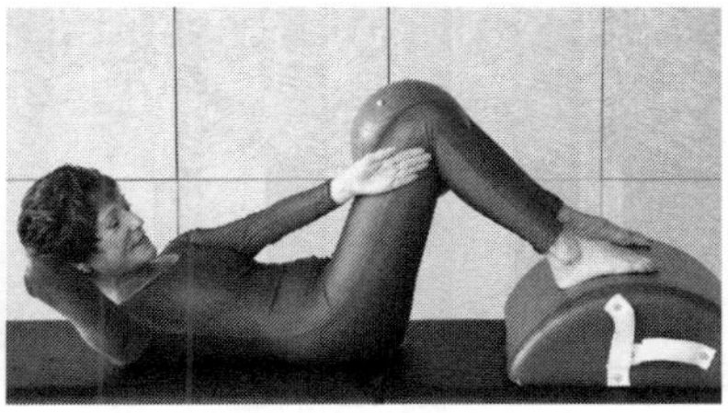

Crisscross
Page 98

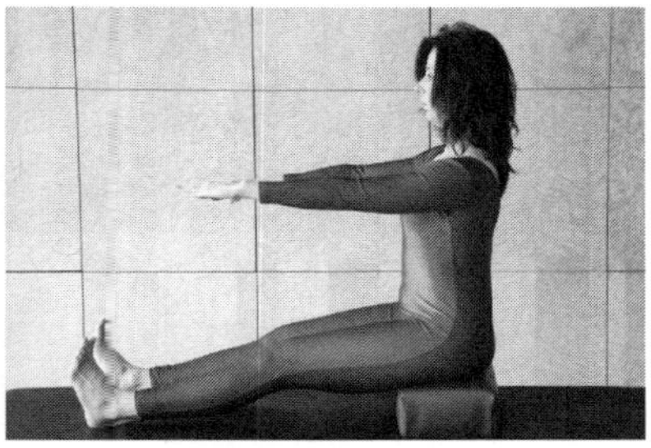

Spine stretch forward
Page 104

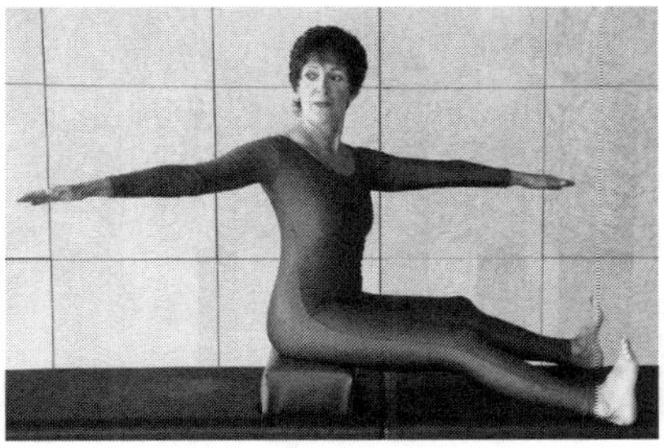

Saw
Page 107

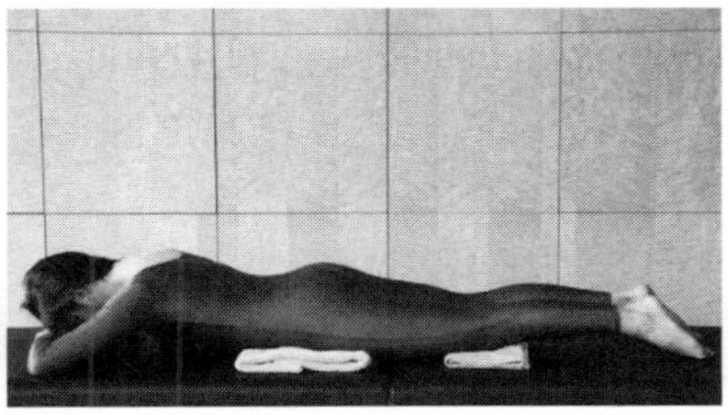

Swan prep
Page 111

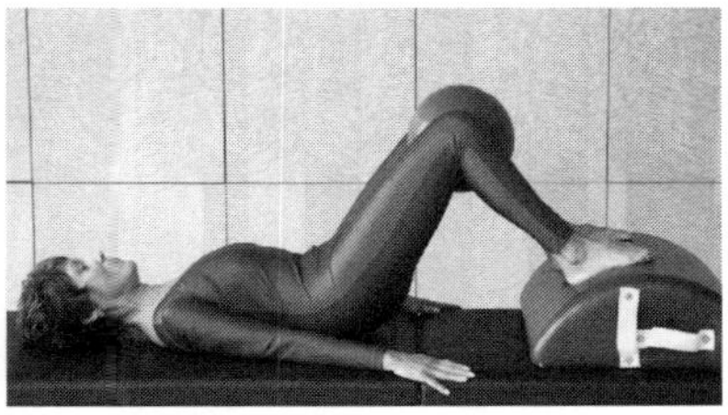

Shoulder bridge (modified), roll up to waist
Page 117

(continued)

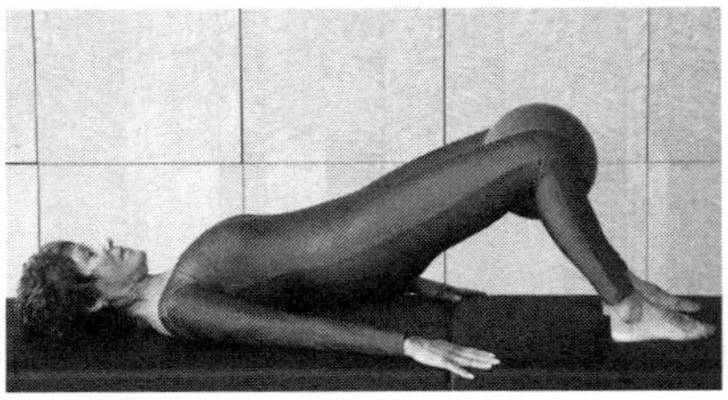
Shoulder bridge (modified), roll up to shoulder blades
Page 117

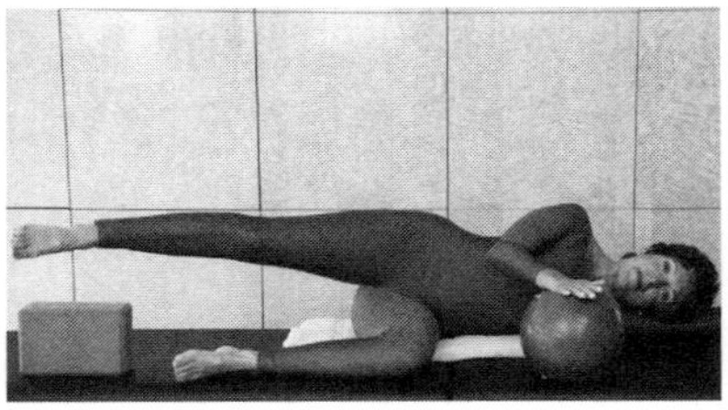
SKS, up and down
Page 270

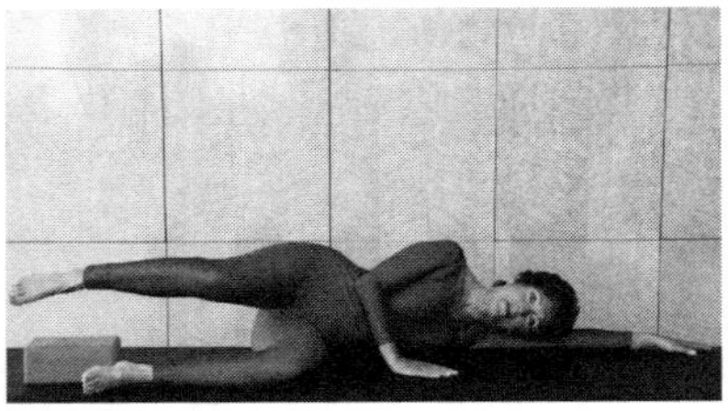
SKS, front and back
Page 274

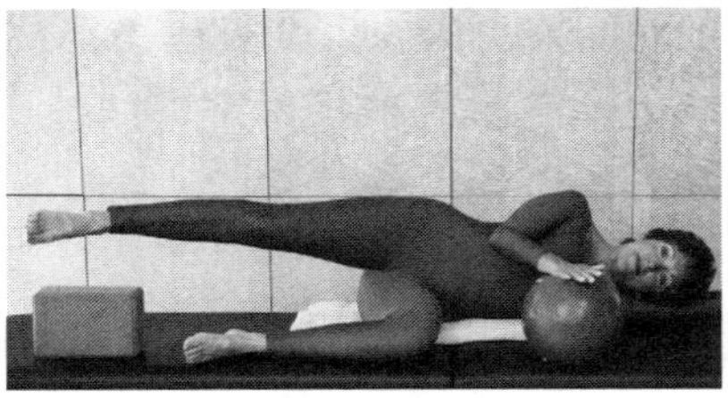
SKS, little circle
Page 278

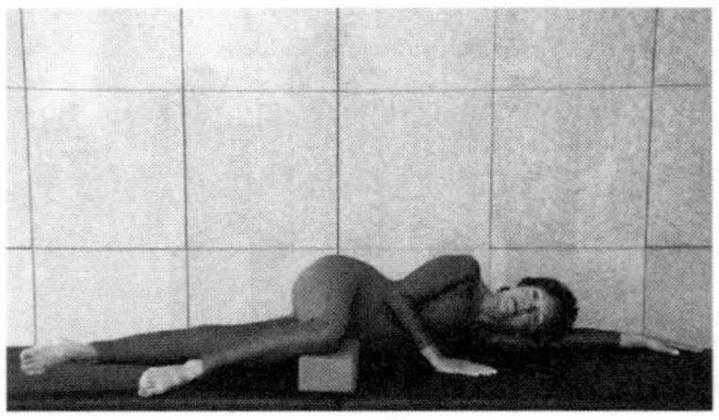
SKS, inner-thigh lift
Page 298

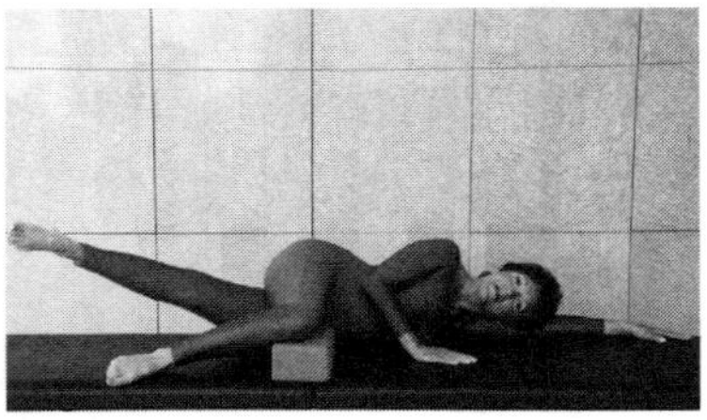
SKS, inner-thigh circle
Page 299

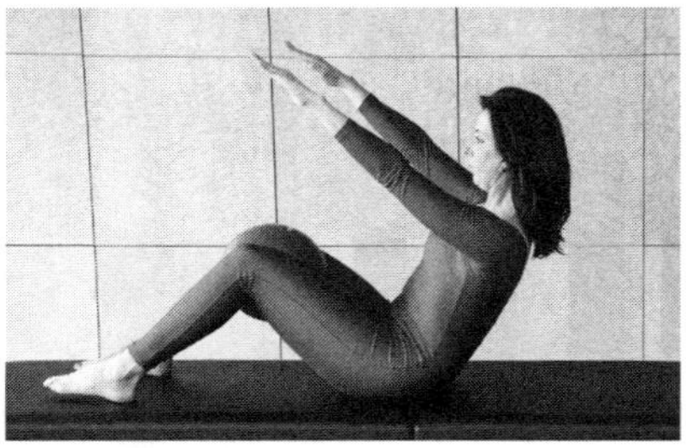
Teaser prep 1
Page 121

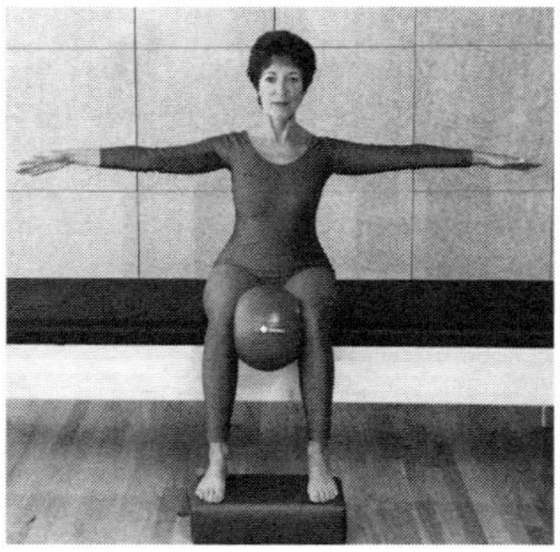
Side stretch
Page 129

Total Hip Replacement (Arthroplasty): Program Sequence for 3 Months Postop

Case scenario continued: A 50-year-old female with osteoarthritis of the hip underwent a scheduled THA 3 months ago and is now ready for a specified Pilates mat program for 3 to 6 months postop. She completed a preoperative Pilates program and a 6 weeks to 3 months postop Pilates mat program.

Exercises: 30

Approximate time: 50 minutes

Pre-Pilates Exercises

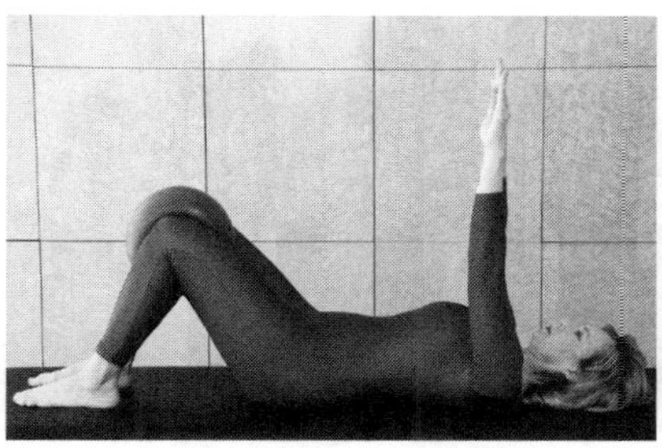

Abdominal prep
Page 48

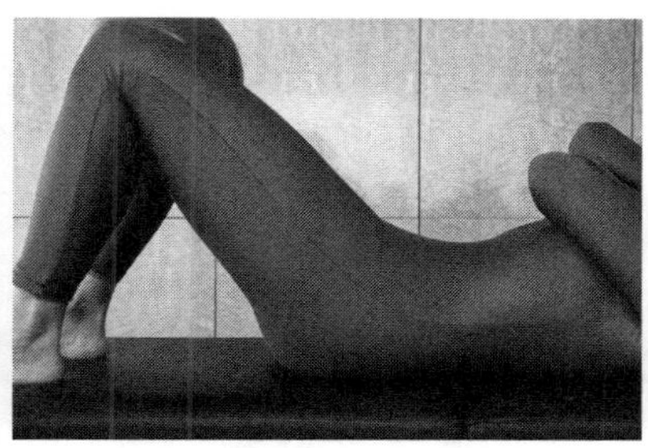

Pelvic curl
Page 45

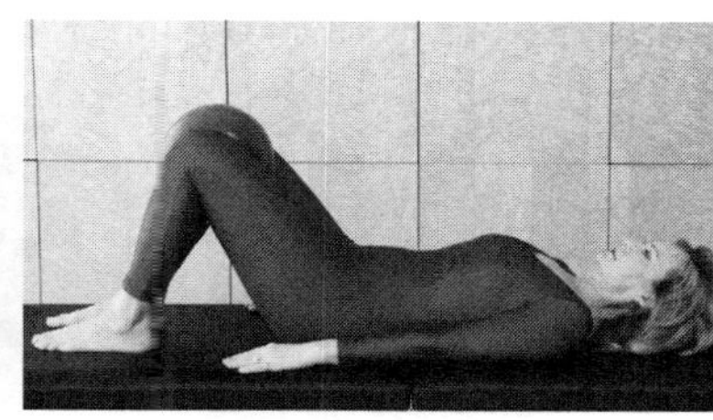

Adductor squeeze
Page 52

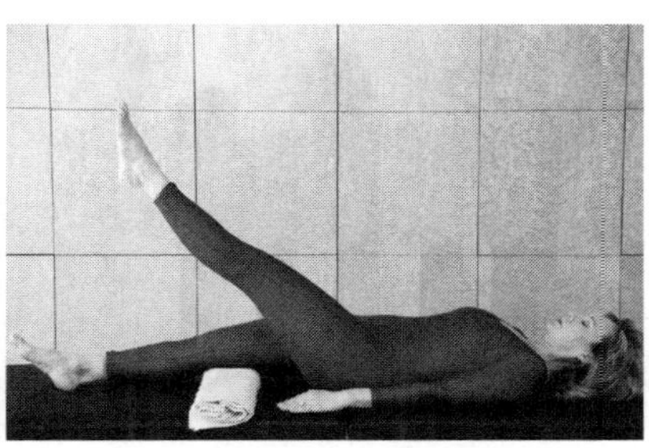

Supine leg lift, version one
Page 53

(continued)

Pilates Exercises

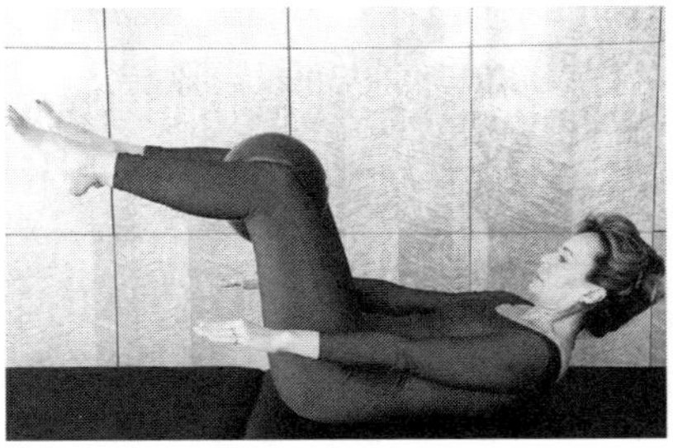

Hundred
Page 135

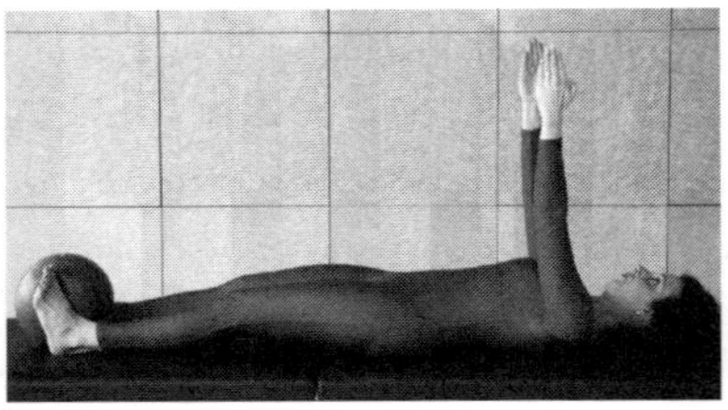

Roll-up
Page 143

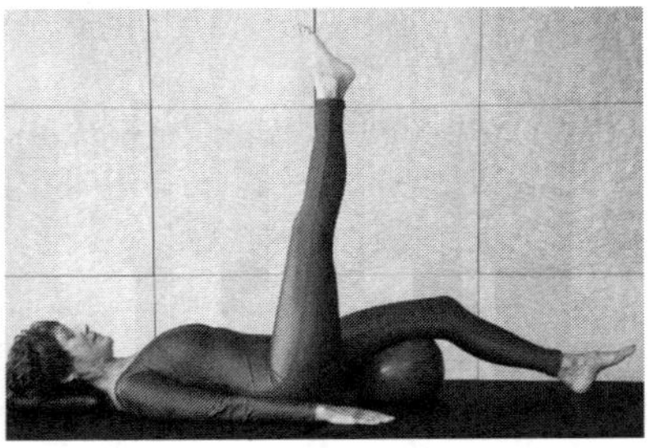

Single-leg circle
Page 152

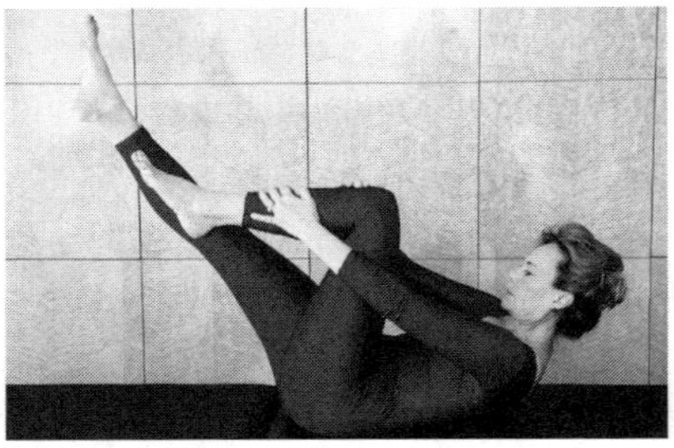

Single-leg stretch
Page 160

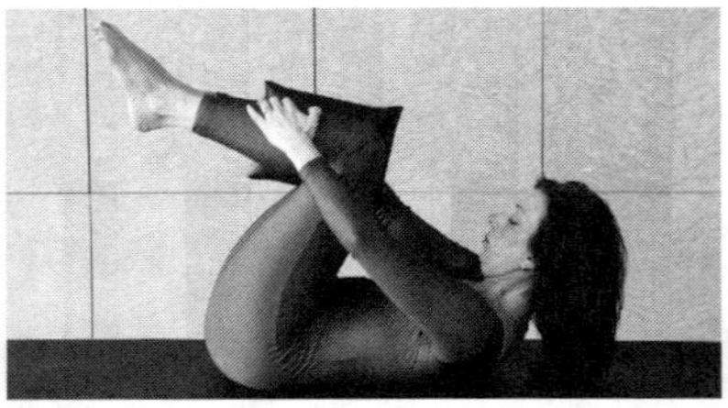

Double-leg stretch
Page 163

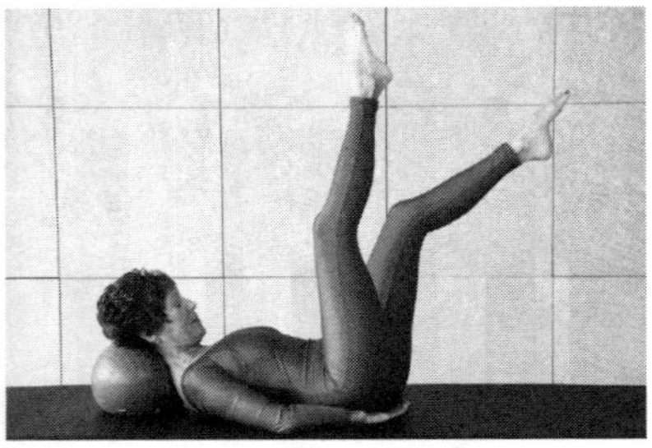

Scissors, 6 weeks
to 3 months postop version
Page 92

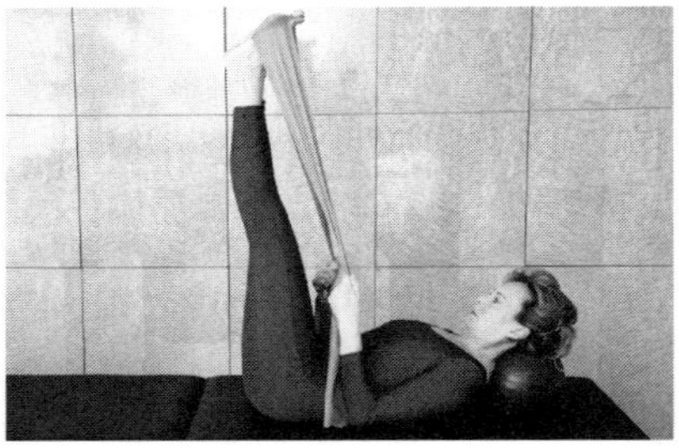

Lower lift
Page 172

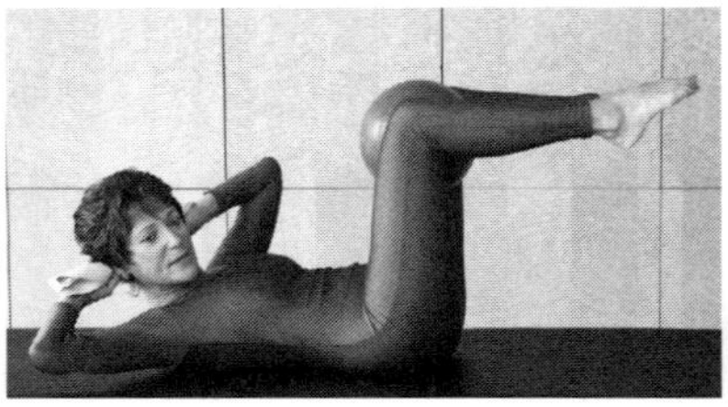

Crisscross, 6 weeks to 3
months postop version
Page 101

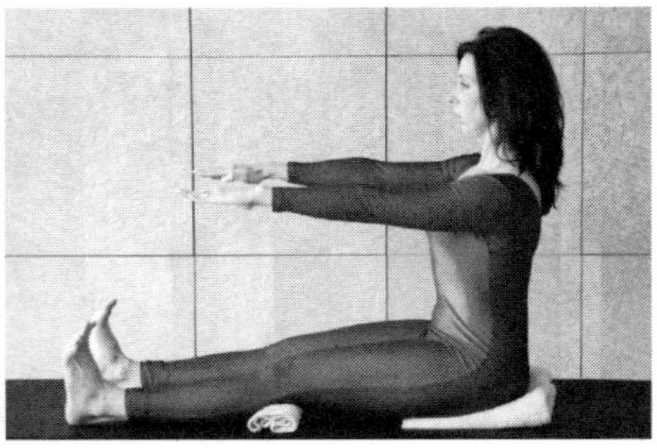

Spine stretch forward
Page 177

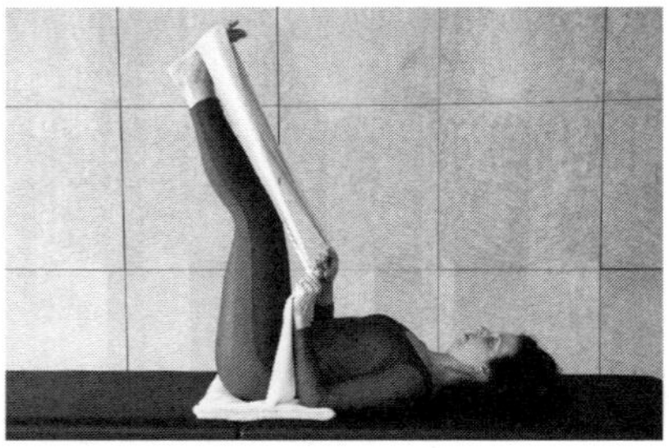

Corkscrew
Page 183

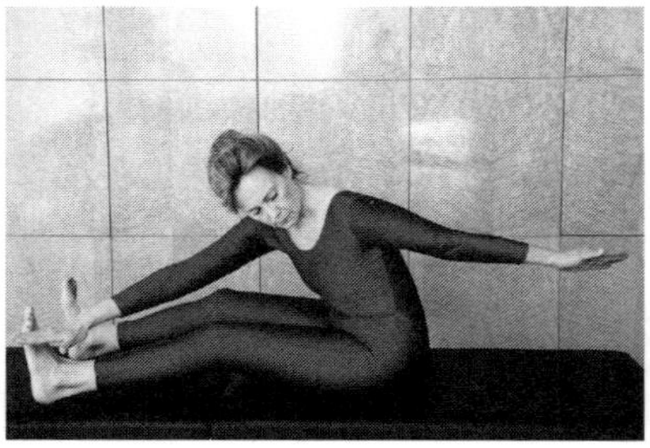

Saw
Page 187

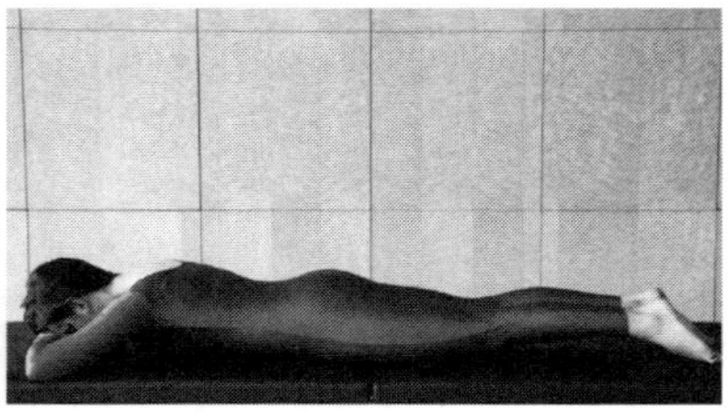

Swan prep
Page 191

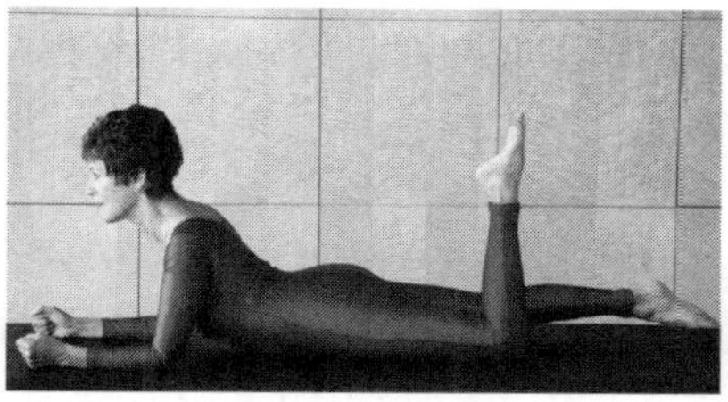

Single-leg kick
Page 196

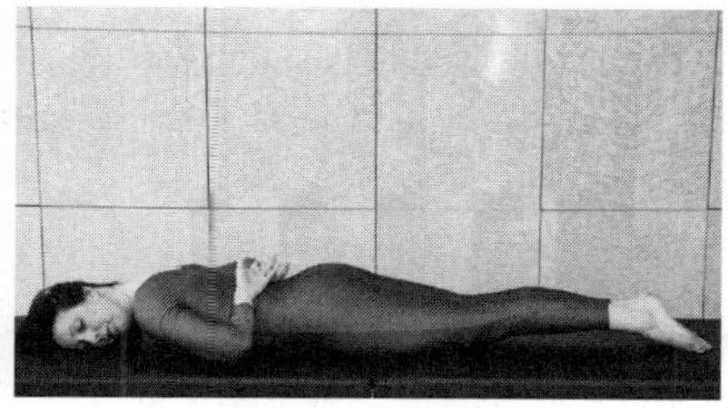

Double-leg kick
Page 198

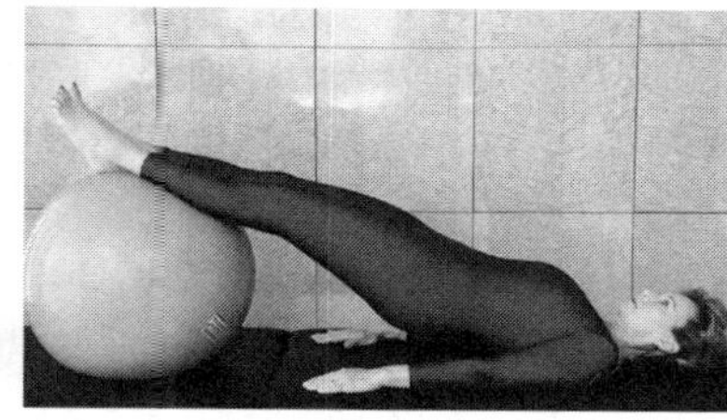

Shoulder bridge
Page 214

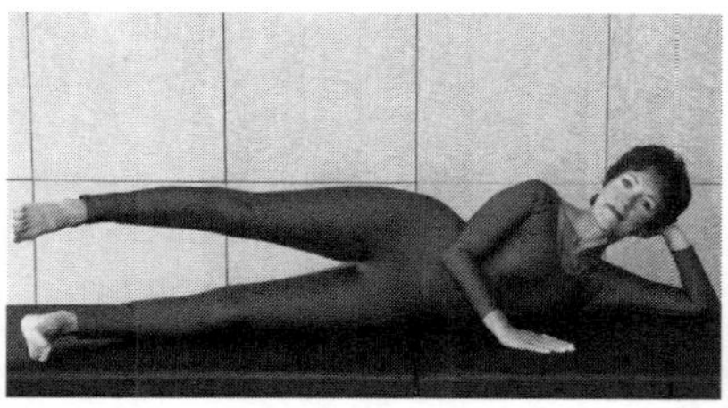

SKS, up and down
Page 272

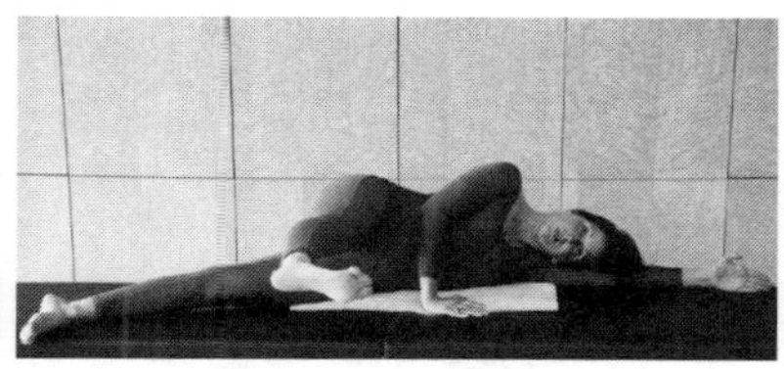

SKS, front and back
Page 277

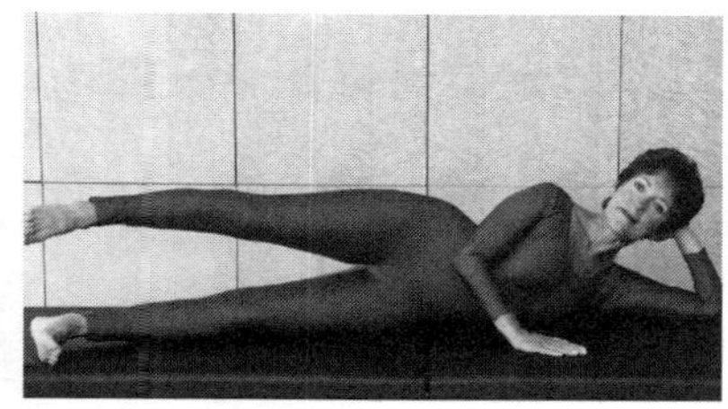

SKS, little circle
Page 279

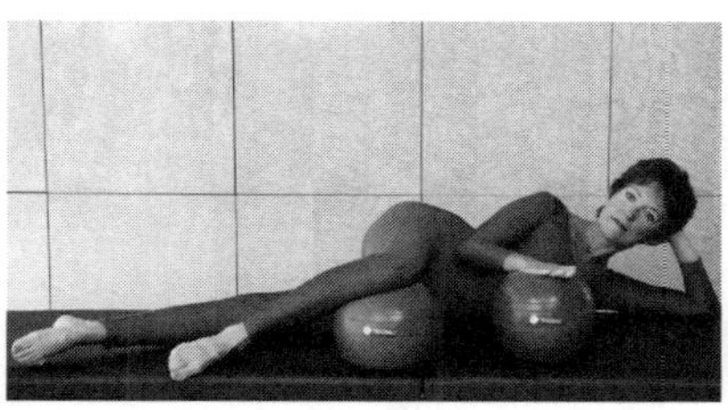

SKS, inner-thigh lift and circle
Page 300

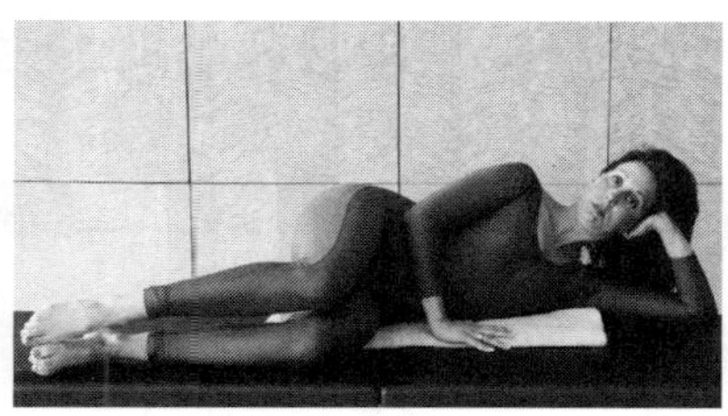

SKS, 90° bent-knee lift and lower
Page 308

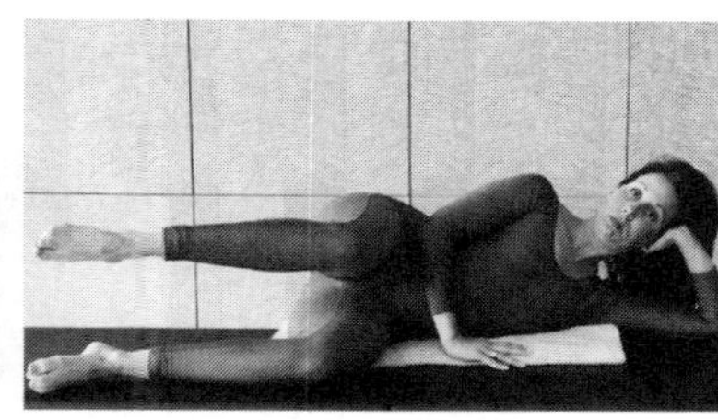

SKS, 90° bent-knee circle
Page 309

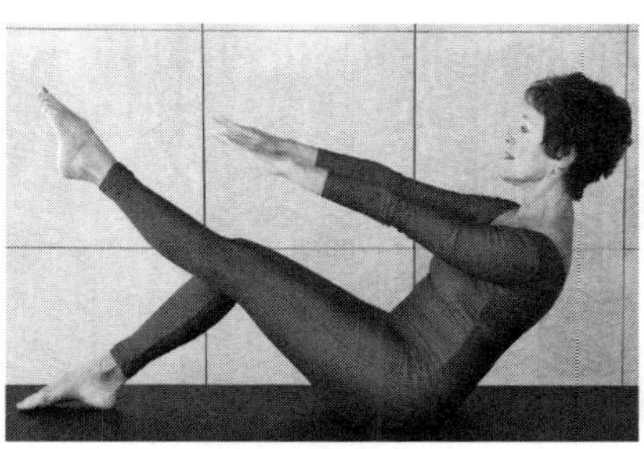

Teaser prep 2
Page 219

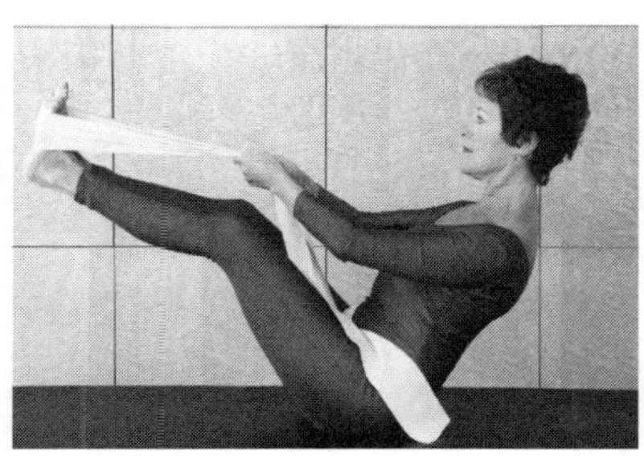

Teaser 2
Page 228

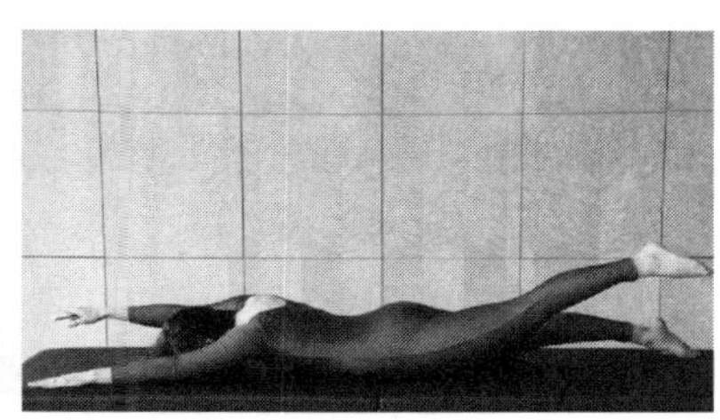

Swimming prep
Page 238

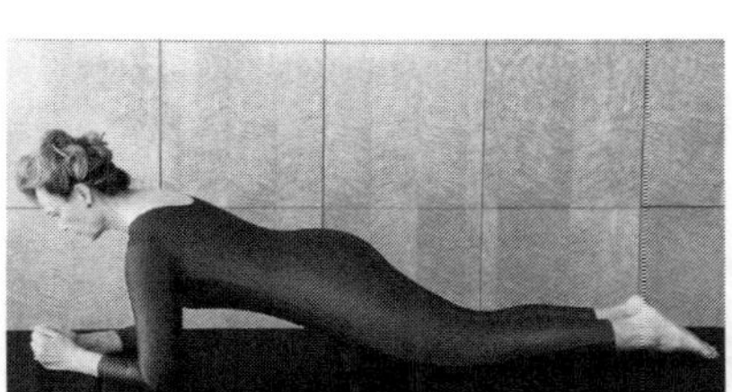

Serratus push-up (modified)
Page 251

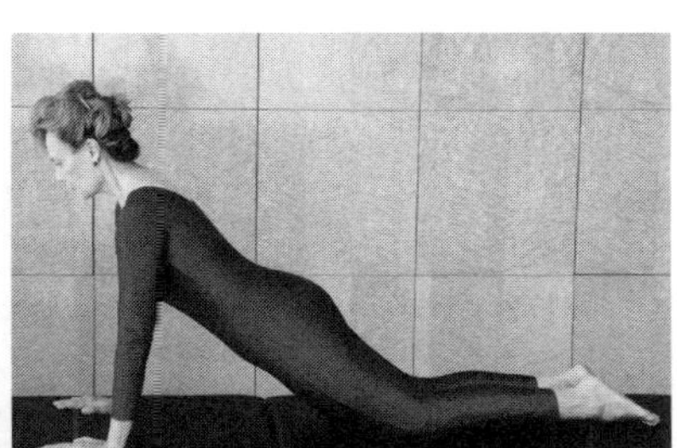

Push-up (modified)
Page 257

Total Hip Replacement (Arthroplasty): Program Sequence for 6 Months Postop

Case scenario continued: A 50-year-old female with osteoarthritis of the hip underwent a scheduled THA 6 months ago and is now ready to work toward the ideal expression of the Pilates mat exercises by following a specified Pilates mat program for 6 months postop. She performed Pilates exercises for 3 days a week preoperatively and has been performing Pilates exercises since 6 weeks postoperatively.

Exercises: 38

Approximate time: 50 minutes

Pre-Pilates Exercises

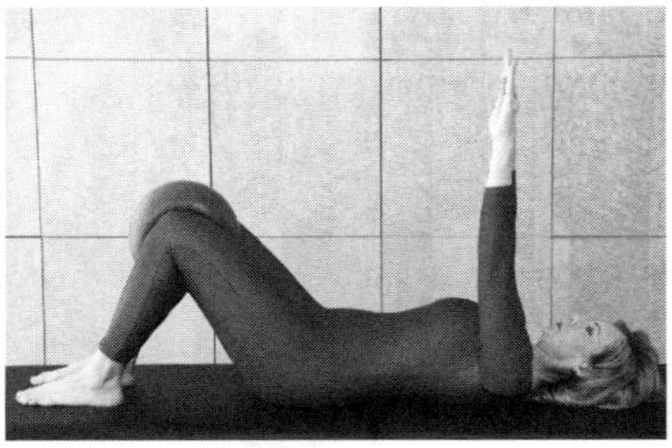

Abdominal prep
Page 48

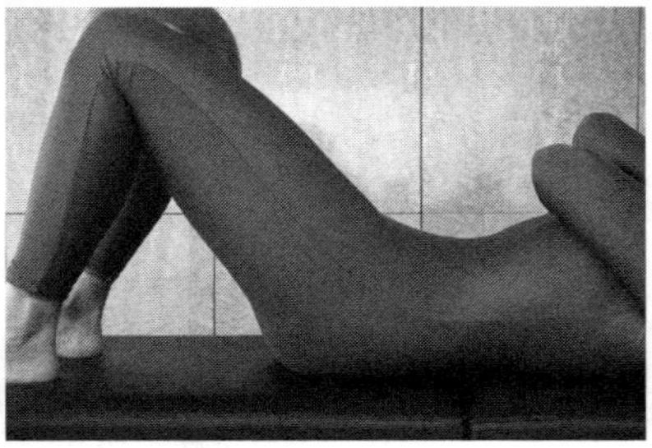

Pelvic curl
Page 45

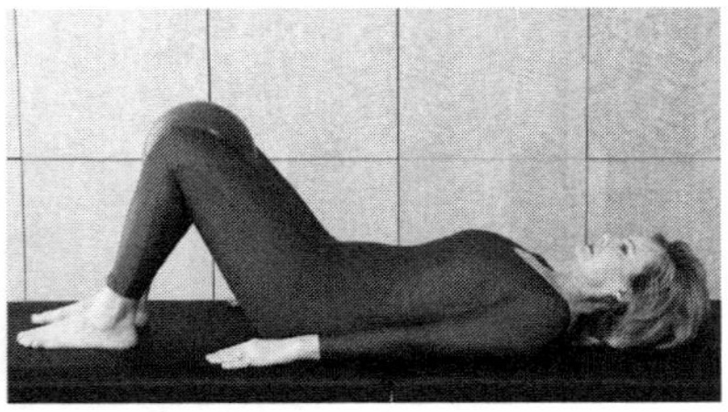

Adductor squeeze
Page 52

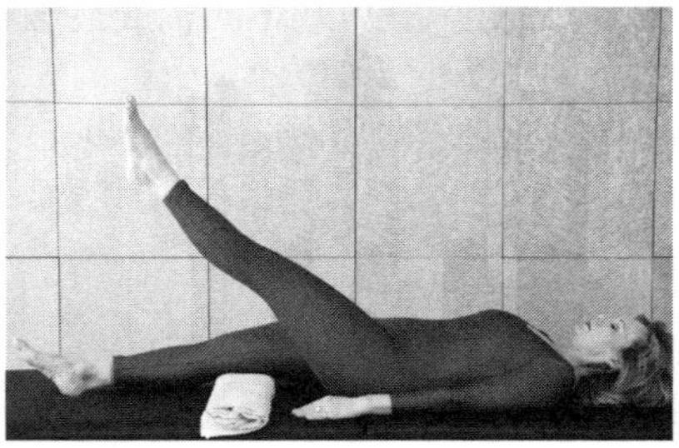

Supine leg lift
Page 53

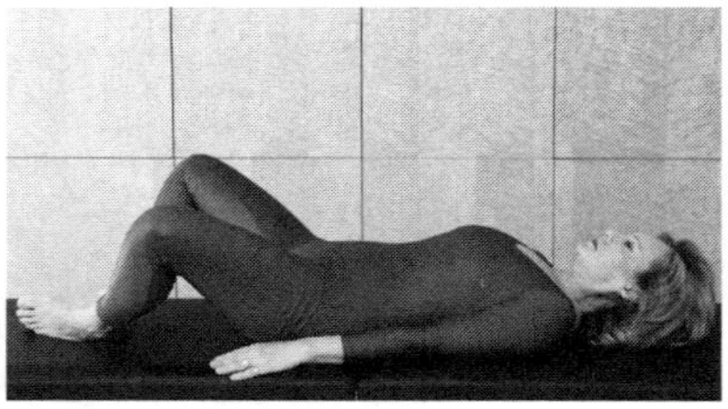

Knee fold
Page 50

Pilates Exercises

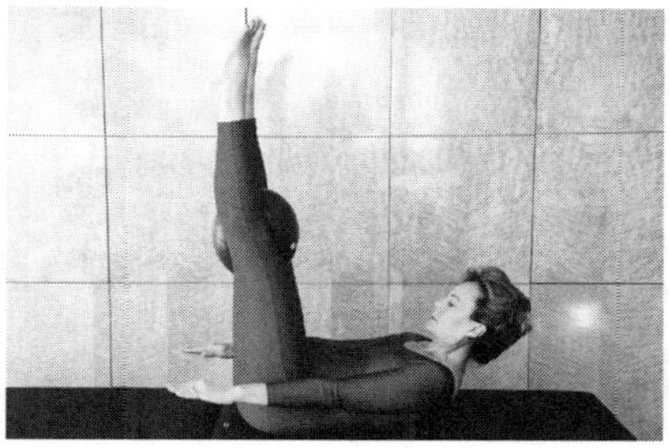

Hundred
Page 137

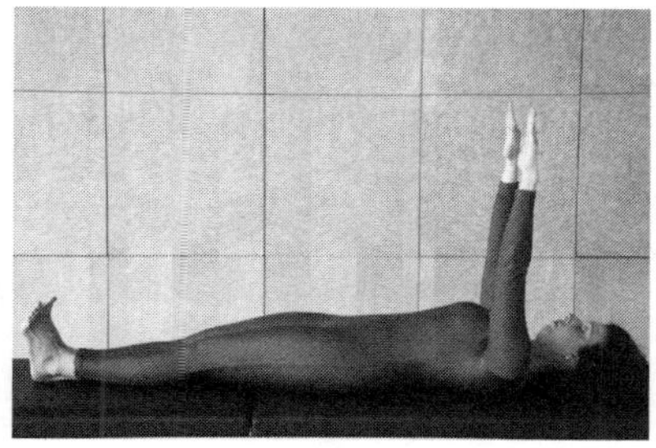

Roll-up
Page 147

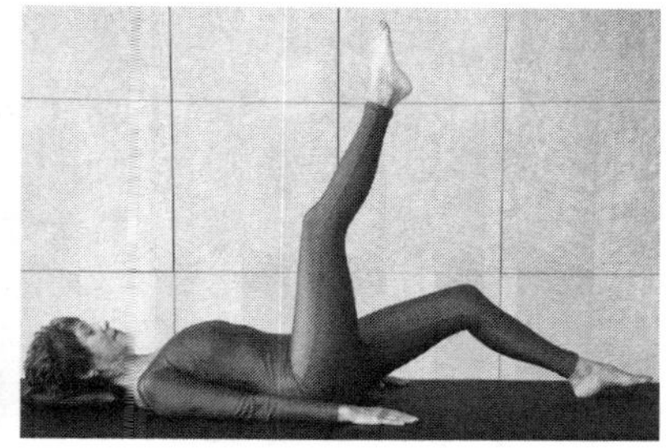

Single-leg circle
Page 152

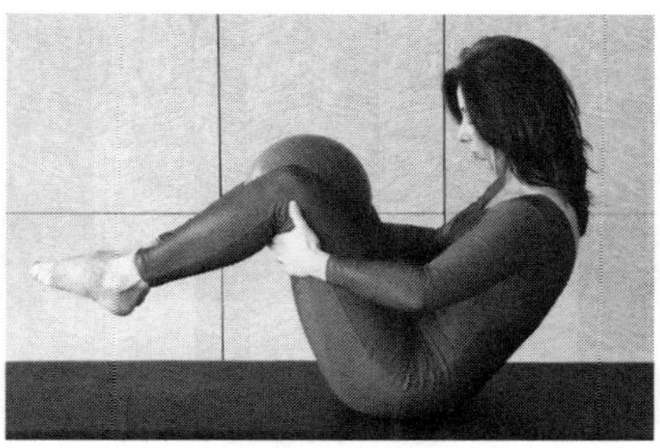

Rolling like a ball
Page 159

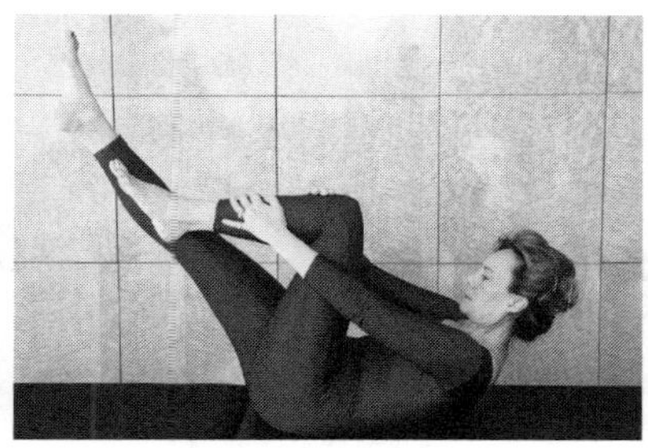

Single-leg stretch
Page 160

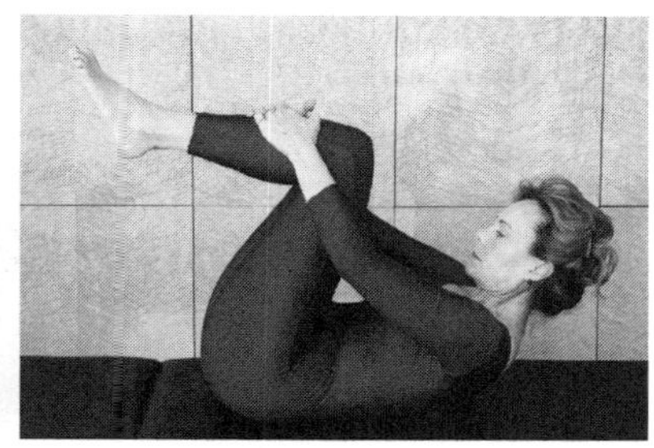

Double-leg stretch
Page 166

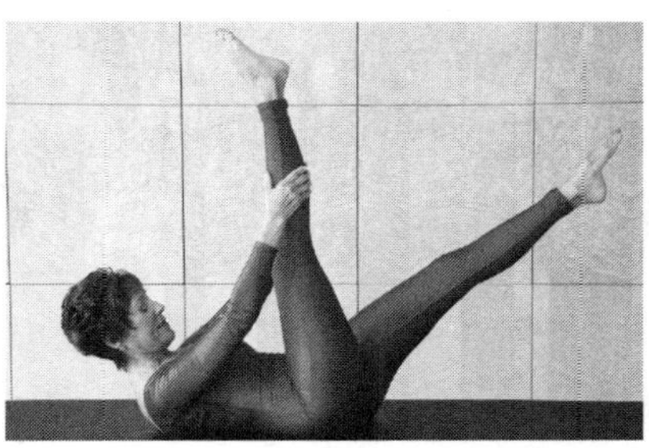

Scissors
Page 168

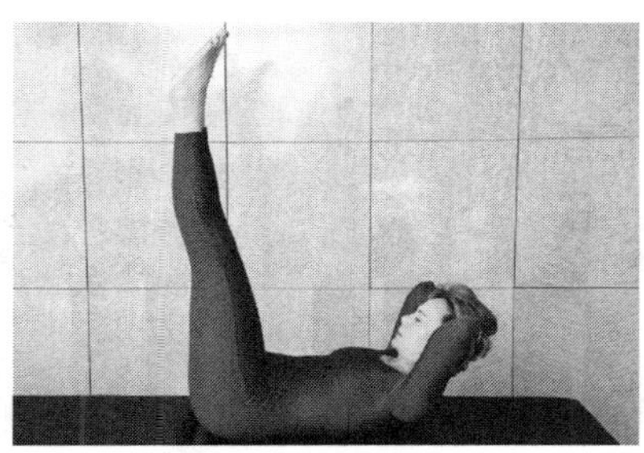

Lower lift
Page 171

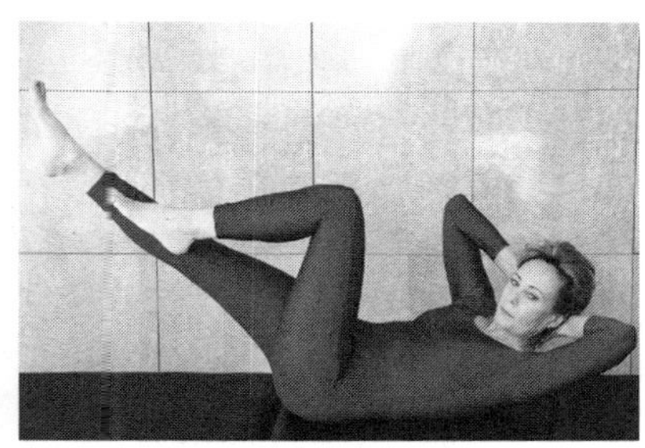

Crisscross
Page 174

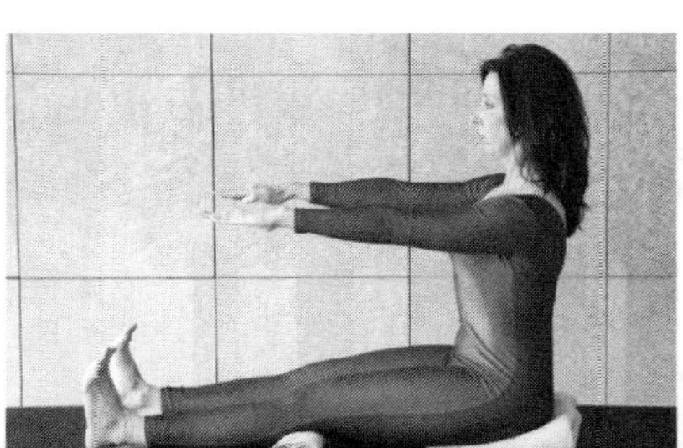

Spine stretch forward
Page 177

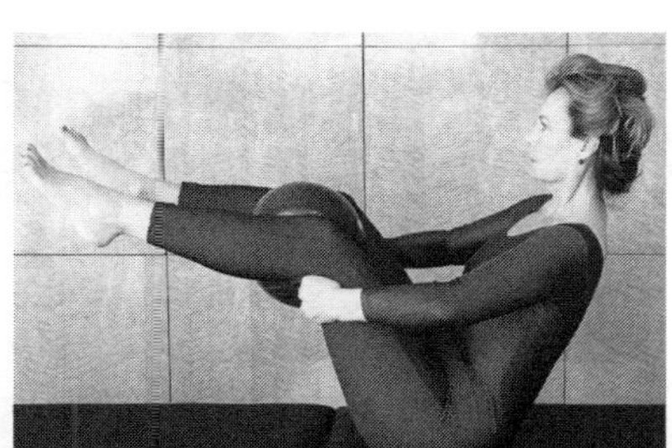

Open-leg rocker
Page 179

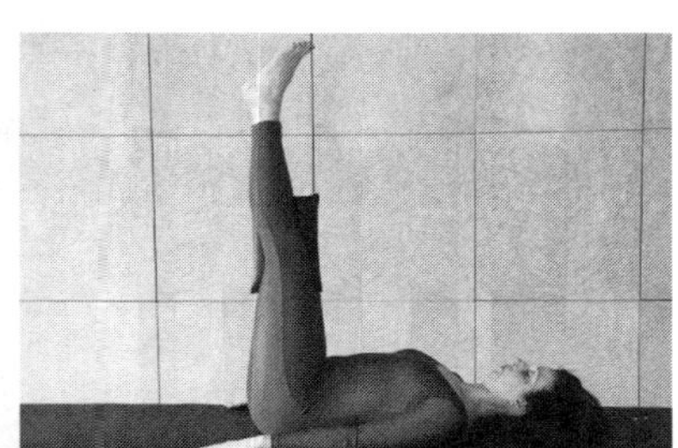

Corkscrew
Page 185

(continued)

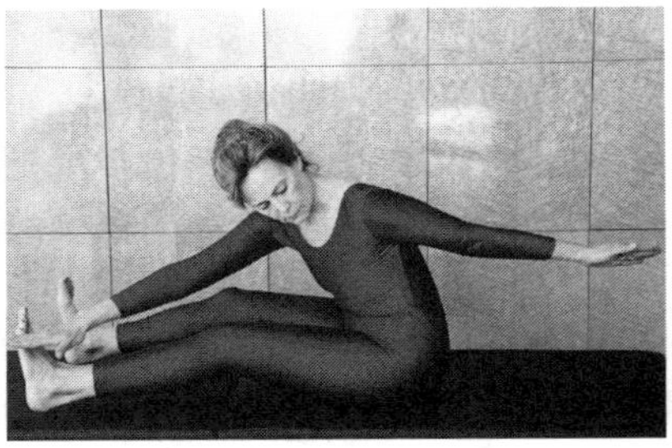

Saw
Page 187

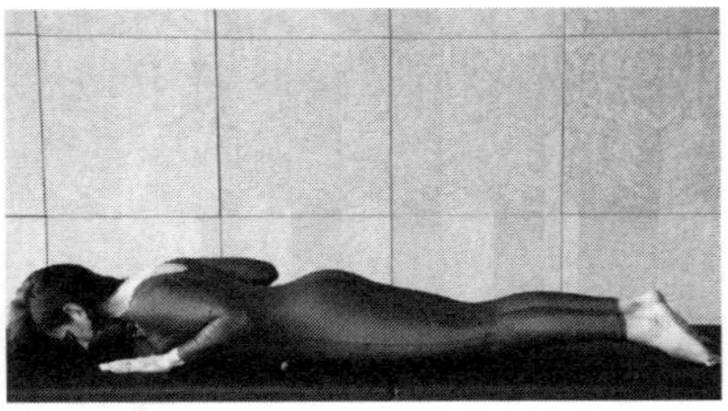

Swan
Page 193

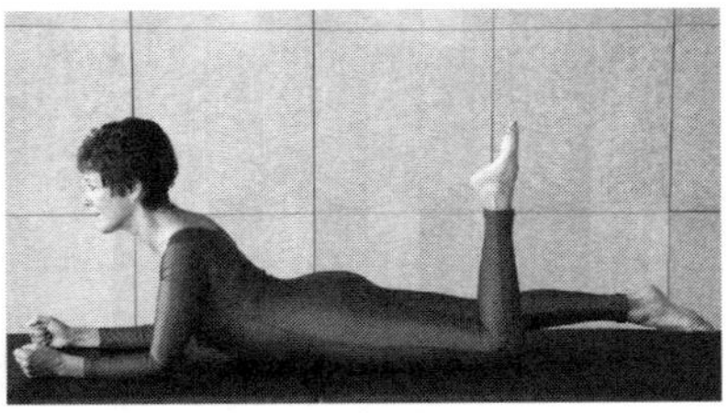

Single-leg kick
Page 196

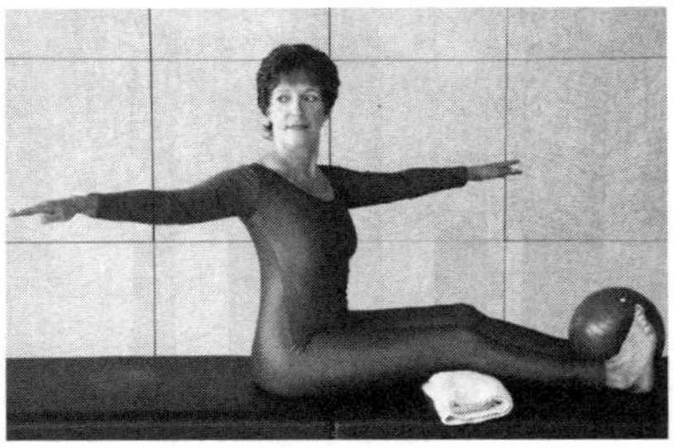

Spine twist
Page 201

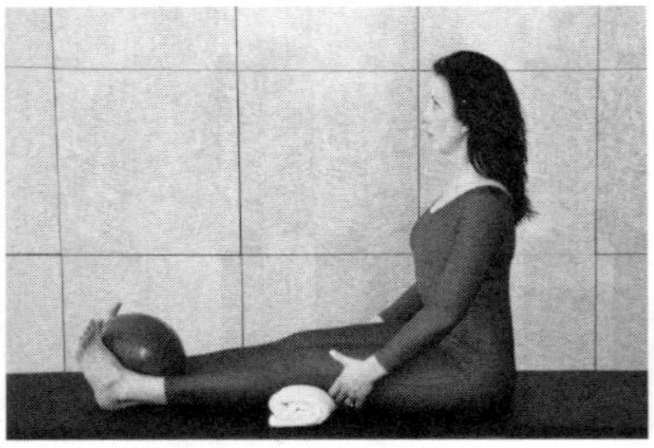

Neck pull (modified), 3 to 6 months postop version
Page 204

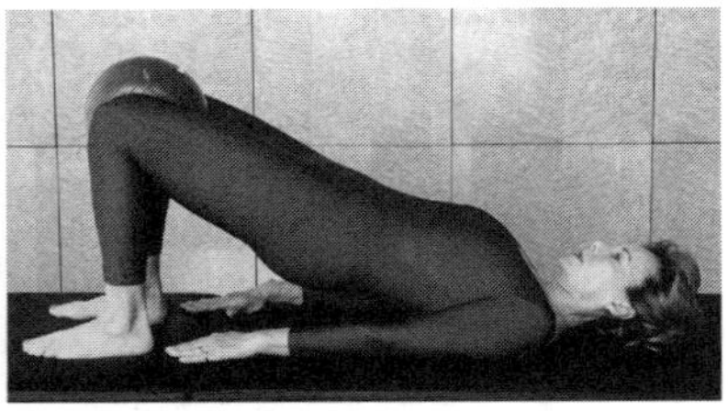

Shoulder bridge
Page 211

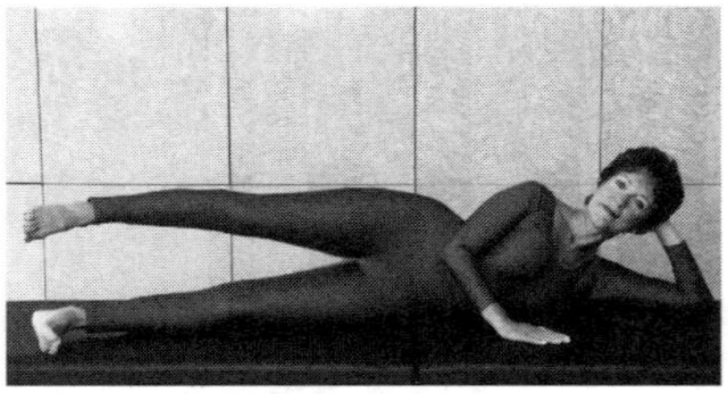

SKS, up and down
Page 272

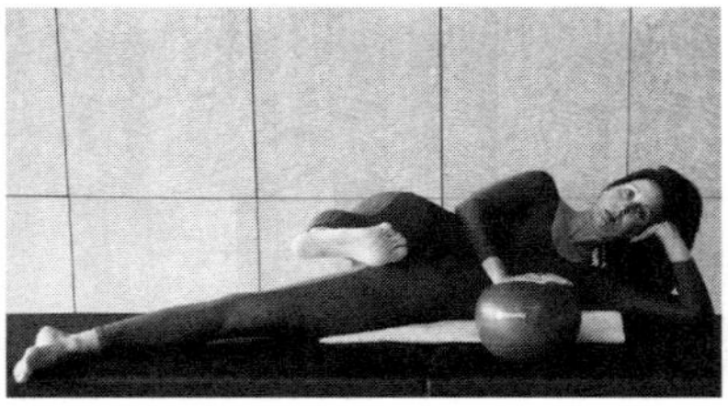

SKS, front and back
Page 276

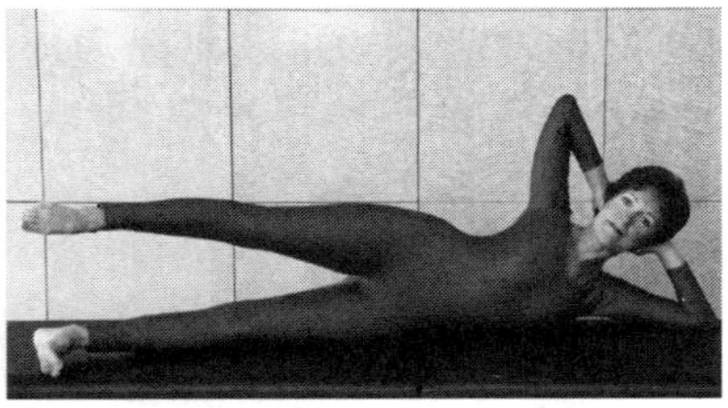

SKS, little circle
Page 279

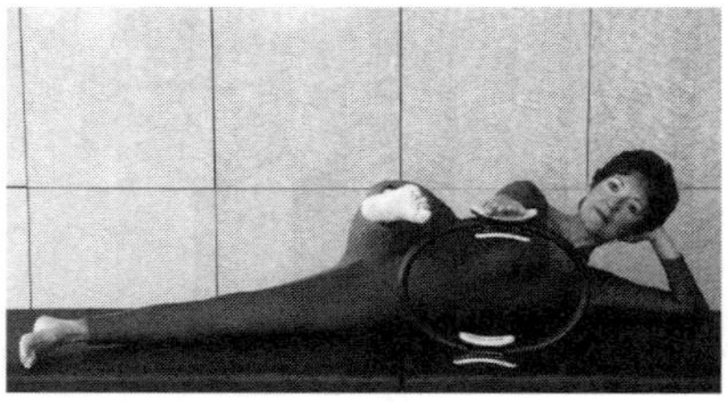

SKS, D-circle
Page 281

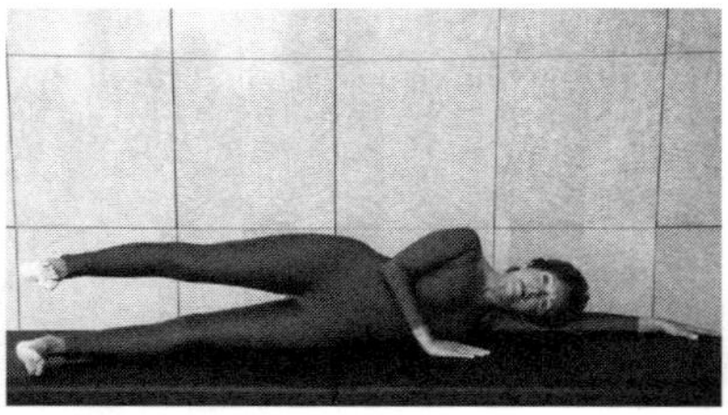

SKS, internal and external rotation, slightly flexed knee (not pictured)
Page 285

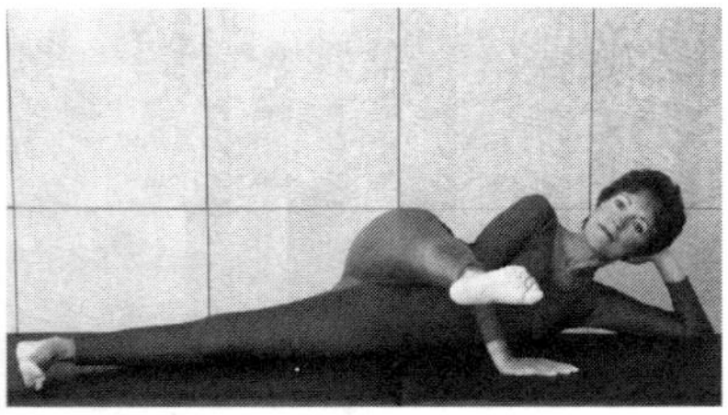

SKS, bicycle
Page 287

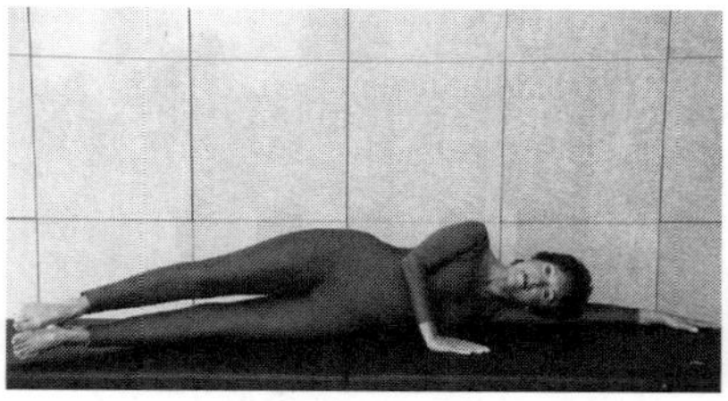

SKS, lift, lift, lower, lower
Page 293

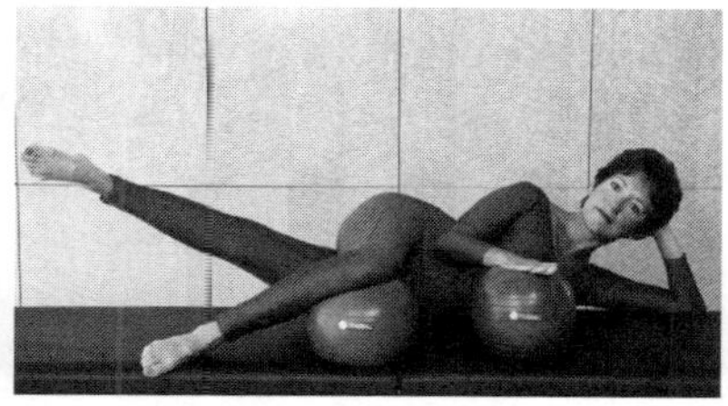

SKS, inner-thigh lift
Page 300

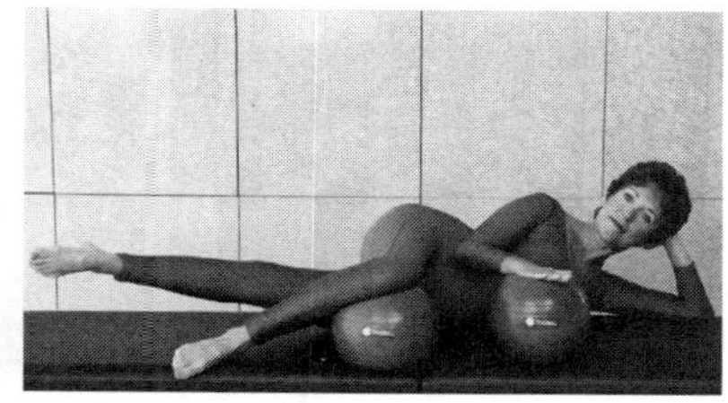

SKS, inner-thigh circle
Page 302

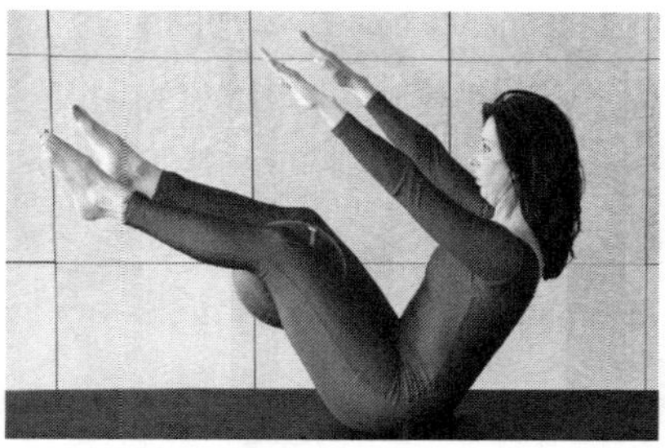

Teaser 1
Page 223

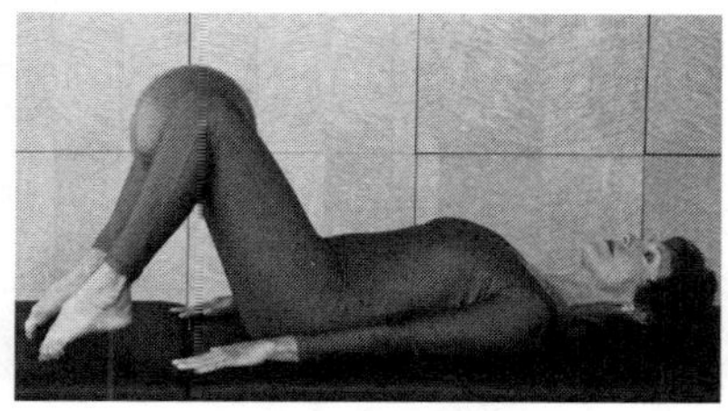

Cancan (modified)
Page 236

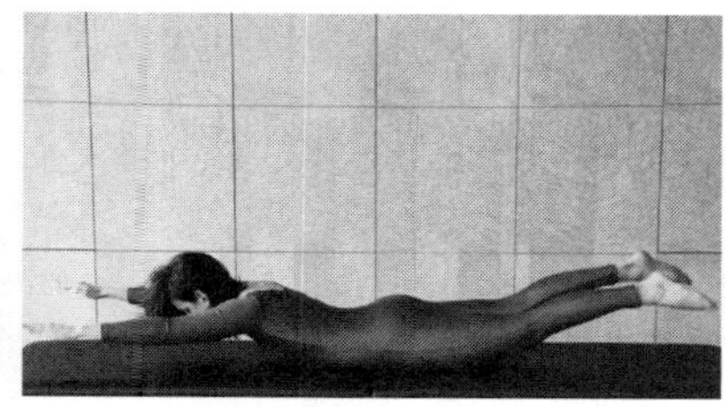

Swimming
Page 239

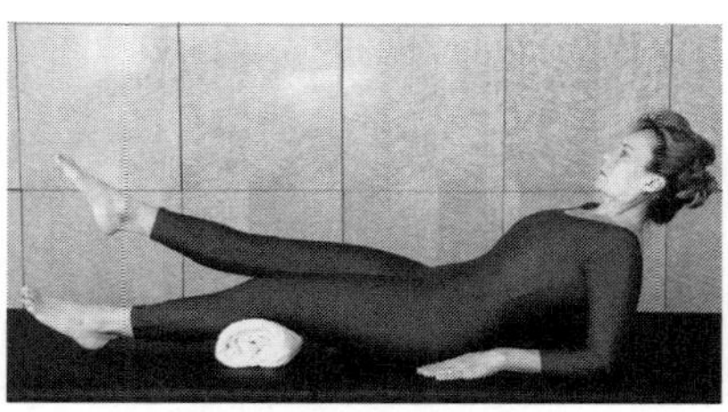

Leg pull (modified)
Page 243

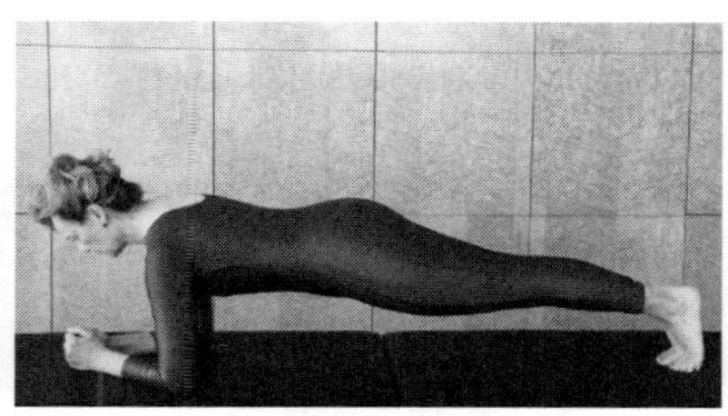

Serratus push-up
Page 254

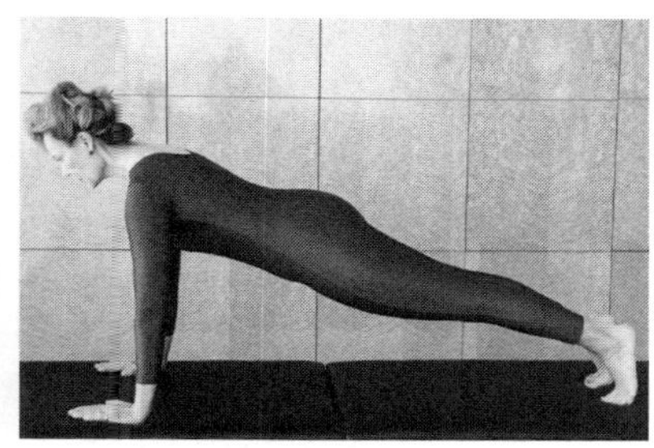

Push-up
Page 260

Glossary

abduction—A movement of a part of the body away from the midline (central axis) of the body. An example is lying supine on the mat and sliding the right leg out away from the midline of the body.

active movement—A voluntary movement that is actively performed by clients. Active movements have special value in that they combine tests of joint range, control, muscle power, and a patient's willingness to perform a movement (Magee 2008).

active movement of the hip, normal ranges—Flexion (in supine position with knee flexed) of 110° to 120°, extension (in prone position with leg extended) of 10° to 15°, abduction (in supine position) of 30° to 50°, adduction (in supine position) of 30°, lateral rotation (in supine, prone, or sitting position) of 40° to 60°, and medial rotation (in supine, prone, or sitting position) of 30° to 40° (Magee 2008).

active movement of the knee, normal ranges—Flexion (in supine position) of 0° to 135° (0° being straight knee), extension (in supine position) of 0° to 15° (in women with hyperextended knees, or genu recurvatum, the active extension can be up to –15°), medial rotation (in non-weight-bearing position) of the tibia on the femur of 20° to 30°, and lateral rotation (in non-weight-bearing position) of the tibia on the femur of 30° to 40° (Magee 2008).

adduction—A movement of a part of the body toward the midline (central axis) of the body. An example is lying supine on the mat and sliding the right leg in toward the midline of the body.

anatomical position—The standard anatomical position is standing upright with the feet parallel, the arms hanging by the sides of the body, and the palms and face directed forward.

antalgic gait—A limp in which a phase of the gait is shortened on the injured side to alleviate the pain experienced when bearing weight on that side.

articulation—A joint or juncture between bones or cartilages. Bones are joined to one another in several ways to permit a great variety of movement. Where free movement is essential, the articulating ends of the bones are shaped and the joint constructed to permit and even facilitate motion.

bursa—A small fluid-filled sac that reduces friction between two structures.

cartilage—Shiny and white connective tissue that covers the articulating surfaces of bones. Cartilage can be damaged by trauma or excessive wear. Rheumatoid arthritis and osteoarthritis are two common diseases that damage cartilage.

concentric contraction—A type of muscle contraction in which the muscle shortens while generating force. A concentric contraction of the hamstrings bends the leg at the knee and moves the heel of the foot toward the buttocks against the force of a spring or weight.

coronal plane—Also known as the *frontal plane*, the coronal plane is any plane perpendicular to the median plane. It divides the body into anterior and posterior parts. Movements in this plane are adduction and abduction and lateral flexion.

crepitation—A dry sound such as that of grating the ends of a fractured bone. Also an audible or palpable crunching movement of tendons or ligaments over bone.

diarthroses joints—Joints, such as the hip and knee joints, in which a small space, or joint cavity, exists between the articulating surfaces of the two bones that form the joint. Because there is a cavity and there is no tissue growing between the articulating surfaces, the surfaces are free to move against one another. A thin layer of hyaline cartilage covers the surfaces of the articulating bones and a sleevelike, fibrous capsule lined with smooth, slippery synovial membrane cases the joint. The capsule contains synovial fluid. The fluid lubricates and provides nutrients to the cartilage. Diarthroses joints are freely movable joints.

disassociation—The act of separating related items or the isolation of movement. For instance, disassociation is needed to keep the pelvis steady on the mat while performing a single-leg circle. The ball (head of the femur) moves freely within the socket (acetabulum) of the hip. Another example is performing a side kick front and back while keeping the torso stable on the mat.

distal—Toward the end of a structure or farther away from the core of the body. Distal is the opposite of proximal.

eccentric contraction—A type of muscle contraction in which the muscle elongates while under tension due to the opposing force being greater than the force generated by the muscle. An eccentric contraction of the hamstrings extends the knee and moves the heel of the foot away from the buttocks while opposing the force of the springs or weights.

extension—A movement in the sagittal plane that takes a part of the body backward in relation to its anatomical position. Examples of extension include the swan, single-leg kick, double-leg kick, and lying prone on the mat with the arms long by the sides of the body and lifted away from the mat. It also means to extend or lengthen on the mat. When performed from the flexed position, extension restores a part to its anatomical position.

external rotation—Also called *lateral rotation*, rotation away from the center of the body.

flexion—A movement in the sagittal plane that takes a part of the body forward in relation to its anatomical position. Flexion decreases the angle between the anterior surfaces of articulated bones. The exception to this rule is the movement at the knee and toe joints; these joints decrease the angle of the posterior surfaces of the articulated bones. Flexing movements are bending or folding movements.

flexion contracture of the hip—A loss of hip range of motion, when compared with normal hip range of motion, most likely due to osteoarthritis, hip disease, or structural issues.

genu valgum—"Knock knees," a lateral displacement of the distal end of the distal bone in the joint (Beil 2005).

genu varum—"Bow legs," a medial displacement of the distal end of the distal bone of the joint (Beil 2005).

Gerby's tubercle—A lateral tubercle of the tibia, located where the tensor fasciae latae and iliotibial band insert.

internal rotation—Also called *medial rotation*, rotation toward the center of the body.

intra-articular—Something that is situated within or occurring within the joint surface. Joints can be classified based on their articulation surfaces. A complex joint (e.g., the knee joint) involves two or more articular surfaces and an articular disc or meniscus.

isometric—An increase in tension without change in muscle length.

kyphosis—A condition characterized by an abnormally increased convexity in the curvature of the thoracic spine as viewed from the side.

ligament—A fibrous connective tissue that connects bone to bone.

lordosis—An abnormally increased concavity in the curvature of the lumbar spine as viewed from the side.

prone—Lying face down on the mat on the belly.

proximal—Near the center of the body or the point of attachment of a structure that is closer to the core of the body. Proximal is the opposite of distal.

range of motion (ROM)—How much movement a part of the body can execute. Joint ROM is the distance and direction a joint can move to its full potential. Joint ROM is affected by the muscles, bones, ligaments, and fascia.

sagittal plane—The median plane of the body; it divides the body into right and left halves. This plane can be represented by drawing a line down the middle of the body from the crown of the head through the belly button and pubic bone and between the legs to the floor. Movements in this plane are flexion and extension.

supine—Lying face up on the mat on your back.

synovial joint—A joint containing a lubricating substance (synovial fluid) and lined with a synovial membrane or capsule.

tendon—A fibrous tissue connecting skeletal muscle to bone.

transverse plane—The plane that divides the body into superior and inferior (upper and lower) parts. Movements in this plane are medial and lateral rotation.

Trendelenburg gait—An abnormal gait associated with a weakness of the hip abductor muscles (gluteus medius and minimus); characterized by a drop in the pelvis on the unaffected side of the body at the moment of the heel strike on the affected side. If there is bilateral weakness of the abductors, the gait shows a side-to-side movement, resulting in a wobbling gait (Magee 2008).

Movement and Cueing Vocabulary

articulation—A movement of the spine in which each vertebra touches the mat one at a time. This is in contrast to moving in one segment (e.g., roll-down on the mat in flexion or swan in extension).

C-curve—The shape of the spine when creating a curl off the sit bones with a deep scoop in the abdominals or rounding the back in flexion (e.g., half roll-down).

core stability—The ability to maintain a neutral spine with the abdominals drawn in and up while performing a Pilates movement.

curl the head, neck, and shoulders up off the mat—In preparation for the supine Pilates abdominal movements, curl the upper body up off the mat to the bottom tips of the shoulder blades, gaze toward the core, and keep a space the size of a tangerine between the chin and the chest.

draw the abdominals in and up—Draw the abdominals in toward the spine. This is best achieved during the exhale of the breath cycle, especially when first learning Pilates. It helps to engage the deep abdominal muscles to hold in the viscera and decrease the abdominal wall. The goal is to engage and activate the obliques and transverse abdominis, which in turn support the back. Other cues are to scoop the abdominals in and up, melt the navel to the spine, and draw the powerhouse in and up.

legs in tabletop position—Lying supine on the mat with the knees and feet up off the mat. The knees are bent to 90° of flexion and the hips are bent to 90° of flexion. The hips are in line with the knees and the knees are in line with the ankles. The shins are parallel to the floor and the thighs are vertical to the wall.

lengthen—This term has several meanings. Working to a full range of motion creates length. In this book the term is used in visual and verbal cues: Lengthen out on the mat, lengthen out of the hip, reach out as if you were trying to touch the wall, feel opposition through lengthening, imagine one arrow of energy pointing through the foot and one pointing through the crown of the head.

lever length—Lever length is adjusted by extending a limb away from the core or shortening a limb to bring it closer to the core. For instance, in the Pilates side kick series, performing the movements with the legs long on the mat lengthens the lever to make a movement more challenging or bending the legs shortens the lever in order to reduce the stress on the joint.

make a diamond with the hands—Position the hands flat on the mat under or in front of the tailbone (toward the feet), with the fingers open and the thumbs and first fingers touching to create a diamond shape.

make a pillow with the hands—Place one hand over the other to create a pillow with the hands. Place the forehead on the pillow (hands).

neutral spine—The position of the spine when the pubic bone and hip bones (anterior superior iliac spine, or ASIS) are on the same plane. The neutral spine is the ideal position of the spine in standing, when the natural curves of the spine work like shock absorbers. For example, when you are lying supine on the mat with the knees bent, hip-distance apart, and parallel, two spaces of the back should not be touching: the back of the neck and the waist (low back).

opposition—To create opposition through movement. Cues are to reach long with the arms as you draw the abdominals in deep in opposition from the reach; lengthen out as if you could touch the wall with your foot, lift the abdominals in and up, and lengthen through your crown in opposition; and as you twist to the right, draw your left hip back in opposition to the twist.

Pilates stance—Standing with the heels together and toes apart so that the feet form a small V. The inner-thigh and gluteal muscles are engaged and the abdominals are drawn in and up.

powerhouse—The core of the body, including but not limited to the transverses abdominis, internal and external obliques, lumbar multificus, pelvic floor, and diaphragm as well as the gluteus maximus, gluteus medius, and quadratus lumborum. Muscles that contribute to core stability via a neurophysiological connection include the hip adductors (Smith 2005).

qualified instructor—An instructor who has earned a diploma or certificate from a school by completing the training hours and all that that entails and completing a final exam at the end of the course.

shoulders drawn back and down—Drawing the shoulders away from the ears as if suspenders were attached to the bottom tips of the shoulder blades and to the hips. Learning to draw the shoulders back and down is important for learning to keep proper alignment while sitting and standing. The shoulders should never be lifted toward the ears and neck.

sit bones—Also called the *sitz bones*, the ischial tuberosity (bent portion of the ischium), or the bones under the flesh that you sit on.

torso stability—Important for many Pilates exercises, the ability to not move a part of the body while another part is challenging it. For example, when performing the lower lift, it is important to draw the abdominals in and up and maintain torso stability as the legs lower away from the core to 45° and lift back up to 90°. The low back should not lift away from the neutral spine as the legs lower and challenge the core musculature. It is important to know your end range in order to maintain the torso stability.

working in neutral spine with the tailbone long on the mat—When performing many of the Pilates exercises, working in a neutral spine is preferred. However, when first learning how to engage the core, beginners often curl their tailbone up, creating a tuck in the lower spine to flatten the back. The goal is to work in a neutral spine to strengthen the natural curves of the back. These curves work as shock absorbers for the spine and provide an environment that places the least amount of stress on the muscles and bones.

Using the Web Resource

An added bonus of *Pilates for Hip and Knee Syndromes and Arthroplasties* is the available web resource material. The web resource provides guidelines, in PDF format, on using all of the Pilates equipment to devise a safe program for clients with hip or knee syndromes or replacements. It outlines what equipment is appropriate to incorporate at the optimal time for rehabilitation. This information is for the fully trained Pilates equipment instructor. In addition, a set of comprehensive resources is included to guide you in finding a qualified Pilates training program and a qualified Pilates instructor. The Web resource can be accessed at www.HumanKinetics.com/PilatesForHipAndKneeSyndromesAndArthroplasties.

Bibliography

American Sports Data. www.americansportsdata.com; 2008.

Anthony CKN. *Textbook of Anatomy and Phsiology.* St. Louis: Mosby; 1971.

Archibeck MJ. Soft-tissue disorders about the hip. In: Callaghan JJ, Rosenberg AG, Rubash HE, eds. *The Adult Hip.* Vol 1. 2nd ed. Philadelphia: Lippincott Williams & Wilkins; 2007:598-604.

Berger RA, Jacobs JJ, Meneghini RM, Della Valle C, Paprosky W, Rosenberg AG. Rapid rehabilitation and recovery with minimally invasive total hip arthroplasty. *Clin Orthop and Relat Res.* 2004;429:239-247.

Biel A. *Trail Guide to the Body.* 3rd ed. Boulder, CO: Books of Discovery; 2005.

Bird PA, Oakley SP, Shnier R, Kirkham BW. Prospective evaluation of magnetic resonance imaging and physical examination findings in patients with greater trochanteric pain syndrome. *Arthritis Rheum.* 2001;44(9):2138-2145.

Brosseau L, MacLeay L, Robinson V, Wells G, Tugwell P. Intensity of exercise for the treatment of osteoarthritis. *Cochrane Database Syst Rev.* 2003;2:CD004259.

Brugioni DJ, Falkel J. *Total Knee Replacement and Rehabilitation.* Alameda, CA: Hunter House; 2004.

Calais-Germain B. *Anatomy of Movement.* Seattle: Eastland Press; 1993, 2007.

Calais-Germain B. *Anatomy of Movement.* Seattle: Eastland Press; 2007:192-255.

Ege Rasmussen KJ, Fano N. Trochanteric bursitis. Treatment by corticosteroid injection. *Scand J Rheumatol.* 1985;14(4):417-420.

Franklin E. *Dynamic Alignment Through Imagery.* Champaign, IL: Human Kinetics; 1996.

Frintze M, Voogt T. *Pilates Triadball Manual.* Minneapolis, MN: Orthopedic Physical Therapy Products; 2009.

Grindulis KA. Rheumatoid iliopsoas bursitis. *J Rheumatol.* 1986;13(5):988.

Heaton K, Dorr LD. Surgical release of iliopsoas tendon for groin pain after total hip arthroplasty. *J Arthroplasty.* 2002;17(6):779-781.

Herman E. *Pilates Cadillac* San Fransisco: Ellie Herman Books; 2006.

Herman E. *Pilates Workbook on the Ball.* Berkeley, CA: Ulysses Press; 2004.

Johnston CA, Lindsay DM, Wiley JP. Treatment of iliopsoas syndrome with a hip rotation strengthening program: A retrospective case series. *J Orthop Sports Phys Ther.* 1999;29(4):218-224.

Johnston CA, Wiley JP, Lindsay DM, Wiseman DA. Iliopsoas bursitis and tendinitis. A review. *Sports Med.* 1998;25(4):271-283.

Klein GR, Levine BR, Hozack WJ, Strauss EJ, D'Antonio JA, Macaulay W, Di Cesare PE. Return to athletic activity after total hip arthroplasty. Consensus guidelines based on a survey of the Hip Society and American Association of Hip and Knee Surgeons. *J Arthroplasty.* 2007;22(2):171-175.

Kurtz S, Mowat F, Ong K, Chan N, Lau E, Halpern M. Prevalence of primary and revision total hip and knee arthroplasty in the United States from 1990 through 2002. *J Bone Joint Surg Am.* 2005;87(7):1487-1497.

Kurtz S, Ong K, Lau E, Mowat F, Halpern M. Projections of primary and revision hip and knee arthroplasty in the United States from 2005 to 2030. *J Bone Joint Surg Am.* 2007;89(4):780-785.

Kurtz SM, Ong KL, Schmier J, Kurtz SM, Ong KL, Schmier J, Mowat F, Saleh K, Dybvik E, Kärrholm J, Garellick G, Havelin LI, Furnes O, Malchau H, Lau E. Future clinical and economic impact of revision total hip and knee arthroplasty. *J Bone Joint Surg Am.* 2007;89(suppl 3):144-151.

Lachiewicz PF, Kauk JR. Anterior iliopsoas impingement and tendinitis after total hip arthroplasty. *J Am Acad Orthop Surg.* 2009;17(6):337-344.

Levine B, Kaplanek B, Scafura D, Jaffe WL. Rehabilitation after total hip and knee arthroplasty: A new regimen using Pilates training. *Bull NYU Hosp Jt Dis.* 2007;65(2):120-125.

Levine BR, Jaffe WJ, Kaplanek BA. Pilates training for use in rehabilitation after total hip and knee arthroplasty: A preliminary report. *Clin Orthop and Relat Res.* 2009;467(6):1468-1475.

Magee DJ. *Orthopedic Physical Assessment.* 5th ed. St. Louis: Saunders; 2008:659-843.

Mullins MM, Norbury W, Dowell JK, Heywood-Waddington M. Thirty-year results of a prospective study of Charnley total hip arthroplasty by the posterior approach. *J Arthroplasty.* 2007;22(6):833-839.

Pilates J, Miller JM. *Return to Life Through Contrology.* Miami, FL: Pilates Method Alliance; 1945:15-32.

Pilates Method Alliance. *The PMA Pilates Certification Exam Study Guide.* Miami, FL: Pilates Method Alliance; 2005:17-18.

Pilot P, Bogie R, Draijer WF, Verburg AD, Van Os JJ, Kuipers H. Experience in the first four years of rapid recovery: Is it safe? *Injury.* 2006;37(suppl 5):S37-40.

Shbeeb MI, Matteson EL. Trochanteric bursitis (greater trochanter pain syndrome). *Mayo Clin Proc.* 1996;71(6):565-569.

Siller B. *The Pilates Body.* New York: Broadway Books; 2000:1-5.

Smith ESK. *Pilates for Rehab: A Guidebook to Integrating Pilates in Patient Care.* Minneapolis: OPTP; 2005.

Toohey AK, LaSalle TL, Martinez S, Polisson RP. Iliopsoas bursitis: Clinical features, radiographic findings, and disease associations. *Semin Arthritis Rheum.* 1990;20(1):41-47.

Ungaro A. *The Pilates Promise.* New York: DK; 2004:12-13.

Wroblewski BM, Fleming PA, Siney PD. Charnley low-frictional torque arthroplasty of the hip. 20-to-30 year results. *J Bone Joint Surg Br.* 1999;81(3):427-430.

Wunderbaldinger P, Bremer C, Schellenberger E, Cejna M, Turetschek K, Kainberger F. Imaging features of iliopsoas bursitis. *Eur Radiol.* 2002;12(2):409-415.

About the Authors

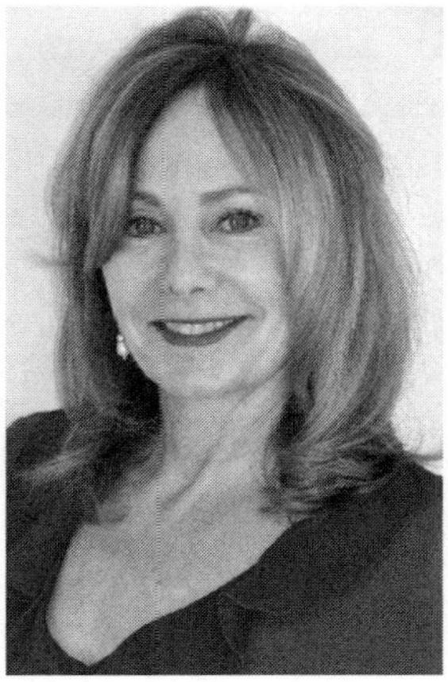

Courtesy of Beth Kaplanek

Beth A. Kaplanek, RN, BSN, is a Pilates instructor and practitioner of Pilates for rehabilitation at the Pilates Center of Long Island in Huntington, New York. Kaplanek served for 20 years as a registered nurse working in various capacities in emergency room care, operating room care, intensive care, drug counseling and rehabilitation, and hospice care.

After undergoing a hip replacement in 2001, Kaplanek began using Pilates as a form of low-impact exercise and strength and flexibility training. Encouraged by her physician's positive prognosis, she began researching how the Pilates method could be modified and used by people with hip or knee conditions and replacements. Kaplanek's research with Dr. Levine and Dr. Jaffe regarding Pilates as a form of postoperative rehabilitation has been published in the *Bulletin of the NYU Hospital for Joint Diseases* and *Clinical Orthopaedics and Related Research*.

Kaplanek resides in Lloyd Harbor, New York, and Coconut Grove, Florida. In her free time she enjoys designing jewelry, hiking, exercising, and attending vintage car road rallies.

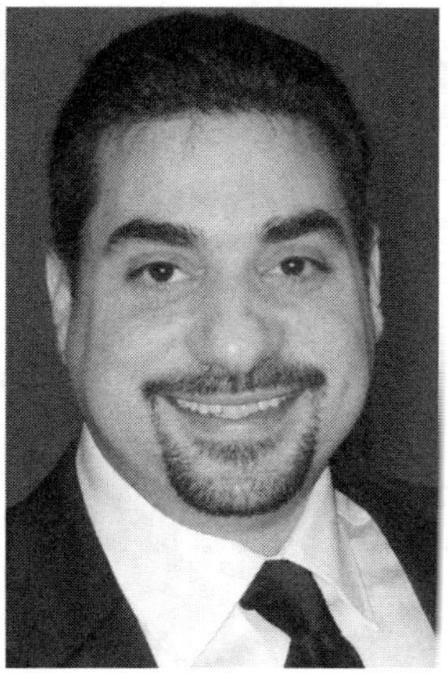

Courtesy of Brett Levine

Brett R. Levine, MD, MS, is board certified in orthopaedic surgery with a subspecialty in adult reconstruction. He is a physician and assistant professor at Rush University Medical Center in Chicago, where he specializes in complex revision hip and knee reconstruction. He also serves as clinical instructor and research coordinator for residents, fellows, and medical students.

His areas of research interest include porous biomaterials, revision hip and knee techniques and technology, metal ion levels and hypersensitivity in metal–metal bearings, cementless TKA, and digital templating accuracy. He serves on editorial boards of *Hospital Physician, Journal of Clinical Rehabilitative Tissue Engineering Research, Clinical Orthopaedics and Related Research, Orthopedics, Journal of Knee Surgery, ACTA Biomaterial*, and the *Bulletin of the NYU Hospital for Joint Diseases*. He is a member of the Mid-America Orthopaedic Association and a fellow of the American Academy of Orthopaedic Surgeons. Levine also serves as chair of the Adult Reconstruction Instructional Course Subcommittee for the American Academy of Orthopaedic Surgeons and is the editor for the *Rush Year in Review*.

Levine resides with his wife, Kari, and their two children in Elmhurst, Illinois. In his free time he enjoys reading, repairing and restoring classic automobiles, and staying physically active through exercise and sports.

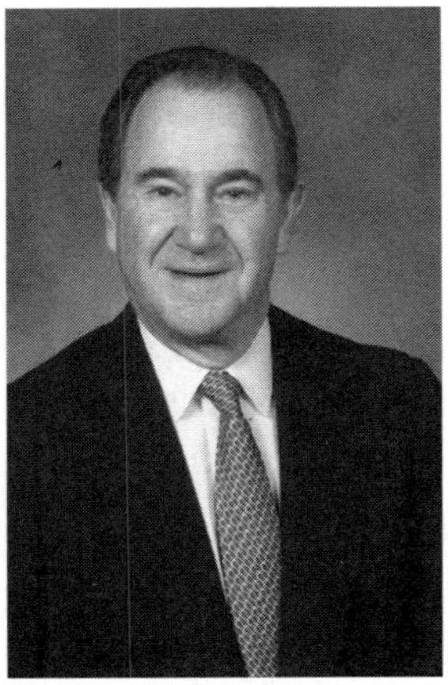

Courtesy of William Jaffe

William L. Jaffe, MD, is a clinical professor and the vice chairman of the department of orthopaedic surgery at New York University Hospital for Joint Diseases in New York City. Jaffe is also an attending orthopaedic surgeon at Bellevue Hospital Center in New York.

Jaffe has served as editor in chief of the *Bulletin of the Hospital for Joint Diseases Orthopaedic Institute* and editor for the *Mediguide to Orthopaedics*. He serves on the editorial boards for the *Journal of Arthroplasty* and *Orthopaedic Section eMedicine* as well as the medical advisory board for Osteonics Corporation in Allendale, New Jersey. He is a consultant in orthopaedic surgery for the University Grants Committee of the Research Grants Council for the Hong Kong government.

Jaffe is a fellow of the American College of Surgeons and the American Academy of Orthopaedic Surgeons. He holds membership in the American Orthopaedic Association, New York State Medical Society, New York County Medical Society, New York Academy of Medicine, Low Friction Arthroplasty Society, and Eastern Orthopaedic Association. In both 1992 and 1995, Jaffe was the recipient of Professor of the Year award from the Hospital for Joint Diseases Orthopaedic Residency Program. Jaffe was chosen as one of the 50 Most Positive Doctors in America in 1996. He resides in New York City.

Hip and Knee Anatomy

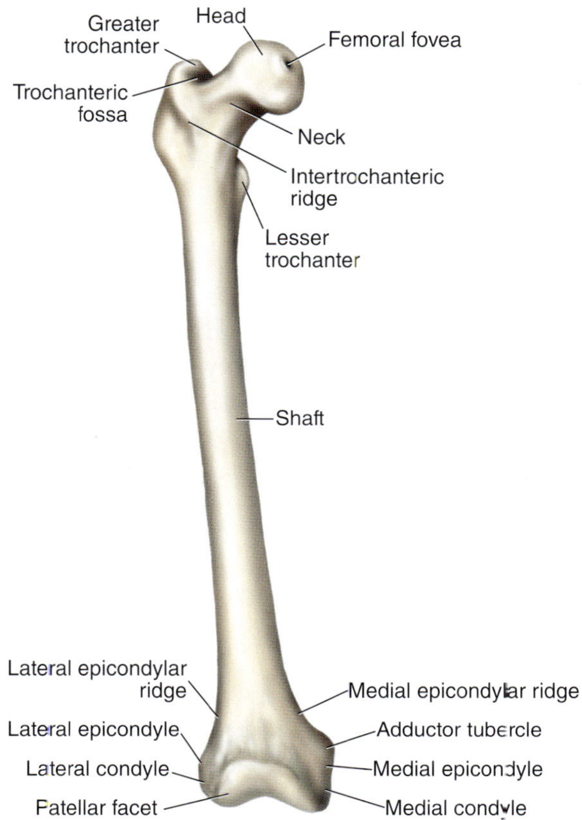

Femur, anterior view.

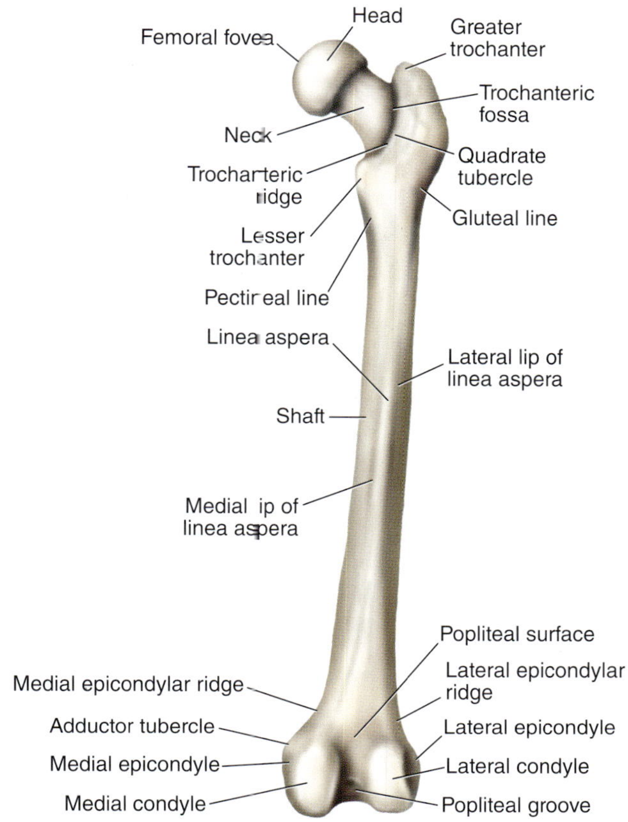

Femur, posterior view.

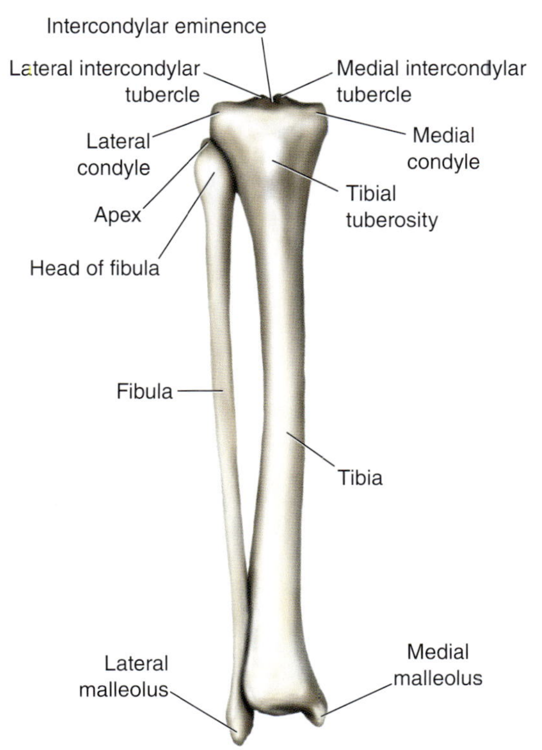

Tibia and fibulia, anterior view.

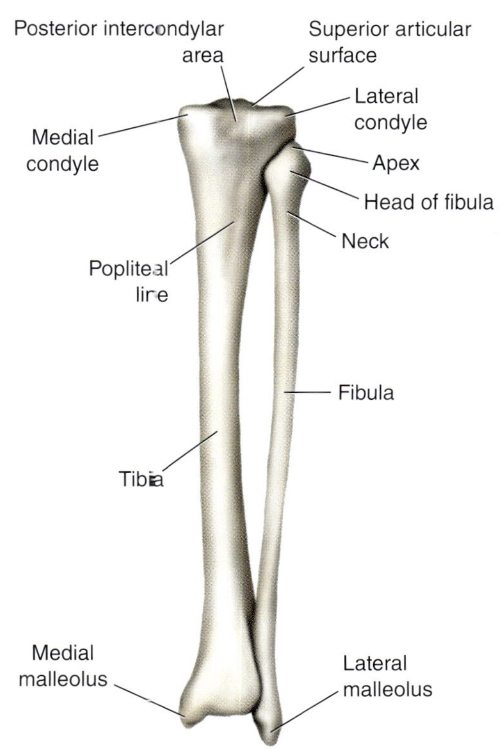

Tibia and fibulia, posterior view.

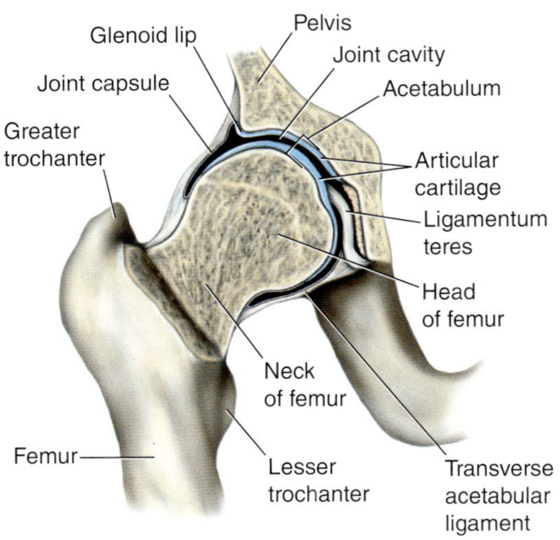

Longitudinal section of the hip joint.

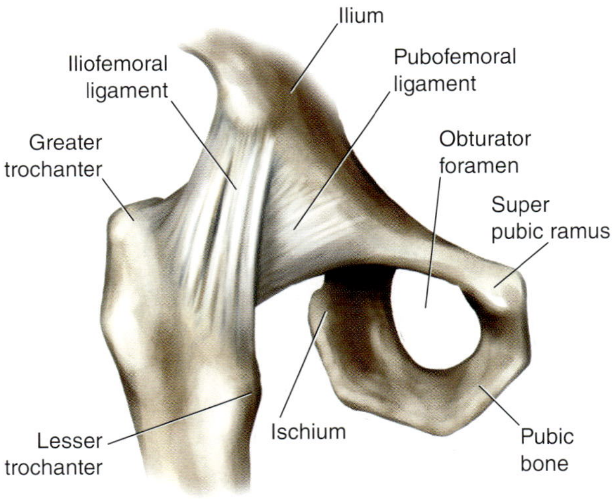

Iliofemoral and pubofemoral ligaments, anterior view.

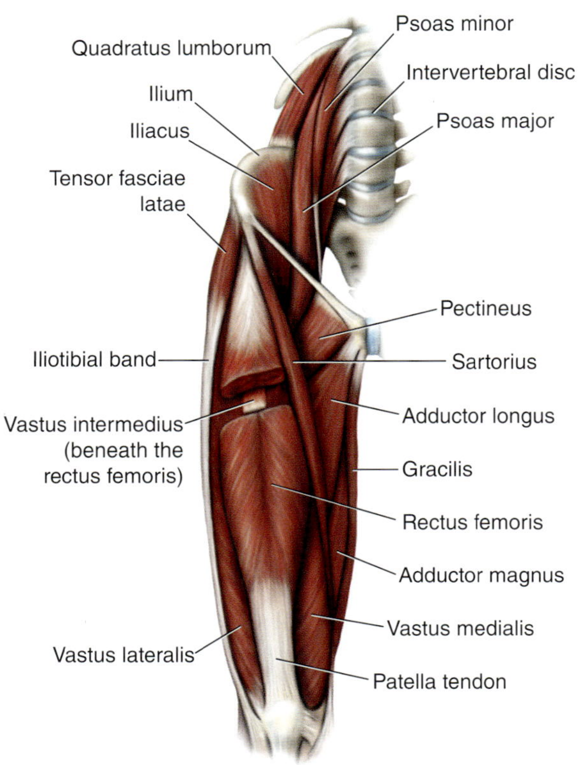

Anterior muscles of the hip.

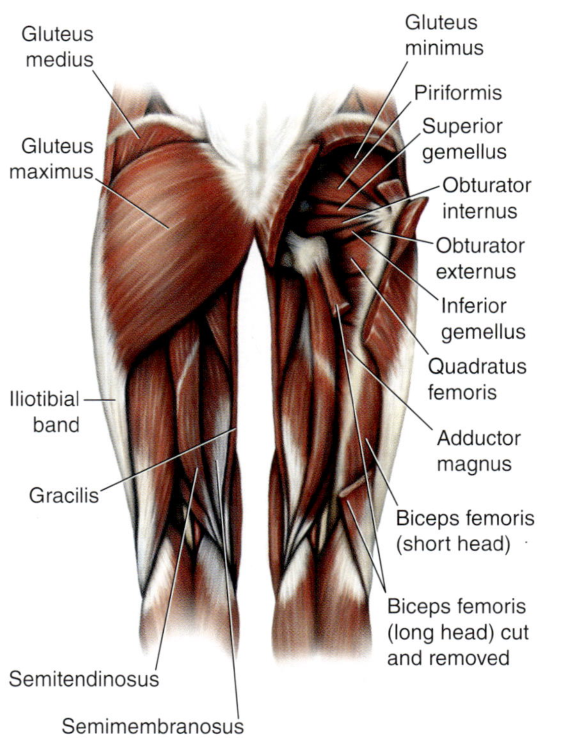

Posterior muscles of the hip.

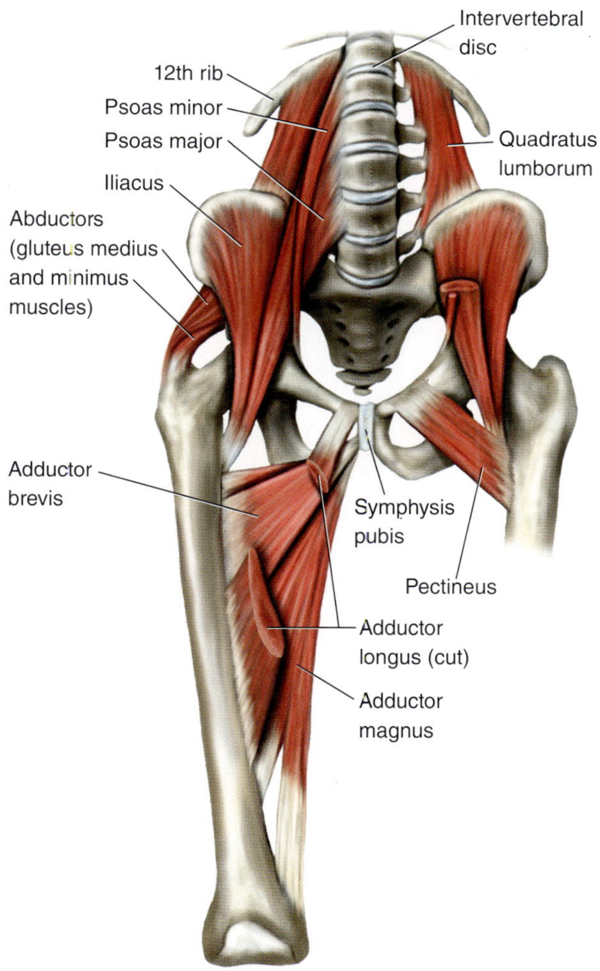

Psoas major, psoas minor, and iliacus.

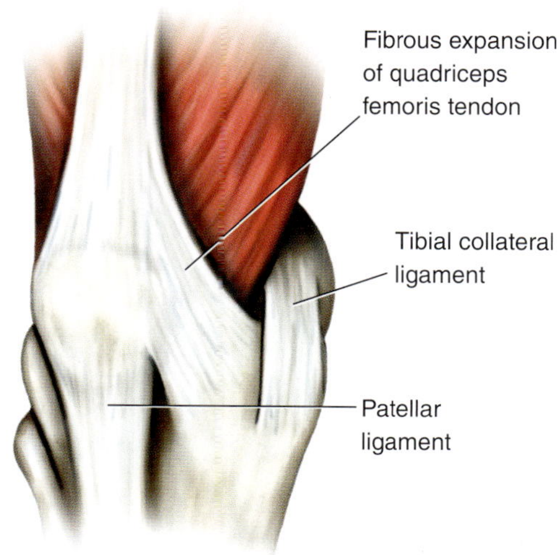

Ligaments of the knee, anterior view.

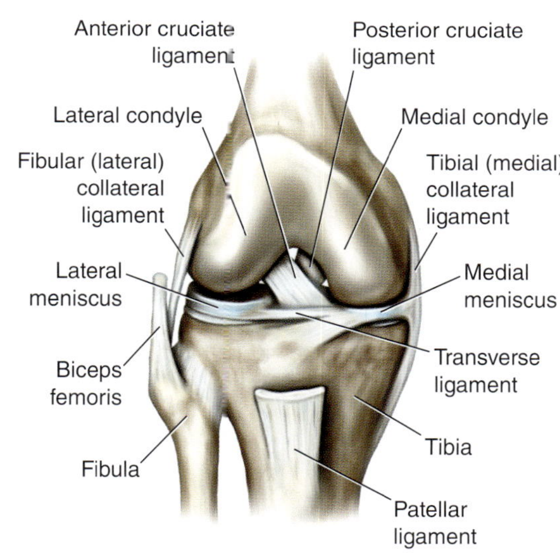

Ligaments of the knee, anterior view.

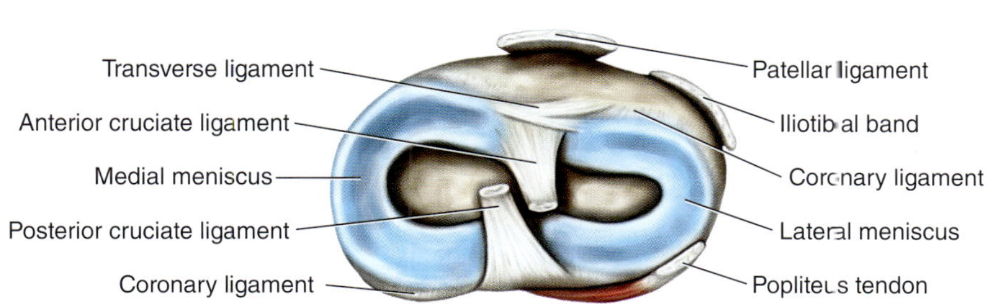

Ligaments of the knee, superior view.

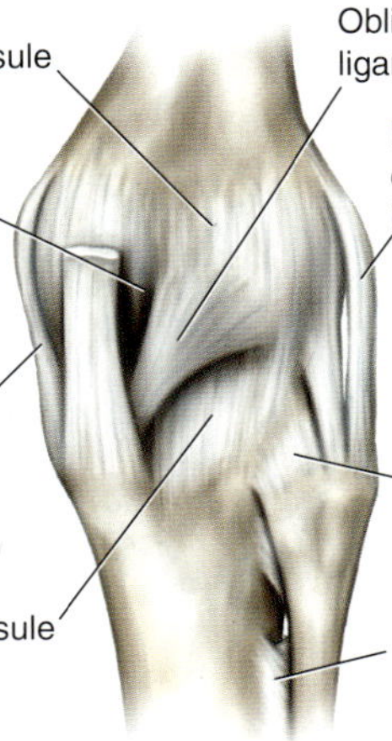

Ligaments of the knee, posterior view.

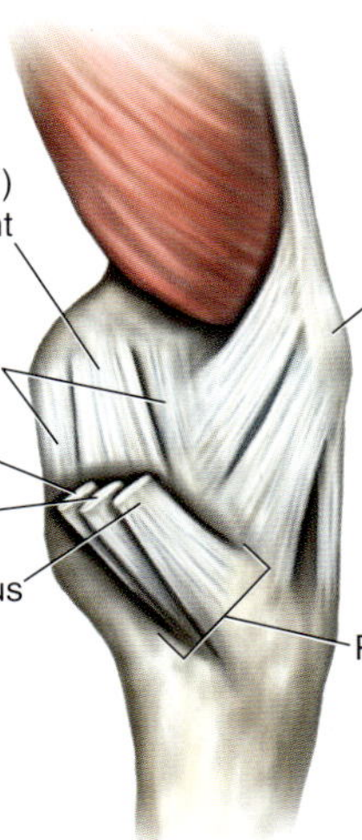

Pes anserinus.

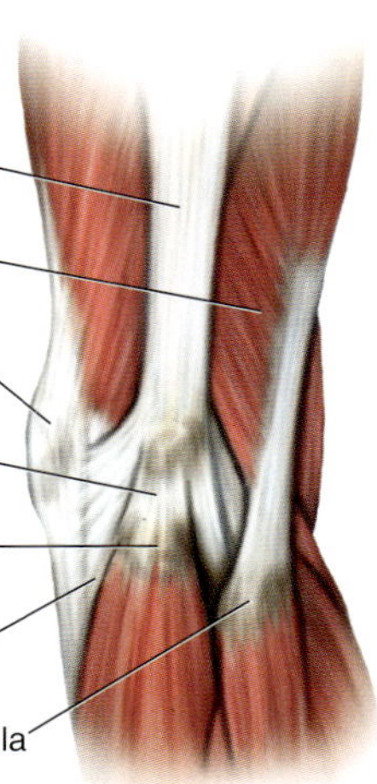

Gerdy's tubercle and iliotibial band.

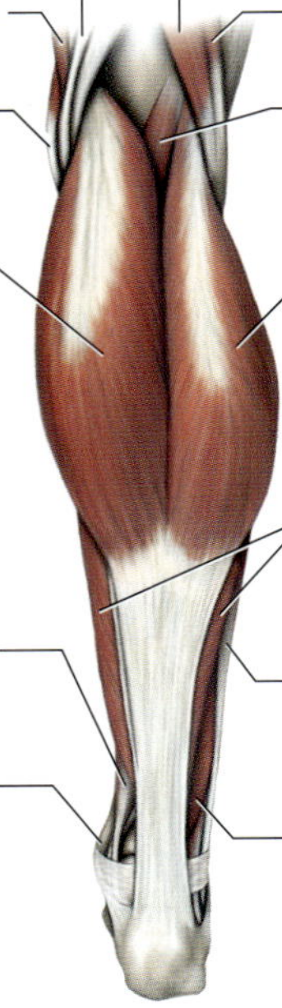

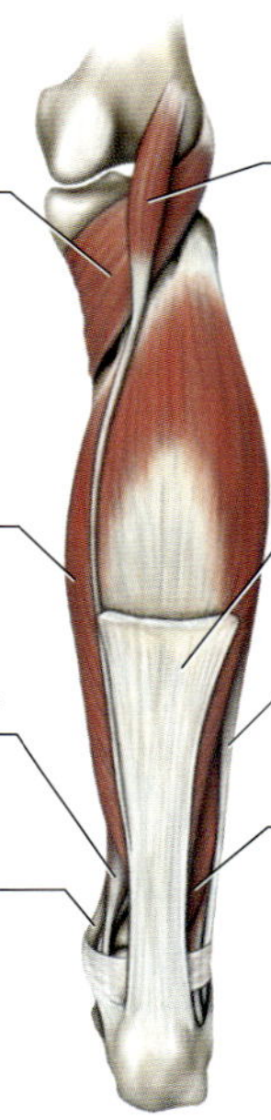

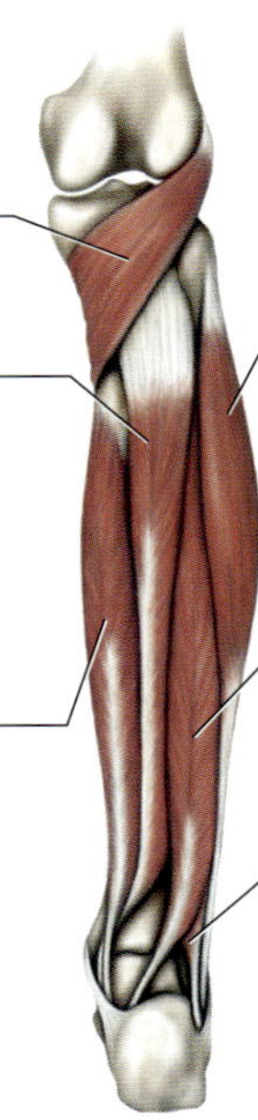

Posterior muscles of the knee and lower leg.

The art in this insert is reprinted from R. Behnke, 2005, *Kinetic anatomy,* 2nd ed. (Champaign, IL: Human Kinetics), 175, 176, 177, 178, 180, 192, 193, 194, 195, 201, 202.